Ounces	
8	9	10	11	12	13	14	15		
227	255	283	312	340	369	397	425	0	Pounds
680	709	737	765	794	822	850	879	1	
1134	1162	1191	1219	1247	1276	1304	1332	2	
1588	1616	1644	1673	1701	1729	1758	1786	3	
2041	2070	2098	2126	2155	2183	2211	2240	4	
2495	2523	2551	2580	2608	2637	2665	2693	5	
2948	2977	3005	3033	3062	3090	3118	3147	6	
3402	3430	3459	3487	3515	3544	3572	3600	7	
3856	3884	3912	3941	3969	3997	4026	4054	8	
4309	4337	4366	4394	4423	4451	4479	4508	9	
4763	4791	4819	4848	4876	4904	4933	4961	10	
5216	5245	5273	5301	5330	5358	5386	5415	11	
5670	5698	5727	5755	5783	5812	5840	5868	12	
6123	6152	6180	6209	6237	6265	6294	6322	13	
6577	6605	6634	6662	6690	6719	6747	6776	14	
7030	7059	7087	7115	7144	7172	7201	7228	15	
7484	7512	7541	7569	7597	7626	7654	7682	16	
7938	7966	7994	8023	8051	8079	8108	8136	17	
8391	8420	8448	8476	8504	8533	8561	8590	18	
8845	8873	8902	8930	8958	8987	9015	9043	19	
9298	9327	9355	9383	9412	9440	9469	9497	20	
9752	9780	9809	9837	9865	9894	9922	9950	21	
10206	10234	10262	10291	10319	10347	10376	10404	22	
8	9	10	11	12	13	14	15		
								Ounces	

**DIAGNOSIS AND MANAGEMENT OF THE
FETUS AND NEONATE AT RISK**

a guide for team care

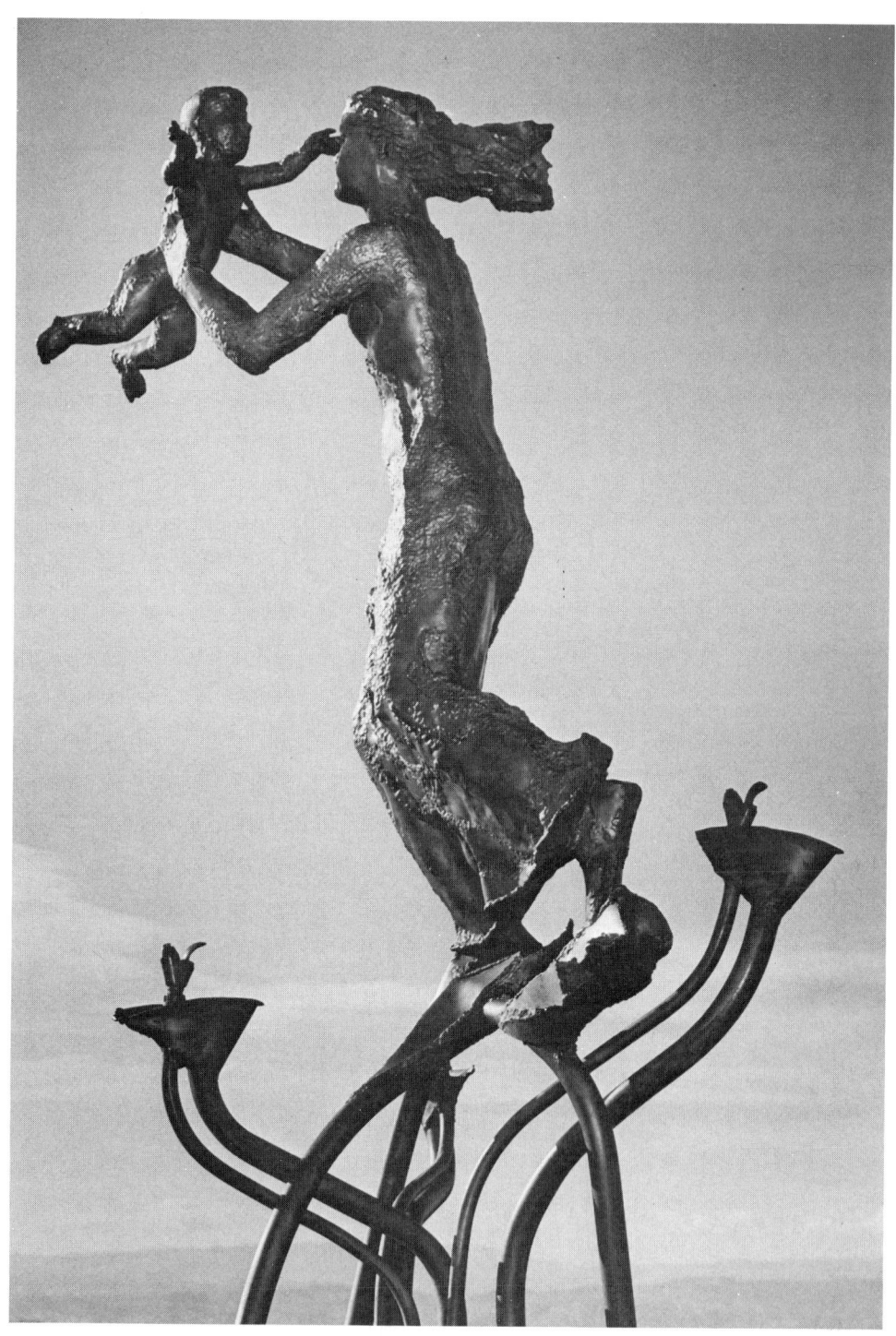

MOTHER AND CHILD

by Frederick Littman in Council Crest Park, Portland, Oregon

DIAGNOSIS AND MANAGEMENT OF THE FETUS AND NEONATE AT RISK   a guide for team care

MARTIN L. PERNOLL, M.D.
Chairman and C.J. Miller Professor,
Department of Obstetrics and Gynecology,
Tulane University School of Medicine,
New Orleans, Louisiana

GERDA I. BENDA, M.D.
Associate Professor of Pediatrics,
Oregon Health Sciences University,
School of Medicine;
Director, Follow-up Clinic,
Neonatal Intensive Care Center,
Doernbecher Memorial Hospital for Children,
Portland, Oregon

S. GORHAM BABSON, M.D.
Emeritus Professor of Pediatrics
and Former Director of
Neonatal Intensive Care Center,
Doernbecher Memorial Hospital for Children,
Oregon Health Sciences University,
School of Medicine,
Portland, Oregon

With the assistance of
KATHERINE SIMPSON, R.N.
Neonatal Nurse Clinician,
Doernbecher Memorial Hospital for Children,
Oregon Health Sciences University,
Portland, Oregon

FIFTH EDITION
With 70 illustrations

The C.V. Mosby Company
ST. LOUIS • WASHINGTON, D.C. • TORONTO • 1986

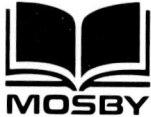

A TRADITION OF PUBLISHING EXCELLENCE

Editor: Carol Trumbold
Assistant editor: Anne Gunter
Manuscript editor: Liz Williams
Design: Diane Beasley
Production: Celeste Clingan

FIFTH EDITION

Copyright © 1986 by The C.V. Mosby Company

All rights reserved. No part of this publication may be reproduced, stored in a retrieval system, or transmitted, in any form or by any means, electronic, mechanical, photocopying, recording, or otherwise, without prior written permission from the publisher.

Previous editions copyrighted 1966, 1971, 1975, 1980

Printed in the United States of America

The C.V. Mosby Company
11830 Westline Industrial Drive, St. Louis, Missouri 63146

Library of Congress Cataloging-in-Publication Data

Babson, S. Gorham (Sydney Gorham)
  Diagnosis and management of the fetus and neonate at risk.

  On t.p. of 4th ed., Babson's name appeared first.
  Includes bibliographies and index.
  1. Neonatal intensive care. 2. Infants (Newborn)—Diseases. 3. Pregnancy, Complications of. 4. Infants (Premature) I. Pernoll, Martin L., 1939-   . II. Benda, Gerda I. III. Title. [DNLM: 1. Infant, Newborn, Diseases—therapy. 2. Infant, Premature, Diseases—therapy. 3. Intensive Care units, Neonatal. 4. Pregnancy Complications—therapy. WS 410 B116p]
RJ253.5.B3   1986   618.92'01   86-5449
ISBN 0-8016-0434-6

T/MV/MV 9 8 7 6 5 4 3 2 1

Preface

The *Primer on Prematurity and High-Risk Pregnancy*, the first edition of this series, was prefaced with comments indicating that the objective of the book was to provide a concise source of information for physicians and nurses who care for the high-risk pregnant mother and the premature infant. Evolutionary changes in subsequent editions broadened that objective to include all risk infants. However, the basic intent to furnish a concise source of information for the health care providers caring for the risk pregnancy and risk fetus-neonate remains the motivation for undertaking this edition (the fifth). Central to this objective is our continued dedication to the concepts of team care and regionalization of care for those individuals negotiating (hopefully unscathed) that most hazardous period of life, the perinatal interval.

Vast changes have occurred in possibilities for perinatal health care during the two decades since the first edition was published (1966). Technological advances in maternal, fetal, and neonatal care have occurred at an unprecedented rate, and there has been a marked decline in perinatal mortality. Save for those perinates below 26 weeks of gestational age, the likelihood of intact survival has materially increased for each weight group. Nearly all disease states exhibit similar decreases in ability to place the perinate at jeopardy. Nonetheless, the most important ingredients in care remain human concern, communication, interpretation, and organization.

In the United States, unfortunately, the health teams necessary to provide these vital services are faced with external constraints that threaten their current ability to function, while limiting their ability to achieve scientific progress at the rate at which we have all become accustomed. Three of the more serious constraints are economic restrictions, a hostile medicolegal climate, and a decline in research funding.

The first problem particularly threatens health care provided to the poor. A deprived population may require more care to achieve the same results, but efforts ensuring that this care is provided are cost-effective in our areas of concern. Denying adequate funding for perinatal care to this segment of the population will increase rather than decrease health care expenditures, in addition to causing a staggering loss of human potential.

The medicolegal crisis threatens everyone's health care and has become evident in those regions of the United States that are experiencing a dearth of obstetrician-gynecologists because of overwhelming malpractice insurance premiums. While no easy answers to this phenomenon exist, the problem is expanding into alarming issues of cost and access to health care.

Research, mentioned last but no less important, is the lifeblood of progress. Indeed, there is direct correlation between the rapid progress of the last decades and the substantial research support that was extended. With proposed major cutbacks in funding, the converse situation is likely to emerge.

These problems are not dealt with in our text, since solutions lie in disciplines beyond the scope of our current efforts; however, the public must be made aware of these issues, and resolutions must be sought at every level. Indeed, health care providers may necessarily have to increase their involvement in local and national efforts to this effect.

The text's direction retains its firm roots in obstetric and neonatal medical information, with focus on an ever-widening bridge of perinatal information. To accomodate new data and yet remain concise, nearly every chapter has been extensively rewritten, although the format remains unchanged. This fifth edition also witnesses further evolutionary change among its authors. Although less involved in technical details, Dr. S. Gorham Babson, neonatologist, has provided his usual superb editorial efforts, and while not an extensive participant in this edition, Dr. Ralph C. Benson, obstetrician, has provided valuable consultation for several of the presented issues.

Although both would modestly object, we dedicate our efforts in the continuation of this series to these two remarkable gentlemen who wrote the first edition. Both Drs. Benson and Babson have been a constant source of inspiration to the many generations of those in all medical disciplines who have been fortunate enough to come into contact with them. Their unselfish efforts and concern for the continuity of care for the perinate have been well matched by their dedication, knowledge, intellectual expertise, and total commitment to give of themselves to others. Their gentility, courtesy, and ability to work together constitute a model worthy of emulation. Thus it is with gratitude, admiration, and a great deal of love that this book is dedicated to them.

M. L. Pernoll
Gerda I. Benda

Contents

Section I DIAGNOSIS AND MANAGEMENT OF THE HIGH-RISK FETUS AND NEONATE

1 What is a risk perinate? 1

Definition of perinatal jeopardy, 2
General factors inimical to pregnancy (which may require special guidance), 2
Social, cultural, and economic factors that influence perinatal morbidity and mortality, 7

2 Standard prenatal care and identification of specific factors, 10

Standard prenatal care, 10
Factors relating to intrauterine jeopardy, 11
Factors placing the newborn at increased jeopardy, 12
Noxious habits, 14
Paternal influences, 16
Miscellaneous factors, 16
Method of identification of specific risk factors, 16

3 Genetic and congenital defects, 21

Chromosomal aberrations and genetic transmissions, 21
Early fetal development and growth, 22
Mutagenesis and teratogenesis, 24
Antenatal diagnosis, 28

4 Longitudinal assessment of fetal health: detection of risk factors, 31

Fetal growth, 31
Clinical parameters of pregnancy duration, 31
Determination of fetal lie, presenting part, and position, 36
Laboratory parameters of fetal growth, 36
Laboratory parameters of fetal well-being, 38
Other methods of determining fetal maturity, 42
Determination of fetal death, 44

5 Indicators of fetal jeopardy, 45

Indications for electronic fetal monitoring in labor, 45
Methods of electronic fetal monitoring, 46
Normal fetal heart rate, 46
Abnormalities of FHR, 46
Periodic heart rate changes, 48
Interpretation of FHR patterns, 51
Pitfalls of electronic fetal monitoring, 51
Confirmation of fetal compromise (biochemical monitoring by fetal scalp blood sampling), 52
Treatment of fetal distress from interpretation of FHR patterns, 54
Antepartum testing, 54
Fetal biophysical profile, 59
FHR tracings in fetuses with congenital anomalies, 59

6 Assessment of labor, 60

Clinical parameters, 60
Fetal nursing care, 68

7 Delivery of the fetus at risk, 70

Which perinates are at risk? 70
Team care in the birth room, 70
General considerations for management of perinatal jeopardy, 72
Analgesia and anesthesia, 72
Cesarean section delivery, 79
Other operative delivery methods, 80
Induction of labor, 80
Specific risk situations, 84

8 Initial care of the infant in the birth room, 87

Initial care of all infants, 87
Cardiovascular and respiratory changes at birth, 90

9 Resuscitation and stabilization of the depressed infant, 93

Equipment and drugs needed in the delivery room, 93
Ventilation for the nonbreathing infant, 94
Continued apnea with assisted ventilation, 94
Circulatory and metabolic support, 94
Continued respiratory difficulty from birth, 95
Increasing cyanosis, 95

10 Techniques of resuscitation and stabilization, 97

Laryngoscopy and endotracheal intubation, 97
Methods of assisted ventilation, 99
Umbilical vessel catheterization, 99
Techniques of catheterization, 100

11 Classification into risk categories at birth, 103

What are the risk groups? 103
Assessment by weight and gestation, 103
Use of body measurements in evaluation of risk groups, 105

12 Infants at medium risk and their specific care, 108

Infants who justify medium-risk care, 108
Preterm infants (33 to 37 weeks of gestational age—1,500 to 2,750 gm), 110
Postterm infants (42 weeks or more of gestational age), 110
Large-for-gestational-age infants, 110
Small-for-gestational-age (SGA) neonates, 111
Hypoglycemia, 111
Problems developing that may require transfer to regional center, 111

13 Transport of the high-risk perinate, 114

Fetal transport, 114
Neonatal transport, 114
Training of transport nurses, 119

14 Intensive care of high-risk infants, 120

Nursery facilities, 120
Nursery regulations for control of infections, 122
Temperature control, 122
Humidification, 124
Monitoring heart rate and respiration, 125
Details of care, 127
Parent-infant relationships, 131
Criteria for discharge from the intensive care unit, 131
Responsibilities of the community health nurse, 132
Responsibilities of the social worker, 132
Special advice for the mother, 133
Responsibilities of the neonatal nurse, 134
Procedures, 134

15 Parenteral administration of fluid and electrolytes, 138

Glucose, water, and electrolytes for short-term needs, 138
Routes of infusion, 139
Homeostatic imbalance, 139

16 Nutritional requirements and oral feeding of the low birth weight infant, 141

Water balance and calories, 141
Nutritional requirements, 142
Feeding plans, 145
Feeding techniques, 147
Necrotizing enterocolitis, 149

17 Total parenteral nutrition, 153

Candidates for parenteral nutrition, 153
Sources of major nutrients, 153
Techniques of care and use, 155
Hazards in the use of parenteral nutrition, 157

18 Untimely termination of pregnancy, 159

Premature labor, 159
Premature rupture of membranes, 166
Incompetent cervix, 171
Prolonged pregnancy, 173
Meconium in the amniotic fluid, 175

19 Disproportionate fetouterine growth, 177

Growth-retarded fetus, 177
Small-for-dates neonates, 179
Overgrown, or large fetus, 181
Hydramnios and oligohydramnios, 183

20 Multiple pregnancy, 185

Incidence and associations, 185
Identification by clinical associations and observation, 186
Diagnosis by laboratory procedures, 187
Special care during pregnancy, 188
Special considerations for delivery, 188
Special perinatal considerations, 191
Complications and sequelae, 192

21 Hypertensive states in pregnancy, 196

Diagnostic criteria, 196
Classification, 197
Clinical states, 197
Laboratory studies, 199
Treatment, 200
General charting and laboratory studies, 205
Complications, 206
Prognosis, 206
Prevention, 207
Neonatal care, 207

22 Late pregnancy hemorrhage, 208

Cervical and vaginal lesions, 208
Coagulopathies, 208
Placental and uterine bleeding, 209
General considerations, 210
Placenta previa, 216
Circumvallate or circummarginate placenta (extrachorial placenta), 218
Vasa previa, 219

Section II SERIOUS OBSTETRIC PROBLEMS AND THE PERINATE

23 Malpresentation and cord accidents, 220

Breech, 220
Other malpresentations, 226
Prolapse of umbilical cord, 226
Velamentous insertion of cord and vasa previa, 227

24 Diabetes mellitus, 229

Classification, 230
Effects of pregnancy on diabetes mellitus, 230
Effects of diabetes mellitus on pregnancy, 230
Detection of diabetes, 231
Management, 232

25 Infections of the perinate, 236

Period of exposure, 236
Bacterial septicemia and other severe infections, 237
Minor infections, 239
Infections with group B beta-hemolytic streptococci, 239
Viral and other congenital infections, 240

Section III SPECIFIC PROBLEMS OF THE NEONATE

26 The very low birth weight baby, 249

General considerations, 249
Approaches to prevention, 249
Specific problems of the small neonate, 250

27 Identification and management of respiratory problems, 252

Recognition of respiratory distress, 252
General management of respiratory distress, 253
Methods of ventilatory assistance, 256
General guidelines in mechanical ventilation, 260
Complications arising from oxygen therapy and mechanical ventilation, 262
Causes of respiratory distress in the neonate, 266

28 Neonatal hyperbilirubinemia and prevention of kernicterus, 275

Conditions associated with increased bilirubin levels, 275
When to investigate clinical jaundice, 276
Diagnostic approach to excessive jaundice and hyperbilirubinemia, 276
Erythroblastosis fetalis, 276
Kernicterus, 277
Phototherapy, 278
Exchange transfusion, 279

29 Cardiovascular problems, 282

Cyanosis, 282
Cardiac failure, 283
Shock, 284
Paroxysmal supraventricular tachycardia (PST or PAT), 286
Patent ductus arteriosus (PDA), 286

30 Serious neurologic disorders, 288

Central nervous system (CNS) disorders, 288
Periventricular and intraventricular hemorrhage, 289
Hydrocephalus and microcephalus, 290

31 Hematologic problems, 293

Anemia, 293
Neonatal hyperviscosity, 294
Bleeding or skin hemorrhage, 295

32 Metabolic problems, 297

Hypoglycemia of the newborn, 297
Hyperglycemia, 299
Hyponatremia, 300
Hypernatremia, 300
Hypocalcemia, 300
Hypomagnesemia, 301
Hypermagnesemia, 301

33 Major congenital anomalies and developmental defects, 303

Anomalies associated with respiratory distress at birth, 303
Cyanosis and congenital heart disease, 306
Intestinal obstruction, 306
Abdominal wall defects, 309
Multiple congenital defects, 310
Metabolic, endocrine, and miscellaneous defects, 310
Summary, 312

34 Perinatal mortality, 313

Fetal mortality, 313
Neonatal mortality, 313
Low birth weight infants and mortality, 314
Summary, 315

Section IV PERINATAL OUTCOME

35 Growth and development of the low birth weight infant: neurologic deficits, 317

Neonatal growth and development, 317
Postnatal growth and development, 319
Neurologic and intellectual deficits, 319
Child abuse, 321
Longitudinal assessments, 321

36 Regionalization and guidelines for perinatal care, 323

Levels of care, 323
Small community or rural hospital (primary care), 323
Larger community hospitals for continuing special care (intermediary care), 325
Regional care centers (tertiary care), 326

Section V PREVENTION

37 Prevention of high-risk pregnancies, 329

Socioeconomic improvement, 330
Sociomedical measures, 330
Obstetric measures, 330
Prevention of unwanted pregnancy—to be welcome and wellborn, 332

Appendixes

A Definitions and terms, 334
B Equipment for endotracheal intubation and umbilical vessel catheterization, 335
C Neonatal emergency transport equipment, 336
D Newborn transfer record, 338
E Neonatal transfer log, 340
F Respiratory flow sheet for all infants receiving oxygen or assisted ventilation, 341
G Drug dosages, 342
H Screening of all pregnancies, 343

DIAGNOSIS AND MANAGEMENT OF THE FETUS AND NEONATE AT RISK

a guide for team care

Section I DIAGNOSIS AND MANAGEMENT OF THE HIGH-RISK FETUS AND NEONATE

1

What is a risk perinate?

Between 5 and 10 million conceptions occur yearly in the United States. Of these, 2 to 3 million are early spontaneous abortions. This loss may be fortuitous because as many as half of these conceptuses demonstrate on study aberrations of chromosome structure or number. Others may suffer from fetal viremia such as rubella or from damage by unidentified pathogens. Nearly 1 million pregnancies are legally or illegally terminated each year.

Of the more than 3.7 million pregnancies each year that reach 20 weeks of gestation, nearly 30,000 result in fetuses that die before delivery. Almost the same number of neonates succumb in the first month of life after birth. Another 30,000 have severe (but often correctable) congenital malformations, although one quarter of these lesions are ultimately lethal. Complications of pregnancy and delivery will contribute heavily to the conditions of at least 90,000 who will be mentally retarded (IQ of 70 or below) and another 150,000 who will have great difficulty in school because they are "poor learners." These handicapped individuals will be unable to compete fully in our increasingly complex society.

Once viability is reached, perinatal death and permanent damage measured in terms of years of loss of life and productive living exceeds death and serious damage caused by other major catastrophes, for example, cardiovascular disease, cancer, or accidents. Indeed, yearly perinatal deaths exceed all other causes of death combined until 55 years of age. Despite marked improvement in perinatal care, prevention of morbidity during this interval remains an urgent problem.

Other factors also contribute to making perinatal safety more pressing at present. For example, sweeping social changes have altered the size of families. Until recently, large families were in vogue, and death or perinatal wastage was unfortunate but not considered a major tragedy. Today, the majority of families consist of one to three children, and current concepts stress quality of life. Deliberate family planning is increasing, and abortion is being used to terminate unintended pregnancies. Every child is increasingly becoming a wanted child. Consequently, the health care worker is asked, with intensified urgency, to protect the individual from damage before, during, and after birth. Moreover, advances along many scientific fronts have afforded knowledge for the achievement of perinatal health care far beyond what was previously available. Indeed, the last two decades have witnessed the introduction and acceptance of risk assessment, clinical ultrasonography, antenatal diagnosis, electronic fetal monitoring, and physiologic maturity testing, to mention just a few of the advances. Why, then, have we not made more progress in decreasing the human suffering and disability that have their genesis in fetal or neonatal life?

Part of the answer may lie in our lack of an educational approach to preventing perinatal health problems. Indeed, the responsibility for reproductive education in the United States is not clearly spelled out, and young adults continue to have little valid information on which to base important reproductive decisions. The increased rate of very low birth weight infants born to younger mothers causes the neonatal mortality to be higher in this than other maternal age groups. While social and economic, as well as educational, factors sharply affect pregnancy health and the utilization of available health care, much of the morbidity and mortality that occurs in the perinatal period could be prevented if current knowledge were promptly applied.

The purpose of this book may be stated simply. We propose to review modern management of commonly encountered perinatal problems in continuity (maternal, fetal, and neonatal) to help the reader acquire practical information necessary for patient care. The comments are directed to the health care team involved in direct patient care, primarily the medical practitioner, the house officer, and the involved nursing staff. We hope that this effort encourages greater application of current knowledge by the various professions to benefit the patient. To provide perinatal safety, it is mandatory to identify those at risk and provide the specific care necessary to prevent death or damage.

DEFINITION OF PERINATAL JEOPARDY

Perinatal jeopardy is the hazard of death or disability that occurs during human growth and development from viability until 28 days after birth. The risk may be subdivided into general influences and specific factors. This division allows better delineation of those factors related to perinatal risk.

GENERAL FACTORS INIMICAL TO PREGNANCY (WHICH MAY REQUIRE SPECIAL GUIDANCE)
Malnutrition

Increased nutritional requirements during pregnancy are multiple. The stress of pregnancy, as well as other intrinsic and extrinsic factors, can be only roughly appraised. Unfortunately, extrapolation from animal studies is in most instances merely suggestive, and therefore much is still unknown about nutrition in pregnancy. However a review of what is known provides a practical basis for recommendations or actions.

WEIGHT GAIN

Pregnancy accounts for about 24 lb of weight gain during gestation. A steady weight gain of 0.5 to 1 lb/wk is recommended. Obviously, one should not attempt corrections on a crash basis, especially during the first or last trimesters, to avoid harm to the fetus. A considerably underweight gravida may do well to gain more than 24 lb, and even in the obese, it may be wise to allow a 20 to 30 lb weight gain. If attempts are made to help the patient reach her ideal weight for height, they should be conducted postpartum and preferably not while the patient is lactating.

More than one third of the total weight gain of 24 lb (11 kg) during a term pregnancy represents fetal weight: approximately 7.7 lb (3,500 gm). The placenta, amniotic fluid, and uterine weight each account for between 1.4 and 2 lb (650 and 900 gm). Increased interstitial fluid and blood volume contribute approximately 2.7 and 4 lb (1,200 and 1,800 gm), respectively. Breast enlargement adds at least 0.9 lb (400 gm). The remaining 3.5 lb (1,640 gm), otherwise unspecified, represents fat and other maternal stores.

Standard weight for height is given in Table 1-1, which applies to women of small, medium, and large body builds who are 25 years of age or older. For patients less than 25 years old, deduct 1 lb for each year. For the young adolescent, however, individualized assessment is necessary, especially if maximal growth has not yet been achieved.

Proper weight gain does not guarantee optimal nutrition. In general, about 4 lb of weight

Table 1-1. Standard weight for height of women

Height feet	inches	Small frame	Medium frame	Large frame
4	10	102-111	109-121	118-131
4	11	103-113	111-123	120-134
5	0	104-115	113-126	122-137
5	1	106-118	115-129	125-140
5	2	108-121	118-132	128-143
5	3	111-124	121-135	131-147
5	4	114-127	124-138	134-151
5	5	117-130	127-141	137-155
5	6	120-133	130-144	140-159
5	7	123-136	133-147	143-163
5	8	126-139	136-150	146-167
5	9	129-142	139-153	149-170
5	10	132-145	142-156	152-173
5	11	135-148	145-159	155-176
6	0	138-151	148-162	158-179

Source of basic data: 1979 Build Study, Society of Actuaries and Association of Life Insurance Medical Directors of America, 1980.

gain in the first trimester, 10 to 12 lb in the second, and 8 to 10 lb in the last are reasonable. Nevertheless, a gain of more than 2 to 3 lb/mo in the last 3 to 4 months suggests fluid retention and may presage a developing toxemia of pregnancy.

ENERGY

The suggested optimal caloric (more than 36 kcal/kg body weight) intake is listed in Table 1-2. Few individuals are capable of counting calories consistently, nor are they generally willing to be specific. Nonetheless, caloric intake and weight gain or loss are rough correlates. Hence adequacy of caloric intake can be estimated by trends in body weight. However, a number of other variables influence trends in body weight, including the basal metabolic rate, lean body mass, and physical activity of the individual, as well as the stage of pregnancy.

Poor maternal nutrition may be a contributing cause of abnormal bleeding and spontaneous premature labor and delivery. The underweight gravida is more likely to deliver early. Moreover, preeclampsia and eclampsia are probably the result, at least in part, of nutritional (most likely protein) deficiency.

The popular belief that intrauterine growth can be satisfactorily maintained despite maternal deprivation is no longer tenable as a generality. The mother's health and that of her offspring depend in large measure on the quality and, to a lesser degree, the quantity of her food. It is known that the fetus normally doubles its weight during the last 8 weeks of pregnancy; this fetal weight gain may be reduced significantly by a starvation regimen.

NUTRIENTS

At least 50 nutrients are believed to be essential nutritional needs of the gravid woman. These needs vary with each individual patient's requirements during the numerous phases of pregnancy and puerperium. If pregnancy is complicated by colitis, for example, amounts and types of food have to be modified accordingly. Fetal growth and maintenance are a greater nutritional challenge than normal recovery postnatally. Lactation naturally adds another dimension.

Table 1-2. Recommended daily dietary allowances for nonpregnant, pregnant, and lactating women

	Recommended daily allowances for women						
	Nonpregnant (age in years)					Pregnant	Lactating
	11-14	15-18	19-22	23-50	51+		
Energy (kcal)	2,400	2,100	2,100	2,000	1,800	+300	+500
Protein (gm)	44	48	46	46	46	+30	+20
Fat-soluble vitamins							
Vitamin A activity (RE)	800	800	800	800	800	1,000	1,200
(IU)	4,000	4,000	4,000	4,000	4,000	5,000	6,000
Vitamin D (IU)	400	400	400			400	400
Vitamin E activity (IU)	12	12	12	12	12	15	15
Water-soluble vitamins							
Ascorbic acid (mg)	45	45	45	45	45	60	80
Folacin (μg)	400	400	400	400	400	800	600
Niacin (mg)	16	14	14	13	12	+2	+4
Riboflavin (mg)	1.3	1.4	1.4	1.2	1.1	+0.3	+0.5
Thiamin (mg)	1.2	1.1	1.1	1.0	1.0	+0.3	+0.3
Vitamin B_6 (mg)	1.6	2.0	2.0	2.0	2.0	2.5	2.5
Vitamin B_{12} (μg)	3.0	3.0	3.0	3.0	3.0	4.0	4.0
Minerals							
Calcium (mg)	1,200	1,200	800	800	800	1,200	1,200
Phosphorus (mg)	1,200	1,200	800	800	800	1,200	1,200
Iodine (μg)	115	115	100	100	80	125	150
Iron (mg)	18	18	18	18	10	+18	18
Magnesium (mg)	300	300	300	300	300	450	450
Zinc (mg)	15	15	15	15	15	20	25

The National Academy of Sciences-National Research Council (Table 1-2) has suggested the optimal nutritional requirements of proteins, together with 16 other food requirements of the pregnant woman.

The importance of protein in the anabolism of pregnancy always is emphasized, but the implication that carbohydrates and fats are of little importance, especially since patients may reduce intake of these to reduce excess weight, is unfortunate. Protein insufficiency can develop, even with adequate protein ingestion, if insufficient calories are available because a large portion of the amino acids in the protein will be deaminated for energy needs. Brief semistarvation (less than 1,500 calories) may reduce body proteins, enzymes, and even hormones. If starvation is extended for weeks or months, fluid retention and weight gain will be noted. Misinterpretations by the obstetrician may lead to an even stricter diet. By and large, reduction of the caloric intake below 1,500 calories for any length of time is unwise during pregnancy because of probable fetal deprivation.

SAMPLE DIET

A good pregnancy diet is deceptively simple. Mores or lack of knowledge, money, or motivation are a few of the reasons the pregnant woman does not receive a well-balanced, high-protein, high-vitamin, high-mineral diet. Excessive carbohydrates, especially sweets, should be limited. Following are the *daily* basic food requirements in pregnancy and lactation:

1. One quart (4 glasses) or more of milk (any kind: whole milk, buttermilk, low fat, skim, or powdered skim milk)
2. Two eggs
3. One or two servings of fish, liver, chicken, lean beef, lamb, or pork, or any kind of cheese
4. One or two good servings of fresh, green, leafy vegetables: mustard, collard, or turnip greens or spinach, lettuce, or cabbage
5. Two or three slices of whole wheat bread
6. A piece of citrus fruit or a glass of lemon, lime, orange, or grapefruit juice
7. One pat of margarine, vitamin A enriched

The pregnant woman should also include the following in her diet:

1. A serving of whole-grain cereal: Wheatena, Cream of Wheat, farina, oatmeal, or granola, four times a week
2. A yellow or red vegetable five times a week
3. Liver once a week
4. Whole baked potato three times a week

For years the notion has persisted that too much table salt or sodium-containing preparations are at least a contributory cause of toxemia. Granted that the preeclamptic patient may not efficiently excrete sodium once the disorder has developed, there is no convincing evidence that the sodium ion is the culprit. "Everything in moderation" still is an excellent maxim. With good diet, especially one with ample protein, the sodium problem usually will take care of itself.

Indeed, patients will fare better if the health care provider stresses good diet rather than total weight gain. Many women become so self-conscious and self critical of poundage that they go on harmful crash diets, take drastic purges, or exhaust themselves in exercise fads. The positive approach of stressing essential foods in reasonable portions rarely has to be critical or accusatory, and patients are more relaxed and cooperative.

Edema is also a bogey during pregnancy. Dependent or physiologic edema occurs in well-nourished, healthy women because of mild circulatory stasis. It is especially common in warm weather, and rest periods and elevation of legs suffice for relief. This type of edema is a sign of neither cardiac nor renal disease nor toxemia of pregnancy. It is not an indication for diuretic therapy. In contrast, generalized or pathologic edema reflects a disease process. This abnormality, often attributable to heart or kidney failure or toxemia of pregnancy, cannot be prevented by diuretics, which may be indicated, however, in the treatment of selected patients. Be this as it may, thiazide diuretics are extremely potent and may cause serious maternal or fetal complications, even when used discriminatingly.

MATERNAL NUTRITIONAL RISK IDENTIFICATION

High-risk obstetric patients needing special dietary (and medical) counseling include women with the following:

1. Anemia (hemoglobin level of less than 9.5 gm, hematocrit reading of 30% and other chronic metabolic disorders, i.e., diabetes

mellitus, thyroid dysfunction, colitis, and cardiovascular and renal disease)
2. A weight 10% under or more than 20% over the standard for height and age at the onset of pregnancy and considerable gain or any loss during gestation
3. A history of serious obstetric complications in a previous pregnancy or sequentially in several prior pregnancies: repeated abortion, toxemia of pregnancy, premature separation of the placenta, low birth weight babies, or a short interval between pregnancies
4. Socioeconomic problems: adolescents, the poor, and those not knowledgeable about the selection, storage, and preparation of food
5. Concurrent obstetric complications: diabetes mellitus, preeclampsia, multiple pregnancy, ulcerative colitis, or hyperemesis gravidarum
6. Intrauterine growth retardation (detected and/or verified by ultrasonography)

FETUS AND NUTRITION

Attempts to assess the effect of maternal nutrition on the outcome of pregnancy have been only partially successful, but fetal growth and development and the function of the placenta obviously are dependent on the type and amount of food metabolized.

Many complications of pregnancy are directly or indirectly caused by inadequate diet and may reflect the lifelong nutritional experience of the gravida as well as shorter-term dietary deficiency. They include iron- and vitamin-deficiency anemias, infection, probably toxemia of pregnancy, and certain instances of obstetric hemorrhage. Prepregnant nutrition, as assessed by weight, and pregnancy gain strongly affect fetal growth. Poor nutrition may be the primary cause of low birth weight infants throughout the world, particularly those in the weight range of 2,000 to 2,500 gm, most of whom are mature at birth. The possibility that normal central nervous system development may be impaired by poor nutrition emphasizes the urgent need for proper food intake during gestation. A favorable nutritional state before conception and in the first trimester, before most prenatal care has started, is often disregarded as a vital need for the fetus. It is proposed by Drillien that poor environment during the mother's childhood is still restrictive of fetal growth of her progeny, even after improvement in her social and economic status.

Prepregnant weight is directly related to birth weight and inversely related to the percentage of low birth weight infants in women delivered at term. (See Table 1-3.)

Weight gain during pregnancy is also related to increased fetal size at birth, with a fall in the percentage of low birth weight infants concomitant with increasing maternal weight gain (Table 1-4). An exception may occur when weight loss has occurred during pregnancy. A suggested explanation is the inclusion of a proportionately larger number of obese women who lose weight during pregnancy whose tendency toward increased fetal weight is only partially blunted by severe dietary control. Women with low prepregnant weight (under

Table 1-3. Association between prepregnancy weight, birth weight, and percentage of low birth weight infants

Prepregnancy weight (lb)	Mean birth weight	Birth weight below 2,501 gm (%)
<100	3,144	4.9
100-119	3,285	2.7
120-139	3,427	1.9
140-159	3,531	0.4
160-179	3,625	0.8
≥180	3,776	0.7

From Eastman, N.J., and Jackson, E.: Weight relationships in pregnancy, Obstet. Gynecol. Survey **23**:1003, 1968.

Table 1-4. Association between maternal weight gain, birth weight, and percentage of low birth weight infants

Weight gain	Mean birth weight	Birth weight below 2,501 gm (%)
Loss	3,360	3.3
0-10	3,278	4.4
11-20	3,301	3.1
21-30	3,426	1.2
31-40	3,562	0.7
≥41	3,636	0.5

From Eastman, N.J., and Jackson, E.: Weight relationships in pregnancy, Obstet. Gynecol. Survey **23**:1003, 1968.

120 lb) and limited pregnancy weight gain (under 11 lb) produce a high incidence of low weight newborns. These infants have a much higher neonatal mortality. Such women should be identified early in pregnancy (or before) and given helpful specific nutritional advice and longitudinal observation.

More liberal diets for average women during pregnancies, with emphasis on quality of food rather than quantity of calories, particularly in those requiring weight limitation, should improve fetal health and size. Although larger babies may be stronger babies, excessive size is related to increased likelihood of dystocia, fetal distress, and birth trauma.

In summary:
1. Faulty maternal nutrition, including vitamin and mineral lack, has an adverse effect on fertility, embryogenesis, and fetal growth.
2. Undernutrition and overrestricted weight gain in the mother increase the incidence of low birth weight infants and perinatal mortality.
3. Close spacing of pregnancies may deplete nutritional stores to the disadvantage of subsequent progeny.
4. The mother's health and that of her offspring depend in large measure on the quality rather than the quantity of her food intake.

VITAMIN AND MINERAL SUPPLEMENTATION

Many investigators have challenged the routine administration of minerals and vitamins (except possibly iron and folic acid) during pregnancy. Certainly indiscriminate nutritional supplementation has never been a replacement for sound nutritional practice. One must conclude at present that routine supplementation of dietary vitamins and minerals is a questionable necessity. However, the risk for complications of supplementation at or near the recommended daily dietary allowances is extraordinarily low. Thus, for the gravida with potential deficiencies, regardless of cause, supplementation appears only sound practice. Indeed, recent evidence indicates that initiating routine prenatal vitamin and mineral supplementation 3 months before the onset of pregnancy significantly decreases the incidence of neural tube defects.

"Megadose" vitamin or mineral supplementation should be avoided during pregnancy. Vitamins A, D, and K (in extraordinary amounts) have demonstrated teratogenic activity. Moreover, the toxic effects of iodine, iron, and aluminum have long been known. Thus only sound evidence of deficiency or other need should be the criterion to exceed recommended daily allowances.

Emotional stress

Childbirth still causes much needless fear and anxiety among women. Many obstetric disorders are emotionally induced or are aggravated by psychologic factors.

The antenatal period offers a unique opportunity to study and treat fears, anxieties, and conflicts related to gestation, parturition, and motherhood. It also affords an ideal opportunity for an educational experience designed to prepare parents not only for childbirth but for the demanding tasks of child rearing. Better understanding and the formation and acceptance of healthy attitudes can make an invaluable contribution to the mental health and happiness of the mother-to-be and her family. Toward that end, childbirth educators might consider more emphasis on the parents' role in rearing children in our complex society. Counseling will do much to prevent and treat many troublesome psychic or somatic complications. Severe problems will require consultation and definitive therapy.

Generally, if circumstances allow, a mother and father gain a special attachment for their baby during pregnancy, while in labor and delivery, and when on the maternity floor. What happens when a newborn is removed to a nursery for high-risk infants? Babies who remain in an incubator for a long time may become rejected, even if they were wanted. One patient said, "I feel like I never had him; he's almost no one to me."

Because emotional stress is a serious problem for many obstetric patients and their husbands, it is important that the health care provider recognize and meet their needs. These individuals may require frequent counseling and direction.

There seems to be no substitute for a good interpersonal relationship between health care providers and the patient. They must have the ability to counsel the mother *and* the father.

The physician may represent an authority figure, and fear of judgment and punishment may enter the picture. The physician should not ask, "Have you been taking the iron pills?" He or she should inquire, "Are you having any trouble taking iron pills?"

Severe, prolonged tension from any cause may alter the fetal environment or the hormonal balance in the delicate maternal-placental-fetal relationship and thus impair fetal development. Pregnancy may come as a surprise, and when the fetus is unwanted sufficient stress in the mother may interfere with pregnancy health. The mother's emotions may affect fetal health in other ways: rejection may be the basis for chain-smoking, excessive intake of tranquilizers or other drugs, variations in food intake, and reduced interest in prenatal care or personal health. In extreme cases the mother may try to take her life or that of the fetus.

SOCIAL, CULTURAL, AND ECONOMIC FACTORS THAT INFLUENCE PERINATAL MORBIDITY AND MORTALITY

The many social factors that place certain neonates at greater risk are interrelated. Ignorance, poverty, and disinterest in the pregnancy are far too prevalent. Specific factors appearing to be related to low birth weight infants follow.

Accidental pregnancy and irresponsible parenthood

Of all the problems that beset the world, unplanned, unexpected pregnancy is one of the most critical. The majority of such pregnancies, particularly in the lower socioeconomic sector of the population, are unwanted and often rejected by one or both parents. These pregnant women, especially if unwed or teenagers, often neglect antenatal care and leave advice unheeded. Whereas many mothers are unconcerned about the outcome, others hope to abort or pray for the birth of a stillborn baby. The high incidence of ill-timed and undesired pregnancies is one reason the United States has an unfavorable position relative to other so-called advanced countries in regard to infant mortality. In any event, the world's birth rate has far outstripped the death rate now that death control has become more efficient than birth control. At the present rate of growth there will be over 6 billion persons in the world by the year 2000.

Race

Racial difference may be a factor in the proportion of smaller infants born in a comparative population. Blacks have a much greater percentage of low birth weight infants compared with whites, particularly in lower weight categories, as shown in Table 1-5. Differences in socioeconomic opportunities may explain much of the disparity. This factor may not be the only one, however, because low birth weight rates of American Indians, persons of very low socioeconomic status, also are similar to those of white U.S. citizens.

Because of the regionalization and general availability of perinatal care, neonatal mortality rates for white and Indian Americans are now similar (Table 1-5). The rate for black Americans, however, is double that of these other groups. Although neonatal mortality for each weight-specific group below 2,500 gm is higher for black infants, black mothers have two to three times the percentage of live-born infants weighing under 1,500 gm than do white mothers. This weight group is responsible for most neonatal mortality. However, postneonatal mortality is considerably higher in both black and Indian than in white infants, suggesting that socioeconomic factors influence mortality

Table 1-5. The racial factor in low birth weight and infant mortality in the United States (1980)

Race	Live births	% Under 1,500 gm	% 1,500-2,499 gm	Neonatal mortality*	Postneonatal mortality
American Indian	36,797	0.9	5.5	6.9	6.3
Black	589,616	2.4	10.1	14.1	7.3
White	2,898,732	0.9	4.8	7.5	3.5

*Rate per 1,000 live births.
From National Center for Health Statistics: Vital statistics of the United States: mortality, vol. 2, U.S. Department of Health and Human Services, 1980.

more after infants have left the hospitals where born. In contrast, it is of interest that Chinese- and Japanese-American infants have an infant mortality one third that of blacks and two thirds that of whites in the United States.

Occupational and educational states: social class

Occupation of the father is related to profound differences in the incidence of prematurity and infant mortality. In Table 1-6 the advantages that the infants of farmers and professional people have over the infants of farm laborers and unmarried mothers are clearly evident. The farmer's limited access to medical care is more than compensated for by an apparently healthier life. Other observations include the following:
1. The incidence of prematurity and perinatal death is increased with menial occupational states (Table 1-6).
2. Ward patients in many hospitals have a more than 50% higher incidence of low birth weight infants than do private patients of the same race in the same institution.
3. College women have half as many low birth weight infants as those with only a grade school education.

Whether these differences are attributable to better pregnancy planning, or differences in living conditions, personal habits, or faulty nutrition remains unanswered, but all of these factors seem to be important.

Teenage and unwed parents

The pregnant teenage girl, whether married or not, presents a serious problem. She and her partner usually are emotionally and intellectually immature and often are unable to cope with the difficult social, economic, and educational problems created by the pregnancy. The following observations generally apply to teenage and unwed parents and their offspring:
1. A greater proportion of births out of wedlock occur in young parents.
2. Teenage marriage, particularly after conception, is notably unstable and usually ends in dissolution.
3. The percentage of infants weighing under 1,500 gm born to teenagers is more than 50% higher than the percentage born to women over 25 years of age.
4. Perinatal mortality in children of the unwed is almost twice that of children of married women.
5. Postneonatal mortality of infants born to mothers under 20 years of age is three times higher than mortality for infants born to mothers over 24 years of age.
6. Children born to teenage mothers require

Table 1-6. Births and infant deaths as recorded on birth and death certificates classified by occupation of father and ranked by premature birth rate, Oregon, 1966

	Number	Percent of total	Premature infants*		Infant death rate for state
			Birth rate†	Death rate	
Farmer	946	2.7	33.8	4.2	8.5
Professional	4,423	12.6	49.1	9.5	15.6
Clerical	1,414	4.0	55.3	9.2	17.7
Sales	2,208	6.3	60.2	8.6	14.0
Managers	2,730	7.8	60.4	11.4	17.6
Craftsmen	4,740	13.5	61.2	12.9	22.2
Operatives	4,972	14.2	66.6	12.7	22.1
Other	1,509	4.3	67.6	13.3	21.2
Laborers	8,647	24.7	71.8	12.0	23.1
Service workers	1,154	3.3	78.3	15.6	27.7
Farm laborers	590	1.7	88.1	25.4	37.3
Illegitimate births‡	1,720	4.9	93.6	19.2	33.7
STATE TOTAL AND RATES	35,053	100.0	64.8	12.1	21.1

From Kernek, C., Osterud, H., and Anderson, B.: Patterns of prematurity in Oregon, Northwest Med. 65:639, 1966.
*In this table premature infants include all births under 5 lb 8 oz.
†All birth and death rates are based on 1,000 live births.
‡Illegitimate births are included for completeness.

hospitalization more than twice as often as those born to older women.

Hence teenage pregnancy is a serious handicap to family fulfillment and solidity and to the achievement of independence. Restriction of the developmental potential of children born out of wedlock or to very young parents is likely, whereas children born to more mature parents generally perform better in school, demonstrate superior emotional balance, and enjoy greater family contentment.

Certainly being a teenager does not inevitably cause compromised pregnancy outcome. It has been convincingly demonstrated that teenagers in special care programs or situations can achieve nearly the same low rates of perinatal morbidity and mortality as the general population. The most successful programs have been multifaceted, stressing social, nutritional, psychologic, and medical assistance for the young gravida. Additionally, being a single parent does not place the more mature, well-motivated, and financially secure gravida at discernibly higher risk than the comparable married woman. However, if this type of parent has long purposefully deferred childbearing (for career or other reasons) and her age now places her at increased risk for chromosomal defects in the offspring, she should receive counseling and possibly antenatal genetic diagnosis (see Chapter 3).

In summary, it seems clear that many factors predisposing fetuses to prematurity are related to educational disadvantage and economic insecurity and result in the pregnant woman not receiving adequate care, diet, or rest. In addition, most high-risk mothers appear to be under stress and to lack family support.

BIBLIOGRAPHY

Babson, S.G., and Clarke, N.G.: Relationship between death and maternal age, J. Pediatr. **103**:391, 1983.

Baruffi, G., Strobino, D.M., and Dellinger, W.S., Jr.: Definitions of high risk in pregnancy and evaluation of their predictive validity, Am. J. Obstet. Gynecol. **148**:781, 1984

Brewer, T.H.: Human maternal-fetal nutrition, Obstet. Gynecol. **40**:868, 1972.

Elliot, K., and Knight, J., editors: Size at birth (Ciba Foundation Symposium), New York, 1974, Excerpta Medica.

Emerson, J.K., et al.: Caloric cost of normal pregnancy, Obstet. Gynecol. **40**:786, 1972.

Gold, E.M.: Interconceptional nutrition, J. Am. Diet. Assoc. **55**:27, 1969.

Gruenwald, P., Funakawa, H., Mitani, S., et al.: Influence of environmental factors on foetal growth in man, Lancet **1**:1026, 1967.

Guzick, D.S., Daikoku, N.H., and Kaltreider, D.F.: Predictability of pregnancy outcome in preterm delivery, Obstet. Gynecol. **63**:645, 1984.

Hendricks, C.H.: Delivery patterns and reproductive efficiency among groups of differing socio-economic status and ethnic origins, Am. J. Obstet. Gynecol. **97**:608, 1967.

Kaminetsky, H.A., Langer, A., Baker, H., et al.: Effect of nutrition in teenage gravidas on pregnancy and status of the neonate, I. Nutritional profile, Am. J. Obstet. Gynecol. **115**:639, 1973.

Kitay, J.Z.: Folic acid deficiency in pregnancy, Mod. Med. **38**:77, 1970.

Lechtig, A., Habicht, J.P., Delgado, H., et al.: Effect of food supplementation during pregnancy on birthweight, Pediatrics **56**:508, 1975.

Levine, M.G., Holroyde, J., Woods, J.R., Jr., et al.: Birth trauma: incidence and predisposing factors, Obstet. Gynecol. **63**:792, 1984.

Low, J.A., Galbraith, R.S., Muir, D.W., et al.: Factors associated with motor and cognitive deficits in children after intrapartum fetal hypoxia, Am. J. Obstet. Gynecol. **148**:533, 1984.

Low, J.A., Galbraith, R.S., Muir, D.W., et al.: The predictive significance of biologic risk factors for deficits in children of a high-risk population, Am. J. Obstet. Gynecol. **145**:1059, 1983.

Miller, H.C., Hassanein, K., Chin, T.D., et al.: Socioeconomic factors in relation to fetal growth in white infants, J. Pediatr. **89**:638, 1976.

Moghissi, K.S., and Evans, T.N.: Nutritional impacts on women, Hagerstown, Md., 1977, Harper & Row, Publishers.

Murthy, L.S., Agarwal, K.N., and Khanna, S.: Placental morphometric and morphological alterations in maternal undernutrition, Am. J. Obstet. Gynecol. **124**:641, 1976.

Phillips, C., and Johnson, N.E.: Impact of quality of diet and other factors on birth weight of infants, Am. J. Clin. Nutr. **30**:215, 1977.

Pitkin, R.M.: Nutritional support in obstetrics and gynecology, Clin. Obstet. Gynecol. **19**:489, 1976.

Smilkstein, G., Helsper-Lucas, A., Ashworth, C., et al.: Prediction of pregnancy complications: an application of the biopsychosocial model, Soc. Sci. Med. **18**:315, 1984.

Stein, Z., Susser, M., Saenger, G., et al: Nutrition and mental performance, Science **178**:708, 1972.

Taylor, B., Wadsworth, J., and Bulter, N.R.: Teenage mothers: admission to hospital and accidents in first 5 years, Arch. Dis. Child. **58**:6, 1983.

Taylor, R.D., and Swartout, J.W.: Biochemical survey of protein efficiency during pregnancy in urban women, Obstet. Gynecol. **29**:244, 1967.

Wallace, H.M.: Selected aspects of perinatal casualties: looking ahead nationally, Clin. Pediatr. **17**:213, 1979.

Whitelaw, A.G.L.: Influence of maternal obesity on subcutaneous fat in the newborn, Br. Med. J. **1**:985, 1976.

2
Standard prenatal care and identification of specific factors

Ideally, each woman contemplating pregnancy (or preferably the couple) should have a preconceptual evaluation to establish by history, physical examination, and indicated laboratory studies the patient's fitness for undertaking a pregnancy. If the history and physical evaluations are essentially negative, laboratory evaluation may consist of nothing more than a complete blood count, a serology test for syphilis, a rubella antibody titer, a urine analysis, and a Pap smear. Obviously in more complex cases additional evaluation is necessary.

This preconceptual visit is also an ideal time to stress the necessity of refraining from smoking, from using ethanol, over-the-counter or prescription drugs not approved by the physician, illicit drugs and other potential teratogens or mutagens. Additionally, the visit provides an opportunity to discuss proper diet, exercise programs or correction of any physical abnormalities that may be necessary. It may also be good to have the patient begin a regimen of prenatal vitamins for 3 months prior to the planned conception.

Unfortunately, few women utilize this preconceptual option, and care usually starts after pregnancy is under way. However, if a gravida participates in prenatal care only, identification and treatment of problems that may threaten the patient or her fetus can still be accomplished. Thus antenatal care is actually a screening procedure to differentiate those at jeopardy (high risk) from those in little danger (low risk). For that system to be effective, it must be based on an uncompromising search for those factors that may endanger the pregnancy. Although several risk-scoring protocols have been proposed, evidence is unconvincing that an increase in precision occurs as a result of their use.

This chapter outlines a routine antenatal care program designed to search for risk factors. Once identified, endangered individuals require highly specialized care, which will be discussed in later chapters.

STANDARD PRENATAL CARE

Pregnancy is a multifactorial dynamic state. The following steps are essential for discrimination of patients at high, moderate, or low risk:
1. A careful screening history
2. A general and specific physical examination designed to identify risk factors
3. Routine laboratory screening
4. Individually indicated maternal laboratory evaluation
5. Careful fetal assessment during the course of pregnancy
6. Specialized studies to ascertain fetal well-being or fetal maturity

Standard records

Concise, problem-oriented obstetric records are necessary to document the progress of each pregnancy. Standard chart forms vary considerably in format and amount of information contained. The record system currently recommended by the American College of Obstetricians and Gynecologists and commercially distributed by the Hollister Company is most satisfactory. These forms are designed for screening of specific risk factors and indicate the data base for the first as well as subsequent visits.

Additional information that may be of marked value but is not formatted on the records is a three-generation pedigree and careful work history (detailing potential mutagen/teratogen exposure or other potentially harmful practices) for both prospective parents. This should be performed on the initial prenatal visit.

Standard antenatal visits

Following is a standard schedule of prenatal office visits:

Weeks of gestation	Frequency of visits
0-32	Once every 4 weeks
32-36	Once every 2 weeks
36-delivery	One a week

At each visit the physician should query the patient about her general health and answer any complaints or questions she may have. Additionally, weight, blood pressure, abdominal examination by Leopold's maneuvers, fundal height measurement, rate and location of fetal heart tones, and examination of the urine for protein and glucose should be recorded each visit. All of these should be reviewed in relationship to the findings of the previous visit so that a beneficial trend can be ascertained.

Routine laboratory screening

Laboratory tests assist in detection or confirmation of the presence of certain risk factors. Other special examinations may be indicated by aberrations discovered through the screening process. The following studies should be obtained as early in pregnancy as possible and some (indicated in italics) should be repeated at 24 to 28 weeks and again at 32 to 36 weeks:

1. *Hematocrit and hemoglobin*
2. White blood count
3. Differential white blood count
4. Urinalysis
5. Culture of urine (with bacterial sensitivities if there are at least 10^5 bacteria/ml)
6. Serologic test for syphilis
7. Rubella antibody titer
8. Toxoplasmosis antibody titer (repeat near term if at first negative)
9. Blood grouping and Rh determination
10. *Screening test for antibodies* (Hemantigen or comparable screening test) (see Appendix H)
11. Papanicolaou smear
12. *Cervical culture for* Neisseria gonorrhoeae

Additionally, some authors recommend routine glucose (fasting or 2-hour post-prandial) screening. Other screening tools include serum alpha fetoprotein measurement and ultrasonography, which appear to have favorable risk/benefit ratios when carefully applied. The serum alpha fetoprotein measurement is best obtained at 17 weeks and the sonogram in the first half of the second trimester.

Other essentials of standard prenatal care, including individually indicated laboratory evaluation, close and comprehensive fetal assessment, and special studies to ascertain fetal well-being, are discussed in later chapters.

FACTORS RELATING TO INTRAUTERINE JEOPARDY

The mother may have a serious health problem, obstetric disorders, poor social environment, or biologic handicap—all potentially inimical to perinatal health. Some fetuses may be damaged early, others late; many infants will be born before their due date or be unusually small for gestational age. A few will have grown too large or will have remained in utero too long; each situation has its special hazards.

Women likely to have a higher perinatal mortality or morbidity during pregnancy must be identified. Completely unexpected complications are rare when thorough evaluation and careful longitudinal observation have been employed and significant variations are recognized and problems are treated during pregnancy and anticipated at delivery. The obstetric nurse, public health nurse, and social worker should complement physician and clinic care in promoting maternal and fetal health, especially during illness, when the family is under stress, or when social conditions are poor.

A list* of maternal high-risk factors contributing to perinatal mortality and morbidity in infants and children is presented here. About 10% to 20% of women fall into these groupings, which account for over half the fetal and neonatal deaths.

---

*Modified from Wigglesworth, R.: "At risk" registers, Dev. Med. Child Neurol. **10:**679, 1968.

1. Family history of serious hereditary and familial abnormalities, e.g., osteogenesis imperfecta or mongolism
2. History of prematurity or small-for-dates birth of self or most recent child
3. Significant maternal congenital anomalies involving the central nervous system, heart, or skeletal system; pulmonary abnormalities; also blood dyscrasias, including anemia (hematocrit under 32%)
4. Severe social problem, e.g., teenage pregnancy, drug addiction, or absence of father
5. Long delayed or absent prenatal care
6. Age under 18 or over 35 years
7. Height under 60 inches and prepregnant weight of less than 20% under or over standards for weight and height
8. Fifth or subsequent pregnancy, especially when gravida is over 35 years of age
9. Conception within 3 months of previous pregnancy
10. History of prolonged infertility or drug or hormone treatment
11. Teratogenic viral illness in the first trimester; extensive exposure to radiation
12. Stressful events, e.g., severe emotional tensions, hyperemesis gravidarum, general anesthesia, shock, or critical accidents
13. Habit of heavy smoking
14. Alcohol consumption or other substance abuse
15. Obstetric complications, past or present, e.g., toxemia, placental separation, isoimmunization, hydramnios, or amniotic fluid leak
16. Multiple pregnancy
17. Fetus that fails to grow normally or is disparate in size from that expected
18. Minimal/no weight gain or extraordinary weight gain
19. Abnormal presentation, e.g., breech, transverse, unengaged presenting part at term
20. Fetus over 42 weeks' gestational age

Demographic studies have identified special maternal and fetal complications that are related significantly to fetal and neonatal death. Tables 2-1 and 2-2 present data from the British Perinatal Mortality Survey that indicate the incidence of specific complications and the perinatal mortality according to each diagnosis.

Although these data are now over 25 years old and were collected before many current diagnostic and therapeutic tools were available, they are nonetheless useful, for they indicate what can be expected without proper intervention. In Table 2-2 breech presentation, premature separation of the placenta, toxemia, twinning, and urinary tract infection are associated with over 60% of fetal and 50% of neonatal mortality. Today much of this perinatal mortality, and the morbidity in survivors, can be avoided by skillful diagnosis and available therapy.

Some of these disorders, for example, eclampsia or nephritis, although uncommon, represent an extremely high attrition, as much as 40% of total perinatal mortality. For twins (about 1.4% to 1.6% of births in the United States) perinatal mortality is about 11% (four times that for pregnancy in general). Obviously, in the presence of potential fetal and neonatal jeopardy, patients will require special care to prevent morbidity and mortality.

FACTORS PLACING THE NEWBORN AT INCREASED JEOPARDY

The incidence of congenital anomalies, premature birth, cerebral palsy, and mental retardation is related to and often caused by undesirable antecedents (preceding delivery and even conception). Identification of harmful influences and their avoidance or neutralization must be the goals of everyone interested in obstetrics, pediatrics, and public health. Some deleterious factors remain unknown; others may be known to exist but thus far defy elimination; but many can be identified and controlled.

After delivery, additional environmental factors may either augment or reduce the ultimate capabilities of the offspring. The following associations during the immediate birthing interval place the infant at increased risk and therefore require special care and observation:
1. Maternal history of risk factors during previous pregnancy, particularly
    a. Prolonged rupture of membranes
    b. Abnormal presentation and delivery
    c. Prolonged, difficult labor, or precipitous delivery
    d. Prolapsed cord
2. Birth asphyxia as suggested by
    a. Fetal heart rate fluctuations
    b. Meconium staining, particularly aspiration

Table 2-1. High-risk pregnancy and related hospital perinatal mortality

Cause of death	Incidence/1,000 total births*	Stillbirths/1,000 total births	Live-born infants, deaths/1,000 total births	Perinatal mortality/1,000 total births
Breech (single)	36.5	3.4	3.1	6.5
Premature separation of placenta	12.6	2.7	1.6	4.3
Twin birth	22.7	0.8	1.4	2.2
Preeclampsia (grade 1)	34.8	1.5	0.5	2.0
Hydramnios	4.7	0.8	1.0	1.8
Urinary tract infection	32.7	0.7	0.7	1.4
Preeclampsia (grade 2)	6.2	0.9	0.4	1.3
Placenta previa	5.7	0.4	0.8	1.2
Prolapsed cord	4.8	0.9	0.3	1.2
Diabetes mellitus	6.0	0.4	0.6	1.0
Hypertension and proteinuria	13.9	0.7	0.1	0.8
Pyelonephritis	6.3	0.2	0.2	0.4
Phlebitis	5.7	0.3	0.1	0.4
Eclampsia	0.8	0.2	0.1	0.3
TOTAL HOSPITAL PERINATAL MORTALITY		16.1	14.9	31.0

From Butler, N.R., and Bonham, D.G.: British perinatal mortality survey, 1958, perinatal mortality report of the survey under auspices of the National Birthday Trust Fund, vol. 1, Edinburgh, 1963, E. & S. Livingstone, Ltd.
*30,765 total births.

Table 2-2. High-risk pregnancy and mortality according to diagnosis

Diagnosis	Incidence/1,000 total births	Mortality (%)		
		Stillbirths	Live births	Totals
Eclampsia	0.8	28.0	12.0	40.0
Hydramnios	4.7	17.2	22.1	39.3
Premature separation of placenta	12.6	21.2	12.7	33.9
Prolapsed cord	4.8	19.7	6.1	25.8
Preeclampsia (grade 2)	6.2	14.7	6.8	21.5
Placenta previa	5.7	7.5	13.8	21.3
Breech (single)	36.5	9.2	8.5	17.7
Diabetes mellitus	6.0	6.0	9.2	15.2
Twin birth	22.7	4.3	6.3	10.6
Hypertension and proteinuria	13.9	5.4	0.7	6.1
Preeclampsia (grade 1)	34.8	4.2	1.5	5.7
Urinary tract infection	32.7	2.1	2.1	4.2
ALL HOSPITALIZED PATIENTS	30,765	1.6	1.5	3.1

From Butler, N.R., and Bonham, D.G.: British perinatal mortality survey, 1958, perinatal mortality report of the survey under auspices of the National Birthday Trust Fund, vol. 1, Edinburgh, 1963, E. & S. Livingstone, Ltd.

    c. Fetal acidosis (pH below 7.2)
    d. Apgar scores below 7, particularly if present at 5 minutes
3. Preterm birth (before 38 weeks)
4. Postterm birth (after 42 weeks) with evidence of fetal wasting
5. Small-for-dates infants (below 5th percentile)
6. Large-for-dates infants (above 95th percentile), especially the large preterm infant
7. Any respiratory distress or apnea
8. Obvious congenital anomalies
9. Convulsions, limpness, or difficulty in sucking or swallowing
10. Distention or vomiting
11. Anemia (less than 45% hematocrit) or bleeding diathesis
12. Jaundice during first 24 hours or bilirubin levels above 15 mg/100 ml

The identification of unexpected neonatal problems and classification by weight/gestation parameters are discussed in Chapter 11. Regionalization of neonatal care and the levels of care necessary for infants at varying degrees of risk are discussed in Chapter 36.

The significance of the enormous morbidity and mortality during the perinatal interval of life cannot be overemphasized. Although perinatal mortality has been reduced in the United States to 20 deaths per 1,000 live-born infants (Fig. 34-1), the risk of death is still relatively high. One must live beyond 60 years of age to expect a similar death rate. Dramatic as the mortality is, it represents just the tip of the iceberg; the larger proportion is the morbidity incurred during this interval of life, when as many as 1 out of every 20 Americans is to a greater or lesser degree impaired for the remainder of his life.

NOXIOUS HABITS

Certain personal habits, often bordering on addiction, create great perinatal risk. Maternal habits with most hazard for the fetus and neonate are drug addiction, smoking, and alcohol abuse.

Effects of maternal drug addiction on the fetus and neonate

Occasional withdrawal reactions have been reported in infants of mothers who excessively use such drugs as barbiturates, alcohol, or amphetamines. Serious reactions are seen in neonates (approximately 85% of those exposed) whose mothers are addicted to heroin or treated with methadone. Almost 50% of pregnancies of women addicted to these narcotics result in low birth weight infants—not necessarily preterm.

I. Possible factors contributing to the greater incidence among drug-addicted mothers of low birth weight infants
 A. Acute infections in the mother, often resulting in premature onset of labor
 B. Poor maternal nutrition, leading to fetal undergrowth
 C. Direct influence of the drug on the fetus (based on animal experiments)
II. Diagnosis of withdrawal reaction
 Symptoms usually occur within 24 hours but can begin as late as 2 to 3 weeks after birth, especially if methadone was taken by the mother. Symptoms vary from mild to severe and may last for several weeks.
 A. Signs commonly seen
 1. Hypertonicity
 2. Irritability and high-pitched cry
 3. Tremors
 4. Vomiting
 5. Diarrhea
 B. Signs occasionally present
 1. Tachypnea
 2. Elevation of temperature
 3. Convulsions
III. Treatment of withdrawal
 Treatment of the infant suffering from narcotic withdrawal is primarily supportive and directed toward lessening the infant's irritability. Swaddling the baby, keeping him in a quiet environment, and disturbing him as little possible is often helpful. Demand feeding the infant also will reduce constant crying.
 While many infants can be so managed, about half of those with symptoms of withdrawal will need pharmacologic therapy. Drugs of choice are:
 A. Phenobarbital
 This drug is especially useful when irritability and crying are major symptoms. Starting doses range between 10 to 15 mg/kg/day followed by a maintenance dose of 5 mg/kg/day, preferably given by mouth, but also parenterally when indicated. Dosage should be tapered slowly after infant has remained asymptomatic for several days.
 B. Paregoric
 This drug has been used especially for infants with gastrointestinal symptoms, such as diarrhea. However, it not only acts as an antispasmodic but also will calm irritability. The dose of paregoric is 0.2 to 0.5 ml every 3 to 4 hours. Again, drug dosage is tapered slowly once symptoms have subsided, for 1 or 2 days.

Infants not able to tolerate feedings may need to be given parenteral fluids temporarily until their conditions improve. Close attention should be given to blood glucose homeostasis by intermittent screening tests.

Infants who exhibit symptoms of withdrawal should be observed in the nursery until they can be managed at home without difficulty and are no longer in need of pharmacologic therapy. Close follow-up of such infants after discharge from the hospital is indicated to detect possible recurrence of withdrawal symptoms, to ensure the infants receive proper nutrition, and to meet the social needs of both the parents and their baby. Involvement of a social worker and community health nurse should be part of the discharge planning for these infants. Although long-term prognosis seems favorable overall, some reports indicate a possible risk of sudden infant death syndrome (SIDS) and later learning disability.

Maternal smoking during pregnancy

The detrimental effect of cigarette smoking on the fetus is now clear. Although nicotine, carbon monoxide, and tars have been held responsible, smoking, like excessive eating or drinking, can also be considered a reflection of stress. Recent studies suggest smoking increases the proportion of hemoglobin bound to carbon monoxide reducing the oxygen-carrying capacity of the blood. The following associations have been shown in controlled studies:

1. Fetal weight is reduced by at least 200 gm on the average, with a significant increase in the incidence of low birth weight infants.
2. Mortality is higher, particularly during fetal life (Fig. 2-1).
3. Chances of spontaneous abortion increase.

A distressing factor is the additional detrimental effect smoking has on conditions affecting placental perfusion, such as has been shown to apply to the hypertensive gravida.

The conclusions of the British Perinatal Mortality Survey (Fig. 2-1) indicate that smoking is prejudicial to fetal health. Consequently, the probable survival of fetuses of mothers in high-risk categories who smoke is further reduced.

Every effort should be made to discourage smoking during pregnancy, even though smoking may be the result of tensions.

Alcohol abuse

Alcohol is a teratogen. Maternal ethanol abuse during gestation creates a readily identifiable syndrome. Moreover, the frequency of affected children may reach 5 per 1,000 live births, making this the most frequent identifiable te-

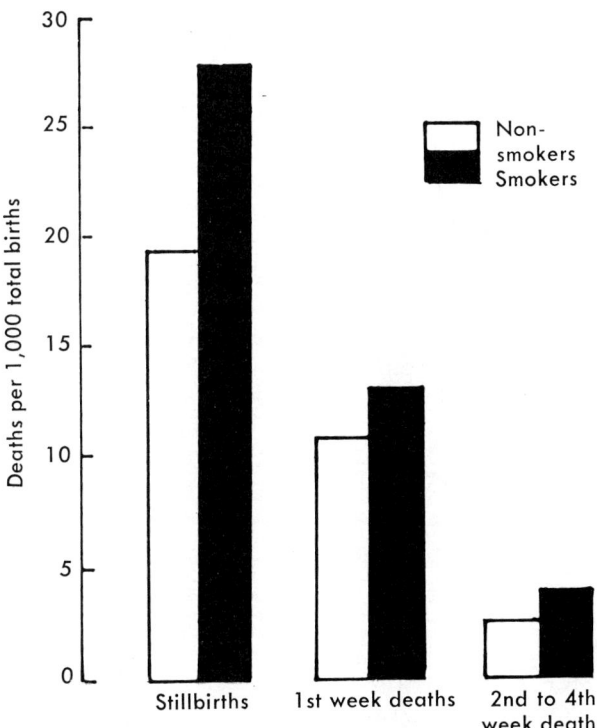

Fig. 2-1. Stillbirth and early and late neonatal mortality by maternal smoking habit. (From Butler, N.R., and Alberman, E.D., editors: Perinatal problems. The second report of the 1958 British Perinatal Mortality Survey, Edinburgh and London, 1969, E. & S. Livingstone, Ltd.)

ratogen. Syndrome identification depends on alterations in brain function, growth, and facial appearance.

The threshold amount of ethanol necessary to cause fetal damage is unknown, and no safe level of ethanol consumption or safe time of gestation for consumption can be established. Certainly chronic consumption of 90 ml of absolute ethanol or more per day (the equivalent of 6 drinks) is known to be associated with fetal anomalies. Fetal alcohol syndrome is discussed in greater detail in Chapter 3.

PATERNAL INFLUENCES

The paternal role in prematurity and high-risk pregnancy is largely theoretical and is yet to be clarified.

1. Higher paternal age has been related to increased incidence of still-born infants and infants having a congenital abnormality. However, maternal age is also higher than the mean in most of these cases, which suggests that paternal age is still an uncertain factor in reproductive wastage.
2. The inheritance of Rh-positive genes from the father by the fetus may result in erythroblastosis fetalis when the mother is Rh-negative.
3. Chronic alcoholism and diabetes mellitus in the father may affect fetal development adversely.

MISCELLANEOUS FACTORS

1. High altitude exposure may result in small-for-dates babies and perhaps developmental anomaly.
2. Hormonal insufficiency indicated by low or inappropriately falling chorionic gonadotropin and pregnanediol levels is a poor prognostic sign for the fetus.
3. Genetic influences often impair fetal development.
4. Extraordinary maternal exercise may contribute to decreased uterine blood flow and therefore compromise fetal growth.

In summary, normal development of the fetus is threatened by a myriad of factors, both singly and in combination. Many are obstetric in nature in that maternal complications play a threatening role. More are environmental factors such as unfavorable social conditions, educational handicaps, or nutritional deficits inimical to optimal fetal health. Interaction between many of these factors occurs and adversely affects perinatal mortality and the conditions of survivors.

Improvement in fetal health care (both medical and environmental) is an obligation of the community and a right of the patient. Solutions for social, economic, and educational deficiencies are current challenges. Pregnancy by choice rather than chance promises to be most relevant in improving the quality of life for the fetus as well as the later condition of the child. Perinatal death and neurologic sequelae will be reduced, and the chain of succeeding generations of physically and emotionally deprived children may be broken.

METHOD OF IDENTIFICATION OF SPECIFIC RISK FACTORS

Certain checkpoints must be used in the continuum of antenatal care to guarantee that all risks are identified and treated appropriately. We employ the following checkpoints:

1. Initial screening
2. Prenatal visit screening
3. Intrapartum screening
   a. On admission to hospital
   b. On admission to obstetric intensive care area
4. Delivery evaluation
   a. Neonatal
   b. Maternal
5. Postpartum evaluation
   a. Neonatal
   b. Maternal

Although a totally exhaustive cataloging of each risk factor is not practical, patients at risk are then defined by the following criteria at each checkpoint:

I. Initial screening
   Biologic and marital factors
   A. High risk
      1. Maternal age of 15 years or less
      2. Maternal age of 35 years or more
      3. Paternal age of 53 years or more
      4. A known genetic abnormality in either parent or a close relative
      5. Massive obesity or marked (less than 10% standard weight for height) malnutrition
   B. Moderate risk
      1. Maternal age 16 to 19 years

2. Maternal age 30 to 34 years
3. Single marital status
4. Nonwhite (if underprivileged)
5. Obesity (more than 20% of standard weight for height) (Table 1-1)
6. Malnutrition (less than 10% standard weight for height)
7. Short stature (60 inches or less)

Obstetric history
A. High risk
   1. Previously diagnosed genital tract anomalies
      a. Incompetent cervix
      b. Cervical malformation
      c. Uterine malformation
   2. Two or more previous abortions
   3. Previous stillborn or neonatal loss
   4. Two previous premature labors or low birth weight infants (less than 2,500 gm)
   5. Two excessively large previous infants (more than 4.000 gm)
   6. Uterine leiomyomas (5 cm or more or submucus in location)
   7. Ovarian mass
   8. Parity of eight or more
   9. Previous infant with isoimmunization
   10. History of eclampsia
   11. Previous infant with
      a. Known or suspected genetic or familial disorders
      b. Congenital anomaly
   12. History of previous need for special neonatal-infant care or birth-damaged infant
   13. Medical indications for termination of a previous pregnancy
   14. Previous
      a. Breech birth
      b. Abruptio placentae
      c. Placenta previa
B. Moderate risk
   1. Previous premature labor, low birth weight infant (less than 2,500 gm), or abortion
   2. One excessively large infant (more than 4,000 gm)
   3. Previous operative deliveries
      a. Cesarean section
      b. Midforceps delivery
      c. Breech extraction
   4. Previous prolonged labor or significant dystocia
   5. Possible fetopelvic disproportion
   6. Previous severe emotional problems associated with pregnancy or delivery
   7. Previous uterine or cervical operations
   8. Primigravida
   9. Parity of five to eight
   10. Previous infertility
   11. Prior ABO incompatibility
   12. Prior fetal malpresentation
   13. Previous history of endometriosis
   14. Pregnancy occurring 3 months or less after last delivery

Medical and surgical history
A. High risk
   1. Moderate to severe chronic hypertension
   2. Moderate to severe renal disease
   3. Severe heart disease (classes II to IV, history of congestive heart failure, or previous cardiac or vascular surgery)
   4. Diabetes (classes B to F)
   5. Previous endocrine ablation
   6. Abnormal cervical cytologic condition
   7. Sickle-cell disease
   8. Drug addiction or alcoholism
   9. Alcohol abuse (either chronic or episodic)
   10. Pulmonary disease (including history of tuberculosis or PPD test revealing a diameter of more than 1 cm)
   11. Malignancy
   12. Gastrointestinal or liver disease
   13. Connective tissue disease
   14. Previous thrombosis or pulmonary embolism
   15. Neurologic disease
B. Moderate risk
   1. Mild chronic hypertension
   2. Mild renal disease
   3. Mild heart disease (class I)
   4. History of mild hypertensive states of pregnancy
   5. History of pyelonephritis

6. Diabetes (class A) or family history of diabetes
7. Thyroid disease
8. Positive serology findings
9. Excessive use of drugs
10. Emotional problems
11. Sickle-cell trait
12. Epilepsy

II. Prenatal visit screening
Early pregnancy
A. High risk
1. Failure of uterine growth or disproportionate uterine growth
2. Exposure to teratogens
   a. Radiation
   b. Infection
   c. Chemicals
3. Pregnancy complicated by isoimmunization
4. Need for antenatal genetic diagnosis
5. Severe anemia (9 gm or less hemoglobin
6. Pregnancy with an intrauterine device in place

B. Moderate risk
1. Unresponsive urinary tract infection
2. Suspected ectopic pregnancy
3. Suspected missed abortion
4. Severe hyperemesis gravidarum
5. Positive VDRL test
6. Positive gonorrhea screening
7. Anemia not responsive to iron treatment
8. Viral illness
9. Vaginal bleeding
10. Mild anemia (9 to 10.9 gm hemoglobin)

Late pregnancy
A. High risk
1. Failure of uterine growth or disproportionate uterine growth
2. Severe anemia (less than 9 gm hemoglobin)
3. More than 42½ weeks' gestation
4. Severe preeclampsia
5. Eclampsia
6. Breech if vaginal delivery is planned
7. Moderate to severe isoimmunization (necessitating intrauterine transfusion or neonatal exchange transfusion)
8. Placenta previa
9. Hydramnios or oligohydramnios
10. Antepartum fetal death
11. Thromboembolic disease
12. Premature labor (less than 37 weeks' gestation)
13. Premature rupture of membranes (less than 38 weeks' gestation) and/or prolonged rupture of membranes
14. Tumor or other obstruction of the birth canal
15. Abruptio placentae
16. Chronic or acute pyelonephritis
17. Multiple gestation
18. Abnormal:
    a. Nonstress test
    b. Contraction stress test
    c. Biometric testing
    d. Falling estriols
19. Diabetes

B. Moderate risk
1. Hypertensive states of pregnancy (mild)
2. Breech if cesarean section is planned
3. Uncertain presentations
4. Need for fetal maturity studies
5. Postdate pregnancy (41 to 42½ weeks)
6. Induction of labor
7. Suspected fetopelvic disproportion at term
8. Floating presentations 2 weeks or less from the estimated date of confinement

III. Intrapartum screening (secondary on admission to hospital or tertiary on admission to obstetric intensive care area)
A. High risk
1. Previous factors indicative of high risk
2. Severe preeclampsia or eclampsia
3. Hydramnios or oligohydramnios
4. Amnionitis
5. Rupture of membranes for over 24 hours

6. Uterine rupture
7. Placenta previa
8. Abruptio placentae
9. Meconium staining of amniotic fluid
10. Abnormal presentation (including breech)
11. Multiple gestation
12. Fetal weight less than 2,000 gm
13. Fetal weight more than 4,000 gm
14. Fetal distress as determined by pH or fetal heart rate
15. Prolapsed cord
16. Fetal presenting part not descending with labor
17. Shoulder dystocia
18. Evidence of maternal distress
19. Immature or intermediate fetal status as determined by lecithin/sphingomyelin ratio, rapid surfactant test, or absent or trace PG
20. Vasa previa

B. Moderate risk
1. Mild hypertensive states of pregnancy
2. Premature rupture of membranes more than 12 hours before labor
3. Primary dysfunctional labor
4. Secondary arrest of dilatation
5. Medical therapy
   a. Tocolytics
   b. Magnesium sulfate
   c. Barbiturates
   d. Narcotics
6. Labor longer than 20 hours
7. Second stage of labor longer than 1 hour
8. Clinically small pelvis
9. Medical induction of labor
10. Precipitous labor (less than 3 hours)
11. Elective induction
12. Prolonged latent phase
13. Uterine tetany
14. Oxytocin (Pitocin) augmentation
15. Marginal separation of placenta
16. Operative forceps
17. Vacuum extraction
18. General anesthesia
19. Any abnormality of maternal vital signs
20. Abnormal uterine contractions

IV. Postnatal criteria for risk
Postnatally the patient's vital signs, uterine tone, lochia, and so forth are observed carefully for the first 6 to 8 hours post partum.

A. Specific factors placing the mother at high risk include
1. Hemorrhage
2. Infection
3. Abnormal vital signs
4. Traumatic delivery

B. The infant is observed briefly in the delivery room, and an initial screening physical examination is completed. Approximately 5% of infants born are at sufficient risk to require being transferred to a neonatal intensive care unit. Another 20% are at medium risk and should receive special care. They include infants who are disproportionate in weight and length according to gestational indexes especially those who are light for length (ponderal index of less than 2.25). The following criteria are used to select high-risk infants for admission to neonatal intensive care units (tertiary centers):
1. Continuing or developing signs of respiratory distress
2. Asphyxiation (Apgar score of less than 6 at 5 minutes)
3. Less than 33 weeks' gestational age
4. Weight of less than 1,500 gm
5. Cyanosis, heart failure, or other signs of possible cardiovascular disease
6. Major congenital malformations requiring surgery or investigation
7. Convulsions, sepsis, hemorrhagic diathesis, or shock
8. Meconium aspiration syndrome
9. Apnea

C. Moderate risk for infants requiring special care at the medium-risk level
1. Dysmaturity
2. Prematurity (1,500 to 2,500 gm)

3. Apgar score of 4 to 6 at 1 minute
4. Feeding problems
5. Multiple birth
6. Transient tachypnea
7. Hypoglycemia
8. Hypocalcemia
9. Hypomagnesemia or hypermagnesemia
10. Hyperbilirubinemia
11. Failure to gain weight
12. Jitteriness or hyperactivity with specific causes
13. Central nervous system depression
14. Anemia

BIBLIOGRAPHY

American Academy of Pediatrics, Committee on Drugs: Neonatal drug withdrawal, Pediatrics **72:**895, 1983.

Anderson, J.M.: High-risk groups—definitions and identifications, N. Engl. J. Med. **273:**308, 1965

Butler, N.R., and Bonham, D.G.: British perinatal mortality survey, 1958, perinatal mortality report of the survey under auspices of the National Birthday Trust Fund, vol. 1, Edinburgh, 1963, E. & S. Livingstone, Ltd.

Clarren, S.K., and Smith, D.W.: The fetal alcohol syndrome, N. Engl. J. Med. **298:**1063, 1978.

Davies, D.P., and Abernethy, M.: Cigarette smoking in pregnancy: associations with maternal weight gain and fetal growth, Lancet **1:**385, 1976.

Finnegan, L.P.: In utero opiate dependency and sudden infant death syndrome, Clin. Perinatol. **6:**163, 1979.

Gold, E.M.: Identification of the high risk fetus, Clin. Obstet. Gynecol. **11:**1069, 1968.

Haxton, M.J., and Bell, J.: Fetal anatomical abnormalities and other associated factors in middle-trimester abortion and their relevance to patient counselling, Br. J. Obstet. Gynaecol. **90:**501, 1983.

Jacobson, H.N., and Reid, D.E.: A pattern of comprehensive maternal and child care, II. N. Engl. J. Med. **271:**302, 1964.

Kandall, S.R., and Garner, L.M.: Late presentation of drug withdrawal symptoms in newborns, Am. J. Dis. Child. **127:**58, 1974.

King, C.R., Pernoll, M.L., and Prescott, G.: Reproductive wastage, Obstet. Gynecol. Annu. **11:**59, 1982.

Kline, J., Stein, Z.A., Susser, M., et al.: Smoking a risk factor for spontaneous abortion, N. Engl. J. Med. **297:**793, 1977.

Larsonn, G.: Prevention of fetal alcohol effects (an antenatal program for early detection of pregnancies at risk), Acta. Obstet. Gynecol. Scand. **62:**171, 1983.

Lewis, B.V., and Nash, P.J.: Pregnancy in patients under 16 years, Br. Med. J. **2:**733, 1967.

Lilford, R.J., and Chard, T: Problems and pitfalls of risk assessment in antenatal care, Br. J. Obstet. Gynecol. **90:**507, 1983.

Miller, H.C., Hassanein, K., Chin, T.D., et al.: Socioeconomic factors in relation to fetal growth in white infants, J. Pediatr. **89:**638, 1976.

Myer, M.B., and Tonascia, J. A.: Maternal smoking, pregnancy complications and perinatal mortality, Am. J. Obstet. Gynecol. **128:**494, 1977.

Niswander, K. R., and Gordon, M.: The women and their pregnancies, Philadelphia, 1972, W.B. Saunders Co.

Reddy, A.M., Harpes, R.G., and Stern, G.: Observations on heroin and methadone withdrawal in the newborn, Pediatrics **48:**353, 1971.

Rosen, T.S. and Johnson, H.L.: Children of methadone maintained mothers: follow-up to 18 months of age, J. Pediatr. **101:**192, 1982.

Russell, C.S., Taylor, R., and Maddison, R.N.: Some effects of smoking in pregnancy, J. Obstet. Gynaec. Brit. Comm. **73:**742, 1966.

Russell, J.K.: Pregnancy in the young teenager, Lancet **1:**365, 1969.

Terris, M., and Gold, E.M.: An epidemiologic study of prematurity, I and II. Am. J. Obstet. Gynecol. **103:**358, 1969.

Tracy, T., and Miller, G.D.: Obstetric problems of the massively obese, Obstet. Gynecol. **33:**204, 1969.

Von der Ahe, C.V.: The unwed teenage mother Am. J. Obstet. Gynecol. **104:**279, 1969.

Wright, A.D., et al.: Spontaneous abortions and diabetes mellitus, Postgrad. Med. J. **59:**295, 1983.

Yerushalmy, J.: Mother's cigarette smoking and survival of the infant, Am. J. Obstet. Gynecol. **88:**505, 1964.

Zackler, J., Andelman, S.L., and Bauer, F.: Young adolescent as an obstetric risk, Am. J. Obstet. Gynecol. **103:**305, 1969.

Zelson, C., Lee, S.J., and Casalino, M.: Neonatal narcotic addiction, N. Engl. J. Med. **289:**1216, 1973.

3

Genetic and congenital defects

Significant deleterious deviations from normal standards of structure and function (malformations, anomalies, or defects) occur with regularity in human reproduction. Indeed, approximately 3% to 7% of newborns have malformations serious enough to require treatment. Although a number of agents are believed to be responsible for these abnormalities (e.g., irradiation, viruses, gases and drugs), causes for the majority of defects unfortunately remain unclear. Indeed, the inherent risk of a "natural" aberration occurring in the complex reproductive process is unknown. Estimates of etiologic associations are as follows:

Maternal metabolic imbalance	1%-2%
Infections	2%-3%
Chromosomal aberrations (new mutations)	3%-5%
Drugs and environmental agents	4%-5%
Known genetic transmission	20%
Unknown	60%-70%

CHROMOSOMAL ABERRATIONS AND GENETIC TRANSMISSIONS

Chromosomal aberrations involve alterations in both number and morphology. The numerical abnormalities are the result of nondisjunction. Nondisjunction is a failure of the double chromosomal complement to be equally divided between the two daughter cells. Therefore one cell has an extra chromosome and the other is missing the homologous chromosome. This may result in trisomy (an extra chromosome) or monosomy (a missing chromosome) after combination with a normal gamete. Postzygotic nondisjunction results in a mosaic (cells of two or more different chromosomal constitutions).

Aberrations of morphology may relate to chromosomal breakage. For example, Bloom's dwarfism and Fanconi's anemia both show an increased incidence of chromosomal breakage. The most common morphologic aberration is translocation. However, deletion may also occur.

If these changes occur in sex chromosomes, a spectrum of sex chromosomal abnormalities results. These include Turner's syndrome (gonadal female dysgenesis), triple or tetra X syndrome, Klinefelter's syndrome (seminiferous tubule dysgenesis), true hermaphroditism, pure gonadal dysgenesis, or familial XY gonadal dysgenesis.

In autosomes, more common diseases are Down's syndrome, trisomy 18 syndrome, trisomy 13 syndrome, cri-du-chat (cat-cry) syndrome, and trisomy-8 mosaicism.

The risk of aneuploidy is most commonly encountered in cases of advancing maternal age (Table 3-1). However, the risk is not confined to such cases. Paternal age becomes a factor warranting investigation at 53 years of age.

Fortunately, devastating genetic aberrations in newborns are relatively uncommon, with certain notable exceptions. However, cytogenetic studies of spontaneously aborted human fetuses reveal 30% to 50% of all first- and second-trimester losses to be chromosomally abnormal. Indeed, 5% to 10% of all human conceptuses may have chromosomal abnormalities, and at least 95% of these are aborted. A great number of the abnormalities are numerical.

The genetically transmitted processes are described by their mendelian inheritance pattern.

Table 3-1. Maternal age and fetal chromosomal abnormalities

Incidence of Down's syndrome at birth*	Maternal age	Incidence of Down's syndrome at second trimester†,‡		Incidence of total aneuploidies at second trimester†,‡	
1/1682	15-19				
1/1352	20-24				
1/1133	25-29				
1/885	30				
1/826	31				
1/725	32				
1/592	33				
1/465	34				
1/365	35 ⎫	0	1/143	1/104	1/66
1/287	36 ⎭				
1/225	37 ⎫	1/128	1/100	1/48	1/54
1/176	38 ⎭				
1/139	39 ⎫	1/149	1/45	1/75	1/35
1/109	40 ⎭				
1/85	41 ⎫	1/32	1/41	1/23	1/31
1/67	42 ⎭				
1/53	43 ⎫	1/18	1/18	1/14	1/10
1/41	44 ⎭				
1/32	45				
1/25	46				

*Hook, E.B., and Lindsjo, A.: Down syndrome in live births by single year maternal age interval in a Swedish study: comparison with results from a New York study, Am. J. Hum. Genet. **30:**19, 1978.
†Hook, E.B.: Differences between rates trisomy 21 Down syndrome (DS) and other chromosomal abnormality diagnosis in live births and in cell culture 2nd trimester amniocentesis: suggested explanations for genetic counseling and program planning, Birth Defects, **14:**249, 1978.
‡Golbus, M., Laughman, W., et al.: Prenatal genetic diagnosis in 3000 amniocenteses, New Engl. J. Med. **300:**157, 1979.

Thus, they are classified as being autosomal dominant, autosomal recessive, sex-linked, sex-limited, or of polygenic inheritance. Examples of dominantly inherited autosomal diseases are achondroplasia, Ehlers-Danlos syndrome, hereditary spherocytosis, Huntington's chorea, Marfan's syndrome, neurofibromatosis, osteogenesis imperfecta, retinoblastoma, and tuberous sclerosis.

Examples of recessively inherited autosomal diseases are albinism, galactosemia, Gaucher's disease, Hurler's syndrome, maple syrup urine disease, phenylketonuria, sickle-cell anemia, thalassemia, and Wilson's disease. A sex-linked dominant inherited disease is vitamin D–resistant rickets (some types). Recessively inherited conditions include color blindness, glucose-6-phosphate dehydrogenase deficiency (G6PD), hemophilia A, hemophilia B, muscular dystrophy of Duchenne, and Lesch-Nyhan syndrome.

Many diseases are multifactorial in origin. Some cases are believed to represent a spectrum of interaction between the genotype and its environment. In other instances there may be several possible causes for the same disease or process. These conditions are more difficult to describe genetically and pose challenges for genetic counseling. Examples of such conditions include cleft palate, spina bifida, and pyloric stenosis.

Inborn errors of metabolism are usually inherited as autosomal recessives. They are a rare but serious group of diseases, many of which are detectable by antenatal genetic diagnosis.

EARLY FETAL DEVELOPMENT AND GROWTH

The reproductive process can be adversely affected at any of its several stages by a number of agents or processes. The clinician is most frequently faced with questions relating to potential defects occurring as a result of exposure to various agents during fetal development and growth. To improve understanding of the sig-

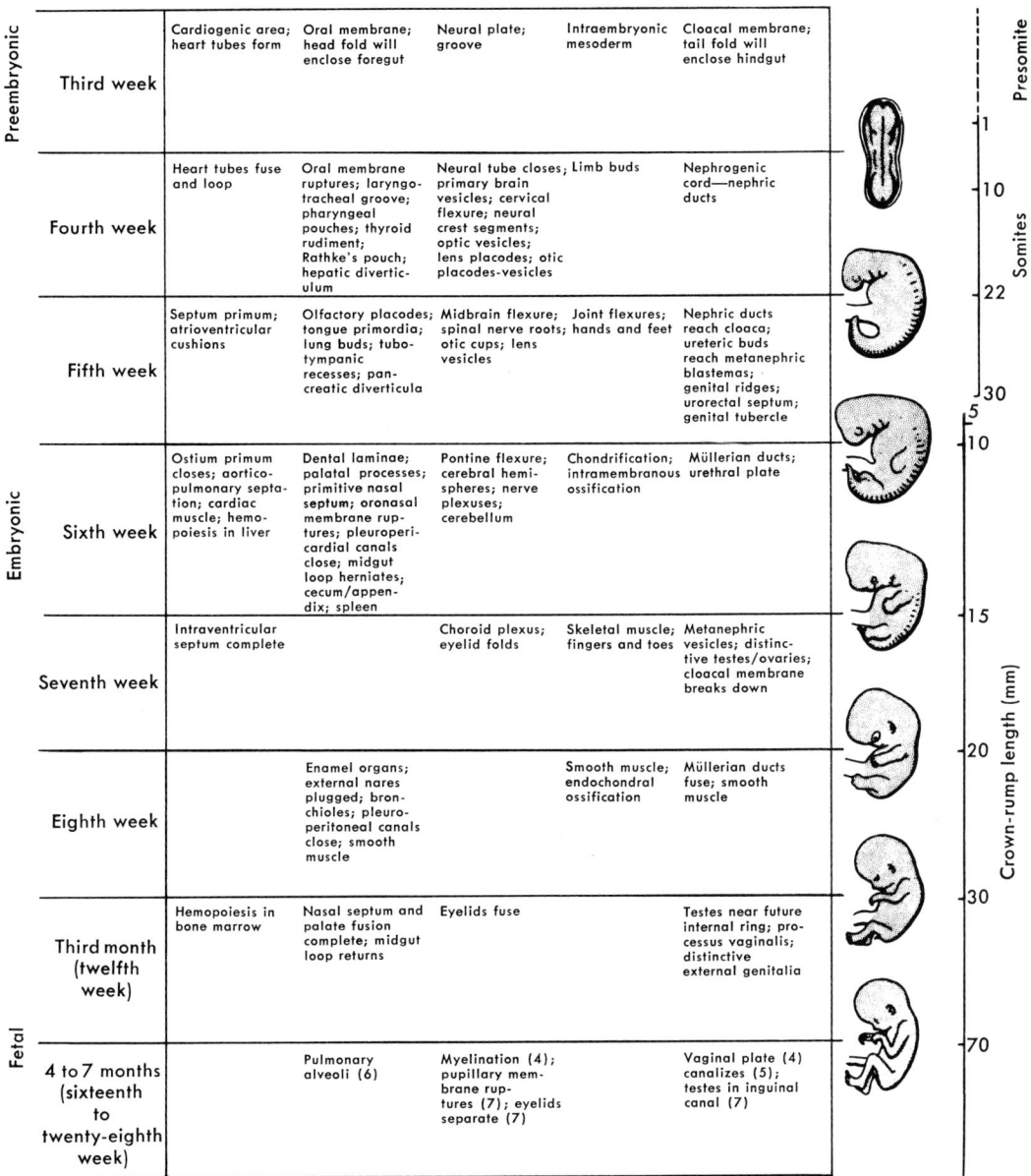

Fig. 3-1. Organogenesis. (From Williams, P.L., Wendell-Smith, C.P., and Treadgold, S.: Basic human embryology, London, 1966, Pitman Medical Publishing Co., Ltd.)

nificance of deviations from established norms, it is necessary to describe the different phases of fetal development and growth. Terminologies to express these phases overlap, and none has been demonstrated superior. Although the following terminology differs from that used in Fig. 3-1 and in Table 3-2, the relationship between susceptibility to defect from exposure to teratogenic agents and the stage of development at the time of exposure can still be appreciated.

The *ovular phase* comprises the first 4 weeks after fertilization. In that period there occurs a series of rapid mitotic divisions (cleavage) that result in the formation of a blastula. Next a blastocyst is formed, and organ anlagen are relatively positioned by the process of gastrulation.

Table 3-2. Potential adverse effects and malformations related to time of insult

Week since ovulation	Period	Potential adverse effect or malformation
1	Zygote	Abortion
2-7	Embryo	Fetal wastage
		Structural malformations (see specific defects below)
		Carcinogenesis
		Severe intrauterine growth retardation
3	Embryo	Ectopia cordis
		Omphalocele
		Ectomelia
		Sympodia
4	Embryo	Omphalocele
		Ectomelia
		Tracheoesophageal fistula
		Hemivertebra
5	Embryo	Tracheoesophageal fistula
		Hemivertebra
		Nuclear cataract
		Microphthalmia
		Facial clefts
		Carpal or pedal ablation
6	Embryo	Microphthalmia
		Carpal or pedal ablation
		Cleft lip
		Agnathia
		Lenticular cataract
		Congenital heart disease
		Gross cardiac septal and/or aortic anomalies
7	Embryo	Congenital heart disease
		Intrarventricular septal defects
		Pulmonary stenosis
		Digital ablation
		Cleft palate
		Micrognathia
		Epicanthus
		Brachycephaly
8	Fetus	Congenital heart disease
		Epicanthus
		Brachycephaly
		Persistent ostium primum
		Nasal bone ablation
		Digital stunting
9-40	Fetus	Central nervous system anomalies
		Behavioral disorders
		Functional abnormalities
		Reproductive system defects
		Intrauterine growth retardation

The *embryonic phase* extends from approximately the end of the fourth week until between the eighth and eleventh weeks. During this interval the organ systems develop from their primordia. This phase is characterized by considerable growth and differentiation. The sequence of organogenesis is shown in Fig. 3-1.

The *fetal phase* is the interval from completion of organogenesis until delivery. This time is characterized by growth and development. Natural events or insults that will irrevocably alter that individual's life may occur at any phase. However, the time of occurrence of such events will determine the extent of the insult. For example, in monozygotic twinning timing of division has a dramatic and profound influence on subsequent development.

1. Division prior to the fifth day (prior to the morula stage) results in separate or fused placentas, two chorions, and two amnions.
2. Division from the fifth to the tenth days (after trophoblast differentiation but before amnion formation) results in a single placenta, a common chorion, and one amnion.
3. Division from the tenth to the fourteenth days (after amnion differentiation) results in monochorionic, monoamnionic twinning, an unusual condition.

Furthermore, incomplete monozygous segmentation between the eighth and fourteenth days results in conjoined "Siamese" twins. When cleavage is further postponed, incomplete twinning may occur.

Table 3-2 relates malformations to time of insult. This information may be of assistance in counseling a patient concerning the possibility of malformation from various potentially injurious events or agents.

MUTAGENESIS AND TERATOGENESIS

Agents that create defects are known as *mutagens* or *teratogens*. A mutagen is a chemical or physical agent that induces genetic mutation. A teratogen is an agent or factor that causes the production of physical defects in the developing product of conception. One difference between the two is whether the defect occurs in a somatic cell or a germ cell. In the latter a permanent transmissable change in the character of an offspring from those of its parents is induced (a mutation), whereas in teratogenesis only that particular offspring will be affected. Mutagens must involve macromolecular or micromolecular change in germ cell DNA, whereas teratogenic change may be evoked by a number of mechanisms including mutations, chromosomal nondisjunction and breaks, mitotic interference, altered nucleic acid integrity or function, lack of precursors and substrates necessary for biosynthesis, alteration of energy sources, enzyme inhibitors, osmolar imbalance, and altered membrane characteristics. Fortunately, maternal metabolic diseases having potential to create fetal defects are relatively few and usually amenable to screening procedures. Well-known examples of these disease states include maternal diabetes mellitus, hyperthyroidism, hypothyroidism, and phenylketonuria.

Recognition of teratogenic agents in humans requires that certain criteria be employed. Wilson has suggested using the following:

1. Abrupt increase in incidence of a particular defect or association of defects (syndrome)
2. Coincidence of this increase with a known environmental change (for example, widespread use of a new drug)
3. Known exposure to the environmental change early in pregnancy yielding characteristically defective infants
4. Absence of other factors common to all pregnancies yielding infants with the characteristic defect or defects

The relationship between exposure to a potential mutagen or teratogen and creation of a defect is influenced by many factors. For example, access of the adverse influence to developing tissue depends on the nature of the influence and its interaction with the maternal organism, its transport to the fetus, its interaction with the fetus, and certain reparative phenomena. Factors that may influence a chemical's capability to induce alteration in germ or somatic cellular DNA are detailed below.

1. Gross host factors limiting amount of agent to which DNA is exposed
   a. Absorption
   b. Penetration
   c. Transport
   d. Activation
   e. Inactivation
   f. Excretion
2. Local host factors influencing outcome
   a. Removal of mutated cells
   b. pH
   c. Temperature
3. Genetic mechanisms potentially influencing outcome
   a. Condensations of nuclear membrane
   b. Condensation of chromosomes

Table 3-3. Perinatal viral infections (see also Chapter 25)

Maternal viral disease	Fetal or newborn effect
Coxsackievirus B disease	Meningoencephalitis, myocarditis, and hepatitis
Cytomegalovirus disease	Viruria, hepatosplenomegaly, hepatitis, occasionally transient thrombocytopenia, microcephaly, chorioretinitis, intracerebral calcifications, deafness, visual deficits, portal fibrosis, and mental retardation
Hepatitis	Hepatitis
Herpes	Nonfatal predominantly cutaneous infection, generalized herpes, encephalitis, fulminating disseminated visceral disease, mental retardation, microcephaly with intracranial calcifications, retinal dysphasia, microphthalmus, and neurologic deficits
Influenza	Various malformations
Mumps	Fetal death, various malformations, and possible endocardial fibroelastosis
Poliomyelitis	Abortion, "rag-doll syndrome," spinal or bulbar poliomyelitis
Rubella	Abortion, "blueberry-muffin babies," malformations (microcephaly, cataracts, chorioretinitis, deafness, heart defects), thrombocytopenia, hemolytic anemia, hepatosplenomegaly, pneumonitis, hepatitis, osteomyelitis, encephalitis, mental retardation
Rubeola	Abortion, stillbirth, congenital measles
Vaccinia	Abortion, clinical vaccinia
Herpes zoster	Abortion, stillbirth, prematurity, chickenpox or shingles
Variola	Abortion, stillbirth, and clinical smallpox
Western equine encephalitis	Encephalitis

c. Production of specific nucleotide kinases and DNA replicase (avoids incorporation of wrong nucleotides into DNA)
d. Excision of wrong bases and repair
e. Repair of single-stranded lesions
f. Repair of double-stranded lesions
g. Recombination

Table 3-3 demonstrates many of the perinatal viral infections with sequelae. Currently, it is believed the perinatal infections contributing to most morbidity and mortality are those of the so-called TORCH group (toxoplasmosis, rubella, cytomegalovirus, and herpes). However, syphilis must still be considered a preventable contributor. The effects of these infections are believed to be separate and distinct from the general alterations that occur with severe maternal infections (hyperpyrexia and possible metabolic derangements). The general alterations frequently precipitate premature labor. Moreover, certain infections carry a much greater maternal mortality, thus leading to fetal mortality or morbidity. An example of this extreme form of fetal compromise is influenza.

Table 3-4 illustrates some of the compounds or medicaments with proved, suspected, or possible mutagenic or teratogenic effects.

The maximum dose of ionizing radiation believed to be relatively safe for the embryo has been stated by the National Committee on Radiation Protection to be 10 rads. There is suggestive evidence of an increased incidence of leukemia by 10 years of age if exposure is more than 15 rads. For purpose of comparison, a routine chest x-ray examination with current image enhancement should not exceed 0.03 rads.

Table 3-4. Human fetotoxic compounds

Maternal exposure	Fetal or neonatal effect
Established fetotoxicity	
(definite evidence of increased defects or deaths)	
Alcohol (ethanol)	Mental retardation, microcephaly, poor coordination, hypotonia, infantile irritability, childhood hyperactivity, prenatal and postnatal growth deficiency, diminished adipose tissue, short palpebral fissures, short upturned nose with hypoplastic philtrum, hypoplastic maxilla, thinned upper vermilion, retrognathia in infancy, micrognathia or relative prognathia in adolescence
Antibiotics	
Chloramphenicol	Gray syndrome, neonatal death (not reported if gravida alone received drug)
Chloroquine	Death, deafness, retinal hemorrhage
Erythromycin	Possible hepatic injury
Nitrofurantoin	Megaloblastic anemia, G6PD deficiency
Novobiocin	Hyperbilirubinemia
Quinine, quinidine	Possible ototoxicity, thrombocytopenia
Streptomycin	Nerve deafness
Sulfonamides	Kernicterus caused by competition with bilirubin for albumin-binding sites
Tetracyclines	Inhibition of bone growth, enamel pigmentation or hypoplasia, congenital cataracts
Antineoplastic agents	Abortion, fetal malformations
Aminopterin	
6-Mercaptopurine	
Busulfan (Myleran)	
Chlorambucil (Leukeran)	
Colchicine	
Cyclophosphamide	
Methotrexate	
Androgenic hormones	Masculinization of fetus
Antithyroid agents	Goiter, occasional hypothyroidism
Propylthiouracil	
Methimazole	
Potassium iodide	
Benzene	Various malformations
Cadmium	Various malformations

Table 3-4. Human fetotoxic compounds—cont'd

Maternal exposure	Fetal or neonatal effect
Established fetotoxicity—cont'd	
(definite evidence of increased defects or deaths)	
Coumarins	Fetal death, hemorrhage, calcifications
Diethylstilbestrol	Vaginal adenosis, uterine, cervical, and vaginal malformations, clear cell carcinoma
Lead	Abortion, various malformations, growth retardation (also causes decreased fertility)
Mercury	Abortion, cerebral palsy, microcephaly, variable malformations, growth retardation
Oral contraceptives	Anomalies of genitalia, limb-reduction defects
Progestins	Central nervous system and genitalia abnormalities
Radioiodine	Early in gestation causes various anomalies; later in gestation causes congenital hypothyroidism
Smoking	Fetal growth retardation, increased perinatal deaths, decreased fetal oxygenation
Thalidomide	Phocomelia, fetal death
Warfarin	Chondrodysplasia punctata, various anomalies
Suspected fetotoxicity	
(apparently increased deaths or disability)	
Anesthetic gases	Abortion, stillbirths, various malformations
Antidiabetics	
Chlorpropamide	Fetal death, prolonged neonatal hypoglycemia
Tolbutamide	Possible teratogenic effects
Narcotics	Neonatal addiction with subsequent withdrawal reaction (no evidence of mutagenesis or teratogenesis)
Neurotropic-anorectic agents	Various malformations
Phenytoin	Cleft lip, cleft palate, microcephaly, congenital limb defects
Quinine	Limb reduction defects, congenital deafness
Reserpine	Neonatal nasal congestion, congenital lung cysts
Thiazides	Thrombocytopenia
Vitamins	
Vitamin A	Congenital anomalies
Vitamin D	Supravalvular aortic stenosis, elfin facies, mental retardation
Vitamin K	Hyperbilirubinemia, kernicterus
Possible embryotoxicity	
(suggestive animal studies, suggestive but limited human data)	
Caffeine	Intrauterine growth retardation
Carbaryl	Various congenital defects (possible reduced fertility)
Carbon disulfide	Teratogenesis
Chlorcyclizine (Perazil)	Case reports of anomalies
Chlordane	Possible mutagenesis
Cyclizine (Marezine)	Various anomalies in case reports
Diazepam (Valium)	Various anomalies
Ethylene oxide	Possible teratogenesis
INH (isoniazid preparations)	Various anomalies
Insulin	Caudal regression syndrome, various anomalies
Kepone	Reduced male fertility, effect on female unknown
Librium	Various anomalies
Lithium	Case reports of anomalies and increased malformation rates
Meclizine	Case reports of anomalies
Meprobamate	Various anomalies from early pregnancy exposure
PCB (polychlorinated biphenyls)	Increased abortions (also decreased fertility)
Phenmetrazine (Preludin)	Case reports of anomalies
Phenothiazines	Cardiovascular anomalies
Salicylates	Possible bleeding diatheses, prolongation of gestation
Trichloroethylene	Mutagenic and teratogenic
Trimethadione	Various anomalies
Vinyl chloride	Possible mutagenesis

ANTENATAL DIAGNOSIS

Intrauterine diagnosis of many disease processes that may result in a seriously deformed or mentally deficient child is now feasible by amniocentesis and subsequent studies. Nonetheless, there are definite risks to prenatal diagnosis (the two most common being hemorrhage and infection). Therefore a number of prerequisites for patient selection must be established.

Prerequisites for patient selection

1. The pregnancy must be at high risk for a specific disease process.
2. There must be a specific demonstrable chromosome or biochemical marker that will reliably indicate a fetus affected with that disease.
3. The chromosome or biochemical marker must be demonstrable early enough in gestation to permit reasonable options.
4. The available treatment and prognosis of the disorder must be known.
5. The risk of complications from amniocentesis must be less than the hazards of the disease.

In practice, these prerequisites are usually fulfilled by any of the following:

1. A previous child or close relative with Down's syndrome or other chromosomal disorders
2. Advanced maternal age (35 years of age or older) or great anxiety regarding anomalies in a somewhat younger mother (33 years of age)
3. The significant likelihood that a child will have one of the following inherited metabolic disorders, which are now amenable to antenatal diagnosis*:

Acatalasia
Argininosuccinicaciduria
Chédiak-Steinbrinck-Higashi syndrome
Citrullinemia
Congenital erythropoietic porphyria
Fabray's disease
Fucosidosis
Galactosemia
Gaucher's disease
Glucose-6-phosphate dehydrogenase deficiency
Glycogen storage diseases (types 2 to 4)
GM_1 gangliosidoses (types 1 and 2)
GM_2 gangliosidoses (types 1 to 3)
Homocystinuria
Hyperlysinemia
Hypervalinemia
I-cell disease
Ketotic hyperglycemia
Krabbe's disease
Lesch-Nyhan syndrome
Lysosomal acid phosphatase deficiency
Mannosidosis
Maple syrup urine disease
Metachromatic leukodystrophy
Methylmalonic aciduria
Mucopolysaccharidoses (types 1 to 6)
Niemann-Pick disease
Ornithine-α-keto acid transaminase deficiency
Orotic aciduria
Pyruvate decarboxylase deficiency
Refsum's disease
Xeroderma pigmentosum

4. A previous child or sibling with a severe sex-linked recessive disease (e.g., the Duchenne type of muscular dystrophy)
5. A previous child with a neural tube defect

Certain requirements for providing intrauterine diagnosis must be met. Only those with experience should undertake this service, which can be provided only by a team composed of, at minimum, an obstetrician experienced in amniocentesis, a medical genetics group with biochemical and cytogenetic expertise who have proper counseling capability, and a full range of professional referrals.

Timing

Amniocentesis is most frequently accomplished between 14 and 16 weeks of gestation. Timing is based on the relative amount of amniotic fluid available and the number of cells in the fluid. Most experts recommend transabdominal amniocentesis, which is generally performed as an outpatient procedure after thorough explanation of the risks as well as advantages and options. Ultrasonography is increasingly being used to "map" the area and thus decrease the possibility of transplacental bleeding because of injury. The usual procedure follows:

1. Use ultrasonography to locate placenta, examine and measure the viable fetus and identify site for needle placement where there is maximal opportunity to obtain amniotic fluid with minimal risk.
2. Prepare abdomen with tincture of iodine.
3. Drape the sterile area.
4. Infiltrate skin and subcutaneous tissues with 1 ml of 1% procaine.
5. Insert 3½-inch 22-gauge disposable spinal needle into uterine cavity.
6. Remove stylet and aspirate amniotic fluid, filling two 10 ml plastic syringes.

---

*This is an incomplete list. Since the diseases amenable to antenatal diagnosis are increasing, one would be wise to consult the nearest genetic center for specific information before counseling the family about a specific process.

Risks

The exact risk of amniocentesis for both the patient and the fetus are unknown at present, but short-term and intermediate complications are fortunately uncommon (less than 1% in most reported series).

Limitations

Prenatal diagnosis still has numerous limitations. Consequently, counseling regarding interruption or continuation of pregnancy should consider the following:

1. Diagnosis of metabolic diseases from amniotic fluid or from uncultured or cultured amniotic fluid cells has been made in relatively few cases for each disease, so the procedure must be considered quasi-experimental.
2. Culturing amniotic fluid cells is a tedious and complex process. Mean time from amniocentesis to results is approximately 19 days. This waiting interval is emotionally difficult for families, and when more complex biochemical analyses are required, diagnosis may take 4 to 8 weeks.
3. Usually only one specific disease process can be investigated in each case.
4. Many autosomal dominant diseases, such as Huntington's chorea and Marfan's syndrome, are not currently amenable to prenatal diagnosis or medical treatment.

Because the capability for diagnosis is increasing rapidly, one should check with a genetics center regarding newer specific analyses before counseling patients.

Chorionic villi sampling

Although most women currently receive antenatal diagnosis by undergoing amniocentesis, a new method of obtaining diagnostic genetic information about the developing fetus, chorionic villi sampling (CVS), appears to be very promising. Because the chorion originates from the same cell(s) as the fetus and is also growing very actively, it usually provides adequate numbers of cells (from the cytotrophoblast) in proper phase of development for standard cytogenetic analysis. Thus the time-consuming step of cell culture may be avoided for many conditions. However, should cell culture be necessary (e.g., for biochemical disorders) it may be performed from the material sampled. CVS may be accomplished earlier than amniocentesis (during postmenstrual weeks 8 to 12). Earlier testing and more rapid results may be beneficial if pregnancy termination is indicated, which may be accomplished more safely during the first trimester (in contrast to second trimester termination necessitated by amniocentesis antenatal diagnosis).

Indications for CVS and those for antenatal diagnosis by amniocentesis are the same, with the exception of detection of neural tube defects. Detection of the open neural tube defect

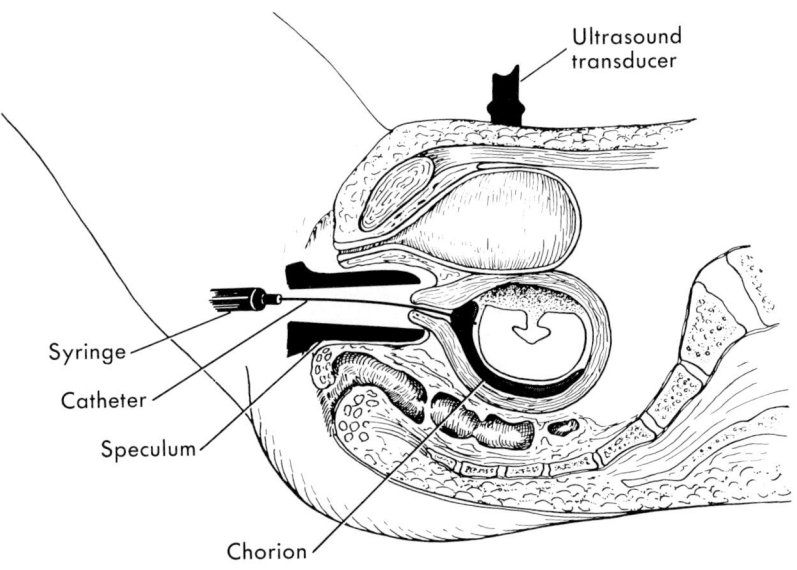

Fig. 3-2. Chorionic villi sampling (CVS).

depends on the alpha fetoprotein measurement, which is obtained from either the maternal serum or the amniotic fluid. Therefore CVS is not effective for diagnosis of this condition.

CVS is performed as an outpatient procedure between postmenstrual weeks 9 and 10, but it may be done as early as the eighth or as late as the twelfth postmenstrual week. Because timing for the procedure is critical it is often desirable to obtain an earlier ultrasonic scan to time the procedure correctly. The procedure is always immediately preceded by ultrasonic evaluation of the uterus, placenta, and fetus.

Following the ultrasonic evaluation, the woman is placed in the dorsal lithotomy position and the cervix exposed using a speculum. The vagina and cervix are cleansed using an antiseptic. Under continuous abdominal ultrasonic monitor and guidance, a sterile thin plastic catheter (Trophocan CVS catheter, 26 cm length, available through Portex, Inc. Wilmington, MA) with a malleable metal stylet is curved to the proper shape to reach the chorion, and gently inserted through the cervix (Fig. 3-2). After the chorion is reached (as confirmed by ultrasonography), the metal stylet is removed and a syringe with nutrient fluid (RPMI) is attached. Gentle suction is applied while the catheter is withdrawn with the trapped portions of chorion. No anesthesic is used and women generally report little discomfort.

Exact data concerning the level of risks of CVS is not available because the total number done is still small, and (as with many technical procedures) the complications are expected to decrease in direct relationship to increasing experience. However, the limited experience available to date indicates that potential maternal-fetal complications include rupture of membranes, infection, abortion, intrauterine death, uterine cramping, and vaginal bleeding. Indeed, approximately one third of all patients with continuing pregnancies experience vaginal bleeding after the procedure. Additionally, the syncytiotrophoblast has a great number of mosaic cells. Thus in the laboratory it must be carefully separated from other tissues so that the results accurately reflect the fetal genotype. The procedure is still considered investigational and must be performed in centers fully prepared for the investigational protocol that includes reporting problems, follow-up of the continuing pregnancies, and accurate data compilation.

BIBLIOGRAPHY

Apgar, V., and Gause, R.W.: Teratology, Med. World News **11**:59, 1970.

Berry, C.L., Poswillo, R.K., et al.: Teratology trends and applications, New York, 1975, Springer-Verlag New York, Inc.

Butcher, R.L., and Page, R.D.: Introductory remarks: environmental and endogenous hazards to the female reproductive system, Environ. Health Perspect. **38**:35, 1981.

Cohlan, S.Q.: Fetal and neonatal hazards from drugs administered during pregnancy, N.Y. J. Med. **64**:493, 1964.

Gardiner, H., Clark, C., et al.: Spontaneous abortion and fetal abnormality in subsequent pregnancy, Br. Med. J. **1**:1016, 1978.

Golbus, M.S.: Teratology for the obstetrician: current status, Obstet. Gynecol. **55**:269, 1980.

Golbus, M.S., Loughman, W.D., Epstein, C.J., et al.: Prenatal genetic diagnosis in 3000 amniocenteses, N. Engl. J. Med. **300**:157, 1979.

Heller, M.B., Terdiman, J.F., and Pasternanck, B.S.: A procedure for calculating the gonadal x-ray dose in diagnostic radiography, Br. J. Radiol. **39**:686, 1966.

Hill, R.M., Verinand, W.M., Hornig, M.G., et al.: Infants exposed in utero to antiepileptic drugs, Am. J. Dis. Child. **127**:645, 1974

Jones, K.L., Smith, D.W., Streissguth, A.P., et al.: Outcome in offspring of chronic alcoholic women, Lancet **1**:1076, 1974

King, C.R., Pernoll, M.L., and Prescott, G.: Reproductive wastage, Obstet. Gynecol. Annu. **59**: 1982

Nora, J.J., Nora, A.H., Sommerville, R.J., et al.: Maternal exposure to potential teratogens, JAMA **202**:1065, 1967.

Pernoll, M.L., King, C.R., and Prescott, G.: Genetics for the clinical obstetrician-gynecologist, Obstet. Gynecol. Annu. 1, 1980.

Rao, K.S., and Schwetz, B.A.: Reproductive toxicity of environmental agents, Annu. Rev. Public Health **3**:1, 1982.

Smith, D.W.: Recognizable patterns of human malformation, ed. 2, Philadelphia, 1976, W.B. Saunders Co.

4

Longitudinal assessment of fetal health: detection of risk factors

FETAL GROWTH

Since growth in the healthy fetus apparently proceeds in a demonstrable fashion, deviations from this pattern of growth for any fetus may be of clinical significance. Fig. 4-1 illustrates growth patterns and the associated morbidity factors when fetal growth deviates above the 90th percentile or below the 10th percentile. The type of problem shown depends on the timing and type of insult. Interference with development, for example, chromosomal defects or rubella, may be demonstrable throughout gestation, whereas interference with growth has a variable onset that depends on the complication. Nutritional impairment usually is imposed after midpregnancy, whereas multiple pregnancy, toxemia, placental insufficiency, and postmaturity have variable times of onset of effects.

Fetal growth charts have become valuable as a reference even though at present the data used can show only the distribution of measurements of many who were born prematurely, rather than longitudinal data on the presumably healthier population that is delivered at term.

Fig. 4-2 shows the fetal growth curves of a Denver population. The Denver curves are primarily representative of a population of low socioeconomic background and are reduced in comparison to the Portland curves (Fig. 4-1), which apply to white, middle-class, private patients. The former were born above a 5,000-foot altitude, and the latter were born at virtual sea level. The Denver grid may be more applicable to general populations but, as such, does not reflect optimal fetal growth. The slowing of fetal growth toward the end of the last trimester of pregnancy is a result of the restriction imposed by the fetal environment rather than a declining growth potential. Thus this slowing of growth of the fetus is subject, to some extent, to nutrition. The adequacy of the placenta, the health of the mother, and the nutrition available to the fetus determine the timing of this slowing of fetal growth. In a sequential study of Japanese babies, Gruenwald and colleagues show that improvement in the socioeconomic state of the population increases the weight of infants at term. Linear growth of fetuses during World War II continued only until 35 or 36 weeks of gestation, whereas by 1963-1964, fetal growth continued unchecked to 38 weeks. Similar differences may explain the Denver/Portland comparisons of growth in weight.

When precise measurements of the fetus can be plotted longitudinally against normal growth curves, the physician has a powerful tool to access the physiologic well-being of the perinate. There are clinically applicable techniques for these determinations.

CLINICAL PARAMETERS OF PREGNANCY DURATION
Estimation of fetal age

The duration of pregnancy, more specifically fetal age, has become increasingly important in the determination of fetal prognosis and specific

32 *Diagnosis and management of the high-risk fetus and neonate*

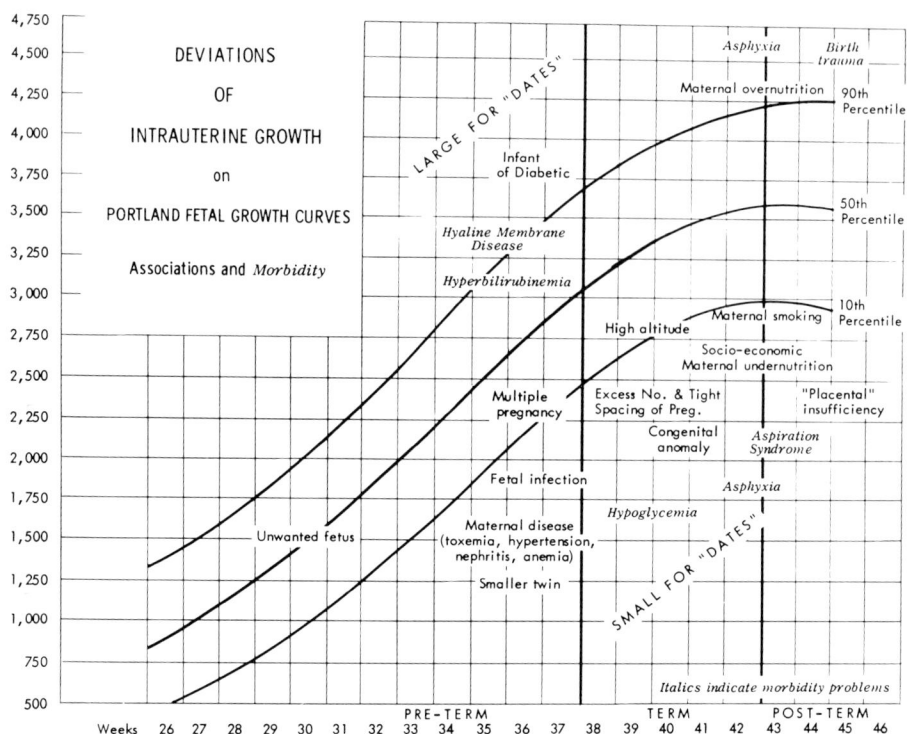

Fig. 4-1. Important associations and morbidity factors of accelerated or reduced fetal growth above the 90th percentile and below the 10th percentile for gestational age using the Portland curves. Fetal growth data obtained from 40,000 single, white, middle-class infants born near sea level.

requirements of nursery care after birth. The principal reason is the enhanced accuracy of ultrasonography in these determinations and the accumulated knowledge concerning how fetuses of various sizes respond to modern neonatal care.

Certainly, a number of conditions are associated with the untimely termination of pregnancy. Toxemia of pregnancy and previous cesarean section each account for about a fourth of all early terminations of pregnancy, whereas isoimmunization and diabetes mellitus each make up approximately one fifth of inductions for early delivery. Obviously, when termination of a pregnancy is not urgently indicated, the physician should delay until fetal maturity has been reached. If compelling reasons exist for premature delivery or intervention, however, all parties must be apprised of the problems to be faced.

Despite vast increases in precision no single method of determining fetal age or maturity is precise enough to substantiate a clinical decision. Several procedures, together with an accurate obstetric history and physical examination, increase the accuracy of the estimation of gestational age. One should first use the simplest and safest methods and progress to more intricate and variable procedures if equivocal results are obtained initially. Regrettably, even when these methods are used, data are still scant regarding complications of pregnancy such as toxemia, erythroblastosis, and diabetes, for which early delivery may be required.

CALCULATION OF PREGNANCY DURATION FROM LAST MENSTRUAL PERIOD

An important estimate of gestational age is calculated from the first day of the last menstrual period. This span of time is actually the menstrual age, but it is used synonymously with gestational age, even though conception probably did not occur until approximately 2 weeks later. The time interval is best expressed in

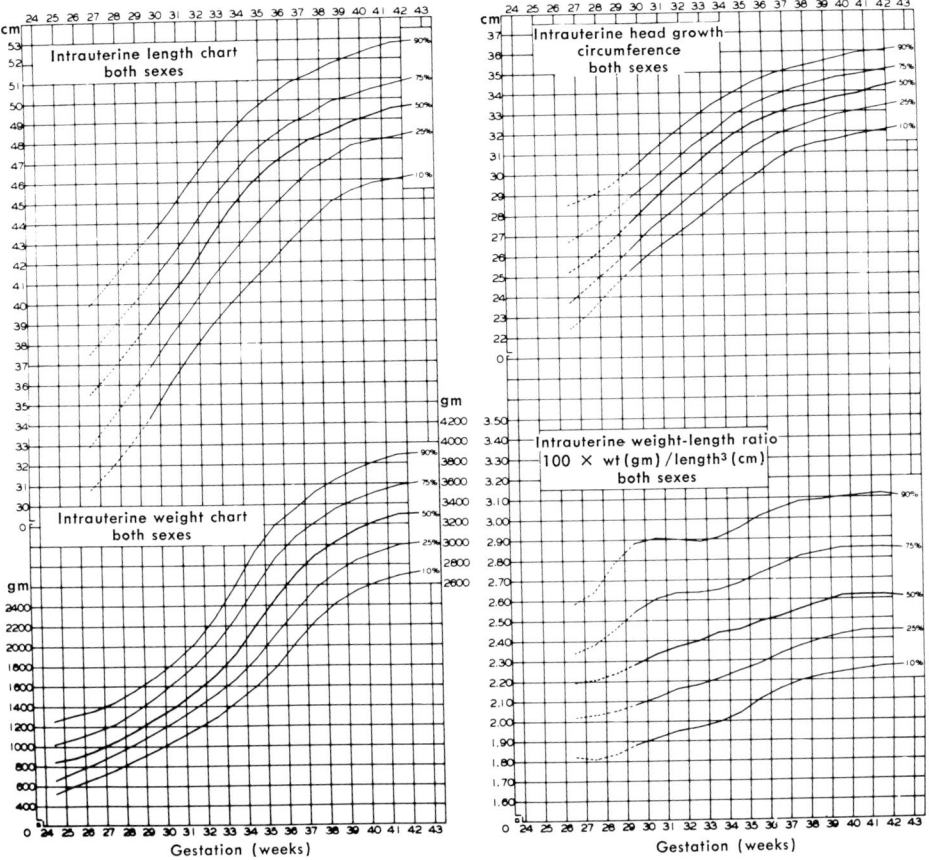

Fig. 4-2. Weight, height, and head circumference of living infants born after 24 weeks' gestation graphed as percentiles. (From Lubchenco, L.O., Hansman, M., and Boyd, E.: Pediatrics 37:403, 1966.)

whole weeks rather than as a mixed number of days. The World Health Organization has recommended the use of "completed weeks" rather than rounding to the nearest week.

Numerous problems must be considered when one calculates the duration of gestation from the first day of the last menstrual period (LMP):

1. Many women fail to record their menstrual dates.
2. Menstrual cycles are often irregular and variable.
3. Pregnancies may follow in close sequence without menstruation occurring between gestations.
4. Postconceptual bleeding may be confused with menstruation.
5. Ovulation that occurs during the cycle immediately after cessation of ovulation-inhibition methods of contraception may be delayed.

These factors may affect the accuracy of calculations in 10% to 40% of women, depending on the population observed. The physician who considers menstrual age questionable must estimate gestational age. This can be done prenatally with increasing accuracy. Indeed, even if dates are considered to be accurate, it is prudent to use other objective data to confirm gestational age.

BASAL BODY TEMPERATURE RECORD OR SINGLE COITUS

If a reliable basal body temperature record is available, or if an isolated intercourse can be dated, the precise onset of pregnancy can be documented. Such a range record may be invaluable; however, it may still be unwise to base a clinical decision on this parameter alone.

Measurement of uterine size

The most frequently used clinical parameter for estimation of fetal well-being is serial abdominal measurement of the height of the uterine fundus.

    I. Height of fundus in relation to anatomic landmarks

        The anteverted fundus is palpable just above the symphysis pubis at 10 to 12 weeks' gestation. It is halfway between the symphysis and the umbilicus at approximately 15 weeks. These and other relationships of the height of the fundus on the abdominal wall are demonstrated in Fig. 4-3.

    II. Mensuration of fundal height

        Because landmarks are less useful in estimation of the duration of pregnancy during the second half of pregnancy, various calculations involving the direct measurement of fundal height have been advocated. One popular approach is *McDonald's maneuver* (Fig. 4-3). It is performed by measurement with a flexible tape from the anterosuperior margin of the symphysis pubis over the circumference of the uterus to its uppermost extent. This distance then allows calculation of the duration of gestation: height of fundus in centimeters $\times$ 8/7 = weeks of pregnancy. Although not an exact indicator of fetal age, serial measurements assist in documenting fetal growth.

    III. Correlations of uterine fundal measurement with fetal weight

        R.W. Johnson devised a formula for estimating the weight of the fetus.

$n = 12$, when the station of the fetal head is below the level of the ischial spines
$n = 11$, if the presenting part is above the level of the ischial spines
l is added to n for patients over 200 lb
k = constant (155)

Then

(fundal measurement in cm) $- n \times k$ = approximate fetal weight in gm

Again, this is only an approximation, and only 50% of fetuses will be within 240 gm of the calculated weight; moreover, the calculation applies only to vertex presentations.

    IV. Girth measurements

        Measurements of abdominal circumference taken at the umbilicus with the patient in the supine position also provide a reproducible method for detecting increase, constancy, or decrease of uterine size. Girth measurement is particularly useful in abnormal conditions when used in conjunction with fundal height measurement.

    V. Correlations of abnormal serial measurements

        A. Unexpectedly large measurements
            1. Incorrect date of last menstrual period or of conception
            2. Multiple gestation
            3. Hydramnios
            4. Tumor
            5. Ascites
            6. Massive obesity
            7. Molar gestation

        B. Unusually small measurements
            1. Incorrect date of last menstrual period or of conception
            2. Intrauterine death
            3. Oligohydramnios
            4. Fetal anomaly
            5. Fetal undergrowth
            6. Missed abortion
            7. Molar gestation

Fetal heart tones

Identification of the fetal heart, which constitutes positive proof of fetal life, may be accomplished by electronic detection or fetoscopy.

    1. Electronic detection

        Ultrasonic devices, either scanners or those using the Doppler principle, may detect the fetal heartbeat as early as the eighth or ninth week of gestation. Later in pregnancy these devices may pick up not only fetal heart tones but may document the circulation of fetal blood within large vessels. Equipment of this type is particularly useful early in pregnancy to prove the presence of fetal life, to rule out molar

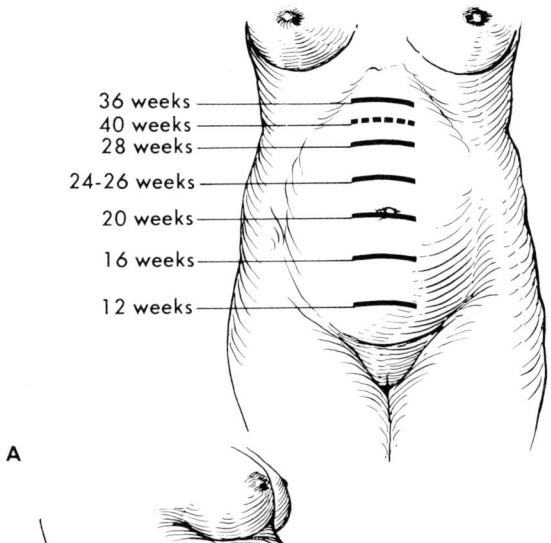
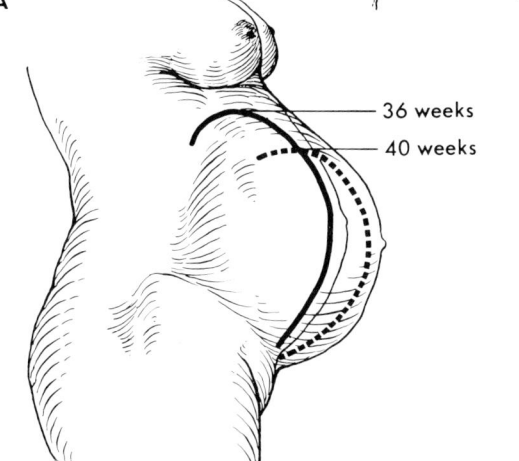
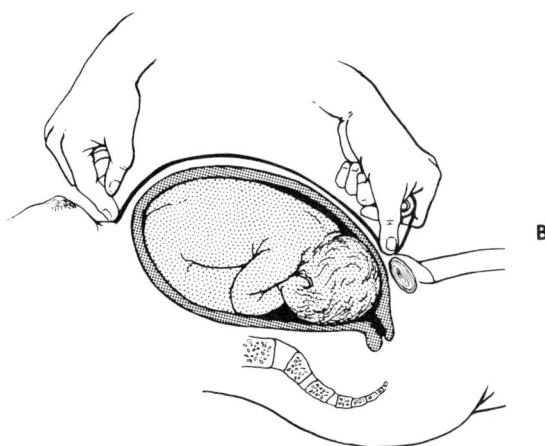

Fig. 4-3. A, Relationship of the uterine fundus to landmarks on the abdominal wall. **B,** Demonstration of McDonald's method of measurement. (From Benson, R.C.: Handbook of obstetrics and gynecology, ed. 4, Los Altos, Calif., 1971, Lange Medical Publications.)

gestations, and to confirm or reject clinical diagnosis of multiple gestations. In later pregnancy, such devices are very useful in cases of hydramnios, multiple gestation, massive obesity, and other states in which auscultation is unsatisfactory.

2. Fetoscopy

Because the range of sound in which fetal heart tones are best heard involves bone conduction, the head fetoscope generally is a reliable stethoscopic instrument. With use of the fetoscope, fetal heart tones can generally first be heard between 18 and 22 weeks of gestation. Because the fetal heart is heard best over the back of the fetus on its left side, the point of maximum intensity of the fetal heartbeat may be used to corroborate impressions gained by Leopold's maneuvers concerning fetal lie and presenting part. For example, if fetal heart tones are heard best in the area above the umbilicus on the right side, it is a reasonable presumption that the fetus is presenting breech, with the back to the mother's right side. Fetal heart rate will gradually slow during the course of pregnancy, but the rate is not a reliable index of the length of gestation.

Fetal motion

Maternal perception of fetal movement, termed "quickening," may provide an additional estimate for the duration of pregnancy. Quickening usually is noted at 20 weeks in the primigravida and 14 to 18 weeks in the multigravida.

On the combined abdominopelvic examination about the sixteenth week, fetal parts may be palpable. At about the same time, active fetal movement can be seen or palpated by the examiner. Passive fetal movement may be noted even earlier in pregnancy by internal ballottement, or palpable bobbing during vaginal examination. This evidence of pregnancy is only presumptive, however.

DETERMINATION OF FETAL LIE, PRESENTING PART, AND POSITION

In the second half of the pregnancy, systematic examination of the abdomen generally should reveal the intrauterine relationship of the fetus. It should be recorded at each visit and is generally accomplished by the four maneuvers of Leopold. These maneuvers are illustrated in Fig. 4-4 and are designed to determine the following:
1. Fetal poles and uterine fundus
2. Side to which the fetal back is directed
3. Part of the fetus that overlies the pelvic inlet
4. Side of the cephalic prominence
5. Depth of the presenting part in the pelvis

Rigorous application of these maneuvers at each patient visit may allow early determination and favorable management of breech, multiple gestation, hydramnios, malpresentation, and compound presentation.

LABORATORY PARAMETERS OF FETAL GROWTH
Ultrasonography

Assessment of fetal growth on the basis of serial measurements of head, femur, abdomen, or other parts made by use of ultrasonography is the simplest and most reliable method of determining fetal progress. Fetal age, for example, is quite predictable from serial biparietal diameters obtained during the late first, the second, and early third trimesters (Table 4-1). There is less correlation in late gestation. All parameters are likely to be less accurate if measured on just one occasion. Estimation of fetal weight, although far less accurate, is also possible.

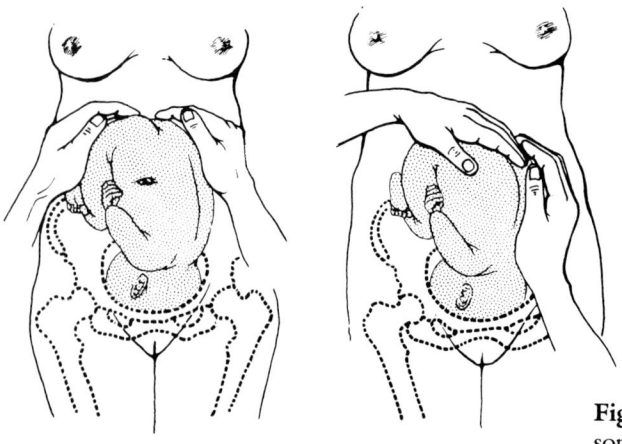
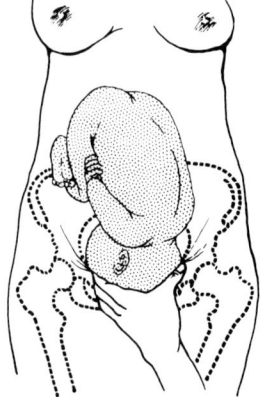
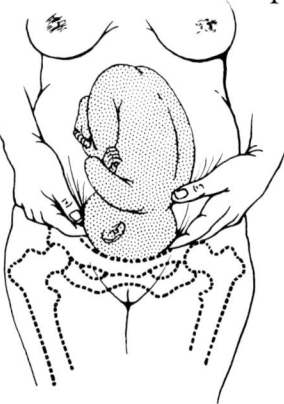

Fig. 4-4. Four maneuvers of Leopold. (From Benson, R.C.: Handbook of obstetrics and gynecology, ed. 4, Los Altos, Calif., 1971, Lange Medical Publications.)

Table 4-1. Ultrasonic estimation of fetal weight and maturity

Biparietal diameter (cm)	Weight gm	Weight lb/oz	Weeks of gestation	Biparietal diameter (cm)	Weight gm	Weight lb/oz	Weeks of gestation
1.0	NA	NA	9	6.0	660.4	1 8	22.5
1.1	NA	NA	9	6.1	737.6	1 10	26.0
1.2	NA	NA	9.5	6.2	814.8	1 13	26.0
1.3	NA	NA	10.0	6.3	892.1	2	26.5
1.4	NA	NA	10.0	6.4	969.3	2 2	27.0
1.5	NA	NA	10.5	6.5	1,046.5	2 5	27.0
1.6	NA	NA	11.0	6.6	1,123.7	2 8	27.5
1.7	NA	NA	11.0	6.7	1,200.9	2 10	28.0
1.8	NA	NA	11.5	6.8	1,278.2	2 13	28.0
1.9	NA	NA	12.0	6.9	1,355.4	3	28.5
2.0	NA	NA	12.0	7.0	1,432.6	3 3	29.0
2.1	NA	NA	12.5	7.1	1,509.8	3 5	29.0
2.2	NA	NA	13.0	7.2	1,587.0	3 8	29.5
2.3	NA	NA	13.0	7.3	1,664.3	3 11	29.5
2.4	NA	NA	13.5	7.4	1,741.5	3 14	30.0
2.5	NA	NA	14.0	7.5	1,818.7	4	30.5
2.6	NA	NA	14.0	7.6	1,895.9	4 3	30.8
2.7	NA	NA	14.5	7.7	1,973.1	4 5	31.0
2.8	NA	NA	15.0	7.8	2,050.4	4 8	31.7
2.9	NA	NA	15.0	7.9	2,127.6	4 11	32.0
3.0	NA	NA	15.5	8.0	2,204.8	4 14	32.7
3.1	NA	NA	16.0	8.1	2,282.0	5	33.0
3.2	NA	NA	16.0	8.2	2,359.2	5 3	33.6
3.3	NA	NA	16.5	8.3	2,436.5	5 6	34.0
3.4	NA	NA	17.0	8.4	2,513.7	5 8	34.6
3.5	NA	NA	17.0	8.5	2,590.9	5 11	35.0
3.6	NA	NA	17.5	8.6	2,668.1	5 14	35.5
3.7	NA	NA	18.0	8.7	2,745.3	6	36.0
3.8	NA	NA	18.0	8.8	2,822.6	6 3	36.5
3.9	NA	NA	18.5	8.9	2,899.8	6 6	37.0
4.0	NA	NA	19.0	9.0	2,977.0	6 8	37.4
4.1	NA	NA	19.0	9.1	3,054.2	6 11	38.0
4.2	NA	NA	19.5	9.2	3,131.4	6 14	38.4
4.3	NA	NA	20.0	9.3	3,208.7	7 2	39.0
4.4	NA	NA	20.0	9.4	3,285.9	7 3	39.0
4.5	NA	NA	20.5	9.5	3,363.1	7 6	39.8
4.6	NA	NA	21.0	9.6	3,440.3	7 10	40.0
4.7	NA	NA	21.0	9.7	3,517.5	7 11	40.8
4.8	NA	NA	21.5	9.8	3,594.8	7 14	41.0
4.9	NA	NA	22.0	9.9	3,672.0	8 2	41.7
5.0	NA	NA	22.0	10.0	3,749.2	8 3	NA
5.1	NA	NA	22.5	10.1	3,826.4	8 6	NA
5.2	42.6	2	23.0	10.2	3,903.6	8 10	NA
5.3	119.9	5	23.0	10.3	3,980.9	8 13	NA
5.4	197.1	6	23.5	10.4	4,058.1	8 14	NA
5.5	274.3	10	24.0	10.5	4,135.3	9 2	NA
5.6	351.5	13	24.0	10.6	4,212.5	9 5	NA
5.7	428.7	14	24.5				
5.8	514.9	1 2	25.0				
5.9	583.2	1 5	25.0				

Courtesy Timothy G. Lee, M.D., Chief, Section of Ultrasound, Department of Diagnostic Radiology, University of Oregon Health Science Center.

Although some have reported ultrasonic thoracic measurement to be inaccurate, others have found that one third of small-for-dates fetuses have a proportionally reduced growth rate that may be noted earlier in the thoracic measurement than in measurement of the biparietal diameter of the head.

Ultrasonographic examination is safe and reliable and can be used repeatedly throughout pregnancy when indicated. It may be useful for the following:
1. Appraisal of fetal growth
2. Localization of placenta
3. Assessment of volumetric growth of the placenta
4. Diagnosis of molar gestation
5. Identification of multiple gestation
6. Detection of certain fetal abnormalities (e.g., anencephaly, hydrocephaly, certain meningomyeloceles, and other defects)
7. Diagnosis of fetal death
8. Confirmation of fetal lie, presenting part, position, and tone
9. Identification of compound presentations
10. Detection of oligohydramnios or polyhydramnios
11. Direction of sample obtainment for antenatal genetic diagnosis by amniocentesis or chorionic villi sampling
12. Assistance in determination of fetal well-being (e.g., the biophysical profile, see Chapter 5)

The role of ultrasonography as a screening device that should be applied routinely in pregnancy is currently debatable, and the Consensus Conference of the National Institute of Health did not indicate that utilization was desirable. However, because of the number of risk states discoverable and the apparent safety of short-term diagnostic ultrasonography, its use as a routine screening tool appears to be gaining advocates.

Radiography

Ultrasonography generally is greatly superior to radiography for visualization and mensuration of both bony and soft tissues. Additionally it is much safer. Therefore fetal radiography is not often indicated for fetal mensuration. However, it may be useful in detection or evaluation of certain defects (e.g., bony dysplasias and dwarfism).

Radiologic examinations during pregnancy may expose the fetus and mother to undesirable amounts of radiation. Nonetheless, the consequences of such exposure must be contrasted with the need for precision to ensure proper obstetric management.

LABORATORY PARAMETERS OF FETAL WELL-BEING
Biochemical testing
HUMAN CHORIONIC GONADOTROPIN (HCG)

Human chorionic gonadotropin, a protein hormone, is produced by the syncytiotrophoblast. Detection and measurement of HCG is of practical importance for diagnosis of pregnancy and evaluation of possible trophoblastic disease. The most sensitive method for measuring HCG is by radioimmunoassay. Although a test with this degree of sensitivity is important in prognosis of choriocarcinoma, immunologic tests employing hemagglutination, inhibition, or latex agglutination are usually satisfactory for diagnosis of pregnancy. Radioimmunoassay techniques may demonstrate HCG as early as 24 hours after implantation, but the more commonly employed urinary tests for pregnancy are usually not reliable until about 42 days after the first day of the last menstrual period. The hormone peaks at 60 to 70 days of gestation, followed by a slow fall to a relatively steady titer at 100 to 130 days. Pregnancy tests have not been useful in prognosis or for routine fetal evaluation. There is a significant incidence of both false-negative and false-positive results with immunologic pregnancy tests.

ESTRIOL

The biosynthesis of the steroid hormone estriol depends on an intact maternal-fetal placental unit. Urinary estriol determinations are meaningful only if they are determined serially in the latter half of the same pregnancy. A normal range may indicate that the fetus is not in immediate danger; nonetheless, low (less than 4mg/24hr) or significantly decreased estriol excretion has been associated with fetal disease and even impending death. Estriol values may be useful in assessment of fetal well-being in pregnancies complicated by diabetes mellitus, hypertension, eclamptogenic toxemia, placental insufficiency (including postmaturity), and suspected intrauterine fetal demise. Estriol excretion is decreased in cases of fetal anencephaly and in gravidas taking large doses of corticosteroids or taking medications such as ampicillin or chlorothiazide diuretics, in those who have severe anemia or severe rental disease, and in those who live at high altitudes. In contrast, urinary estriol is elevated in normal multiple gestation.

Neonatal apnea, noticeable cyanosis, or gross neurologic abnormality may be associated with reduced urinary estriol excretion. A drop of 40% from a previously obtained value is indicative of fetal distress and warrants assessment and possible intervention. Table 4-2 details average estriol excretion in normal pregnancy.

Several conspiring factors make estriol determinations more difficult and less accurate than desirable. Serial (and often numerous) tests are usually necessary, and it is often difficult to obtain patient compliance for numerous 12- or 24-hour urines. To complicate this problem, there is wide circadian variation in serum measurements, and to be of value samples must be obtained at the same time of day after the patient has been at similar metabolic conditions. The test is also complex, and there is a wide range of normal values. In addition, correlation with fetal outcome is less accurate than desirable.

These problems have led to attempts to correlate estriol with other measurable indices (e.g., creatinine), but it has gradually become evident that estriol determinations are an indirect reflection of fetal well-being and that a great deal of compromise may occur before estriol production is altered. Thus attention has recently been directed more toward biometric measurements.

HUMAN PLACENTAL LACTOGEN (HPL)

Human placental lactogen is also called human chorionic somatomammotropin (HCS). HPL is a protein hormone produced by the syncytiotrophoblast. Generally, this hormone is measured by radioimmunoassay. HPL values equal to or less than 4 μg/ml of maternal serum after 30 weeks of gestation are abnormally low. After the first day post partum, HPL is no longer detectable in the serum. HPL levels may identify a pregnancy that is compromised by placental insufficiency because of vascular disease, hypertension, preeclampsia, pyelonephritis, essential hypertension, lupus erythematosus, or glomerulonephritis.

OTHER MEANS OF BIOCHEMICAL TESTING

Heat-stable alkaline phosphatase, diamine oxidase, cystine aminopeptidase (oxytocinase), and pregnanediol may become valid methods for assessing fetal viability. However, these determinations are not yet recommended for routine clinical use.

Physiologic maturity determination

Physiologic maturity determination by means of amniotic fluid testing has proved to be exceed-

Table 4-2. Average estriol excretion in normal pregnancy

Gestation (weeks)	Mean estriol excretion (mg/24 hr)	Standard deviation (mg)	Number of subjects
6	0.05		3
7	0.06		3
8	0.09		4
9	0.15	0.079	7
10	0.16	0.085	7
11	0.23	0.255	7
12	0.28	0.153	8
13	0.58	0.249	9
14	0.70	0.354	10
15	1.15	0.425	7
16	1.95	0.760	8
17	2.40	0.775	10
18	3.65	0.899	15
19	4.36	1.339	29
20	5.59	1.932	31
21	6.70	2.256	11
22	7.59	1.904	9
23	9.36	2.221	12
24	10.04	2.144	11
25	10.57	3.228	11
26	12.98	1.612	11
27	13.75	2.100	10
28	12.96	3.465	19
29	14.67	3.266	42
30	15.21	3.490	41
31	15.24	3.604	18
32	17.51	4.265	11
33	18.12	4.197	15
34	18.82	3.571	16
35	22.55	3.040	15
36	23.39	3.928	19
37	28.61	7.652	24
38	31.33	6.565	42
39	33.34	9.373	46
40	34.49	9.352	25
41	33.22	7.935	16

From Klopper, A., and Billewicz, W.: Urinary excretion of estriol and pregnanediol during normal pregnancy, J. Obstet. Gynaec. Brit. Comm. **70:**1024, 1963.

ingly useful when premature termination of pregnancy threatens, when gestation is prolonged (over 42 weeks), and when fetal survival may depend on early delivery in complicating disease states.

Amniocentesis may be performed as early in pregnancy as one believes there is a reasonable chance of fetal survival. Care should be taken to perform the amniocentesis either behind the fetal neck or below the presenting part (toward the cervix). Real-time or sector scan ultrasonography is invaluable in detailing where amniocentesis is best accomplished. If blood is encountered, one should determine whether it is of fetal or maternal origin. Kleihauer's stain is useful for this purpose.

The various amniotic fluid tests for determining physiologic maturity are detailed below.

I. Rapid surfactant test
A rapid test for surfactant in amniotic fluid to assess the risk of respiratory distress syndrome was described by Clements and colleagues in 1972. This test is extremely important because it may be performed by a competent laboratory or physician with minimal effort and equipment, and it has a high degree of reproducibility.
A. Reagents
1. 0.9% sodium chloride (9 gm/L distilled water)
2. 95% ethanol
B. Equipment
1. Centrifuge
2. Vortex mixer
3. Two 14 × 100 mm tubes
4. Two No. 0 rubber stoppers
5. Two 1 ml and one 2 ml pipettes
6. Test tube rack
7. Pipette bulb
C. Procedure
1. Centrifuge amniotic fluid at 2,000 rpm for 10 minutes immediately after drawing sample to settle particulate matter.
2. Drawing with pipette from the "clear" supernatant, place 1 ml into 14 × 100 ml tube and 0.5 ml into the other.
3. Add 0.5 ml saline to the second tube.
4. Add 1 ml 95% ethanol to each tube, stopper, and shake (Vortex), setting at 5-6 for 15 seconds.
5. Immediately place tubes upright in test tube rack and let them sit for 15 minutes. A ring of bubbles completely around the meniscus after 15 minutes is a positive test result.
6. Determine fetal maturity using Table 4-3.

Table 4-3. Method of interpretation of fetal lung maturity tests

Predicted fetal status	Lecithin/sphingomyelin ratio	Rapid surfactant test
Mature	≥2.00	Complete ring of bubbles persisting 15 min at 1:1 and 1:2 dilutions
Intermediate	1.50 to 1.99	Complete ring of bubbles persisting 15 min at 1:1 dilution only
Immature	<1.50	Incomplete ring of bubbles at both dilutions

We have found that fetal lung maturity can be correlated with the results of amniotic fluid analysis (578 samples). The rapid surfactant test was found to be 99% reliable in predicting fetal lung maturity, and it was more reliable in predicting fetal lung immaturity (69%) than was the lecithin/sphingomyelin (L/S) ratio (38%) discussed below. Thus the rapid surfactant test can be used as a primary method for determining fetal pulmonary maturity, and the L/S ratio can be used as an additional indicator of fetal maturity when the rapid surfactant test is intermediate or the sample is contaminated by blood or meconium.

II. Lecithin/sphingomyelin ratio (L/S ratio) A method of determining the relative L/S ratio in amniotic fluid was published by Gluck and coworkers in 1971. Most authorities now agree that the L/S ratio is a useful test for fetal maturity. Nevertheless, there are reports of discrepancies between the results of the test and the clinical status of the infant, particularly when the L/S ratio is in the intermediate range. Moreover, it has been argued that the test is not a reliable index of fetal lung immaturity, as was previously noted (38%). This technique, like the rapid surfactant test, is most commonly used prior to repeat cesarean section and in preeclampsia, isoimmunization, diabetes mellitus, fetal postmaturity, premature rupture of membranes, and potential fetal jeopardy from other causes. The test requires a well-equipped laboratory with capability for thin-layer chromatography. In our hands, the test has been most reproducible if a densitometer is employed. Each laboratory should develop its own standards. The L/S ratio is interpreted as is noted in Table 4-3.

III. Phosphatidylglycerol

Measurement of one component of pulmonary surface active material, phosphatidylglycerol (PG), has been demonstrated to add sensitivity to determination of pulmonary maturation. It is usually measured by biplanar, thin-layer chromatography in a qualitative (present or absent) assay, although both one-dimensional, thin-layer chromatography and more quantitative assays have been proposed.

Although it is most commonly utilized in a panel with an L/S ratio, PG levels can be measured earlier than a mature L/S ratio can be determined, between 28 and 38 weeks, regardless of underlying pregnancy complication. The rate of respiratory distress drops from greater than 85% with an immature L/S ratio with PG absent, to approximately 3.5% when the L/S ratio is immature but PG is present. Thus determination of PG may be invaluable when perinatal high-risk management demands the earliest possible indication of fetal pulmonary maturity. Moreover, there is early appearance of PG after preterm membrane rupture.

IV. Creatinine

Measurement of amniotic fluid creatinine somewhat correlates with fetal gestational age. Unfortunately this determination has the inherent limitations of all the methods listed below because none measures a vital substance necessary for fetal survival. Before 34 weeks of pregnancy it is infrequent to find creatinine levels of more than 2 mg/100 ml, and after 37 weeks it is unusual to encounter less than 2 mg/100 ml (many samples contain 3 to 4 mg/100 ml) of amniotic fluid creatinine.

V. Spectrophotometric analysis

The $\Delta\ OD^{450nm}$ (difference in optical density) in nonisoimmunized patients may also be used to indicate the length of gestation. At less than 35 weeks many are more than 0.01 Δ OD, and if 36 weeks or more, Δ OD is usually 0.

VI. Amniotic fluid osmolarity

In early pregnancy amniotic fluid is virtually isotonic, but near term a decrease in protein concentration and increased chloride ion content, as compared with concentrations in maternal serum or plasma, result in ever-decreasing osmolarity (or freezing-point depression caused by solute concentration). Osmolarity cannot be determined accurately when there has been blood contamination of the amniotic fluid. At term amniotic fluid osmotic pressure of about 250 mOsm/L can be expected. This is 20 to 25 mOsm/L lower than the osmotic pressure of fetal or maternal plasma. A slow but definite fall in osmolarity after 40 weeks then occurs. This pattern of osmolarity is not altered appreciably, except by severe maternal fluid-electrolyte derangement such as might occur in uncontrolled diabetes mellitus or advanced nephritis. Hence decreasing amniotic fluid osmolarity can be equated with advancing gestational age, even in toxemic patients or those with severe isoimmunization. Obviously, several amniocenteses should be done to establish the trend.

VII. Visual inspection

Visual inspection of amniotic fluid may allow certain generalizations. It is yellow or straw colored and slightly turbid early in gestation; as term approaches, it becomes clear and opalescent and has varying amounts of white particulate matter floating in it (vernix). With isoimmunization, it is yellow and slightly turbid. When it contains blood, amniotic fluid is opaque and varying degrees of dark red. Meconium staining is characterized by green-brown coloration and opacity. The yellow-brown "tobacco juice" opaque fluid that accompanies intrauterine death is characteristic.

OTHER METHODS OF DETERMINING FETAL MATURITY

There are a number of qualitative techniques for assessing fetal maturity of which only the more well known are discussed here. The majority of these techniques attempt to provide more rapid analysis, but accuracy appears to suffer from that effort.

1. ΔOD^{650nm}
   Increasing phospholipids in amniotic fluid produce increasing turbidity, which may be measured by spectrophotometry. An absorbance of greater than 0.15 OU at 650 nm indicates fetal lung maturity. The major disadvantages include some false-positive and a large number of false-negative predictions.
2. Fluorescence microviscosity
   While amniotic fluid phospholipids increase as a function of increasing gestation, fluid viscosity decreases as a summation measure of pulmonary surface active material. The critical microviscosity for fetal lung maturity has been determined, but has not been shown to be an accurate indicator.

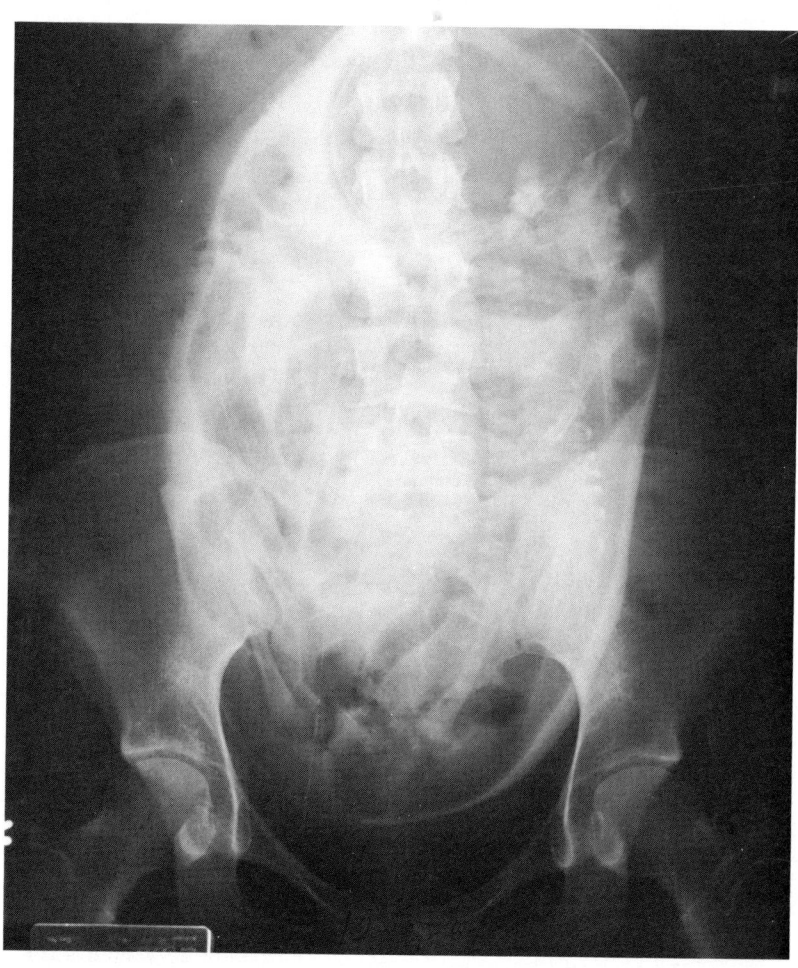

Fig. 4-5. Anteroposterior amniogram showing breech presentation, with placenta on right lateral uterine wall.

Other means of fetal assessment
AMNIOSCOPY

Amnioscopy often identifies the presence of meconium, presumably a sequel to hypoxia or other critical stress. Amnioscopy is relatively easy to accomplish in multiparas near term, but it is satisfactory only occasionally in the primigravida. Amnioscopy is not a widely practiced screening procedure, but it is reportedly of assistance in detection of meconium and in observation of prolonged pregnancy, and pregnancy complicated by maternal hypertension, suspected intrauterine growth retardation, and previous stillbirth. Amnioscopy has several inherent disadvantages. Many cases may not be anatomically suitable for observation, the procedure may rupture the membranes, and the manipulation may cause or further an ascending infection. Moreover, not all fetuses pass meconium, especially when premature, even in the presence of definite hypoxia. The test must be done daily or every few days in questionable cases, the cervix must already be dilated slightly, and the physician must be able to assume that the patient is at or near term.

AMNIOGRAPHY

Amniography employs roentgenography to contrast the soft tissues and skeleton of the fetus, the uterine cavity, and the fetoplacental surface (Figs. 4-5 and 4-6). It is particularly useful in the identification of fetal abnormal-

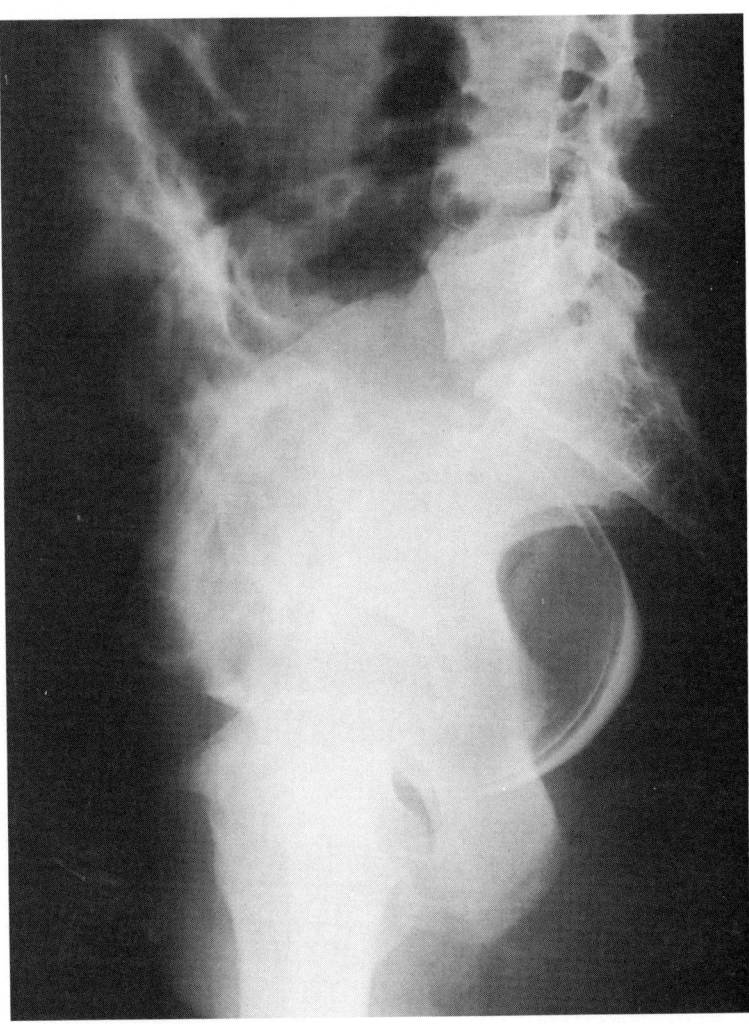

Fig. 4-6. Lateral amniogram showing intact membranes, engaged vertex, and absence of placenta previa.

ities, for example, scalp edema, hydrops, and anomalous development such as gastrointestinal atresia. Amniography facilitates fetal transfusion and may confirm fetal jeopardy or demise.

Iothalamate acid (Angio-Conray) or diatrizoate sodium (Hypaque-M), 75% is the aqueous contrast medium often used. Generally, 10 to 15 ml of amniotic fluid is removed at 22 to 28 weeks and 20 ml from 29 weeks onward, followed by instillation of a similar quantity of the iodine solution.

Opacification of amniotic fluid is seen in the fetal gastrointestinal tract within 15 minutes of injection as early as the twelfth week of pregnancy. Lack of swallowing indicates gastrointestinal obstruction, serious fetal compromise, or death.

Liposoluble contrast media such as iophendylate (Ethiodan) may also be used in amniography. These slightly viscid fluids are absorbed progressively on the vernix and, after 6 to 8 hours, outline the fetal skin clearly, remaining visible on x-ray films for several weeks after injection.

Prior to 38 weeks, the skin and even the fingers, toes, and external genitalia of the fetus are almost completely outlined by iophendylate, 8 ml, injected into the amniotic cavity. Between 38 and 40 weeks, the outlines of the extremities and abdomen become patchy, so that a clear, complete outline is not evident. At term and later, only the outline of the head and back is seen clearly. The gastrointestinal tract of the normal fetus will also contain the liposoluble contrast medium.

DETERMINATION OF FETAL DEATH

Clinically, the subjective diagnosis of fetal death often is suspected when the gravida ceases to appreciate fetal movements. Objectively, cessation of uterine growth or perhaps even regression suggests fetal death. Absence of fetal heart tones may be noted. However, unless the location of the heart is identified and that precise point is observed by real-time or sector scan ultrasonography, absent fetal heartbeat cannot be accepted as a sign of death. Biologic tests are of little value because the placenta may continue to function for a time. X-ray signs of fetal death include overlapping of the fetal cranial bones in a patient not in labor (Spaulding's sign), demonstration of gas in the fetal heart or large vessels, and abnormal angulation of the fetal spine.

BIBLIOGRAPHY

Browne, A.D.H., and Brennan, R.K.: The application value and limitation of amnioscopy, J. Obstet. Gynaec. Brit. Comm. **75**:616, 1968.

Clements, J.A., Platzker, A.C.G., and Tierney, D.F.: Assessment of the risk of the respiratory and distress syndrome by a rapid test for surfactant in amniotic fluid, N. Engl. J. Med. **286**:1077, 1972.

Donald, I.: Sonar in obstetrics and gynecology. In Greenhill, J.B., editor: The year book of obstetrics and gynecology, 1967-1968, Chicago, 1968, Year Book Medical Publishers, Inc.

Farr, V., and Mitchell, R.G.: Estimation of gestational age in the newborn infant, comparison between birth weight and maturity scoring in infants premature by birth, Am. J. Obstet. Gynecol. **103**:380, 1969.

Gluck, L., Kulovich, M.V., Borer, R.C., Jr., et al.: Diagnosis of the respiratory distress syndrome by amniocentesis, Am. J. Obstet. Gynecol. **109**:440, 1971.

Gruenwald, P., Funakawa, H., Mitani, S., et al.: Influence of environmental factors on foetal growth in man, Lancet **1**:1026, 1967.

Hamilton, P.R., Hauschild, D., Broekhuizen, F.F., et al.: Comparison of lecithin: spingomyelin ratio, fluorescence polarization, and phosphatidylglycerol in the amniotic fluid in the prediction of respiratory distress syndrome, Obstet. Gynecol. **63**:52, 1984.

Hellman, L.M., Kobayashi, M., Fillisti, L., et al.: Growth and development of the human fetus prior to the twentieth week of gestation, Am. J. Obstet. Gynecol. **103**:789, 1969.

Keniston, R.C., Pernoll, M.L., Buist, N.R.M., et al.: A prospective evaluation of the lecithin/sphingomyelin ratio and the rapid surfactant test in relation to fetal pulmonary maturity, Am. J. Obstet. Gynecol. **121**:324, 1975.

Loeffler, F.E.: Clinical fetal weight prediction, J. Obstet. Gynaec. Brit. Comm. **74**:675, 1967.

Michie, E.A.: Urinary estriol excretion in pregnancies complicated by suspected retarded intrauterine growth, toxemia, or essential hypertension, J. Obstet, Gynaec. Brit. Comm. **74**:896, 1967.

Miles, P.A., and Pearson, J.W.: Amniotic fluid osmolality in assessing fetal maturity, Obstet. Gynecol. **34**:701, 1969.

Moodley, S., Liu, J.H., Cherkis, R.C., et al.: Fetal pulmonary maturity: relationship between optical density (650nm) to the lecithin/sphingomyelin ratio and phosphatidylglycerol in amniotic fluid, Int. J. Gynaecol. Obstet. **21**:199, 1983.

Semmer, J.R., Traylor, T.R., Linton, E.B., et al.: Amniotic fluid phosphatidylglycerol: a predictor of fetal lung maturity using conventional one-dimensional thin-layer chromatography, South. Med. J. **76**:1257, 1983.

Whittle, M.J., Wilson, A.I., and Whitfield, C.R.: Amniotic fluid phosphatidylglycerol: an early indicator of fetal lung maturity, Br. J. Obstet. Gynaecol. **90**:134, 1983.

Usher, R., and McLean, F.: Intrauterine growth of liveborn Caucasian infants at sea level: standards obtained from measurements of infants born between 25 and 44 weeks of gestation, J. Pediatr. **74**:901, 1969.

5

Indicators of fetal jeopardy

Fetal distress is a symptom complex indicating a critical response to stress. It implies metabolic derangements, including hypoxia and acidosis, which affect essential body functions to the point of temporary or permanent injury or death. Fetal distress may be acute, chronic, or "additive" (see Table 7-1) and may be created by or associated with many diseases or processes. Unfortunately, precise detection of fetal distress, short of fetal death or severe damage, is difficult, and there is obviously still much to be learned. However, certain methods for detection of fetal distress are available, the most commonly employed being monitoring of the fetal heart rate (FHR).

There are several methods of determining FHR, and there is relatively good correlation between certain alterations of FHR and fetal compromise. Moreover, there seems little question today that FHR monitoring is warranted in risk states. However, routine electronic FHR monitoring in labor has been subject to much criticism and debate, for it is not clear that the practice is as effective in the low-risk patient in detailing fetal jeopardy during labor. Nevertheless there is general agreement concerning the urgency for the detection of fetal distress to avoid compromise of successful reproduction. The incidence of unanticipated serious fetal distress during labor ranges from approximately one in 100 to one in 400 deliveries. Further, it has been estimated that five deaths occur for every 1,000 deliveries as a direct result of fetal distress.

Thus health care providers are presented with three choices in caring for low-risk patients. They can employ electronic FHR monitoring, arrange for other suitable (equivalent to electronic) FHR monitoring (e.g., auditory monitoring in a prescribed manner by a well-trained attendant), or run the risk of not detecting fetal distress and having patients suffer its subsequent sequelae.

INDICATIONS FOR ELECTRONIC FETAL MONITORING IN LABOR

Although complete-labor internal monitoring may not be necessary in all cases, certain diseases or processes predispose to fetal distress with sufficient consistency to warrant electronic fetal monitoring. The more common of these conditions are listed below. Neutera's data indicate that the higher the risk category, the greater the chance that fetal monitoring will be effective in detection of fetal distress.

The following are diseases or processes predisposing to fetal problems during labor. The list is designed to be illustrative and is not exhaustive (i.e., there are other indications for electronic fetal monitoring).

Maternal
  Hypertensive states of pregnancy
  Premature labor
  Diabetes mellitus
  Maternal infections
  Maternal cardiac or respiratory insufficiency (e.g., cyanotic maternal heart disease)
  Maternal collagen diseases (e.g., systemic lupus erythematosus)
  Severe maternal anemia
  Previous cesarean section in labor
  Previous stillbirth
  Drug addiction

Fetal
  Prematurity
  Growth retardation
  Isoimmunization
  Malpresentation
  Abnormal antepartum fetal monitoring
  Abnormal FHR (by auscultation) or other abnormalities of intrapartum monitoring
  Multiple gestation
Placental, uterine, or related to cord, membranes, or amniotic fluid
  Prolapsed umbilical cord
  Third trimester bleeding (including abruptio placentae and placenta previa)
  Chorioamnionitis
  Premature or prolonged rupture of membranes
  Meconium-stained amniotic fluid
  Hydramnios or oligohydramnios
  Placental insufficiency
  Failure to progress (prolonged latent phase, protracted labor, or arrested labor)
Other
  Abnormal labor pattern
  Oxytocin administration
  Use of tocolytics

METHODS OF ELECTRONIC FETAL MONITORING

Methods of electronic labor monitoring currently available are as follows:
  I. Fetal heart rate
     A. Indirect
        1. Phonocardiograph
        2. Ultrasonography
        3. Fetal ECG from maternal wall
     B. Direct
        1. Clip
        2. Spiral electrode
        3. Other methods of direct contact
  II. Uterine activity
     A. Intrauterine catheter
     B. Tocodynamometer (strain gauge applied to abdominal wall)

Although the most information is obtained by direct monitoring and an intrauterine catheter, this requires rupture of the membranes and has inherent risks (see pitfalls of electronic fetal monitoring, p. 51). Indirect methods of FHR monitoring used in conjunction with a tocodynamometer are certainly useful for screening and are "noninvasive," although they provide less information. Fig 5-1 schematically demonstrates internal monitoring.

NORMAL FETAL HEART RATE

A normal FHR is between 120 to 160 beats per minute. When electronically monitored in a normal mature fetus, the rate demonstrates fluctuations of approximately 1 to 8 beats per minute, and the fluctuations have a frequency of 3 to 10 cycles per minute. This is referred to as beat-to-beat variability or irregularity. Some have termed the individual beat-to-beat variability in heart rate "short-term variability" and the longer cyclic changes (noted above) "long-term variability."

Beat-to-beat variability is nearly always present in the normal, mature, unmedicated, unnarcotized, and unasphyxiated fetus. Although the exact mechanism for it remains unclear, it has been suggested that this irregularity is created by asynchronous attempts of the two portions of the autonomic nervous system (sympathetic and parasympathetic) to regulate the FHR.

Normal FHR also will occasionally show accelerations that may be related to a fetal movement. These will be discussed later (fetal activity acceleration determinations). With increasing maturity there is also a slowing of the FHR within the normal range noted above.

ABNORMALITIES OF FHR

Aberrations of normal FHR may occur as abnormalities of rate and of beat-to-beat variability or as absence of accelerations with fetal movement. There may also be an abnormality of longer term variability that has been described as a sinusoidal pattern.

Bradycardia

Fetal bradycardia is defined as moderate if it is between 100 to 119 beats per minute and severe if less than 100 beats per minute. Severe fetal bradycardia is unusual and in addition to its relation to hypoxia may be associated with congenital heart block or congenital heart lesions in the fetus. Unless persistent bradycardia is associated with noticeable FHR decelerations, it is not associated with neonatal asphyxia.

Tachycardia

Fetal tachycardia is defined as moderate if it is between 161 to 180 beats per minute and

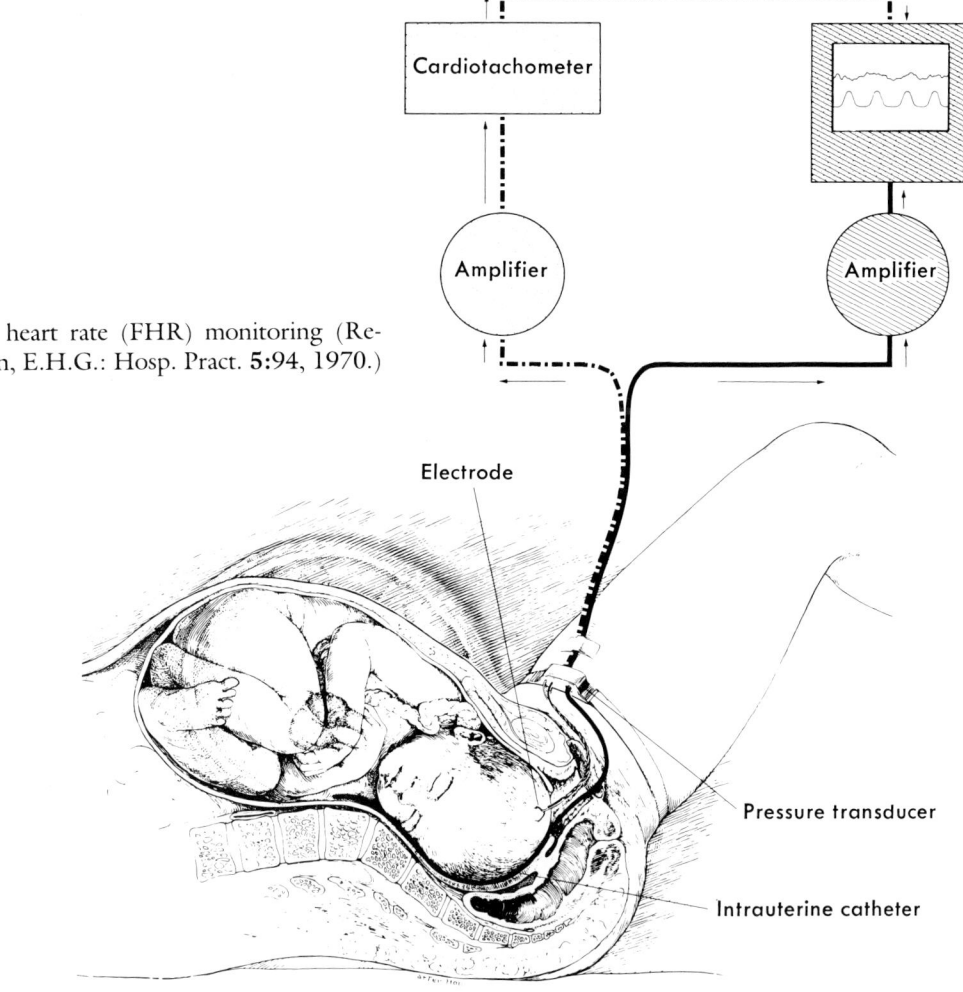

Fig. 5-1. Fetal heart rate (FHR) monitoring (Redrawn from Hon, E.H.G.: Hosp. Pract. **5:**94, 1970.)

severe if more than 180 beats per minute. Fetal tachycardia is associated with fetal immaturity, maternal fever, fetal hypoxia, maternal hyperthyroidism, amnionitis, parasympatholytic drugs, fetal cardiac arrhythmias, fetal hypovolemia, and fetal heart failure. It is more ominous as a predictor of fetal distress when there is absence of beat-to-beat variability, when it is associated with late or prolonged variable deceleration, or when it is associated with FHR irregularity late in the contracting phase of the uterus.

Beat-to-beat variability

Beat-to-beat variability is believed to express fetal reserve; thus its absence is a possible cause for concern. It is usually decreased or absent in immature, asphyxiated, narcotized, tranquilized, or anesthetized fetuses. Additionally, variability is decreased or absent in fetuses with faulty nervous control of the heart, and it is decreased or difficult to detect with fetal tachycardia. Thus absence of beat-to-beat variability may be ominous in the term or near-term fetus, implying altered nervous control of the heart because of anoxia, acidosis, or drug effects.

Hon has suggested classification of variability on the basis of the peak-to-peak fluctuations, thus:

1. No variability—0 to 2 beats/min
2. Minimal—3 to 5 beats/min
3. Average—6 to 10 beats/min
4. Moderate—11 to 25 beats/min
5. Marked (strong)—greater than 25 beats/min

Longer term abnormalities of a cyclic nature

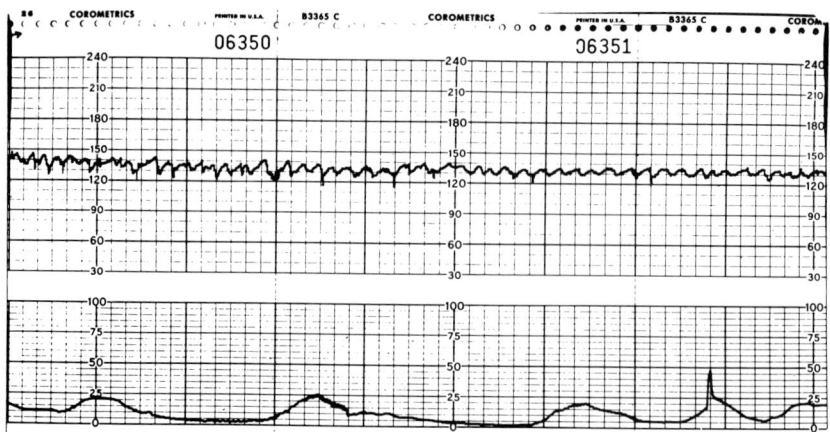

Fig. 5-2. An example of a sinusoidal FHR pattern with normal outcome. Normal beat-to-beat variability is notable.

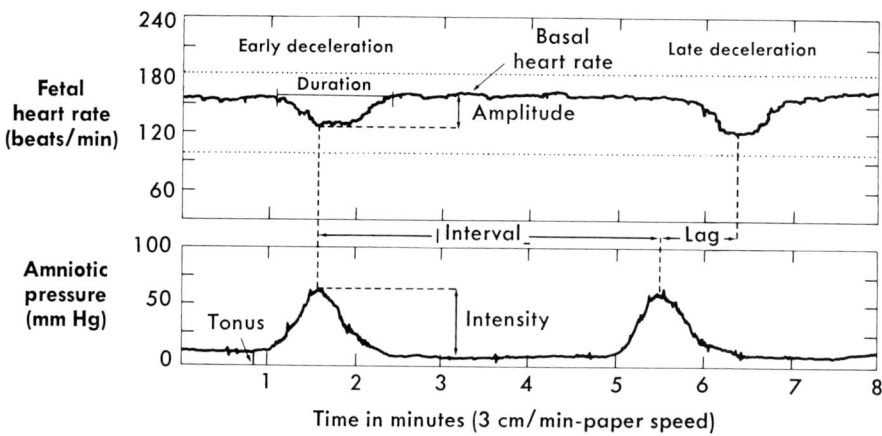

Fig. 5-3. Some of the variables observed in the tracings of the FHR and amniotic fluid pressure (uterine contractions) and their chronologic relationships.

have been termed "sinusoidal" fetal heart patterns and although considered an ominous sign (especially when associated with decreased beat-to-beat variability), they have also been observed in normal fetuses (Fig. 5-2).

PERIODIC HEART RATE CHANGES

Periodic heart rate changes are short-term alterations that occur in relation to stress. Thus, by inference, when stress is not present, the FHR may be termed "baseline" and used as a reference to detect changes. Periodic heart rate observations are usually performed in relation to uterine contractions because labor contractions impose a temporary decrease in uterine blood supply. This may affect fetal oxygenation and transfer of carbon dioxide sufficiently to evoke a demonstrable fetal response, which may indicate fetal status. Useful terminology for understanding and discussing FHR patterns are demonstrated in Fig. 5-3. The several classifications of periodic heart rate changes follow.

Accelerations

Accelerations are transient increases of FHR concomitant with other events. Accelerations are most commonly observed with fetal motion and, when proper criteria are met, indicate fetal well-being. They may also be noted in a number of circumstances when the fetus is stimulated (by sound, direct manipulation, or indirect manipulation) and again are thought to indicate fetal well-being. However, accelerations of FHR may also occur in relation to uterine

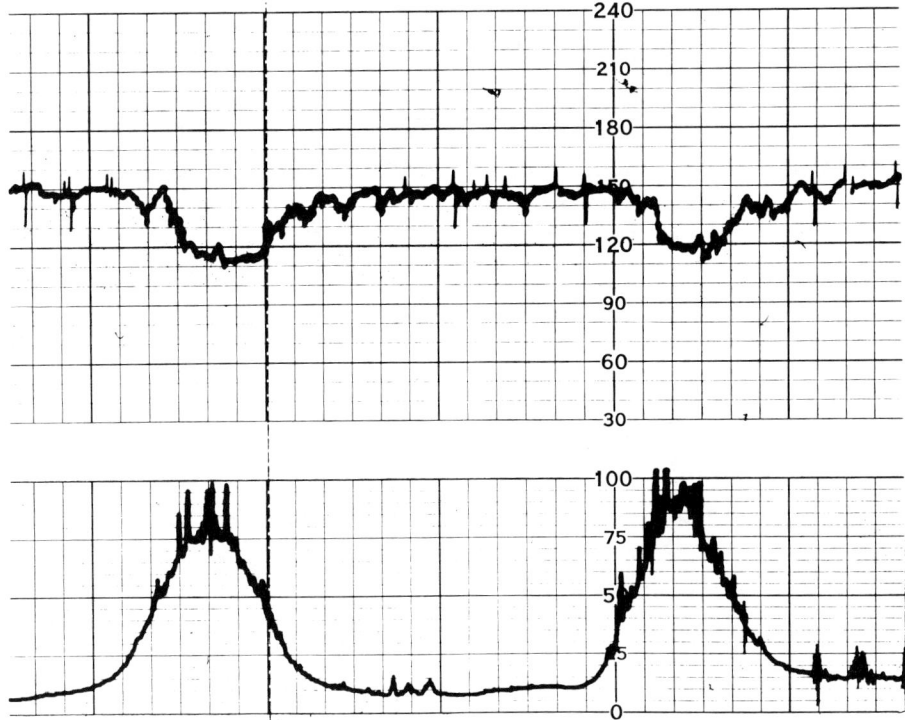

Fig. 5-4. Early deceleration (head compression). Note the early onset of bradycardia, its recovery by the end of the contractions, and the proportionate relationship between the individual patterns and the associated contractions.

contraction. In this circumstance they have been reported as an early indicator of possible fetal compromise; although in Hon's experience, the presence of accelerations, without other abnormalities of FHR pattern, has not been associated with poor clinical outcome or significant changes in fetal acid-base status.

Decelerations

Decelerations are transient decreases of FHR in response to uterine contraction. There are three "pure" types currently known: early, late, and variable.

1. *Early deceleration* is a transient decrease in FHR in response to a uterine contraction. It is believed to be caused by fetal head compression. The curve of the deceleration is of uniform shape, reflecting the intrauterine pressure curve (Fig. 5-4). Amplitude of the deceleration does not exceed 40 beats/min and deceleration normally occurs between 140 and 100 beats/min. An important differentiating characteristic is that recovery of FHR to baseline rate occurs at or before the end of the contraction. This FHR pattern has not been associated with depressed newborns, but it appears to be innocuous.

2. *Late deceleration* is a transient fall in FHR occurring after the uterus has begun to contract. Its curve has a uniform shape, but the deceleration has a later onset than early deceleration and may not cease immediately with the contraction (Fig. 5-5). Late deceleration is believed to be caused by uteroplacental insufficiency and is an ominous sign of fetal distress.

An important difference between early and late deceleration is that late deceleration has its onset late in the uterine contracting phase and FHR does not return to baseline until after cessation of the contraction. It usually occurs between 180 and 120 beats/min but if severe may be 60 or fewer beats/min. It is frequently associated with high-risk pregnancy and with maternal hypotension or uterine hyperactivity. It is critical to note that this most ominous indicator of fetal distress usually occurs in the normal FHR range.

50 *Diagnosis and management of the high-risk fetus and neonate*

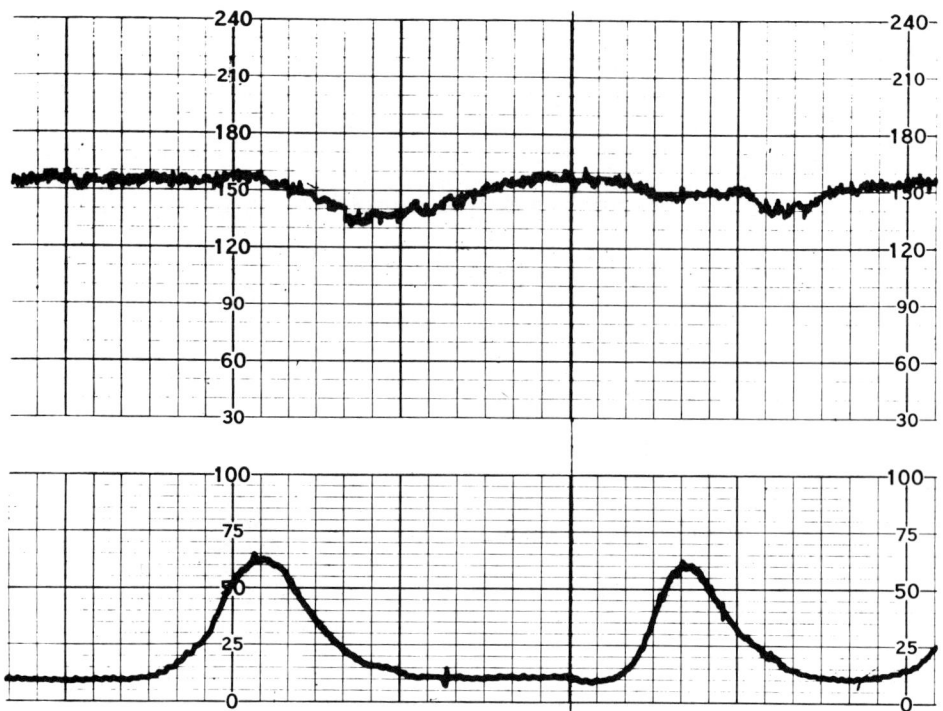

Fig. 5-5. Late deceleration (uteroplacental circulatory insufficiency). Note the late onset, the lag, the delay in recovery, and the proportionate relationship between the individual patterns and the associated contractions *(bottom)*.

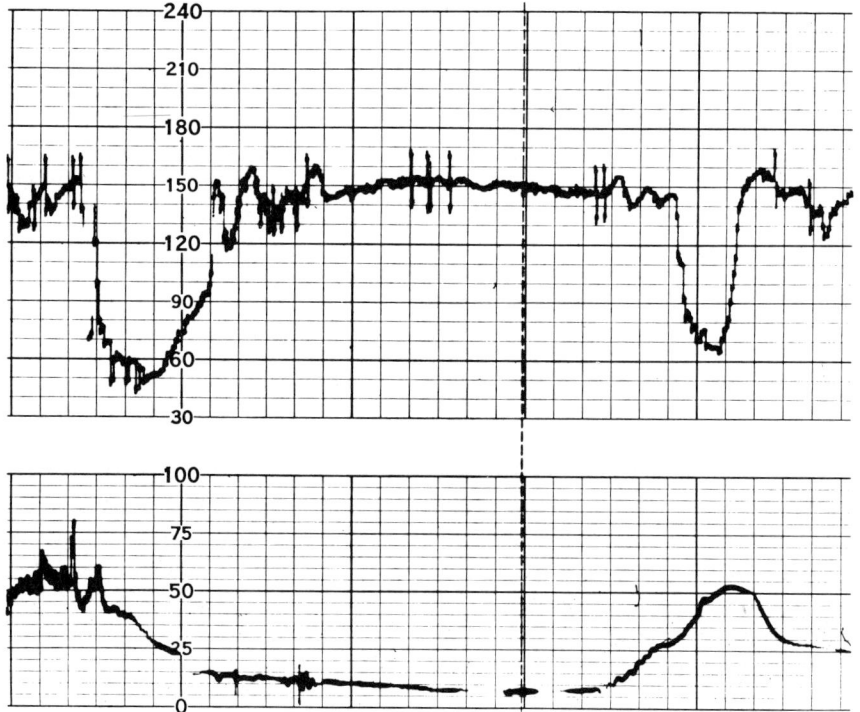

Fig. 5-6. Variable deceleration (cord compression). Note the great variability in onset, depth, shape, and recovery in relation to the uterine contractions.

Moreover, in the severely compromised fetus alteration of FHR may be quite subtle. Therefore complete assessment of the mother and fetus, weighing other risk factors, utilizing other criteria, and taking great care in interpreting this criteria, will yield the greatest correlation with fetal distress.

3. *Variable deceleration* is a transient decrease in FHR that may occur at varying times in relationship to uterine contraction. The pattern is not of uniform shape and varies in intensity (Fig. 5-6). It usually occurs in the range of 140 to 160 beats/min and is believed to be associated with umbilical cord compression. It may be associated with depressed newborns if prolonged and severe (below 90 beats/min for 60 sec or more) but is usually alleviated by maternal position change.

Combined patterns

The full significance of combined patterns is not yet known. Suffice it to note, however, that combinations of those patterns indicative of fetal distress are probably an ominous sign.

INTERPRETATION OF FHR PATTERNS

Interpretation of FHR patterns must be performed in an organized fashion. A useful organization for this analysis (including labor) follows:

    Uterine activity
        Baseline tonus (with intrauterine catheter)
        Contraction
            Amplitude (with intrauterine catheter)
            Frequency
            Duration
    FHR
        Baseline
            Rate
            Beat-to-beat variability (with direct monitoring)
        Periodic changes
            Accelerations
            Decelerations
                Early
                Late
                Variable
        Combined patterns
    Assessment and comments

All FHR pattern interpretation depends on ensemble characteristics. The diagnosis of a given pattern cannot be made on the basis of a single contraction. Current knowledge suggests that electronic fetal monitoring pattern interpretation may be considered in three categories: reassuring, suspicious, or ominous.

Reassuring signs

Signs of fetal well-being observable on electronic fetal monitoring that are reassuring include normal rates and variability, FHR alteration (usually acceleration) with manipulation, stimulation for fetal movement, and lack of variable or late deceleration patterns.

Suspicious signs

Changes that create suspicion of fetal distress include decreased or markedly increased variability, subtle or inconsistent late decelerations, and mild variable decelerations.

Ominous signs

Early signs of fetal compromise that may be ominous include further decreased variability, increased heart rate (in comparison to what it was previously), and variable or late decelerations with normal beat-to-beat variability.

Late signs of fetal compromise include no variability, severe variable and/or late decelerations with minimal variability, bradycardia after a previously normal FHR, or a sinusoidal FHR pattern.

In summary, it is believed that variability expresses fetal reserve and that deceleration waveforms may express the cause of the insult. However, acid-base determinations may be necessary to determine severity of compromise.

PITFALLS OF ELECTRONIC FETAL MONITORING

The major pitfalls to electronic fetal monitoring are listed as follows:

1. *Maternal*
   a. Maternal pH will affect fetal pH and therefore also affect FHR patterns.
   b. In extremely obese patients external monitoring may not be effective.
   c. Uterine perforation may occur with insertion of intrauterine catheters.
   d. Prolonged intrauterine catheterization may enhance the possibility of infection.

e. Improper electrode placement may record maternal heart rate and indeed, even if properly placed on a dead fetus, will record maternal heart rate. If there is maternal tachycardia there is a greater chance of confusing maternal and fetal heart rates.
f. Maternal medication may greatly affect fetal cardiac responses.
g. Monitoring may increase the cost of medical care.
h. Improper interpretation of fetal distress may lead to unwarranted instrumentation or cesarean section.

2. *Fetal*
   a. Rupture of membranes results in an eightfold increase in the incidence of early deceleration.
   b. The external FHR monitor does not accurately depict beat-to-beat variability, and therefore variability may not be determined by external monitoring except with a fetal electrocardiographic monitor.
   c. Low FHRs may be mistaken for the maternal heart rate.
   d. A dead fetus may not be recognized because the mother's heart rate may be recorded.
   e. A breech presentation may require a switch in equipment polarity.
   f. Fetal scalp infections may occur (less than 1%) with direct monitoring. These are usually very limited in extent and respond well to local care.
   g. Prolonged intrauterine catheterization may enhance the risk of infection.
   h. Soft-tissue trauma may occur from improper electrode placement.
   i. Little is currently known about monitoring during the second stage of labor and extreme caution must be applied in interpretation of second-stage monitoring.

CONFIRMATION OF FETAL COMPROMISE (BIOCHEMICAL MONITORING BY FETAL SCALP BLOOD SAMPLING)

With asphyxia, respiratory gas exchange across the placenta falls, accompanied by hypoxia and hypercapnia in the fetus. The result is a combination of respiratory and metabolic acidosis. The latter is enhanced by the accumulation of organic acids, which result from anaerobic metabolism. Acidosis is identified by a falling blood pH. It has been amply demonstrated that considerable reduction in oxygen supply to the fetus may cause a significant rise in basal FHR initially; severe oxygen lack invariably results in bradycardia or arrhythmia or both, and, finally, fetal death.

In complications that impair gaseous exchange (most often of placental or maternal origin), any hypoxia leading to fetal acidosis will threaten cellular metabolism after a variable latent period. Circulation, muscle tone, motility, and respiratory functions may all suffer as a result. The latent period between the onset of hypoxia and the adverse effect on the fetus depends on whether the hypoxia is acute or chronic, the condition of the fetus at the time the complication occurs,* the duration of the metabolic disturbance, and the maturity of the fetus.

Determination of fetal blood pH value in a complicated pregnancy after established labor gives the obstetrician an accurate method (confidence limit for scalp blood is 0.05 pH units, for cord blood, 0.02 pH units) for assessment of severity of fetal distress. A fall in pH value to below 7.25, but remaining above 7.2, is cause for immediate concern and initiation of any therapy that might enhance oxygenation (e.g., administration of maternal oxygen, improving maternal blood volume by positional change or fluid administration). In the nonacidotic mother, a fall in pH to 7.2 or below is an indication to perform delivery immediately by the best means possible.

Although FHR changes and meconium passage show a correlation with fetal asphyxia, they do not indicate degree of distress as accurately as fetal blood pH determination does.

Through the innovative work of Erich Saling, fetal blood sampling has added an important parameter to recognition of the fetus in distress. It is now agreed that pH and blood gas measurements taken under defined conditions truly represent arterial circulation, particularly during the first part of labor.

---

*For example, a fetus that has suffered growth retardation or wasting has reduced glycogen resources for the support of anaerobic metabolism.

I. Indications for fetal blood sampling
   A. Acute problems
      1. Meconium present (vertex presentation)
      2. Unexplained FHR over 160 or under 100 beats/min
      3. Bradycardia that continues for more than 30 seconds after the end of a contraction (late deceleration)
      4. Severe variable deceleration or combination of late and variable deceleration
      5. Combined FHR patterns indicative of distress

      If the first fetal blood sample done at the appearance of these signs is less than 7.25 pH, repeat the test immediately.
   B. Chronic problems

      Moderate or strong toxemia, diabetes mellitus, severe Rh sensitization, and amnionitis, as well as postterm births, dysmaturity, and dystocia; borderline cephalopelvic disproportion, uterine dyskinesia, prolonged labor, oxytocin stimulation, and a history of unexplained prior stillbirth.

      The first fetal blood sample obtained at the onset of labor should be repeated if signs of fetal distress develop. Deliver the fetus at once if pH is less than 7.20 on two successive samples, in the absence of maternal acidosis.
II. Method of obtaining fetal blood
   A. Pass amnioscope and wipe scalp or buttock with antiseptic on gauze.
   B. Apply silicone to allow a drop of blood to remain at incision site.
   C. Nick skin, no more than 2 mm.
   D. Aspirate blood into capillary tube.
   E. Do not remove amnioscope until bleeding has ceased. Determine pH without delay.
III. Advantages of fetal blood sampling
   A. An operative delivery indicated by the usual signs of fetal distress may be avoided if the acid-base balance of the fetus is satisfactory.
   B. Fetal asphyxia of a mild type (pH 7.20 to 7.24) that is only slowly progressive (a substantial majority) can be followed serially every half hour, and if operative intervention becomes necessary, it can be performed under optimal conditions.
   C. Acute and severe reductions in fetal acid-base balance that demand immediate delivery can be detected.
   D. Fetal blood sampling indicates fetal distress, which may not be evident by clinical signs of meconium passage or FHR changes.
   E. Recognition of fetal acidosis will allow early correction at birth by the injection of buffer solution through an umbilical vessel (p. 231). This procedure prevents an aggravated peak of metabolic acidosis, which usually occurs 5 to 10 minutes after delivery and if untreated may intensify the already depressed function of vital centers and contribute to cerebral hemorrhage.
IV. Reasons for discrepancies between level of fetal acidosis as measured by pH and vigor of the newborn at birth
   A. False normal

      In approximately 10% of cases pH may be normal with depressed neonates. This may be the result of perinatal asphyxia that occurs after the sample has been taken, incomplete asphyxial recovery, narcosis, infection, prematurity, trauma, congenital anomalies, or airway obstruction after birth.
   B. False abnormal

      pH may be low with a vigorous neonate in up to 8% of cases. This is usually associated with maternal acidosis or milder states of fetal acidosis in which the fetal central nervous system has not yet been depressed. The etiology of nonasphyxial metabolic acidosis includes supine hypotension, maternal narcosis, amniotomy, and transient fetal bradycardia. Maternal acidosis may be caused by excess muscular activity, starvation, dehydration, a long first stage of labor, a long second stage of labor, and metabolic disease. When the mother is acidotic, fetal scalp pH

indicates fetal acidosis if it is 0.2 pH units below that of the mother.
V. Risks in fetal scalp sampling
Risks to the fetus has been infrequent infection and bleeding. Pressure alone will usually suffice to stop bleeding, but a suture in the scalp may be necessary.

TREATMENT OF FETAL DISTRESS FROM INTERPRETATION OF FHR PATTERNS

Currently the most readily available data concerning fetal status are from FHR patterns, despite the possible desirability of fetal scalp sampling to enhance accurate detection of fetal distress. Therefore the treatment of fetal distress is discussed in relationship to FHR pattern interpretation.

No fetal distress

Short-term early deceleration of the FHR usually indicates innocuous fetal head compression (Fig. 5-4). No therapy is indicated. The consequences of long-term early deceleration are unknown.

Suspicion of fetal distress

Variable FHR deceleration may be from seconds to a minute long; it is a warning that may indicate cord compression (Fig. 5-6), especially with tachycardia of more than 160 beats per minute. FHR does not mirror the uterine contraction curve or the strength of the contractions. If the variable FHR acceleration is confined to the period of uterine contraction, even if associated with noticeable temporary bradycardia, it probably is reflex in nature and not serious.

The patient should be repositioned to one side or the other and the condition treated as fetal distress if improvement does not follow the change of position. Decreased beat-to-beat variability should be closely followed by direct monitoring.

Fetal distress

I. Prolonged or worsening *variable FHR deceleration* (more than 1 minute) with bradycardia of under 100 beats per minute indicates possible cord compression.
   A. Give oxygen, 6 to 7 L/min by mask. Reposition patient.
   B. Begin administration of 10% glucose intravenously.
II. *Late FHR deceleration* (with or without tachycardia) generally identifies uteroplacental circulatory insufficiency and fetal hypoxia (Fig. 5-5). The problem may be critical also if tachycardia and a relatively smooth FHR baseline are present. Therapy is designed to alleviate problems that lead to reduced uteroplacental circulation.
   A. Discontinue oxytocin, if being used.
   B. Administer oxygen at 6 to 8 L/min by mask or nasal prongs.
   C. Correct maternal hypotension.
      1. Place patient in the lateral recumbent position (avoid the supine position).
      2. Administer intravenous fluids rapidly.
   D. Alert the operating room for possible cesarean section.
   E. Consider fetal scalp blood analysis for pH determination.

Critical fetal distress

When the suggested therapy yields no improvement in FHR patterns indicative of definite fetal distress, and there is an abnormal pH on scalp sampling, the condition may be termed "critical fetal distress." Delivery should be effected immediately. If fetal scalp sampling is unavailable or if patterns are of such ominous nature that the waiting interval may jeopardize the fetus, immediate delivery should be performed.

ANTEPARTUM TESTING

In certain risk situations (see p. 45) the severity of the process or disease may be enough to compromise uteroplacental-fetal reserve. When such compromise is suspected, antepartum electronic fetal monitoring may give a gross evaluation of prenatal fetal well-being. Two types of fetal monitoring tests are currently used: the nonstress test (fetal activity-acceleration determination) and the contraction stress test (oxytocin challenge test).

Nonstress testing (NST)

Fetal activity-acceleration determination (FAD) requires simultaneous monitoring of the FHR and determination of fetal movement. Interpretation at 32 weeks or earlier is less certain because accurate data for comparison have not been collected. Clinical indications include the following (among others):

Diabetes mellitus
Hypertensive states of pregnancy
Intrauterine growth retardation
Postmaturity
Previous perinatal loss
Meconium-stained amniotic fluid
   (detected by amniocentesis or amnioscopy)

There are no known contraindications.

PROCEDURE

1. Explain test to gravida.
2. Place patient supine with head elevated 30 degrees to prevent supine hypotension.
3. Monitor blood pressure every 20 minutes and record it on fetal monitoring strips.
4. Record baseline FHR for minimum of 10 minutes, noting rate and uterine contractions.

Acceptable fetal movements are defined by a fetal movement that is palpable to both the mother and an observer palpating or visualizing motion of the abdominal wall. To make an FAD, fetal movement must occur simultaneously with an alteration in heart rate.

If after 10 minutes a fetal movement has not occurred, Leopold's third and fourth maneuvers are used to stimulate the fetus. The test may be discontinued when two fetal movements with concurrent FHR acceleration have occurred within 20 minutes and the FHR acceleration curves have regular configuration. Indeed, recent data indicate that if a single FAD is observed the test may be terminated with little if any loss of accuracy.

If within 20 minutes fewer than two fetal movements occur, 20 or more minutes of monitoring is conducted with continued stimulation at 5-minute intervals. In the presence of a nonreactive test (absence of fetal movements or absence of FHR accelerations) the oxytocin challenge test should be considered.

Care must be exercised in interpretation if testing is done at a time of day when the mother may be hypoglycemic. Experience has shown that if the test is conducted in the first 2 hours after a meal, there are a greater number of fetal movements. Thus it may be necessary to repeat the FAD in a few hours or after the mother has been given fruit juice.

INTERPRETATION

To be judged as *reactive* (Fig. 5-7), the FAD curve must have a smooth, regular configuration and there must be two or more FADs per minutes for the duration of greater than 15

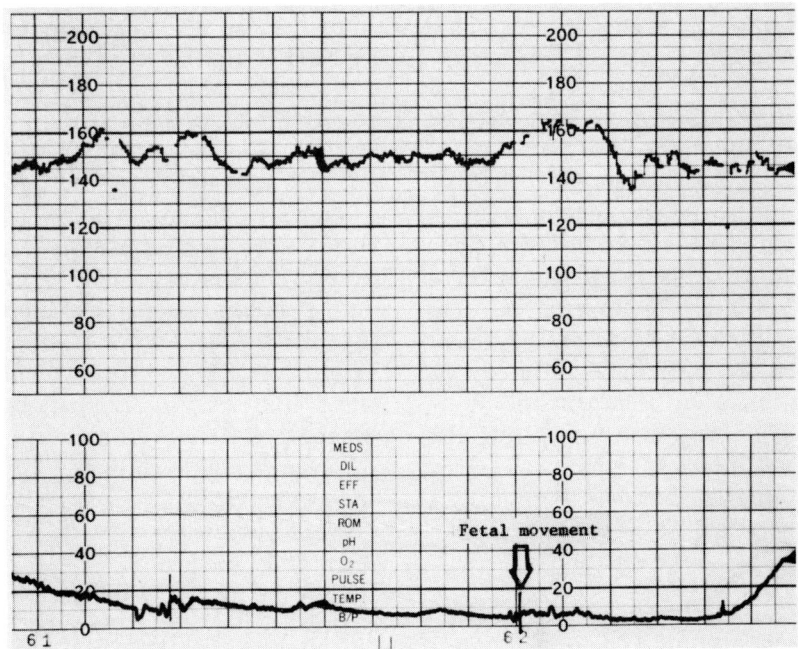

Fig. 5-7. Normal cardiac response to fetal movement demonstrates an acceleration of more than 15 beats lasting more than 15 seconds.

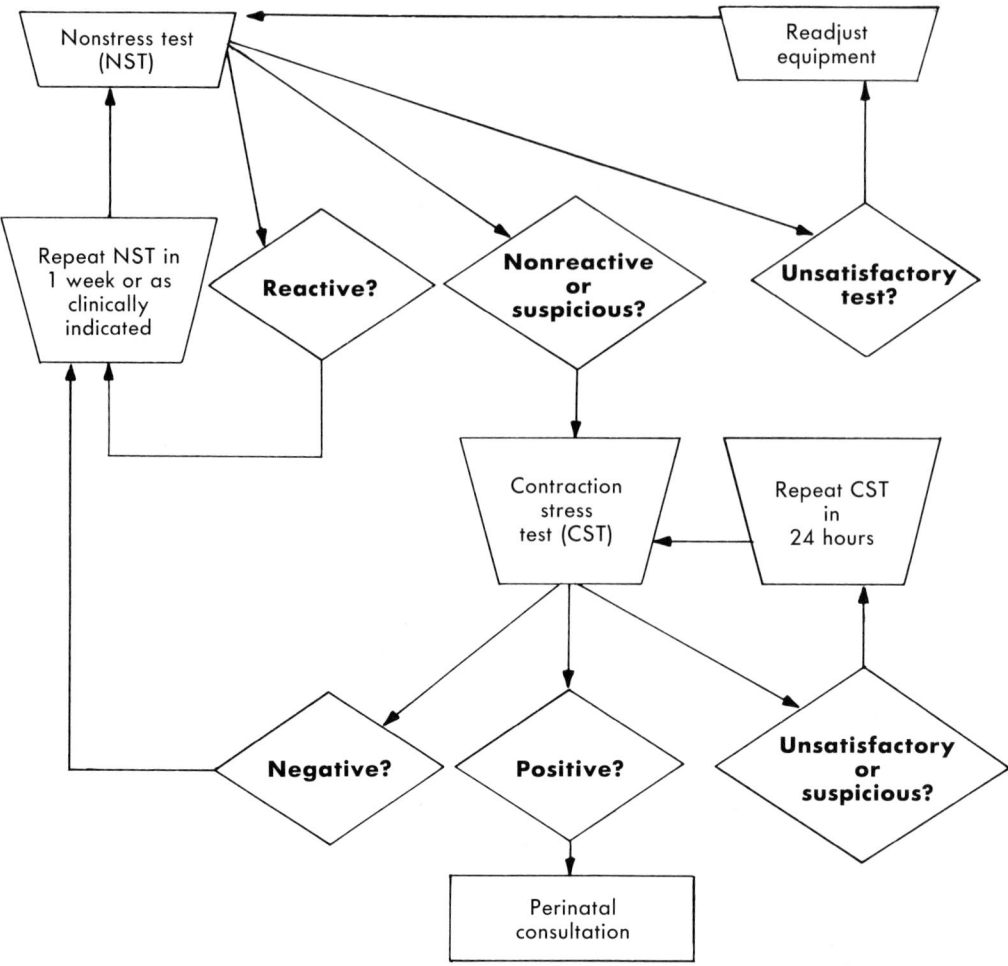

Fig. 5-8. An algorithm for use of nonstress and contraction stress testing.

seconds and an amplitude of more than 15 beats per minute. The *nonreactive* classification includes no fetal activity either spontaneously or with stimulation and/or no demonstrable FHR changes. *Suspicious* classification includes three or fewer fetal movements in 40 minutes of monitoring with a mean duration of less than 15 seconds or longer than 60 seconds without regular configuration. Additionally, the amplitude may be less than 15 beats per minute or not more than 30 beats per minute. If the tracing is not of sufficient quality to allow interpretation, it must be classified as unsatisfactory. The algorithm in Fig. 5-8 is employed in these cases.

Contraction Stress Testing (CST): oxytocin challenge test (OCT)

The oxytocin challenge test (or contraction stress test) constitutes a means of determining the respiratory reserve of the uteroplacental-fetal unit (an external method for the evaluation of the "respiratory" function of the placenta).

The oxytocin challenge test consists of giving the patient intravenous oxytocin by infusion pump sufficient to produce three contractions in a 10-minute period, and simultaneously recording FHR and uterine contractions with an external monitor. (No oxytocin is necessary if three contractions occur spontaneously.) The oxytocin challenge test may be started as early as 32 weeks when clinically indicated. Clinical indications and contraindications are as follows:

Clinical indications
  Diabetes mellitus
  Chronic hypertension
  Pregnancy-induced hypertension
  Intrauterine growth retardation
  Sickle-cell disease
  Maternal cyanotic heart disease

Postmaturity
History of previous stillbirth
Rh sensitization
Meconium-stained amniotic fluid detected by amniocentesis

Contraindications

Risk of premature labor
Premature rupture of membranes
Placenta previa
Previous classical cesarean section
Multiple gestation (where disadvantages of premature labor outweigh advantages)
Incompetent cervix
Cervix with a high Bishop score

PROCEDURE

1. Perform a vaginal examination and conduct Bishop scoring of the cervix (may be omitted if previously performed within 6 hours and there are no signs of labor).
2. Place patient in supine position with head elevated 30 degrees.
3. Check blood pressure initially and then every 15 minutes.
4. Record baseline FHR for 10 minutes, with rate, variability, and uterine contraction pattern being noted. If three contractions with interpretable FHR are obtained during this 10-minute period, do not give oxytocin.
5. Start intravenous infusion of 250 ml D5 Ringers' lactate (dextrose 5% in water). Piggyback with a T-connector 500 ml D5 normal saline with Pitocin and 1 ml Berocca-C.
6. Start oxytocin at 0.5 mU/min and increase amount, depending on response, every 10 minutes until contraction frequency is 3 in 10 minutes. Discontinue oxytocin and record until uterine contractions diminish in frequency and intensity.
7. Consult physician for dose above 10 mU/min (if test is nurse-monitored).
8. Label monitor strip, record blood pressure readings on strip, and discontinue test:
   a. When you have three good contractions in 10 minutes and a negative test
   b. When late decelerations occur, indicating a positive test
   c. If hyperstimulation occurs
   d. If prolonged bradycardia occurs
   e. If test is suspicious
9. If fetal distress is noted:
   a. Stop oxytocin and increase rate of glucose solution.
   b. Turn patient to left side.
   c. Start oxygen at 6 to 7 L/min.
   d. Notify appropriate physicians.

INTERPRETATION OF TEST RESULTS

Negative. There is a uterine contraction frequency of at least 3 in 10 minutes and no late decelerations of FHR with this uterine contraction frequency. There is usually, but not necessarily, a good baseline variability and acceleration with fetal movement.

Positive. Consistent and persistent late decelerations occur repeatedly with most uterine contractions even if the frequency is less than 3 in 10 minutes, and the decelerations are usually but not necessarily associated with a decreased variability of FHR and the absence of FHR acceleration with fetal movement.

Suspicious. Inconsistent but definite late deceleration does not persist with continued uterine contractions and baseline FHR variability is normal or decreased. Acceleration of FHR with fetal movement may be present. The test may be repeated in 24 hours. Patients with falling estriol levels may be retested every 24 hours.

Unsatisfactory. If the quality of the recording is not sufficient to assure that no late deceleration is present, the record is classified as unsatisfactory for interpretation; or if frequency of the uterine contractions achieved is less than 3 in 10 minutes, the test is not considered satisfactory for interpretation. If no response is obtained after 45 to 60 minutes of Pitocin infusion, the test is discontinued and repeated in 24 hours.

Breast Stimulation

Recently, breast stimulation has been used extensively for the contraction stress test. Although not confirmed by testing, breast stimulation presumably causes release of oxytocin from the posterior pituitary, which subsequently initiates uterine contractions. This method of initiating uterine contractions has several advantages over using oxytocin: an intravenous line is not necessary; idiosyncratic oxytocin reactions are eliminated; oxytocin dosage errors cannot occur; it is easily applied; it is less expensive and less time-consuming. Breast stimulation may be expected to produce adequate

Table 5-1. Fetal biophysical profile score

Variable	Score 2	Score 0
1. Fetal reactivity	Presence of 2 or more FHR accelerations of at least 15 beats/min and lasting at least 15 sec and associated with fetal movement in 40 min	No FHR acceleration or fewer than 2 accelerations in 40 min of observation
2. Fetal tone	At least 1 episode of motion of a limb from a position of flexion to extension and a rapid return to flexion	Fetus in position of semi- or full-limb extension with no return to flexion with movement (Absence of fetal movement is counted as absent tone.)
3. Fetal movements	Three or more gross body movements in 30 min of observation (Stimultaneous limb and trunk movements are counted as a single movement.)	Two or fewer gross body movements in 30 min of observation
4. Qualitative amniotic fluid volume	Pocket of amniotic fluid that measures at least 1 cm in 2 perpendicular planes	Largest pocket of amniotic fluid measures <1 cm in 2 perpendicular planes
5. Fetal breathing movements (FBM)	Presence of at least 30 sec of sustained FBM in 30 min of observation	Less than 30 sec of FBM in 30 min

From Manning, F.A., et al.: Am. J. Obstet. Gynecol. **140**:289, 1981.

Table 5-2. Management based on biophysical profile scoring

Score	Recommended management
0-2	Evaluate for immediate delivery. In cases of certain pulmonary immaturity, give steroids and deliver in 48 hr.
4-6	If fetal pulmonary maturity is assured and cervix favorable, deliver. Otherwise repeat scoring in 24 hr. If score of 4 to 6 persists, deliver if fetal pulmonary maturity is certain. Otherwise treat with steroids and deliver in 48 hr.
8-10	Repeat scoring in 1 week. In diabetic (insulin-dependent) and postdates patients, repeat twice weekly. No active intervention is indicated.

From Manning, F.A., et al.: Am. J. Obstet. Gynecol. **140**:289, 1981.

contractions for evaluation in over 90% of patients.

The method of breast stimulation has not yet been standardized. Several methods (all performed by the mother herself) have been suggested: deep breast massage followed by nipple rolling between the fingers; application of lubricant and rolling the nipple between the fingers, with or without gauze; application of warm wash-cloths, with or without nipple stimulation. Stimulation has been applied through clothing and on the bare breast with satisfactory uterine contractions occurring with both methods. It has been suggested as safer to start with one breast and only proceed to bilateral stimulation if unilateral does not produce contractions.

The test is conducted in exactly the same manner as is the oxytocin challenge test; the end points and interpretations are the same, and accuracy is comparable. It is imperative that all of the same precautions be taken with this test and that the test be started with relatively minor stimulation because of a high incidence (as much as 45%) of exaggerated uterine activity. The latter is defined as contractions that occur more than once every 2 minutes or that last more than 90 seconds.

To minimize exaggerated uterine activity, the test should begin with 1 minute of unilateral nipple stimulation and then 3 minutes of observation. If this does not evoke uterine contractions, 5 minutes of unilateral nipple stimulation should follow. If there is still no response, five to ten minutes of bilateral stimulation should be performed. If this does not evoke uterine contractions, the test should be terminated and the oxytocin challenge test used. After nipple stimulation even more care must be taken in application of the oxytocin challenge test, for the stimulation may produce a significant increase in the incidence of prolonged contractions.

FETAL BIOPHYSICAL PROFILE

Manning and coworkers have demonstrated the usefulness of a fetal biophysical profile and scoring system. The hypothesis of their work is that combined observation of separate fetal biophysical activities can significantly improve accuracy in predicting fetal well-being or jeopardy. Using the five observations noted in Table 5-1, they demonstrated decreased false-negative as well as false-positive results when compared to any single test. Table 5-2 indicates suggested management based on biophysical profile scoring. Their data, and that of others, clearly suggest this method may be used effectively to screen and manage high-risk patients.

FHR TRACINGS IN FETUSES WITH CONGENITAL ANOMALIES

More frequently than not, a fetus with congenital malformations will have an abnormal heart rate pattern. The most common abnormal patterns are baseline bradycardia, variable decelerations, baseline tachycardia, and decreased variability. The highest rates (over 80%) of abnormal FHR patterns are in those with multiple malformations and chromosomal aberrations. Over 70% of those with lesions of the central nervous system will exhibit abnormal patterns.

This information makes the biophysical profile even more useful, for many of these defects could be detected antenatally and unnecessary cesarean deliveries based on FHR patterns alone could be prevented.

BIBLIOGRAPHY

Biale, Y., Brawer-Ostrovsky, Y., and Insler, V.: Fetal heart rate tracings in fetuses with congenital malformations, J. Reprod. Med. **30**:43, 1985.

Druzin, M.L., Gratacos, J., Keegan, K.A., et al.: Antepartum fetal heart rate testing: the significance of fetal bradycardia, Am. J. Obstet. Gynecol. **139**:194, 1981.

Freeman, R.K., Garite, T.J., Modanlou, H., et al.: Postdate pregnancy: utilization of contraction stress testing for primary fetal surveillance, Am. J. Obstet. Gynecol. **140**:128, 1981.

Gratacos, J.A., and Paul, R.H.: Antepartum fetal heart rate monitoring: nonstress test versus contraction stress test, Clin. Perinatol. **7**:387, 1980.

Hill, W.C., Moenning, R.K., Katz, M., et al.: Characteristics of uterine activity during the breast stimulation stress test, Obstet. Gynecol. **64**:489, 1984.

Huddleston, J.F., Sutliff, G. and Robinson, D.: Contraction stress test by intermittent nipple stimulation, Obstet. Gynecol. **63**:669, 1984.

Johnson, T.R.B., Jr., Compton, A.A., Rotmensch, J., et al.: Significance of the sinusoidal fetal heart rate pattern, Am. J. Obstet. Gynecol. **139**:446, 1981.

Keegan, K.A., Jr., and Paul, R.H.: Antepartum fetal heart rate testing: the nonstress test as a primary approach, Am. J. Obstet. Gynecol. **136**:75, 1980.

Keegan, K.A., Jr., Paul, R.H., Broussard, P.M., et al.: Antepartum fetal heart rate testing: the nonstress test—an outpatient approach, Am. J. Obstet. Gynecol. **136**:81, 1980.

Lenstrup, C., and Haase, N.: Predictive value of antepartum fetal heart rate non-stress test in high-risk pregnancy, Acta Obstet. Gynecol. Scand. **64**:133, 1985.

Manning, F.A., Baskett, T.F., Morrison, I., et al.: Fetal biophysical profile scoring: a prospective study in 1,184 high-risk patients, Am. J. Obstet. Gynecol. **140**:289, 1981.

Mendenhall, H.W., O'Leary, J.A., and Phillips, K.O.: The nonstress test: the value of a single acceleration in evaluating the fetus at risk, Am. J. Obstet. Gynecol. **136**:87, 1980.

Miyazaki, F.S., and Miyazaki, B.A.: False reactive nonstress tests in postterm pregnancies, Am. J. Obstet. Gynecol. **140**:269, 1981.

Mueller-Heubach, E., Meyers, R.E., and Adamsons, K.: Fetal heart rate and blood pressure during prolonged partial asphyxia in the rhesus monkey, Am. J. Obstet. Gynecol. **137**:48, 1980.

Phelan, J.P.: The nonstress test: a review of 3,000 tests, Am. J. Obstet. Gynecol. **139**:7, 1981.

Spellacy, W.N., Cruz, A.C., Kalra, P.S., et al.: Oxytocin challenge test results compared with simultaneously studied serum human placental lactogen and free estriol levels in high-risk pregnant women, Am. J. Obstet. Gynecol. **135**:917, 1979.

Weingold, A.B., Yonekura, M.L., and O'Kieffe, J.: Nonstress testing, Am. J. Obstet. Gynecol. **138**:195, 1980.

Zanini, B., Paul, R.H., and Huey, J.R.: Intrapartum fetal heart rate: correlation with scalp pH in the preterm fetus, Am. J. Obstet. Gynecol. **136**:43, 1980.

Zuspan, F.P., Quilligan, E.J., Iams, J.D., et al.: Predictors of intrapartum fetal distress: the role of electronic fetal monitoring, Am. J. Obstet. Gynecol. **135**:287, 1979.

6

Assessment of labor

CLINICAL PARAMETERS
General assessment

On admission to the labor and delivery area, every patient must be evaluated for maternal and fetal jeopardy.

I. Review history, physical examinations, laboratory data, course of pregnancy, and nutritional and hydration states.
II. Determine
   A. Time of onset of labor
   B. Presence or absence of bloody show or other vaginal bleeding
   C. Status of fetal membranes (in approximately 10% of all pregnancies membranes rupture prior to the onset of labor)
   D. Temperature, pulse, and blood pressure
   E. Time last food or fluid was taken
   F. Any allergies to medication
   G. Maternal and paternal emotional states
   H. Presence of preexisting risk states.
III. Perform
   A. Brief general physical examination
   B. Palpation of uterus for fetal lie, presenting part, engagement
   C. Assessment of fetal size (Chapter 4)
   D. Pelvic examination (if not contraindicated by abnormality of any of the above) for cervical dilatation, cervical effacement, consistency and position of cervix, fetal presenting part (including station), and position of presenting part
   E. Assessment of pelvic capacity
      Clinical pelvimetry is notoriously inaccurate; however, it is useful as a screening device for those patients who will need more accurate evaluation of their pelvic capacity. One indication for radiographic pelvimetry may be failure to progress in labor. (See Table 6-1.) Other indications for radiographic pelvimetry are as follows:
      1. Fetopelvic disproportion in previous pregnancy
      2. Physical examination indicating
         a. Diagonal conjugate of 11.5 cm or less
         b. Narrow midpelvis (prominent spines and converging side walls)
         c. Narrow intertuberous plane (less than 9 cm) or decreased sum of the intertuberous and posterior sagittal planes (less than 15 cm)
      3. Lack of engagement of fetal head with labor to 5 cm of cervical dilatation (with bowel and bladder empty)
      4. Gravida at term with breech presentation (if vaginal delivery is contemplated)
   F. Auscultation of FHR and point of maximum intensity identified for monitoring
   G. Evaluation of amniotic fluid for meconium
IV. Institute
   A. Urinalysis
      Obtain clean-catch specimen for protein and glucose.
   B. Periodic evaluation of maternal vital

signs (never less than every hour, but frequency depends on situation)
C. Intake and output record
D. Intravenous fluids through a large needle
E. Fetal monitoring for FHR and uterine contractions
F. Other fetal or maternal testing (e.g., scalp sampling, ultrasonography, x-ray pelvimetry, etc.) as indicated
G. Preparation and cleansing of pudendum
H. Enema (optional)
I. Restriction of oral intake
Stomach emptying time is delayed in pregnancy; therefore, should anesthesia be administered or any complication ensue, the hazard of aspiration is greatly enhanced.
J. Lateral positioning if bed rest is ordered
Cardiac output is greatly influenced by the uterus' compressing of the inferior vena cava when patient is in the supine position; the extreme is supine hypotensive syndrome.

Assessment of progress in labor

Labor is defined as the process by which the products of conception are normally delivered. Progress of labor represents an interaction between the forces exerted by the uterus to expel the products of conception (uterine contractions), fetal size, and capacity of the maternal pelvis. Important parameters of labor are progressive effacement and dilatation of the cervix and descent of the presenting part.

I. Differentiation of false labor from true labor (Table 6-2)
Braxton Hicks' contractions, or prodromal labor, may be mistaken for true labor, and the differential diagnosis is exceedingly important.
II. Cervical dilatation and effacement
A. Labor is divided into three stages:
1. The first stage of labor begins with demonstrable progressive dilatation and effacement of the cervix in response to uterine contractions and ends with complete (10 cm) dilatation of the cervix.
2. The second stage of labor begins when the cervix is completely dilated and ends with complete birth of the baby.
3. The third, or placental, stage of labor begins with the birth of the infant and ends with the delivery of the placenta.
B. Evaluation of cervical dilatation allows determination of relative progress in labor. Friedman's data for the mean nulliparous labor and mean multiparous labor are shown in Figs. 6-1 and 6-2. The hours and statistical

Table 6-1. Minimal adequate values for radiographic pelvimetry if fetus is of average or greater size

Planes	Anteroposterior (cm)	Transverse (cm)	Posterosagittal (cm)
Inlet	10.0	12.0	—
Midplane	11.5	9.5	4.0
Outlet	11.5	10.0	7.5

Table 6-2. Differentiation of false labor from true labor

	True labor	False labor
Contraction interval	Regular (gradually shortens)	Irregular (remains irregular)
Contraction duration	Regular	Irregular
Contraction intensity	Gradually increases	Remains same
Discomfort location	Generally in back and abdomen, spreading from back to front in a girdlelike distribution	Located primarily in lower abdomen, rarely in back; however, may be fundal
Effect of exercise	Intensified by walking	Not intensified by walking
Effect of mild sedation	Not affected	Usually relieved

62 *Diagnosis and management of the high-risk fetus and neonate*

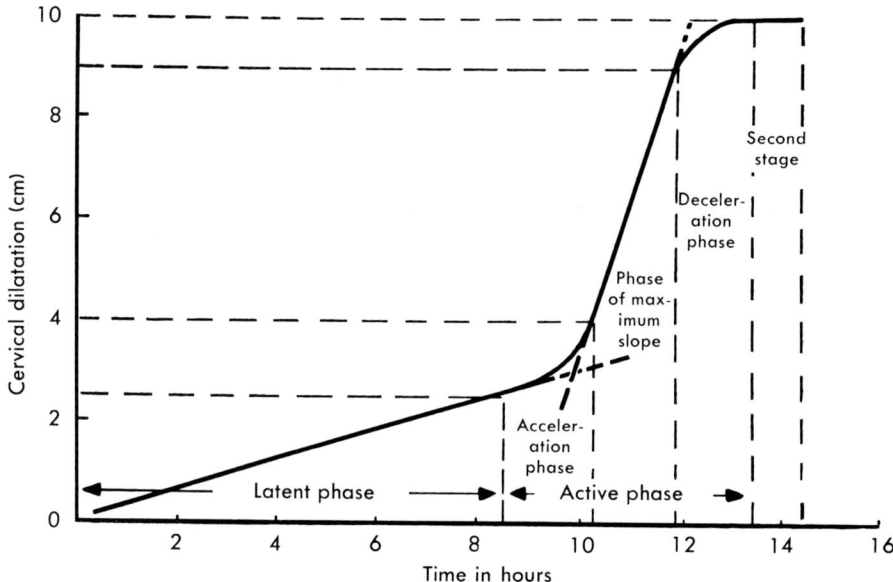

Fig. 6-1. Composite of the patterns of the cervical dilatation—time function based on a study of 500 nulliparas. (From Friedman, E.A.: Obstet. Gynecol. **6:**569, 1955.)

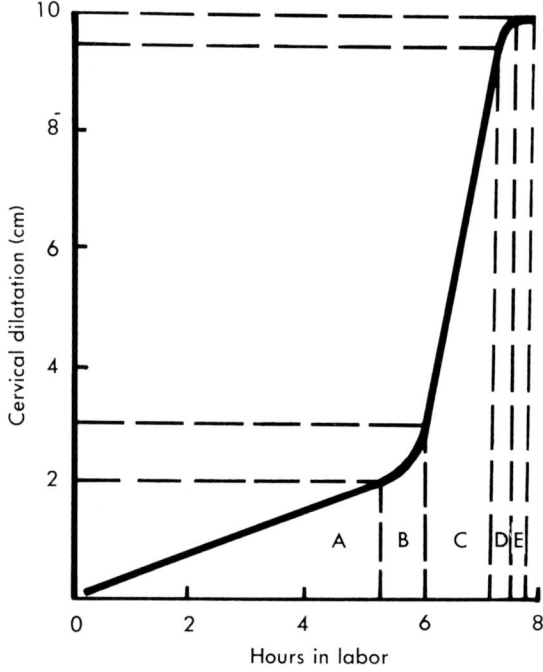

Fig. 6-2. Mean multiparous labor pattern based on a study of a series of 500 multiparas. *A,* Latent phase. *B,* Acceleration phase. *C,* Phase of maximum slope. *D,* Deceleration phase. *E,* Second stage. *B* to *D* is the active phase. (From Friedman, E.A.: Obstet. Gynecol. **8:**692, 1956.)

limits are included in Tables 6-3 and 6-4. Every laboring patient should be evaluated by means of this or similar data. Fig. 6-3 illustrates a management program for the secondary arrest of dilatation-time patterns.

III. Descent of presenting part

Friedman's data for descent of the fetal presenting part are correlated with cervical dilatation and time in Figs. 6-4 and 6-5. Again, these correlative data are extremely important for assessment of progress in labor. Friedman's data demonstrate that the presenting part must be below the level of ischial spines at the onset of the second stage (in both multiparous and nulliparous labor) to fall within two standard deviations of normal.

Special care must be taken in monitoring the risk patient's labor. For example, for the frank breech presentation selected for vaginal delivery the pattern should approximate a normal dilatation pattern, but the fetus may start at a higher station and descend more rapidly. Dysfunctional labor with breech presentation presages the same problems as it does in vertex presentations. The patient who has had a previous cesarean delivery for nonrecidive cause and is undergoing a vaginal birth must be observed closely for signs of uterine rupture (extraordinary pain, often described as tearing, then cessation of pain with uterine relaxation and possible vaginal bleeding).

Assessment of uterine contractions

With true labor the upper portion of the uterus (the active segment, or fundus), which contains a larger percentage of smooth muscle than does the lower segment (the passive segment), exerts forceful contractions. During these contractions there is also some relatively mild contraction of the lower uterine segment. As labor progresses, the active segment becomes progressively thicker and the lower segment progressively thinner.

In the slender gravida it is possible during labor to palpably differentiate between the two uterine segments because the upper segment becomes much firmer than the lower segment. Despite this reassurance that actual labor (as opposed to false labor) is in progress, which allows one to follow the interval and duration of contractions, palpation of the uterus gives no

Table 6-3. Mean nulliparous labor

	Mean	Mode	Median	SD*	SE_m†	Range	Statistical limit‡
Latent phase (hr)	8.6	6.0	7.5	6.0	0.27	1.0-44	20.6
Active phase (hr)	4.9	3.0	4.0	3.4	0.15	0.8-34	11.7
Deceleration (hr)	0.9 (54 min)	0.5	0.8	1.2	0.05	0.0-14	3.3
Maximum slope (cm/hr)	3.0	1.5	2.7	1.9	0.08	12.0- 0.4	1.2
Second stage (hr)	0.95 (57 min)	0.6	0.8	0.8	0.04	0.0- 5.5	2.5

From Friedman, E.A.: Primigravid labor, a graphicostatistical analysis, Obstet. Gynecol. 6:567, 1955.
*Standard deviation, $SD = \sqrt{\Sigma d/N}$; d = deviation from mean.
†Standard error of mean, $SE_m = SD/\sqrt{N}$.
‡Deviation twice standard deviation greater than mean, p = 0.05, except maximum slope, which because of its skew distribution has a lower limit 95 percentile points below the median.

Table 6-4. Mean multiparous labor

	Mean	Mode	Median	SD	SE_m	Range	Statistical limit
Latent phase (hr)	5.3	3.5	4.5	4.1	0.19	0.4-36	13.6
Active phase (hr)	2.2	1.5	1.8	1.5	0.07	0.3-15	5.2
Deceleration (hr)	0.23 (14 min)	0.1	0.2	0.33	0.01	0.0-3.5	0.88 (53 min)
Maximum slope (cm/hr)	5.7	4.5	5.2	3.6	0.16	2.4-0.7	1.5
Second stage (hr)	0.24 (14 min)	0.1	0.2	0.30	0.01	0.0-3.0	0.83 (50 min)

From Friedman, E.A.: Labor in multiparas, a graphicostatistical analysis, Obstet. Gynecol. 8:691, 1956.

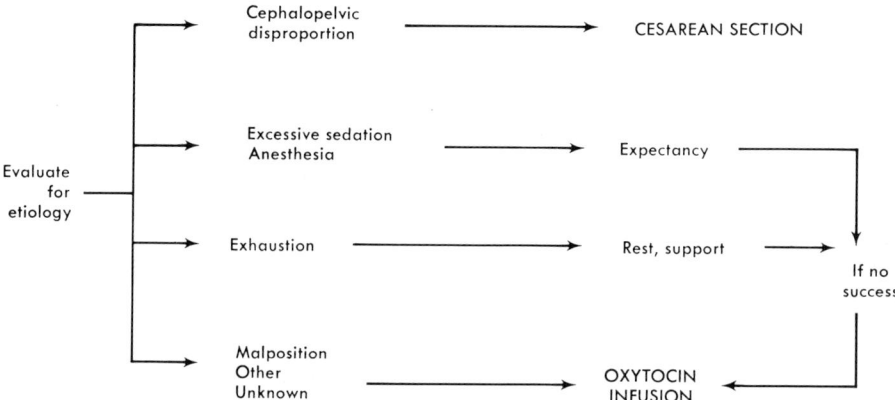

Fig. 6-3. Recommended program of management of patient with secondary arrest of dilatation-time patterns. (From Friedman, E.A.: Bull. Sloane Hosp. Women **9:**20, 1963.)

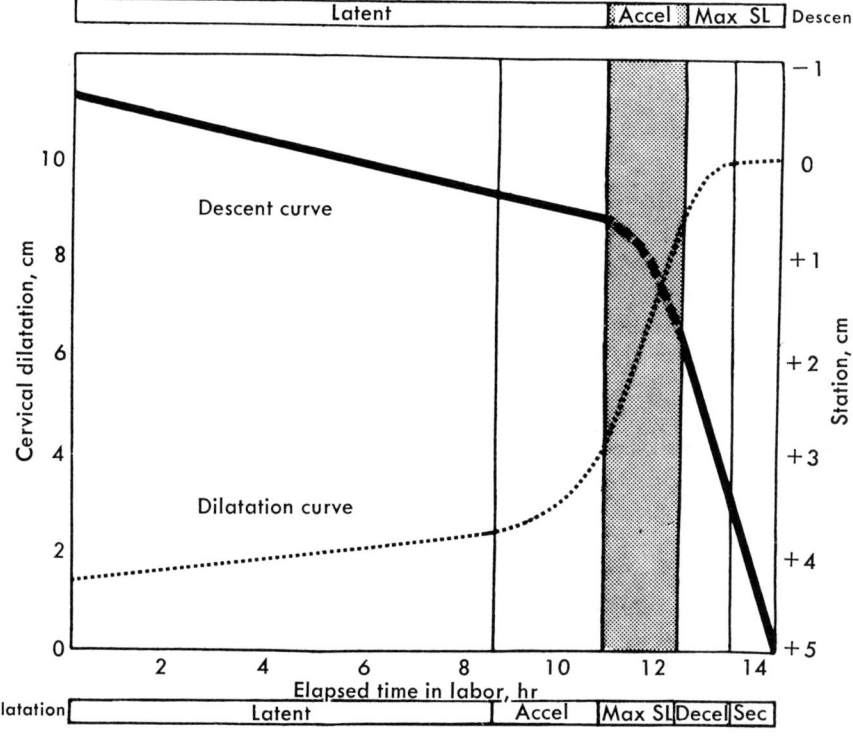

Fig. 6-4. Composites of mean descent versus time *(solid line)* and dilatation versus time *(broken line)* curves for a series of 421 unselected nulliparas. (From Friedman, E.A.: Am. J. Obstet. Gynecol. **93:**525, 1965.)

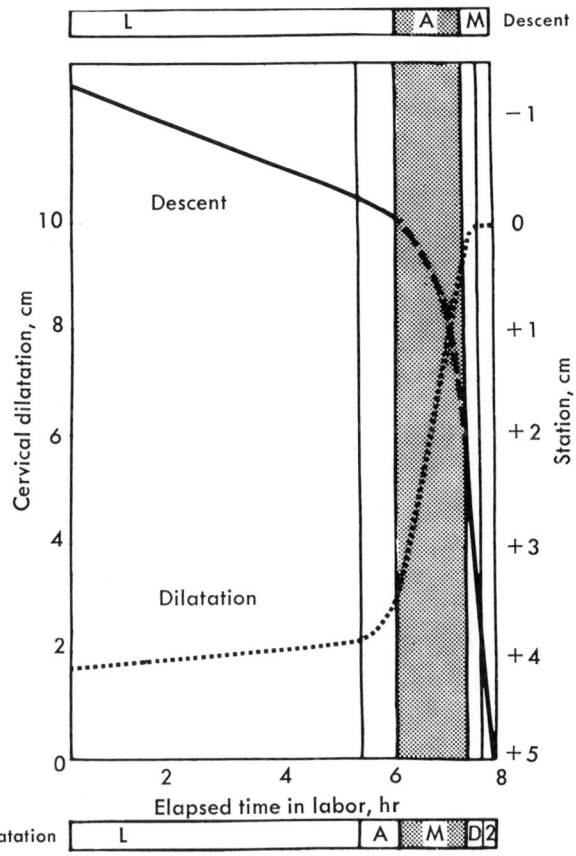

Fig. 6-5. Composite mean curves for descent *(solid line)* and dilatation *(broken line)* for 389 unselected multiparas. *L*, Latent; *A*, Acceleration; *M*, Maximum slope; *D*, Deceleration; *2*, second stage. (From Friedman, E.A., and Sachtleben, M.R.: Am. J. Obstet. Gynecol. **93**:522, 1965.)

information concerning the pressure of uterine contractions.

Pressure of uterine contractions may be measured directly by the intrauterine catheter of an electronic fetal monitor once the membranes have ruptured. Sterile technique is used to insert a plastic catheter guide containing a saline-filled catheter just through the internal cervical os. If placental location is known, the catheter is advanced away from the placental site. Ideally the catheter will lie at midfetal level. The other end of the catheter is connected to a strain-gauge on the monitor and adjusted to the same level as the catheter tip in the uterus.

Most normal active labor exhibits uterine contractions with durations of 30 to 60 seconds at intervals of 3 to 5 minutes. The intensity at the apex of the contraction is usually 50 to 75 mm Hg, and there is complete return to baseline tone (less than 5 mm Hg). It is not uncommon for patients to have more frequent or more forceful contractions. In such circumstances, provided FHR is not affected, they may be considered normal, but careful observation is warranted. Excessive oxytocin stimulation is a common cause of such uterine hyperactivity. Still other normal patients exhibit progressive effacement and dilatation of the cervix with considerably less uterine activity. With uterine hypoactivity and lack of progress in labor, in the absence of contraindications, it is common to employ dilute oxytocin in an attempt to stimulate labor.

It is less common for contractions to last longer than 60 seconds or for baseline tone of the uterus to become elevated. Both situations may occur with abruptio placentae and thus gaseous exchange to and from the fetus is more likely to be decreased. Therefore great care is warranted in observing these cases.

Abnormal labor patterns

Three major groups of abnormalities of labor patterns appear in light of the Friedman data.
1. Prolongation disorders
   This abnormality is usually a prolonged latent phase. By definition, a prolonged latent phase in nulliparas is greater than 20 hours and in multiparas greater than 14 hours. The usual treatment is therapeutic rest. Occasionally oxytocin stimulation is necessary or cesarean section is mandated by urgent problems.
2. Protraction disorders
   There are two types of protraction disorders:
   a. Protracted active phase of dilatation
      This condition is defined as dilatation of less than 1.2 cm/hr in nulliparas and less than 1.5 cm/hr in multiparas. It is usually treated by close observation and support, with cesarean section reserved for standard criteria.
   b. Protracted descent
      Protracted descent occurs when there is descent of less than 1 cm/hr in nulliparas and less than 2 cm/hr in multiparas. It is also treated most commonly by close observation and support. Cesarean delivery is reserved for standard criteria, the most common being fetopelvic disproportion.
3. Arrest disorders
   There are four definable arrest disorders:
   a. Prolonged deceleration phase
      This situation is defined as greater than 3 hours of labor in nulliparas and greater than 1 hour in multiparas without progress in cervical dilatation. Unless fetopelvic disproportion is present, the disorder is best treated by oxytocin augmentation of labor, or rest if the patient is exhausted. With fetopelvic disproportion cesarean delivery may be necessary.
   b. Secondary arrest of dilatation
      A secondary arrest of dilatation is defined as no progress in dilatation for 2 hours in nulliparas or multiparas. It is usually associated with fetopelvic disproportion and cesarean delivery is necessary.
   c. Arrest of descent
      This condition occurs when there is no descent of the presenting part for over 1 hour in either nulliparas or multiparas. It also is frequently associated with fetopelvic disproportion and may necessitate cesarean delivery.
   d. Failure of descent
      Failure of descent occurs when there is no descent during the deceleration phase or second stage of labor. Incidence of fetopelvic disproportion is very high with this disorder and cesarean delivery is usually performed.

Assessment of amniotic fluid

As pregnancy nears term, amniotic fluid volume decreases. It is difficult to quantify proper amounts prospectively, but extremely small amounts of amniotic fluid are clearly a warning sign. With oligohydramnios there is a much greater incidence of variable decelerations (see Chapter 5) caused by cord compression. Oligohydramnios does not preclude vaginal delivery, but it does warrant special observation. Additionally, since oligohydramnios is associated significantly with fetal abnormalities (the most common being obstruction of the fetal urinary tract and renal agenesis) the neonate must be carefully evaluated.

Meconium staining of amniotic fluid in late pregnancy may be an early sign of fetal distress. Fetal death before onset of labor most often is accompanied by the passage of meconium. The few exceptions are probably attributable to fetal death caused by acute compression of the umbilical cord. Meconium passage before the middle of the last trimester or staining of fluid with the premature infant is infrequent perhaps because of the immaturity of the fetal autonomic nervous system in its influence on gastrointestinal activity.

When amniotic fluid is clear at the onset of labor, perinatal mortality is low (less than 1%); when amniotic fluid is stained by meconium, perinatal mortality rises to about 6%. Apgar scores are significantly lower in surviving neonates of the stained fluid group.

Amniotic fluid staining in the last trimester is of such concern that once detected continuous observation of the pregnancy is necessary, with the inclusion of fetal monitoring, measurement of estriol excretion, assessment of fetal age and size, etc., to best determine appropriate timing and method of delivery. Meconium passage before and even during labor, particularly prolonged labor, should alert the obstetrician to a possible emergency and need for a reassessment of management.

I. Incidence of meconium passage (green- or yellow-stained amniotic fluid) in late pregnancy
   A. In a general pregnant population—5% to 10%
   B. In women with no risk factors—1% to 2%
   C. In selected groups of high-risk patients—up to 35%
II. Indications for screening amniotic fluid for meconium passage
   A. Maternal disease, e.g., toxemia, diabetes, hypertension—usually screened at 36 to 37 weeks
   B. Prolonged pregnancy—42 weeks or more
   C. Impaired fetal growth or change in fetal activity
   D. Late or prolonged variable FHR deceleration
III. Methods of evaluating amniotic fluid
   A. Amnioscopy (widely used in Europe)
      This procedure requires practice for reasonable accuracy when minor color changes in amniotic fluid have occurred. If there is doubt, amniocentesis should be performed.
      1. Technique
         a. Slip tubular or cone-shaped amnioscope into the slightly dilated cervix against the membranes.
         b. Focus a light source on the membranes (avoid fiberoptics because of greenish tinge to the light).
         c. Observe for color, meconium, and blood within the amniotic sac.
      2. Complications
         a. Rupture of membranes occurs in approximately 3% of patients.
         b. Occasional minor bleeding may develop but is rarely a serious problem.
         c. Maternal or fetal sepsis can occur but is rare.
   B. Amniocentesis
      This procedure is also important when the fetus is rhesus sensitized or when insufficient fluid escapes from a membrane rupture to determine the color of the amniotic fluid.
      1. Technique (p. 28)
         Fluid obtained is evaluated against a white background.
      2. Complications
         a. Injury to placental vessels with possible fetal exsanguination
         b. Injury to fetus itself

Overactivity of fetus

Threshing or tumultous movements of the fetus have been time-honored signs of fetal distress. Carbon dioxide retention stimulates the fetal respiratory center, and hyperreflexia follows. Brief overactivity of fetus has been reported in cord compression and abruptio placentae. Nevertheless, with progressive hypoxia, fetal depression follows rapidly. Therefore the value of this largely subjective sign of fetal danger is minimal.

Diagnostic aids

I. Indirect monitoring of FHR
   A. Auscultation with traditional stethoscope
      Although electronic recording of the FHR has demonstrated the limitations of the stethoscope, nurses and aides must be trained in its more effective use. An important detail for using it more advantageously is counting the fetal heartbeat throughout and just after a contraction, rather than waiting until the uterus is relaxed.
      The following method is useful for observation of the fetus during labor, particularly when an increased risk to the fetus is present (Whitfield):
      1. Count heartbeats for successive 5-second periods during and after contractions.

2. The lowest 5-second count times 12 gives the approximate depth of bradycardia in beats/min.
3. The number of 5-second periods from the end of contraction to the first count of more than 10 beats, that is, a rate of over 120 beats/min, gives a simple measure of delay in recovery of a uteroplacental insufficiency pattern or the duration of an episode of late deceleration.
4. Any beat-to-beat arrhythmia must be noted.
5. Intervals between observations are shortened if any bradycardia or irregularity is observed.

B. Electronic FHR monitoring by indirect methods

Indirect forms of electronic monitoring are external means of gathering data concerning uterine contractions and FHR patterns. Interpretation is basically the same as that of direct methods. The advantage of indirect monitoring is that it is noninvasive. However, indirect methods have two important limitations: uterine activity is indicated in a qualitative manner and cannot be interpreted quantitatively, and indirect methods all produce FHR patterns that appear to have normal beat-to-beat variability, but this phenomenon is an inherent artifact and does not actually reflect the beat-to-beat variability seen with direct monitoring. Indirect electronic FHR monitoring methods are as follows:
1. Phonocardiography (using an electronic pickup, amplifier, and speaker system)
2. Ultrasonic monitoring (using the Doppler principle)

FETAL NURSING CARE

Intensive nursing care for women in labor must also include zealous guarding of the fetus. Although this may seem entirely logical, the product of pregnancy is too often treated as a casual by-product.

Nursing has always been patient-oriented, but when one considers the parturient, a double responsibility must be assumed, particularly during labor and delivery, when the needs and problems of the fetus become especially demanding. Assessment of fetal well-being during labor demands special training and experience.

The first objective of fetal nursing is maternal homeostasis. Proper physical and psychological support is most important. Information regarding the gravida's past and present health is particularly pertinent because, as in cases of hypothyroidism or toxemia, fetal growth and development may be compromised by a maternal health problem. Specific therapy may have to be initiated, continued, or changed. The nurse must also appreciate the character of labor because dystocia may add another, often cumulative, dimension to other problems.

The change in fetal environment before, during, and after parturition is extreme. The offspring's environment is totally altered. The stresses of labor and delivery induce complex, often critical variations in maternal and fetal physiology. The number of alterations and the degree of change may vary even from minute to minute.

Fetal nursing has always been limited, but new approaches are now feasible, particularly with the general availability of practical, accurate monitoring equipment. Nevertheless the nurse still cannot determine before birth whether the fetus will be pink or blue, sleeping or critically irresponsive, or bathed in clear or meconium-stained amniotic fluid.

The nurse can do much, however, to determine fetal safety or jeopardy, observing and reporting (1) maternal emotional symptoms and (2) signs of fetal embarrassment. The nurse is a vital member of the medical team, even though it is ultimately the physician who must decide whether a particular obstetric management plan should be continued or altered.

Accurate and complete nurse's observations invariably strengthen the physician's judgment. Grave responsibility is carried by the nurse, who may be the only professionally trained person with the obstetric patient, and on whose decisions the life or health of the fetus may depend.

Fetal distress requires special vigilance, particularly in high-risk cases. Moreover, one cannot anticipate crises like cord compression or predict accidents such as concealed partial separation of the placenta. The nurse who is knowledgeable, attentive, and concerned may in fact be a lifesaver.

Prompt detection and reporting of abnormal fetal heart signs often mark the initial steps in fetal rescue. This is especially important because about 50% of perinatal deaths are preventable. Fenton and Steer have stated, "Fetal survival is directly correlated with the time interval between the discovery of the signs of fetal distress and delivery. Thirty minutes is the critical time."

Matousek has suggested the following excellent routine for fetal nursing:
1. Complete observation
   a. Note any unusual fetal activity. Record findings.
   b. Identify and record presence of meconium when membranes rupture. Repeat each time the patient is examined.
   c. Auscultate and record FHR every 10 to 15 minutes in the pregnancy at risk, more often during the second stage of labor, and immediately after rupture of membranes.
   d. Note particularly the duration of any tachycardia or bradycardia that continues after a contraction.
2. Prompt reporting
   Promptly describe unusual signs (hyperactivity, bradycardia, passage of meconium, etc.) to the physician.
3. Complete reporting
   Relate current fetal signs, as well as former pattern, to the following conditions of the fetal environment:
   a. Maternal vital signs
   b. Medications administered, noting amount and time given
   c. Frequency, type, and duration of uterine contractions
   d. Intactness of membranes and presence or absence of meconium
   e. Bleeding, if any, noting amount
   f. Other significant changes in the mother's condition that occur at or near the time of altered fetal signs

BIBLIOGRAPHY

Cohen, W., and Friedman, E.A., editors: Management of labor, Baltimore, 1983, University Park Press.

Huntingford, P.J., Hüter, K.A., and Saling, E., editors: Perinatal medicine, First European Congress, Berlin, Stuttgart, 1969, Georg Thieme Verlag.

Matousek, I.: Fetal nursing during labor, Nurs. Clin. North Am. **3:**307, 1968.

Perinatal factors affecting human development, Washington, D.C., 1969, Scientific Pub. No. 185, Pan-American Health Organization, Pan-American Sanitary Bureau, Regional Office of the World Health Organization.

Whitfield, C.R.: Clinical significance of electronic methods for monitoring the fetal heart. In Huntingford, P.J., Hüter, K.G., and Saling, E., editors: Perinatal medicine, Stuttgart, 1969, Georg Thieme Verlag.

7
Delivery of the fetus at risk

Birth, for the perinate at risk, may be the most damaging event of that individual's life. All too frequently the compromised fetus, surviving by only a narrow margin, will die when the additional hazards of birth are imposed. Moreover, many emergencies relating to blood flow, oxygenation, the uterus, placenta, cord, and bony pelvis, and even relating to the fetus itself, may become evident only during the final stages of labor or the actual delivery process. Hazards may arise from many factors, from combinations of factors, or even from treatment of various diseases or pregnancy complications. Errors of omission, as well as mistakes of commission, may compound misadventures in risk parturition. For example, the stresses imposed by uterine contractions with subsequent decreased uterine blood flow may expose the fetus with an already compromised placental exchange capability (as could be the case when there is maternal chronic hypertension) to hypoxia, acidosis, and possibly even death. There is even further potential for an untoward result if, in a well-meaning attempt to hasten delivery under these circumstances, attendants encourage the mother's natural impulse to "push." The ensuing Valsalva maneuver increases intraabdominal pressure and may further reduce placental blood flow. Thus, before applying various delivery techniques that in most circumstances would be benign, one must detail several critical issues, including which perinates are at risk during labor and how they are detected, who should be present and what supplies or equipment should be available to maximize the risk perinate's chances of intact survival, and which is the best mode of delivery and the proper choice of analgesia and anesthesia. Several common risk situations are discussed to illustrate application of these concepts of risk care to various situations. Finally, because there are continued risk factors to both mother and baby after birth, the major postpartum risk events are also detailed.

WHICH PERINATES ARE AT RISK?

During delivery there is a host of factors that may create jeopardy. Table 7-1 details some of the risks for which patients must be screened during the delivery process.

TEAM CARE IN THE BIRTH ROOM

The organization of a team to meet both maternal and fetal-newborn needs is imperative if beneficial outcomes are to be expected. Clearly the obstetrician must be responsible for assessing the situation, notifying the appropriate individuals, and assembling the team at the appropriate time.

The constituency of the team may vary considerably from situation to situation but in high-risk situations should include the obstetrician, an obstetrical scrub nurse, a circulating nurse for the obstetrical team, a neonatologist, a neonatal nurse, and a circulating nurse for the neonatal team. In many circumstances an anesthesiologist is mandatory, and appropriate assistants must accompany that individual. In some circumstances a second obstetrician is necessary to provide assistance. In still other circumstances, particularly with multiple births or hypovolemic or isoimmunized babies, it is necessary to include a larger neonatal team. Thus it is obvious that team support for mother and

Table 7-1. Perinatal risk associations during delivery

Maternal associations	Fetal associations
Acute emergencies	
Emergencies associated with delivery	
Premature delivery (including small for dates)	Shoulder girdle dystocia
Fetopelvic disproportion	Malpresentations
Postdates (lack of pliability)	Breech
Excessive size (>4,000 gm)	Transverse and other
Maternal lacerations from instrumentation	Fetal trauma from force or instrumentation
	Amnionitis
	Accidental injection of anesthetic into fetoplacental circulation (paracervical or caudal accident)
Sharp reduction of placental perfusion or fetal circulation	
Abruptio placentae	Umbilical cord compression
Hypertonic uterine contractions	Prolapsed cord (occult or overt)
Hypotension (most commonly supine hypotensive syndrome)	Tight or short cord
Uterine rupture	True knot
Inadequate systemic circulation	
Placenta previa	Hemorrhage (velamentous insertion of the cord, other)
Normovolemic hypotension secondary to conduction anesthesia	Congenital anomaly (heart, cord)
Shock (hemorrhagic, septic, anaphylactic)	Cardiac failure (hydrops fetalis, tachyarrhythmias, myocarditis)
Sudden cardiac failure	
Insufficient blood oxygenation	
Severe anemia, hemorrhage	Fetal distress by electronic fetal monitoring
Hypoxia or hypercarbia (as with poorly controlled anesthesia)	Fetal distress by fetal blood (scalp) sampling
Maternal aspiration syndrome	Acute hemolytic crisis (erythroblastosis)
Impaired respiratory efforts (shock lung, bronchospasm)	
Methemoglobinemia	
Chronic factors predisposing to fetal distress with delivery	
"Chronic" states that may be associated with untoward delivery outcome	
Abnormal labor (prolonged, lack of progress, dystocia, induction, precipitate)	Nonreactive fetal activity-acceleration determination
Drug addiction or alcoholism	Positive stress test (oxytocin)
Infectious disease (syphilis, gonorrhea, herpes, hepatitis, rubella)	Immature L/S ratio or rapid surfactant test (RST)
Previous operative delivery if vaginal delivery is planned	Falling estriols
Systemic diseases of heart, lungs, blood, or kidneys	Premature or prolonged rupture of membranes
Endocrine ablation or replacement	Oligohydramnios or polyhydramnios
Medical indications for termination of a previous pregnancy	Previous neonatal loss or stillborn
	Possible malformation including mutagen/teratogen exposure
	Previous history of need for special neonatal infant care or of birth-damaged baby
Moderate reduction of placental perfusion or fetal circulation	
Hypertensive states of pregnancy	Multiple pregnancy (twin-to-twin transfusion, competition for circulation)
Diabetes mellitus	Meconium staining of amniotic fluid
Postmaturity or dysmaturity	Intrauterine growth retardation
Elderly or grand multipara	Dysmaturity
Premature placental aging, intervillous fibrin deposition, etc.	Partial cord compression
Inadequate systemic circulation	
Cardiovascular disease (congenital, acquired)	Congenital cardiovascular disease
	Maternal-fetal transfusion syndrome
Possible insufficient blood oxygenation to tolerate delivery	
Impaired respiratory efficiency (parenchymal or bony thorax disease)	Intrauterine growth retardation
Low oxygen tension (chronic high altitude)	Prolonged labor

baby varies according to their needs. Team members must know what is expected of them and must have practiced their roles. Finally, anticipation of when to assemble the team for maximum patient benefit is mandatory. This requires careful risk assessment and close cooperation at all professional levels.

GENERAL CONSIDERATIONS FOR MANAGEMENT OF PERINATAL JEOPARDY

1. Monitor FHR constantly, and obtain scalp pH when indicated while observing for fetal distress.
2. Obtain frequent maternal pulse and blood pressure (also temperature and respiration, if indicated).
3. Have an intravenous catheter (18 gauge or larger) in place and working. Consider hemodynamic monitoring if there is a possibility of hemorrhage, shock or cardiovascular instability.
4. Avoid or treat maternal hypotension.
   a. Increase intravenous fluids (administer blood if indicated).
   b. Try positional changes to move the uterus off the inferior vena cava. Maintain the lateral recumbent position.
   c. Push the uterus off the inferior vena cava.
   d. Elevate (Trendelenburg) or wrap the legs with elastic supports.
   e. Consider alternative positions for delivery if supine hypotensive syndrome is severe (e.g., Sims).
5. Guarantee maximal maternal and thus fetal oxygenation by administration of oxygen to the gravida.
6. Have type-specific blood available for the mother (also blood products, if necessary) and baby.
7. In addition, the following should be expeditiously arranged or may have been accomplished while the patient was in labor:
   a. Abdomen shaved and scrubbed with povidone-iodine (Betadine) in preparation for possible cesarean section
   b. Elastic (antiembolic) support hose applied
8. A retention catheter and prep set should be ready for immediate insertion should cesarean section become necessary.
9. Perform a pelvic examination to ascertain progress in labor and to check for other possible abnormalities (e.g., cord prolapse, malposition).
10. A team plan for the most atraumatic delivery possible should be developed.

ANALGESIA AND ANESTHESIA

Analgesia and anesthesia for labor and delivery of both normal and risk perinates poses special problems. This is often the most pain the mother has ever experienced, and pain relief may be necessary over an extended interval. Analgesia and anesthesia may also affect the fetus, and if not chosen and administered carefully, can interfere with uterine contractions. In addition, there are physiologic and paraphysiologic alterations that place the mother and baby at greater risk than either would face singly during anesthesia.

Essentials of obstetric anesthesia include:
1. The amount of analgesia necessary to allow the mother psychologic control must not exceed safe limits for her or the fetus.
2. Preservation of fetal homeostasis must be ensured.
3. Both mother and fetus must be adequately monitored to ensure that harm does not befall either.

The use of analgesia and anesthesia for the high-risk patient, especially in premature labor, requires special precautions. Medication poorly chosen or too liberally administered will be seriously depressing, particularly for the fetus that is not mature or is otherwise jeopardized. All the procedures and agents used to relieve the discomforts of labor and delivery have some advantage or desirable characteristic, but none is perfect. Almost universally, the safety factor is deficient, particularly for the premature infant.

Methods preferred for the fetus at risk in premature labor

I. Prepared childbirth or psychoanalgesia
   A. Familiarize the patient before labor (if possible) with relaxing techniques (Lamaze or Read) and the use of her delivery powers to reduce tension and pain (psychoprophylaxis).
   B. Establish rapport and provide emotional support.
   C. Employ reassurance and kindly direction.

D. Use suggestion and reinforcement when possible.

II. Regional anesthesia

Conduction analgesia and anesthesia usually are more desirable than inhalation or parenteral anesthesia.

All regional blocking agents are absorbed rapidly. These anesthetics may intoxicate the fetus when overdosage occurs, with resultant apnea and vascular collapse from medullary depression, bradycardia because of the quinidine-like effect on the myocardium, and convulsions because of cortical excitation. Anesthetics with the amide molecular linkage (lidocaine, mepivacaine, and prilocaine) have a stability that resists enzymatic splitting and rapidly cross the placental barrier intact. In contrast, local anesthetics with an ester bond (procaine, 2-chloroprocaine, and tetracaine) are metabolized in the plasma and placenta and, if the total dose of procaine is less than 8 mg/kg, there is only minor transfer to the fetus. Even with larger doses, procaine is found in the fetus circulation in concentration 40% to 60% lower than in the maternal circulation. Therefore it is a safer obstetric agent despite a shorter duration of action.

III. Paracervical anesthesia

A. Rapid dilatation follows when the cervix is already dilated more than 4 or 5 cm. Labor prior to dilatation of 4 to 5 cm may be slowed by the anesthesia, and other injections may be necessary.

B. Almost immediate, complete relief of pain is achieved until the presenting part distends the lower birth canal, when a pudendal block or other procedure may be indicated.

C. Technique
1. Prepare the mucosal site 2 cm lateral to the cervix, in the vaginal fornix, with antiseptic solution.
2. Insert a 6-inch 20-gauge needle 0.3 to 0.5 cm into the lateral fornix, using an "Iowa trumpet" (Fig. 7-1). After aspiration (to determine that the needle does not lie in a blood vessel) slowly inject 5 ml of 1% procaine *just beneath the mucosa*. Observe the FHR for bradycardia, or wait for several uterine contractions to avoid an anesthetic reaction; then inject the other side.
3. When the presenting part is deeply engaged and the fornices are blocked, inject the drug high in the lateral vaginal walls and again just beneath the mucosa (to retard absorption).

D. Ideally, the anesthetic lasts about 60 minutes, and only a minority of patients will require subsequent paracervical blocks. Cervical dystocia is often overcome, but a temporary reduction in the intensity and duration of contractions may occur.

E. Avoid paracervical block when
1. Excessive uterine bleeding occurs
2. Vaginal or cervical sepsis is present
3. There is known hypersensitivity or previous idiosyncratic reaction
4. It cannot be determined that the needle is correctly placed (e.g., direct injection into the fetus must be guarded against)

F. Complications
1. Hematoma formation
2. Infection
3. Faintness, syncope, or vascular collapse from inadvertent intravenous administration, too rapid absorption, or sensitivity to the anesthetic agent
4. Chemical lumbosacral neuritis
5. Fetal bradycardia, acidosis (Fig. 7-2), and, rarely, cardiac arrest because of rapid absorption of the drug or toxic effect

Paracervical block probably is associated with more rapid drug absorption than most other blocks because of pronounced cervicouterine vascularity. Therefore precautions must be taken with its use:
a. Avoid injection of an anesthetic drug directly into the maternal circulation or into fetal tissues by limiting the volume of the anesthetic agent to 5 ml to each

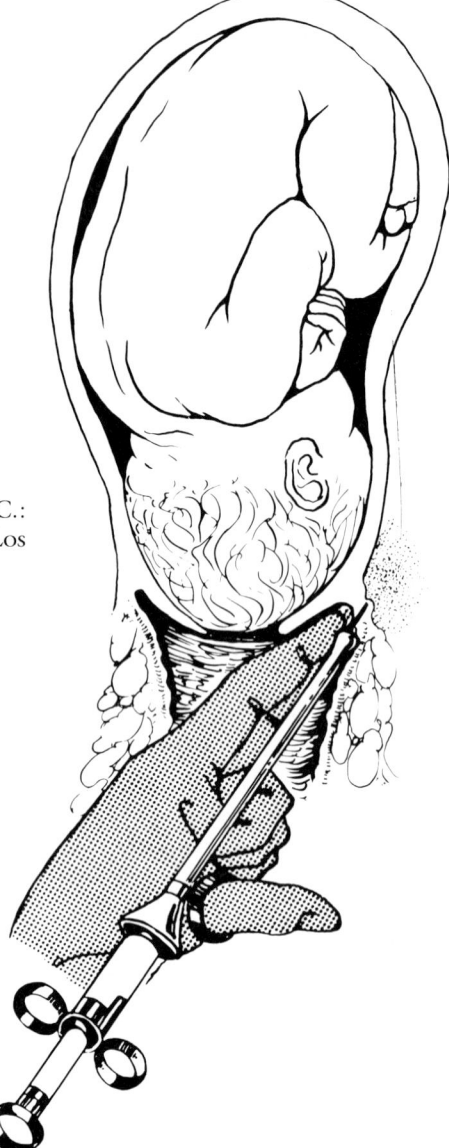

Fig. 7-1. Paracervical block. (From Benson, R.C.: Handbook of obstetrics and gynecology, ed. 4, Los Altos, Calif., 1971, Lange Medical Publications.)

        side of the cervix and placing the drug just beneath the mucosa as a "blister" after first aspirating.
- b. Avoid paracervical block when the fetus may already be hypoxic and acidotic, as in maternal toxemia, diabetes, and possibly postmaturity.
- c. Deny paracervical anesthesia in cases of fetal heart irregularity or after meconium passage in vertex presentation.
- d. Employ constant FHR monitoring in all complicated cases, especially when bradycardia occurs.

IV. Pudendal nerve block
- A. The nerves supplying the lower birth canal are anesthetized by block of the pudendal nerve at the ischial spines.
- B. A transvaginal injection is preferred. A spinal needle is required, and the procedure can be carried out without assistance.
   1. Identify the ischial spines on each side by digital examination through the elastic vagina. Then note the sacrospinous ligament across the sacrospinous notch

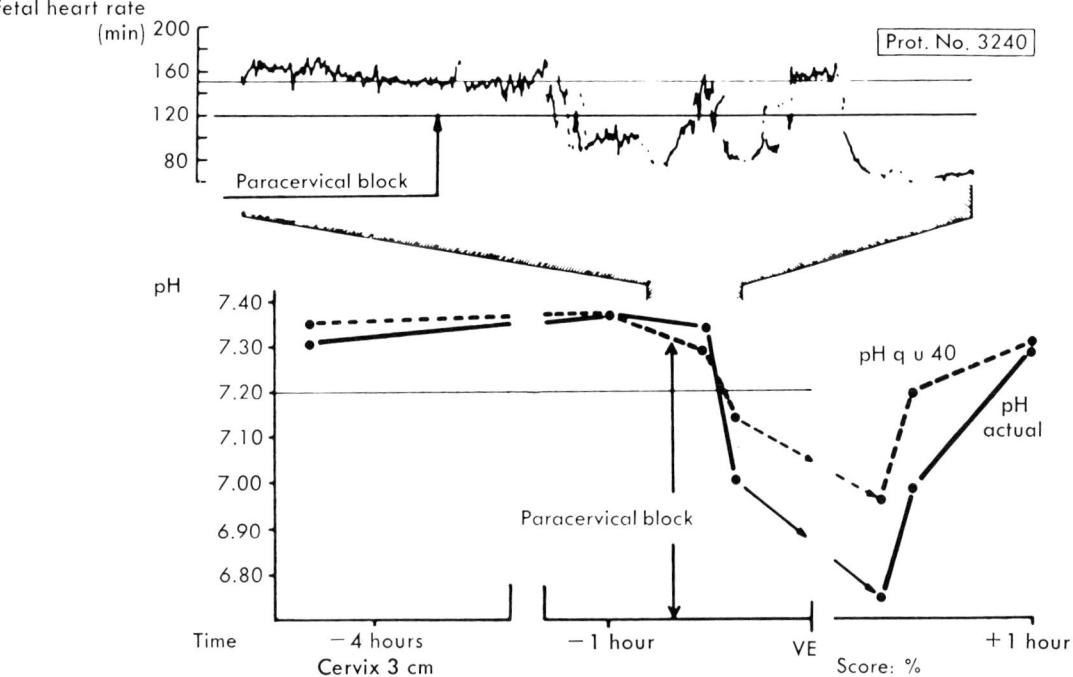

Fig. 7-2. Acute acidosis after paracervical block. (Modified from Käser, O.: Fetal blood sampling. In Huntingford, P.J., Hüter, K.A., and Saling, E., editors: Perinatal medicine, Stuttgart, 1969, Georg Thieme Verlag.)

above and posterior to the spines. The pudendal nerve lies just below the ligament, approximately 1.5 cm medial to the spine.

2. Apply an antiseptic solution to the mucosa of the lateral vaginal wall for about 2 cm inside the introitus. Inject a small amount of 1% procaine or its equivalent at the site of penetration. Advance the needle until the sacrospinous ligament is pierced slightly posterior and medial to the ischial spines.
3. Aspirate. If no blood returns, slowly inject 10 ml of anesthetic solution in the vicinity of each pudendal nerve.

C. A satisfactory block will usually anesthetize the entire vaginal canal, relax the musculature of the introitus, and persist for about 45 minutes. After a 5-minute take, the introitus should gape, and the anus cannot be contracted.

D. *Note:* The inferior pudendal nerve may have an independent origin from the sacral plexus, or it may originate unusually high from the pudendal nerve. Also, the dorsal clitoral nerve may have an anomalous origin. Under these circumstances, additional infiltration of the perirectal and anterior labial regions may be necessary to supplement the pudendal block for satisfactory control of pain at delivery.

V. Lumbar epidural block
Continuous lumbar epidural block, properly carried out in centers with well-trained personnel, is a safe method of anesthesia in the delivery of a jeopardized fetus. It may be selected in certain maternal complications such as congenital or acquired heart disease, pulmonary disorders, some endocrine dysfunctions (diabetes, toxemia, hypertension), and renal or hepatic disease. It may be the best technique for preterm or postterm labor, or cervical dystocia. The low-dosage technique can be augmented, if necessary, to produce anesthesia for cesarean section.

VI. Caudal block
Epidural placement of an anesthetic solution in the caudal canal (caudal block),

although it presents less risk of dural puncture, requires more medication (with attendant fetal risks), and the procedure blocks a larger nerve distribution thus increasing the hazard of hypotension. The anesthetic also may lead to failure of spontaneous internal rotation. Nevertheless, when performed by an experienced practitioner it may be a useful technique.

VII. Spinal block

Maternal hypotension with decreased uterine blood flow is the greatest risk to the fetus when subarachnoid (spinal) block is employed. It is used for alleviation of maternal discomfort only during delivery because it often arrests labor.

VIII. General anesthetics

General anesthetics may be useful adjuncts in certain high-risk cases. One should recall, however, that all the agents are transferred across the placenta and can depress the fetus. General anesthetics may be selected if regional anesthetics are contraindicated or deep uterine relaxation is necessary, for alleviation of constriction rings or relief of tetanic uterine contractions, or when prompt deep anesthesia is necessary.

Medications to be used with caution in high-risk pregnancy

I. Analgesics
   A. The commonly employed analgesics are either narcotic drugs (opiates or synthetic opiates) or inhalants.
   B. Injectable narcotics relieve pain by
      1. Elevating the pain threshold by more than 50% with usual doses
      2. Creating a relaxed, indifferent, or euphoric state
      3. Inducing lethargy or somnolence
   C. The fetus is adversely affected by analgesics because of central nervous system depression, particularly of the respiratory center. Lack of fetal maturity and any maternal medical complications, as well as difficulty during labor and delivery, increase undesirable side effects for the offspring.

   If analgesic medications are necessary, meperidine (often in combination with ataractics) appears to be the safest general parenteral medication currently available. Even so, great care must be taken in evaluating its use with the compromised fetus.

   Depending on the size of the mother and the status of the fetus, 50 to 100 mg of meperidine (especially when given with 25 mg promethazine) may be administered intramuscularly every 3 to 4 hours. More rapid effect may be achieved by giving the agents intravenously (never more than 50 mg meperidine and 25 mg promethazine). Obviously, smaller doses given more frequently are preferable to larger doses.

   Caution: If delivery occurs during the time of maximal effect (45 minutes after intramuscular and 5 minutes after intravenous administration) neonatal respiratory depression may occur. Naloxone (Narcan) 10 µg/kg may be useful in combating this and is usually given in the umbilical vein. Its effects have rapid onset (2 minutes), but they also disappear rapidly (30 minutes) and therefore may require readministration.

II. Sedatives (hypnotics)
   A. These drugs are poor analgesics because they
      1. Reduce reception to suggestion, even in small, moderate doses
      2. Slow mentation and reduce discrimination in large doses
      3. Fail to raise pain threshold
      4. Do not produce amnesia
      5. May slow labor, particularly in large doses, if given too early (in contrast to the meperidine combination noted above which should have no effect on labor)
   B. The likelihood of critical central nervous system depression in the preterm fetus contraindicates use of all sedatives in early termination of labor. These drugs cause periodic apnea or even cessation of fetal movement and do not respond to antagonists.

III. Amnesics (scopolamine and paraldehyde)
   A. Eliminate recent memory
   B. Produce little analgesic effect
   C. Subdue fetal central nervous system (paraldehyde only)

D. Often cause delusions or hallucinations (patients must be restrained, and operative delivery is usually necessary)
   E. Should be used rarely, if at all, in premature labor
IV. Ataractics
   A. Promazine HCL (Sparine), propiomazine HCL (Largon), or hydroxyzine pamoate HCL (Vistaril) may be administered in the usual dosage to patients in premature labor.
   B. They have the following effects:
      1. Reduce maternal anxiety
      2. Suppress nausea and vomiting
      3. Potentiate analgesics
V. Inhalation anesthetics
   A. Agents frequently used (nitrous oxide)
   Nitrous oxide produces analgesia and altered consciousness, but used as a single agent is not a complete anesthetic. Analgesia is usually obtained at levels of 50% (with 50% oxygen); levels exceeding 70% should not be used. Although it may be self-administered as an analgesic, attendants must monitor the maternal airway closely and ensure that aspiration does not occur. Nitrous oxide is much more frequently used in combination with other agents for anesthesia.
   B. Agents less frequently used (halothane, methoxyflurane, enflurane, and ethyl ether)
   The anesthetic agent halothane causes extraordinary uterine relaxation with possible hemorrhage and is therefore generally restricted to very short-term use in only those situations when extreme uterine relaxation is useful (e.g., replacement of the acute inverted uterus). Additionally it has cardiodepressant and hypotensive effects that may contraindicate its use in hypovolemic states.
   In low concentrations, methoxyflurane is a well-tolerated self-administered analgesic. However, extreme care must be exercised because overdose is a major complication. In higher concentrations (anesthetic) it can decrease uterine contractions. It also has a dose-related nephrotoxicity. Thus methoxyflurane has a limited place in either normal or risk obstetric management.
   At analgesic levels enflurane causes unconsciousness. It also has a myometrial depressing effect and a potential for nephrotoxicity. Therefore its obstetric role is limited.
   As an anesthetic agent ethyl ether causes uterine relaxation and deep, prolonged narcosis of the neonate. Therefore it is contraindicated for delivery of the premature or immature fetus or when there is danger of maternal hemorrhage. Because of these effects, plus its extremely explosive nature and unpleasant maternal effects, it is of little use in obstetrics.
   C. Agents used minimally if at all (cyclopropane and trichloroethylene)
   Cyclopropane has two major disadvantages: it is highly explosive, and it causes extreme fetal depression. Thus it is infrequently used.
   Trichloroethylene is no longer available in the United States because it produces toxic products when used in the soda lime closed-circuit anesthesia system. Deaths have been recorded even with self-administration for analgesia.
VI. Parenteral anesthetics
   Thiopental sodium (Pentothal sodium) and thiamylal sodium (Surital) cross the placenta quickly in anesthetic doses. Even 3 to 4 minutes after the start of administration, a premature fetus may have already received so much of the drug that resuscitation may be difficult.
   Moreover, these are poor analgesic agents. Therefore these agents (particularly thiopental sodium) are used in combination to induce obstetric anesthesia. For example, thiopental sodium is injected to induce sleep, succinylcholine is given to achieve muscular paralysis, and, after endotracheal intubation, nitrous oxide and oxygen are administered for ventilation and analgesia.

Anesthesia for cesarean section

A light general anesthetic usually has minimal effect on the baby and at the same time is likely to be safe and comfortable for the mother. A combination of nitrous oxide and a muscle relaxant is an excellent choice for a rapid cesarean section, provided an individual experienced in anesthesiology is available. Following is a successful, light general anesthetic combination:

1. Give up to 300 mg of thiopental sodium for induction of anesthetic but less than 4 mg/kg of body weight shortly before the skin incision.
2. Administer nitrous oxide–oxygen (75%:25%), with reduction in the concentration after about 3 to 4 minutes to a 50%:50% mixture.
3. Administer succinylcholine, 2.5 mg/min in 2 mg/ml dextrose solution (10%), up to 100 mg total.

Regional anesthesia is one of the few methods that will not contribute to depression of the neonate, provided that the maternal blood pressure is kept stable, reasonable amounts of the anesthetic are used, and toxic reactions (for example, convulsions) are avoided. Regional anesthesia will minimize the possibility of maternal aspiration. Unfortunately, maternal complications, such as extreme hypertension or hypotension, and the time required for "fixation" of the anesthetic agent may contraindicate use of spinal or epidural anesthesia.

If delay is hazardous or the fetus's or mother's condition is critical and no anesthesiologist is available, local anesthesia by direct infiltration of 0.5% or 1% procaine, or its equivalent, is an alternative approach to anesthesia for cesarean section.

Procedures that will reduce fetal hazard are as follows:

1. Leave patient in lateral position until skin is prepared.
2. Elevate right hip slightly throughout procedure to lessen possibility of pressure on the inferior vena cava.
3. Give 100% oxygen to the mother by mask when fetal heart tones are decreased or irregular and for 5 minutes before delivery.
4. Make an ample uterine incision.
5. Lift the fetus out through the incision promptly, taking care to prevent fetal aspiration of bloody fluid, and clamp the cord.
6. Transfer the neonate to a waiting physician or a nurse who is experienced in resuscitation and supportive therapy.

Anesthesia for patient in shock

An obstetric patient in shock or threatened with collapse requires a special choice of anesthesia. The physiology involved in hypovolemic shock (hemorrhage), for example, and supportive measures and drugs required in therapy are important to the success of delivery. The patient should be responsive to antishock therapy prior to surgery, but in critical cases a calculated risk must be accepted.

As preoperative medication, atropine sulfate, 0.4 mg, well diluted in normal saline solution, should be given slowly intravenously. Regardless of the anesthetic used, the supine gravida should have the right hip slightly elevated to avoid vascular (caval) obstruction by the pregnant uterus.

Although the choice of anesthetic method may depend on the skill and experience of the anesthesiologist, as well as availability of drugs and equipment, the following procedures have considerable advantages.

Hypovolemic shock. Inhalation anesthesia with maximum oxygen concentration, when nitrous oxide is used, causes no serious electrolyte or metabolic alterations. Certain anesthetics carry serious disadvantages in hypovolemic shock. Hypercarbia (retention of CO_2) is likely when there is inadequate pulmonary ventilation during the use of halothane, cyclopropane, or fluroxene. Moreover, halothane, which causes uterine relaxation, may increase hemorrhage. Spinal or epidural anesthesia often is followed by serious irreversible hypotension.

Septic shock. Thiopental sodium, nitrous oxide, oxygen, and succinylcholine are good choices because fever, vascular collapse, and renal failure complicate the problem. Although succinylcholine is well hydrolized, it does intensify oliguria, which may prolong the effect of the drug.

Neurogenic shock. Shock that follows acute uterine inversion requires an anesthetic such as halothane, which has a rapid induction time and good uterine relaxing capability.

Anaphylactic shock. Oxygen, vasopressor drugs, and corticosteroids are of value preoperatively. Epinephrine by injection or inhalation (spray) is beneficial for relief of bronchospasm. Infiltration anesthesia should be used, if one can assume that there is no sensitivity to local anesthetics.

Cardiogenic shock. Place the patient in Fowler's position with slight elevation of the left hip and use local infiltration for delivery.

CESAREAN SECTION DELIVERY

A cesarean section is often done on an urgent indication when the offspring is not mature or is severely stressed. The indications for cesarean section are varied and before any cesarean section is initiated, a gentle pelvic examination must be performed to ascertain that delivery is not imminent.

1. Fetal distress often is recorded. The problem may be one of hypoxia because of cord compression, premature separation of the placenta, placental insufficiency, etc.
2. Diabetes mellitus—early cesarean section has reduced the high incidence of intrapartal and postnatal death in cases complicated by maternal diabetes. However, cesarean delivery may be unnecessary in many cases if labor is properly monitored.
3. Isoimmunization—cesarean section may avoid irreparable damage to the infant or fetal exodus from icterus gravis or hydrops fetalis in Rh sensitization of the mother when induction of labor is unsuccessful.
4. Prolapse of cord in early labor
5. Herpes labialis or vaginalis complicating labor (procedure must be done within 4 hours of rupture of membranes)
6. Failure to progress in labor despite adequate uterine contractions
7. Fetopelvic disproportion, the most common indication for cesarean section
8. Weakness of the uterine scar after a myomectomy, unification operation, or previous cesarean section; dehiscence (partial or complete) of a prior uterine incision site
9. Placenta previa
10. Abruptio placentae with serious hemorrhage
11. Ruptured uterus (an emergency)
12. Obstructive pelvic tumors
13. Abnormal presentation, that is, transverse, shoulder, posterior face, and often breech presentations* (p. 222)
14. Fulminating eclamptogenic toxemia
15. Maternal complications such as previous vesicovaginal fistula or invasive cervical carcinoma
16. Previous reparative pelvic surgery

An emergency cesarean section obviously is a lifesaving measure for mother or fetus. Technically, operative delivery of the offspring is most desirable within a 5- to 10-minute period. This may not be possible, but expedition is vital. In any event, the surgery must be a successful blend of haste and safety.

1. General considerations
   a. Complications of pregnancy requiring abdominal removal of an infant that is known to be premature occur in 1% to 2% of gravidas.
   b. About 15% of premature infants are subjected to the hazard of cesarean section to avoid the greater risk of remaining in utero until the time of natural delivery.
   c. Between 5% and 10% of elective, repeat cesarean sections are timed inappropriately, and the neonates actually are preterm.
2. Analgesia, anesthesia (p. 77)
3. Precautions
   a. Inaccurate estimation of fetal size or gestational age is the most important single factor in neonatal wastage after elective cesarean section because maturity largely determines survival and normality. More than 10 times as many newborns in the low birth weight category delivered by cesarean section are lost, compared with cesarean delivered term neonates. Morbidity is also much higher in the former group. Therefore, when the expected date of confinement is uncertain, repeat cesarean section is best done only after physiologic maturity testing or as late in pregnancy as possible. Often this will be at the onset of labor.
   b. Even for normal, apparently healthy women, elective cesarean section carries a slight but definite fetal hazard, as contrasted with vaginal birth. Some

problems relate to analgesia-anesthesia, but trauma, atelectasis, and respiratory distress syndrome are also serious complications.

OTHER OPERATIVE DELIVERY METHODS
Forceps delivery

In delivery of a premature baby, instrumentation generally should be avoided. Nevertheless, a skilled physician can assist delivery of a vertex or aftercoming head with proper forceps, achieving an appreciable reduction in perinatal (and maternal) morbidity and neonatal mortality.
1. Obstetric forceps, in the hands of a physician experienced in their use, are effective for
   a. Guidance of the fetus and protection of the offspring and mother
   b. Rotation—usually occiput transverse to occiput anterior
   c. Traction in the pelvic curve
2. The concept of prophylactic (low) forceps delivery embodies prevention of damage to
   a. The fetal central nervous system (from pronounced or extended compression)
   b. The maternal pelvic floor structure (laceration and overstretching during the second stage of delivery procedure)
3. The fetus is eased out, not forced.
4. Prophylactic (low) forceps delivery of a premature infant requires
   a. Complete dilatation of the cervix with vertex on the perineum dilating the introitus
   b. A generous episiotomy
   c. The application of small or light forceps (deep cephalic curve, narrow-shank instruments preferred—Elliott or Tucker-McLean forceps) and slow delivery with minimal traction
5. Delivery of the aftercoming head in breech presentations can be accomplished with maximum safety with Piper or similar forceps while an assistant supports the baby, taking care not to hyperextend the neck.

---

*Many centers, including our own, are tending toward delivery of all breech presentations by cesarean section, regardless of gestation or gravidity.

Vacuum extractor

There are numerous contraindications to vacuum extraction. The device should not be used:
1. For delivery of premature infants (because of the increased risk of damage to more delicate tissues of the scalp and brain)
2. In cases of fetal distress (because too much time elapses to create the vacuum)
3. To accelerate labor before full dilatation (which may lead to tears, dystocia, cephalhematomas, and depressed Apgar scores)
4. In cases of malpresentation or malrotation
5. To attempt delivery of a large infant at high presentation and complete dilatation (high incidence of shoulder girdle dystocia has been reported)

Indeed, the vacuum extractor appears to share with forceps a declining use in modern obstetrics. The indications are relatively the same as for forceps use.

Internal podalic version and extraction

Internal podalic version and extraction is the most dangerous obstetric operation for the undersized (and even mature) infant. This procedure should not be attempted.

INDUCTION OF LABOR

Induction of labor is the initiation of effective uterine contractions by medical or surgical means. In contrast with the need for extension of pregnancy in conditions where intervention would lead to premature delivery, there are disorders that may seriously affect the fetus and lead to death in utero. For example, the obstetrician must not stand idly by while the undersized fetus is being starved or jeopardized by a disease process. The physician must be prepared to rescue the fetus as well as to protect it. Thus, despite what is said about preventing early birth (Chapter 18), purposeful premature delivery may be required to save the life of an infant when an incubator would seem to offer a better environment than the uterus. Maternal or fetal jeopardy mandates the conclusion of pregnancy in 5% to 10% of patients. In such cases physiologic maturity testing is warranted to assist in planning for neonatal care.

Indications

Indications for induction of labor include instances when ending the pregnancy will physically benefit the status of the mother or fetus

and when continuation of the pregnancy will increase the incidence of morbidity and mortality. These indications may include, but are not limited to, the following:
Chorioamnionitis
Hypertensive states of pregnancy
Documented postmaturity (>42 weeks)
Prolonged rupture of membranes with a mature baby
Isoimmunization
Diabetes mellitus
Severe unresolved maternal or fetal infection
Uterine bleeding from partial placenta previa or partial placental separation
Renal insufficiency
Pronounced polyhydramnios (a relative indication, and to be approached with extreme caution)
Fetal death
Anencephaly or other critical anomalies
Complication of pregnancy unresponsive to medical therapy
A known fetal-neonatal complication requiring treatment by a team that cannot respond to meet the imprecise timing of natural labor

Elective induction

Whereas an indicated induction may be justifiable intervention in a pathologic process, an elective induction too often is performed for the convenience of physician or patient. Despite potential risk in an otherwise normal physiologic process, it is occasionally employed in some hospitals in the United States for social, economic, or other nonmedical reasons. The incidence of prematurity after elective induction of labor is at least 5%, with many of these babies developing respiratory disorders with increased mortality and morbidity. The importance of careful assessment of gestational age and physiologic maturity testing in the elective induction patient cannot be overemphasized.

Contraindications to induction

Induction of labor is contraindicated whenever vaginal delivery is undesirable, such as in the following:
Absolute contraindication
Fetopelvic disproportion
Unfavorable presentation (for example, a transverse lie)
Grand multiparity (uterine rupture is a risk)
Total placenta previa
Severe maternal cardiac disease (class 3 or 4)
Hypertonic or dystonic early labor pattern in which a constriction ring or rupture of the uterus may ensue
Poor facilities for stimulation or inadequate supervision of induction
Probable contraindication
Firm closed uneffaced posterior cervix (low Bishop score)
Previous cesarean section or uterine scar (uterine rupture may occur)

Hazards of induction
Fetal
Hypoxia, acidosis, and fetal distress
Premature birth when estimated date of confinement has been grossly miscalculated
Prolapse of cord or cord compression
Infection (e.g., fetal pneumonia, septicemia, or omphalitis after amniotomy)
Precipitous delivery with trauma
Hyperstimulation of uterus by excessive oxytocin can result in fetal hypoxia, fetal death, placental separation, or birth injury
Maternal
Violent labor (hyperstimulation or tetanic contraction)
Premature separation of placenta
Uterine rupture
Cervical laceration
Uterine inertia, prolonged labor
Intrapartum infection
Postpartum hemorrhage
Hypofibrinogenemia
Amniotic fluid embolization
Emotional crisis—fear or anxiety
Water intoxication (large doses or prolonged administration of oxytocin may result in hyponatremia, convulsions, congestive heart failure, and death; to minimize this effect of the drug, oxytocin is usually given in a sodium chloride solution and dosage kept below 45 mU/min)

Procedural recommendations for medical induction

I. The patient should be evaluated by a physician prior to induction of labor.
II. The following should be known or obtained:
   A. Fetal gestational age
   B. Physiologic maturity

Table 7-2. Pelvic score for elective induction

	Score			
	0	1	2	3
Dilatation (cm)	0	1-2	3-4	5-6
Effacement (%)	0-30	40-50	60-70	80+
Station	−3	−2	−1, 0	+1, +2
Cervical consistency	Firm	Medium	Soft	
Cervical position	Posterior	Middle	Anterior	
Elective induction with score of 9+				

From Bishop, E.H.: Obstet. Gynecol. **24**:266, 1964.

  C. Indication for induction
  D. Status of the cervix* (Table 7-2)
  E. Absence of contraindications
  F. Informed consent
 III. The person administering oxytocin (either the physician or other qualified personnel) should be familiar with both maternal and fetal effects and complications. A physician should be immediately available in the event that complications occur.
 IV. Oxytocin, the drug of choice, should be given intravenously, with an infusion pump using a two-bottle setup with the oxytocin being connected piggyback to the primary infusion. The oxytocin connector should be placed as near the intravenous site as possible. A useful technique is noted below:

  The primary intravenous contains 1,000 ml D5W lactated Ringer's solution. The oxytocin infusion contains 10 units of Pitocin in 1,000 ml D5W of NaCl with 2 ml of Berocca C added to clearly mark the oxytocin bottle. They are hung piggyback with a T-connector connected directly to the angiocatheter so that if the oxytocin intravenous infusion is shut off no additional medication remains in the open intravenous line. An infusion pump is used to control the oxytocin flow.

 V. If any other drug or route of oxytocin is used, the physician should be present for the duration of the pharmacologic effect.

 VI. Continuous fetal heart and contraction monitoring should be used and the following should be recorded at 15-minute intervals if electronic fetal monitoring is not employed:
  A. FHR
  B. Frequency and character of contractions
  C. Rate of oxytocin infusion
  D. Maternal blood pressure
 VII. Considerable variations exist in titration regimens for induction of labor with intravenous oxytocin because of individual patient sensitivity. Keep the following considerations in mind:
  A. Patients over 36 weeks' gestation generally require less oxytocin than do those in earlier pregnancy. Start with a low dose (0.2 to 4 mU/min), and titrate each patient individually. A maximum dose of 45 mU/min should not be exceeded.
  B. Approximately 20 minutes is required for the blood level of intravenous oxytocin to stabilize and for the maximum effect of any given dose to be manifest. Wait 15 to 20 minutes between dosage increases, doubling the dose of medication with each increase.
  C. The half-life of oxytocin is approximately 3 minutes; however, pharmacologic effects may last for up to 20 minutes. This short half-life allows for good control and the ability to maintain a consistent blood level with the use of the intravenous medication.
  D. The goal of induction of labor is to stimulate a normal labor pattern,

---

*The Bishop score (Table 7-2) may be used to determine readiness for labor. The most important element is dilatation and the least important is position. Those patients with scores of 9 or greater experienced few failed inductions. With scores of 5 to 8, there are approximately 5% failures, and with a score of less than 5, there are approximately 20% failures.

rather than induce maximal uterine contractions. Attempt to induce one contraction every 3 minutes (with a maximum of one every 2 minutes), with an amplitude of 50 mm Hg (maximum 70 mm Hg) and a duration of 30 to 60 seconds. Induction should continue for a maximum of 6 to 8 hours. If delivery does not occur patient should be made to rest for at least 6 to 8 hours. If process needs to be repeated more than three times, vaginal delivery is unlikely.
    E. Because induction may stimulate endogenous oxytocin release from the pituitary gland, it may be necessary to gradually decrease the rate of intravenous oxytocin to prevent overstimulation.
VIII. Nursing responsibilities
    A. The nurse should provide supportive care by ascertaining whether the patient knows what to expect during the induction. Even though the physician may have explained the procedure to the patient, she may not have heard or may not fully understand what is to be done. If the patient reveals doubts or has questions the nurse should fully explain the procedure and therefore reduce the patient's anxiety level. Often induction of labor is more painful than the normal labor process, and more analgesia may be necessary.
    B. Induction procedure
        Titration. The prime consideration in deciding who should titrate an intravenous induction is not one's title or position, but rather one's qualifications. In an increasing number of institutions, this is the registered nurse. Certainly each hospital needs to develop its own policy in regard to inductions.
        Maintenance. In most instances, nurses prepare the intravenous infusion, maintain it, and monitor the patient's vital signs.
        Hypertonus or hyperstimulation. At the first indication of excessive stimulation, the nurse should shut off the intravenous infusion, place the patient on her side, and administer oxygen. Drugs that relax the uterine musculature should be immediately available. They include amyl nitrate, epinephrine, and drop ether.
    IX. Medications no longer recommended for induction
        A. Intramuscular administration of oxytocin is more dangerous than intravenous administration and is no longer recommended because:
            1. Some patients show an unexpected, strong cumulative response, even to small doses of the drug.
            2. Once a concentrated intramuscular dose is given, it cannot be withdrawn or stopped.
        B. Nasal and buccal forms of oxytocin should not be used because they are less predictable and controllable than is intravenous oxytocin administration.
            1. There is a longer lag period.
            2. They are more difficult to titrate to the patient's needs.
            3. They may cause sudden, unexpected uterine tetany.
        C. Sparteine sulfate, a capricious, potentially dangerous oxytocic, should never be used.

Surgical induction

Indications, contraindications, hazards, and procedural recommendations for medical induction of labor generally apply for surgical induction.
1. Amniotomy
    a. Check the fetal heart tone to be certain of normal rate and rhythm.
    b. Apply gentle pressure to the fundus to encourage engagement of the presenting part.
    c. Introduce forefinger through the cervix to guide a hook or other sharp instrument to the membranes. Rupture the membranes. Put the patient in a low Fowler's position. Allow fluid to drain without displacing the presenting part, or the cord may prolapse. Stripping of membranes is of doubtful value and may be traumatic.

2. Amniocentesis and subsequent injection of prostaglandins or hypertonic saline solution are appropriate only after fetal death.

Combined induction

Medical induction followed by amniotomy may speed labor.

Prognosis for induction

If repeated intensive efforts toward induction are unsuccessful, especially after rupture of the membranes, a cesarean section should be considered.

Amniotomy is the most effective single means of induction of labor, but with it the chance of infection is increased. Medical induction, combined with amniotomy, is even more likely to terminate pregnancy. (Amniotomy may not be necessary and should often be avoided if the patient goes into labor promptly with oxytocic stimulation.)

Induction of labor, including elective induction, carries definite risks for both the mother (principally rupture of the uterus, hemorrhage, and infection) and the fetus (prematurity, infection, hypoxia, precipitous labor and delivery, injury of the central nervous system, and trauma). *The physician must decide whether the hazards of allowing pregnancy to continue will exceed those of induction while considering the possible advantage of cesarean section.*

SPECIFIC RISK SITUATIONS
Breech presentation

A full discussion of the management of breech presentations is presented in Chapter 23.

Multiple gestation

1. The delivery of a multiple gestation is a high-risk event.
2. Cesarean section is being used increasingly when either twin is in a position other than vertex. Recent evidence has dispelled the notion that the second twin is usually smaller; indeed it is usually the larger. Thus delivery may be complicated by a second twin that is in malposition and that may be larger than the first. Should the first twin be breech and the second vertex, the hazard of locking is so great that cesarean section is usually indicated. All monoamniotic twins should be delivered by cesarean section.
3. Electronic fetal monitoring should be employed for both first and second twins for the detection of fetal distress. Should fetal distress occur in the second twin (even if the first is already delivered), it is safer to deliver the baby by cesarean section than to attempt a traumatic instrumented vaginal delivery.
4. Because most multiple pregnancy labors occur prematurely, as little analgesia and anesthesia as possible should be used for delivery.
5. A deep episiotomy is often recommended to shorten the perineal stage of labor and decrease compression of the fetal head. The umbilical cord should be cut immediately after delivery. However, in no circumstances should a cord around the neck of the first twin be cut; it should be manipulated over the head. In numerous circumstances it has been found to be the cord of the second monoamniotic twin. When the cord is cut, it should be identified clearly with a marking clamp.
6. One should perform a vaginal examination immediately after the delivery of the first child to discover the presentation of the second child.
7. Membranes are ruptured in the interval between contractions.
8. The addition of oxytocin will rarely be necessary to augment ineffectual uterine contractions.
9. Various manipulations including version and extraction, should be performed only with *known* fetal deaths.
10. Although operative delivery for the second twin is often indicated when the interval between delivery of the first and second twin exceeds 15 minutes, this is not necessarily the case if one uses electronic fetal monitoring to assess fetal well-being.

Delivery of the preterm infant

The mode of delivery for the preterm infant should be determined by obstetric indications. There is little question that the preterm fetus presenting breech is best delivered by cesarean section.

1. The preterm infant is more susceptible to fetal distress and cerebral trauma; therefore electronic fetal monitoring should be

employed and the progress of labor monitored actively.
2. Minimal analgesia and anesthesia should be used.
3. A generous episiotomy should be used to decrease compression-decompression forces on the fetal head.
4. The use of obstetric forceps, not to exert traction but to cradle the fetal head, may serve to decrease cerebral trauma.
5. In all management, care should be taken to be extremely gentle.
6. The cord should not be clamped until pulsations have stopped, with the baby being kept at or near the placental level. During this interval, care must be taken to ensure that the baby is respiring and does not become chilled.

Meconium-stained amniotic fluid

Meconium in the amniotic fluid may lead to the meconium aspiration syndrome, which has a devastating mortality (approaching 30%). Treatment of the syndrome, once established, is notoriously difficult. Prevention of its occurrence should be attempted by routine suction of the oropharynx when the infant's head is delivered followed by direct laryngoscopy after delivery and suctioning when needed. See p. 97.

Oversized fetuses (see Chapter 12)

The overgrown fetus predisposes to maternal laceration, fetopelvic disproportion, increased cerebral trauma, and shoulder girdle dystocia. Careful prepartum evaluation should reveal the majority of large babies. In many cases cesarean section will be electively employed; however, if the patient's pelvis is adequate, the following steps will prevent or treat shoulder girdle dystocia.
1. When delivery of the head begins an assistant places pressure on the fundus just above the symphysis to orient the shoulders into the oblique plane.
2. If shoulder girdle dystocia appears imminent, a fist should be placed immediately above the symphysis pubis and attempts should be made to rotate the shoulders into the oblique plane.
3. The above failing, a hand should be passed upward along the posterior aspect of the baby and the most easily palpated shoulder should be pushed toward the anterior. These actions should cause the shoulders to decrease in diameter as rotation occurs and also cause rotation into the oblique plane.
4. If the above fails, a hand should be passed into the uterus posteriorly and attempts made to bring the posterior arm down by flexion of the elbow, grasping of the forearm, and delivering. This maneuver, although effective, may lead to fractures of the long bones of the baby's arm and also may create uterine rupture or serious lacerations.
5. If the above steps fail, it has recently been reported that taking the patient's legs out of the stirrups and flexing them at the hip facilitates delivery. The mother may assist in this by placing her hands behind her thighs and pulling the legs into maximal flexion.
6. Finally, if the above steps fail, an effort is made to manually fracture the baby's clavicle by outward displacement. Compression of the infant's chest should be avoided to prevent damage of the brachial plexus or underlying subclavian vein by the broken ends of the clavicle. If this fails, the ultimate solution for cases of shoulder girdle dystocia is cleidotomy.

The following are also indicated in the delivery of the oversized baby:
1. A generous episiotomy
2. No instrumentation until the cervix is fully dilated and the baby is in a deliverable position.

Emergency delivery in the home

Home delivery, never recommended for premature birth or high-risk pregnancy, may be unavoidable; disaster or hostilities may prevent hospitalization. Premature delivery in the home, then, is generally an emergency. The gravida frequently goes into labor well before her expected date of confinement, without warning, and she may deliver abruptly. She usually gives birth unattended by professional personnel, and the infant is thoroughly contaminated. Hence definitive care of both mother and neonate is delayed. If medical personnel can be present at the delivery, the usual precautions in the management of premature labor are observed, even though improvisation is invariably required.

Medical attendants may have equipment and supplies for home delivery with them. In most instances one must use mainly what is at hand: soap and water, a few towels, sheets, kitchen stove heat, kitchen table, and some form of light.

1. Attention to the neonate
   a. Ensure an airway with postural drainage; gently wipe away any pharyngeal materials if suction is not handy.
   b. Use mouth-to-mouth resuscitation if the infant continues to be apneic and has not responded to gentle skin stimulation (p. 99).
   c. Tie the cord with available twine or string and cut it with any cutting edge previously wiped with an antiseptic.
   d. Wrap the infant in a clean towel or blanket and place him in a convenient container, with his mouth to the side.
   e. Place towel-covered hot-water bottles near the infant but not against him.
2. Attention to the mother
   a. Examine the mother for complications such as abnormal bleeding or lacerations.
   b. Transfer the mother to a hospital if any serious medical problems exist.
   c. Determine whether the placenta is intact or abnormal.
   d. Send an unusual placenta to the hospital for study.

BIBLIOGRAPHY

Bradford, W.P., and Gordon, G.: Induction of labor by amniotomy and simultaneous Syntocinon infusion, J. Obstet. Gynaec. Brit. Comm. **75**:698, 1968.

Brown, A.A., Hamlett, J.D., Hibbard, B.M., et al.: Induction of labor by amniotomy and intravenous infusions of oxytocic drugs: comparison between prostaglandins and oxytocin, J. Obstet. Gynaec. Brit. Comm. **80**:111, 1973.

Craig, C.J.T.: Eclampsia and the anesthetist, S. Afr. Med. J. **46**:248, 1972.

Crawford, S.: Maternal mortality associated with anesthesia, Lancet **2**:918, 1972.

Hack, M., Fanaroff, A.A., Klaus, M.H., et al.: Neonatal respiratory distress following elective delivery. A preventable disease? Am. J. Obstet. Gynecol. **126**:43, 1976.

Johnson, W.L., Winter, W.W., Eng. M., et al.: Effect of pudendal, spinal and peridural block anesthesia on the second stage of labor, Am. J. Obstet. Gynecol. **113**:166, 1972.

Lamaze, F., and Vellay, P.: Psychologic analgesia in obstetrics, New York, 1957, Pergamon Press, Inc.

Laros, R.K., Jr., Work, B.A., Jr., and Whitting, W.C.: Amniotomy during the active phase of labor, Obstet. Gynecol. **39**:702, 1972.

Lee, B.O., Major, F.J., and Weingold, A.B.: Ultrasonic determination of fetal maturity at repeat cesarean section, Obstet. Gynecol. **38**:294, 1971.

Lettew, W.L.: Paracervical block in obstetrics, Am. J. Obstet. Gynecol. **113**:1079, 1972.

Lilienthal, C.M., and Ward, J.P.: Medical induction of labor, J. Obstet. Gynaec. Brit. Comm. **78**:317, 1971.

Makowski, E.L.: High risk obstetrics, Clin. Obstet. Gynecol. **21**:285, 1978.

Normington, E.A.M.: A simplified method of Syntocinon infusion following amniotomy, J. Obstet. Gynaec. Brit. Comm. **79**:1108, 1972.

Rutter, P.: Domiciliary midwifery: is it justifiable? A review of over 1,000 cases in general practice, Lancet **2**:7371, 1964.

Schifria, B.S.: Fetal heart rate patterns following epidural anesthesia and oxytocin infusion during labor, J. Obstet. Gynaec. Brit. Comm. **79**:332, 1972.

Schokman, F.C.M., and Correy, J.F.: Pudendal block: assessment of efficacy and area of analgesia, Aust. N.Z.J. Obstet. Gynaecol. **11**:91, 1971.

Shnider, S.M., deLorimier, A.A., Holl, J.W., et al.: Vasopressors in obstetrics. I. Correction of fetal acidosis with ephedrine during spinal hypotension, Am. J. Obstet. Gynecol. **102**:911, 1968.

Turnbull, A.C., and Anderson, A.B.M.: Induction of labor, J. Obstet. Gynaec. Brit. Comm. **74**:849, 1967.

Usubiaga, J.E., La Iuppa, M., Moya, F., et al.: Passage of procaine hydrochloride and para-aminobenzoic acid across the human placenta, Am. J. Obstet. Gynecol. **100**:918, 1968.

Utting, J.E., and Gray, T.C.: Obstetric anesthesia and analgesia, Br. Med. Bull. **24**:80, 1968.

Vasicka, A., Robertazzi, R., Raji, M., et al.: Fetal bradycardia after paracervical block, Obstet. Gynecol. **38**:500, 1971.

Webb, M.J., and Fogarty, A.J.: The timing and dosage of oxytocin in the induction of labor, Aust. N.Z. J. Obstet. Gynaecol. **12**:43, 1972.

Wiese, J.: Induction of labor using small transbuccal doses of Syntocinon, Acta Obstet. Gynecol. Scand. **47**:333, 1968.

Witting, W.C.: A graphic record for monitoring labor induction or stimulation, Obstet. Gynecol. **39**:948, 1972.

Wollman, S.B., and Marx, G.F.: Acute hydration for prevention of hypotension of spinal anesthesia in parturients, Anesthesiology **29**:374, 1968.

8

Initial care of the infant in the birth room

Because up to 20% of potential neonatal problems are still unidentified before birth, all hospitals in which infants are delivered must have sufficient equipment and personnel available for care of any distressed infant until the infant is stabilized or placed in the hands of an experienced transport team. These requirements are especially important for hospitals where babies with known prenatal hazards are delivered. Such hospitals should be set up with on-call perinatal teams prepared to give critical care to the fetus and neonate.

The team of physician, nurse, and respiratory therapist must be capable of expert resuscitation, assisted ventilation, and initial stabilization. Too often advance preparation in terms of both equipment and personnel is not made for the expected delivery of immature infants, most of whom require intubation and positive pressure ventilation in the delivery room. In addition, there must be a predetermined method for contacting a regional neonatal center should consultation or transport of the infant be deemed necessary.

INITIAL CARE OF ALL INFANTS

1. Establish and maintain a clear airway.
    a. Suction the oropharynx and nostrils with a rubber bulb syringe as soon as the head is delivered. When meconium is present, use a Delee trap with a French (Fr) 10 catheter attached for suctioning before the first breath. Right after delivery (unless there is vigorous crying) view the glottis by direct laryngoscopy. If meconium is seen, suction the trachea with a catheter or endotracheal tube.
    b. To avoid aspiration by the neonate, suction the pharynx first and then the nose.
    c. Avoid deep nasal suctioning with a catheter because it may cause reflex bradycardia and laryngospasm.
2. Dry the infant's skin with a prewarmed towel while holding him below the level of the placenta.
3. Clamp the cord after the first breath, or approximately 30 seconds after delivery. At cesarean section, clamp the cord before lifting the infant above the uterus to prevent a backflow of blood into the placenta.
4. Place infant under radiant heat (to prevent cold stress) for further observation if any difficulties were encountered. Otherwise wrap infant in a warm, dry blanket and give him to his mother to encourage bonding.

If the infant shows signs of asphyxia (pallor or bradycardia) at birth or does not breathe within 30 seconds, clamp the cord immediately and move the infant directly to the resuscitation table (Chapter 9).

Physiologic assessment (Apgar scoring)

The scoring method (Table 8-1) introduced by Virginia Apgar in 1952 is still the simplest and most practical method of appraising the condition of the newborn at birth and is extremely useful in predicting the infant's prognosis. It permits a rapid and semiquantitative assessment of five signs of an infant's physiologic state: heart rate by auscultation, respiration from observation of movement of chest wall, color (pallid, cyanotic, or pink), muscle tone from movement of extremities, and reflex activity from a slap on the soles of the feet.

Table 8-1. Evaluation by Apgar score

Sign	Score 0	1 min	5 min	Score 1	1 min	5 min	Score 2	1 min	5 min
Heart rate	Absent			Below 100 beats/min			Over 100 beats/min		
Respiratory effort	Absent			Gasping, irregular			Good		
Muscle tone	Limp			Some flexion			Active motion		
Reflex irritability (slap to feet)	No response			Weak cry			Vigorous cry		
Color	Body pale or blue			Body pink, extremities blue			Completely pink		

1-minute score _____ 5-minute score _____

1. Assessment at 1 minute
   a. A score of 7 to 10 (10 indicates best possible condition) requires no resuscitation and should apply to more than 80% of infants.
   b. Scores of 4 to 6 (approximately 15% of babies) will identify those neonates who are cyanotic and who have irregular respirations and diminished muscle tone; reflex irritability and heart rate (over 100 beats/min) may still be maintained. These scores indicate moderate depression of the neonate who should respond to peripheral stimulation, for example, a sharp slap to the soles of the feet. Nevertheless, sufficient asphyxia may be present to require oxygen by mask at increased pressures (30 to 40 cm H_2O) for a couple of breaths. Should regular respiration not follow, the heart rate fall, or cyanosis persist, one must proceed with full resuscitative efforts. Should heart rate be under 80, proceed immediately with ventilation.
   c. Scores of 0 to 3 (1% to 3% of infants) will reveal severely asphyxiated infants who should be recognized at birth as needing immediate resuscitation. Invariably the heart rate will be under 80 beats/min or inaudible and the infant will be pallid and in shock.
2. Assessment at 5 minutes
Assessment at 1 minute (or before) should identify newborns who require immediate attention. The 5-minute score correlates with neonatal mortality and morbidity. A term infant who has not recovered to have a score of 8 or more, or a preterm infant who remains at 6 or less, is in need of more critical evaluation and closer observation. Such infants should be placed in a special care nursery if not transferred to a neonatal center.

Maintenance of body temperature
(see also Chapter 14)

1. In air-conditioned delivery rooms, cooling jeopardizes the infant at risk by increasing oxygen requirements, accentuating acidosis, and suppressing circulation through the lungs (pulmonary vasoconstriction).
2. Therefore skin temperature should be maintained near 36.5° C (98° F) in these newborns. No infant's temperature should be allowed to drop under 35.5° C (96° F), which can happen easily in air-conditioned delivery rooms.
3. Continuous temperature monitoring with skin thermistor attachment is important for infants requiring prolonged stabilization.

Physical observations in birth room

A brief examination should be performed by a physician, nurse midwife, or perinatal nurse between or after Apgar scoring periods. Prompt knowledge of significant defects or birth injury, overgrowth, undergrowth, or dysmaturity is important, as well as whether or not full term has been reached.

A normal, appropriate for gestation, term infant allows direct transfer to a mother-infant recovery room rather than the observational nursery. Detailed assessment of risk infants and their special needs are discussed in Chapters 11 and 12.

The birth room examination includes the following:
1. External
   a. Note skin color, staining, peeling, and evidence of wasting (dysmaturity).
   b. Observe length of nails and extent of creasing on soles of feet.
   c. Palpate for presence or absence of breast tissue.
   d. Note testicular descent, scrotal rugae, and labial development.
   e. Check nasal patency by occluding one nostril at a time and observing the infant's respiration and color.
2. Chest
   a. Auscultate the heart for rate and quality of sounds and palpate for position of maximum impulse.
   b. Listen with a stethoscope in each axilla for comparison and efficiency of respiratory exchange.
3. Abdomen
   Palpate the liver for consistency and enlargement. Enlargement (3 cm or more below costal margin) of the liver (and spleen) may indicate
   a. Infection—viremia, bacteremia, or sepsis
   b. Cardiac failure
   c. Erythroblastosis fetalis
4. Neurologic examination
   a. Note muscle tone and reflex behavior.
   b. Test the Moro reflex.
   c. Feel the fontanel for fullness or bulging.
5. Supplemental observations
   At least 2% of all infants have significant malformations that are recognizable at birth. The following checks are suggested in all infants, particularly when oligohydramnios or polyhydramnios is present, placental abnormalities including two-vessel cord are noted, or the neonate is small-for-dates.
   a. Inspect for such external defects as misshapen or low-set ears, lymphedema, macroglossia, palatal abnormalities, umbilical defects, variations in the size or shape of the head, spinal column defects, and opacity of the lens or cornea.
   b. Pass a catheter (Fr 10) attached to a DeLee trap through the mouth to establish esophageal patency, and perform gastric aspiration to remove excessive (over 20 ml) and/or green colored fluid suggestive of intestinal obstruction.
   c. Note a protuberant or scaphoid abdomen (diaphragmatic hernia) and organ enlargements or displacements.
   d. Check patency of the anus and rectum and note consistency and color of rectal contents (normally black, sticky meconium).
   e. Observe genitalia for testicular descent and any sexual ambiguity.
   f. Consider multiple anomalies. One major anomaly is often associated with another (25%). Three or more anomalies suggest a chromosomal defect.

Parent-infant bonding (see also Chapter 14)

Infants stable *after* their 5-minute Apgar scoring and physical observations are warmly rewrapped and given to their parents. The opportunities for body and eye contact by the mother and for nursing by the vigorous infant are important in establishing maternal ties to the infant. If the baby is to be placed in an observation or special care nursery, the mother is assured that the infant will be brought to her again when both have recovered from the birth process.

Placental observations

Before the physician or perinatal nurse leaves the birth room, the placenta should be inspected thoroughly, particularly for staining, infection, and infarction, and then weighed. A greenish color on the surface indicates the passage of meconium. The permanency of the stain is related to the length of time of its presence. In prolonged rupture of membranes the danger of perinatal infection is great. Rather than having a normal, steel-blue color, the placental surface appears milky or cloudy, with the underlying vessels less clearly visible. This change in color is the result of migration of polymorphonuclear leukocytes, of which pus is composed. A foul odor indicates more extensive infection. When infection is apparent, a smear and culture of the surfaces of the placenta and of the infant's gastric contents should be carried out. Occasionally a reddish brown or yellowish color of the placenta will indicate hemolytic disease. Brownish granular nodules (amnion nodosum) indicate the likelihood of renal agenesis (Potter's syndrome).

The cord should be observed for the number of vessels, the amount of Wharton's jelly (undernourished infants have less), and the point of attachment. In like-sexed twins, the number of chorionic layers and placental relationship are observed. The placenta, as in other unusual conditions, should be sent for pathologic study. The pathologist should be considered a necessary member of the team in all high-risk pregnancies.

Abnormal placental states, including increases or decreases in amniotic fluid, should be reported to nursery personnel and the physician responsible for the infant's care, as well as recorded on the infant's chart.

CARDIOVASCULAR AND RESPIRATORY CHANGES AT BIRTH
Circulation of the blood before and after birth (Fig. 8-1)

Oxygenated fetal blood is carried by the umbilical vein from the placenta to the inferior vena cava through the liver and ductus venosus. This blood mixes in the inferior vena cava with blood returning from the lower extremities and abdominal viscera, enters the right atrium, and passes through the foramen ovale into the left atrium, where it joins a small amount of blood returning from the lungs by the pulmonary veins. It then flows into the left ventricle and the ascending aorta to supply the head and upper extremities. Blood returns to the right atrium by the superior vena cava and then passes into the right ventricle and into the pulmonary artery. Most of the pulmonary arterial blood flows through the ductus arteriosus; from there part of it supplies the lower extremities and the abdominopelvic viscera through the aorta, and a larger part returns to the placenta by the umbilical arteries.

With the first breath and lung expansion, pulmonary blood flow suddenly increases. Returning blood from the pulmonary veins increases the pressure in the left atrium, resulting in functional closure of the foramen ovale. With increased oxygenation of the blood perfusing it, the ductus gradually constricts, limiting and finally obliterating this second pulmonary bypass, or right-to-left shunt. Decreasing pulmonary vascular resistance lowers pulmonary artery pressure below aortic pressure, causing a reversal of flow through the ductus as long as it remains open (left-to-right shunt). The ductus arteriosus is usually obliterated in the early neonatal period, resulting in the normal, or adult, type of circulation.

Reduced ventilation may, by producing hypoxia and hypercapnia, result in a combined respiratory and metabolic acidosis (augmented by anaerobic metabolism). The combination of acidosis and hypoxia is a powerful vasoconstrictive force in the newborn, except on the ductus arteriosus and umbilical arteries, which tend to remain open as in the fetal state. Pulmonary vasoconstriction leads to an increase in vascular resistance that may on occasion exceed the systemic pressures; under these circumstances a right-to-left shunting through a patent ductus or a patent foramen ovale may occur.

Onset of respiration

The most important adjustment to the extrauterine environment for the infant is the onset of respiration. Air must replace the fluid that fills the airways and alveoli until birth. The process of a vaginal vertex delivery usually squeezes out as much as 20 ml of fluid from the infant's lungs. The remaining fluid probably is absorbed into the vascular and lymphatic bed of the lung through the decrease of pulmonary vascular resistance with the onset of respiration. Delayed onset or inefficient ventilation can retard this process and hinder the establishment of normal pulmonary function, allowing transient tachypnea to develop.

During the first breath the infant develops a negative intrathoracic pressure of 20 to 70 cm of water, drawing in about 40 to 70 cc of air, approximately 20 to 30 cc of which will remain as residual volume. This first breath is frequently followed by a vigorous cry in the undepressed infant as he expires against the closed glottis. After the first few breaths the lungs are almost completely expanded and the pressure is lower than it was at the onset of

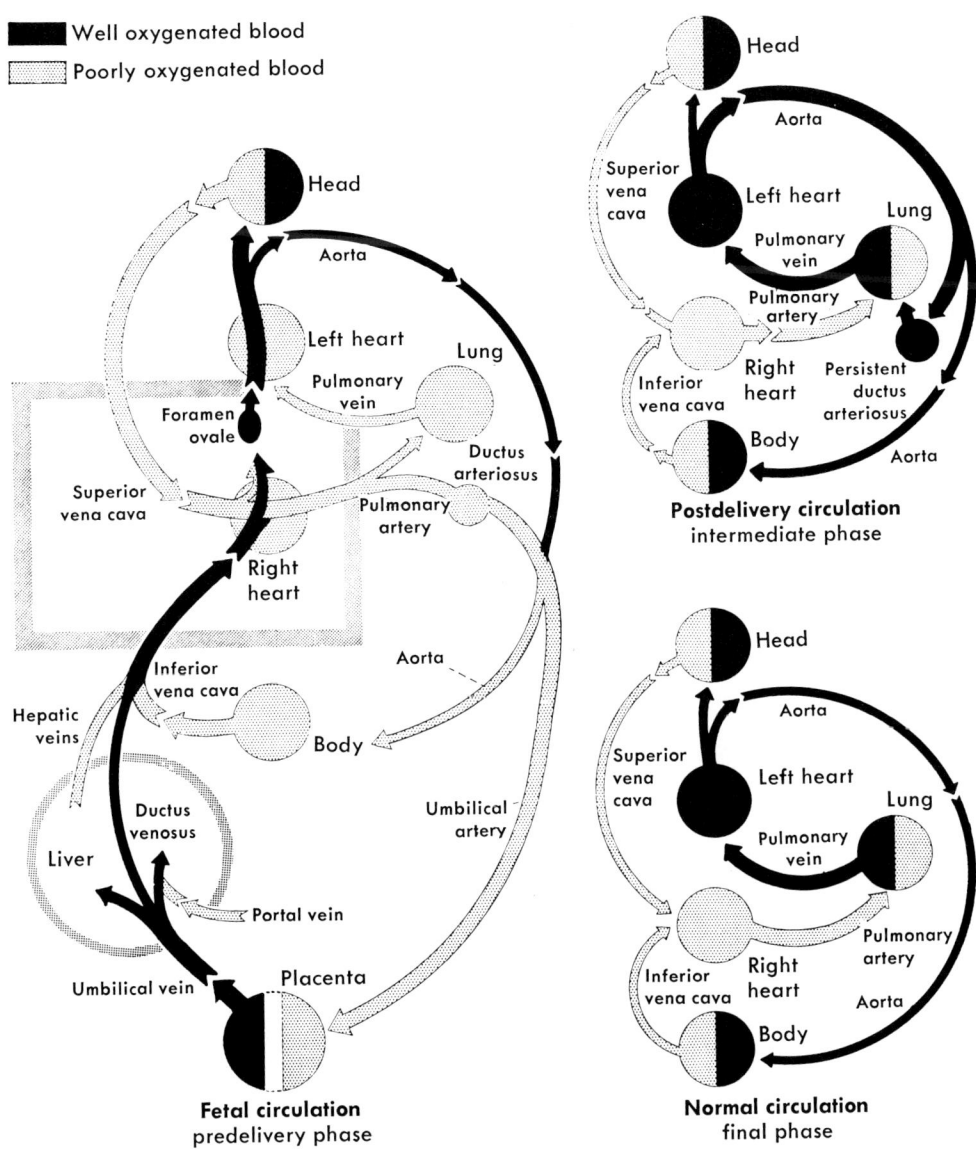

Fig. 8-1. Diagrams of blood circulation before and after birth. (Modified from Benson, R.C., and Griswold, H.E.: Spectrum **10:**80, 1962; courtesy Chas. Pfizer & Co., Inc.)

respiration. The stimuli that provoke the onset of respiration at birth are numerous. Because the interval between birth and the first breath is usually only a few seconds, it is likely that excitation of the respiratory center follows through neurally transmitted impulses from peripherally located receptors. Thermal stimuli seem to be of particular importance here; tactile stimuli and the rise of blood pressure on cord clamping probably play secondary roles.

A significant change of blood gases at birth is another important factor governing the onset of respiration. This stimulus is particularly important for the depressed infant whose respiratory center is less sensitive to peripheral stimuli.

Physiologic aspects of oxygenation

Oxygen is carried in blood in chemical combination with hemoglobin, as well as in physical solution.

At ambient pressures most oxygen is bound to hemoglobin. The quantity is dependent on the partial pressure of oxygen and the hemoglobin-oxygen dissociation curve. This curve for fetal hemoglobin shifts to the left (as compared with the curve for adult hemoglobin). Therefore fetal hemoglobin binds more oxygen at lower pressures, but it also releases less to the tissues.

The oxygen tension in arterial blood not only is dependent on pulmonary function but also is influenced by the degree of venous admixture through shunts. Prolonged breathing of 100% oxygen will correct desaturation secondary to ventilation or diffusion abnormalities and therefore can be useful in differentiating the above causes from significant right-to-left shunts.

The oxygen tension in arterial blood at birth rises rapidly to 60 to 90 mm Hg (somewhat lower for premature infants). Because during the first days of life 20% of cardiac output is shunted right to left, the PA_{O_2} in 100% oxygen will be approximately 440 mm Hg, and not 600 mm Hg as it is in adults. A 50% right-to-left shunt in an infant will prevent the PA_{O_2} from rising above 67 mm Hg even with 100% oxygen.

Placental transfusion

The blood volume of an infant at birth is dependent on the amount of blood received by placental transfusion. The blood volume in the fetus at term averages 66 ml/kg (approximately 78 ml/kg at birth and between 75 and 107 ml/kg at 72 hours, depending on time of cord clamping). As the infant is born, a redistribution of blood takes place between the fetus and the placenta. Blood flow through the umbilical arteries stops approximately 45 seconds after birth, whereas the umbilical vein remains patent longer. The onset of uterine contractions enhances transfer of blood to the infant. Gravity significantly influences transfer of blood between neonate and placenta; elevation of the infant 50 to 60 cm above the level of the placenta for 3 minutes will prevent normal placental transfusion. However, if one places the neonate below the level of the placenta, the process will be accelerated.

The timing of clamping the cord in relation to the above-mentioned factors influences the infant's blood volume and physiologic state.

Infants whose cords have been clamped early often have an initial hypovolemia from redistribution of blood into the expanding pulmonary circuit, lower initial blood pressure, peripheral vasoconstriction, a falling hematocrit and better lung compliance compared with late-clamped infants. Late clamping of the cord tends to cause larger blood volumes, higher initial blood pressures, and a rising hematocrit, as well as occasional respiratory distress caused by reduced lung compliance.

During perinatal asphyxia, a redistribution of blood from the placenta to the fetus seems to take place. It explains the higher plasma and red blood cell volumes of infants with perinatal asphyxia whose cords are clamped early as compared with the plasma and red blood cell volumes in nonstressed neonates.

BIBLIOGRAPHY

Benirschke, K.: Placental causes of maldevelopment. In Berry, C.L., and Poswillo, D., editors: Teratology trends and applications, New York, 1975, Springer-Verlag.

Cordero, L., and Hon, E.H.: Neonatal bradycardia following nasopharyngeal stimulation, J. Pediatr. **78**:441, 1971.

Dahm, L.S., and James, L.S.: Newborn temperature and calculated heat loss in the delivery room, Pediatrics **49**:504, 1972.

Delivoria-Papadopoulos, M., Rončević, N.P. and Oski, F.A.: Postnatal changes in oxygen transport of term, premature and sick infants: the role of red cell 2,3-diphosphoglycerate and adult hemoglobin, Pediatr. Res. **5**:235, 1971.

Desmond, M.M., Rudolph, A.J., and Phitakspraiwan, P.: The transitional nursery care, Pediatr. Clin. North Am. **13**:651, 1966.

Finer, N.N., Robertson, C.M., Richards, R.T., et al.: Hypoxic-ischemic encephalopathy in term neonates: perinatal factors and outcome, J. Pediatr. **98**:112, 1981.

James, L.S., and Adamsons, K.: Respiratory physiology of the fetus and newborn infant, N. Engl. J. Med. **271**:1352, 1954.

Karlberg, P.: The adaptive changes in the immediate postnatal period, with particular reference to respiration, J. Pediatr. **56**:585, 1960.

Nelson, K.B., and Ellenberg, J.H.: Apgar scores as predictors of chronic neurologic disability, Pediatrics **68**:36, 1981.

Prod'hom, L.S., Levison, H., Cherry, R.B., et al.: Adjustment of ventilation, intrapulmonary gas exchange and acid-base balance during the first day of life, Pediatrics **33**:682, 1964.

Saigal, S., O'Neill, A., Surainder, Y., et al.: Placental transfusion and hyperbilirubinemia in the premature, Pediatrics **49**:406, 1972.

Saint-Anne Dargassies, S.: La maturation neurologique du prématuré, Rev. Neurol. **93**:331, 1955.

Strang, L.B.: Uptake of liquid from the lungs at the start of breathing. Development of the lung, Ciba Foundation Symposium, London, 1967, J. & A. Churchill, Ltd.

Yao, A.C., and Lind, J.: Placental transfusion, Am. J. Dis. Child. **127**:128, 1974.

9

Resuscitation and stabilization of the depressed infant

Severely depressed infants present a medical emergency and require immediate resuscitation. They are usually flaccid, pale, and apneic and will respond slightly or not at all to stimulation. The heart rate is usually less than 80 beats/min. There will be hypoxia and significant acidosis.

One must not delay or vacillate in performing resuscitation in what might seem a hopeless situation, for example, Apgar score of 0 at 1 minute. Experience* indicates that if cardiac arrest does not last over 5 minutes or if regular respirations are established within 30 minutes thereafter, prognosis appears to be uniformly good.

Although as many as 3% of infants at birth are severely asphyxiated as revealed by their appearances and low Apgar scores, an almost equal number, without being asphyxiated, remain apneic after birth and need positive pressure ventilation to avoid severe asphyxia. They include the following:
1. The preterm infant (usually weighing under 1,500 gm) whose respiratory center does not respond to usual stimuli because of his immature state
2. Infants depressed from anesthesia, particularly those delivered by cesarean section 20 or more minutes after initiation of anesthesia to the mother
3. Infants whose mothers received narcotics within 2 hours of delivery
4. Infants with congenital anomalies that obstruct or impinge on the airway (see Chapter 33)

There may develop during labor certain events that will forewarn the physician or nurse that delivery of a depressed infant is likely. This will allow time to assemble a perinatal team or additional support. Among these conditions are the following:
1. Abnormal FHR patterns, particularly with fetal acidosis (pH less than 7.2) confirmed by scalp sampling (see Chapter 5)
2. Meconium staining of the amniotic fluid, which may be aspirated by the fetus
3. Vaginal evidence of bleeding from the fetus confirmed by a positive Apt or Kleihauer test indicating fetal hemoglobin
4. Maternal hypotension during cesarean section

EQUIPMENT AND DRUGS NEEDED IN DELIVERY ROOM

Every delivery room should have an area set aside to be used for the initial care of the newborn, preferably allowing 120 square feet of space for this purpose. The "resuscitation island" should be completely equipped so that resuscitative and other maneuvers can be carried out under optimal conditions of light for the physician and warmth for the infant. Oxygen, compressed air, and vacuum outlets should be available. The height of the table on which the infant is placed for immediate care should be sufficient to allow easy intubation of the infant. An overhead radiant heating device is essential.

---

*Thomson, A.J., Searl, M., and Russell, G.: Quality of survival after severe birth asphyxia, Arch. Dis. Child. **52**:620, 1977.

The following is equipment to be used for resuscitation:

1. Rubber bulb syringe
2. Heart rate monitor with needle electrodes
3. Suction catheters Fr 8 and 10 attached to DeLee trap
4. Stethoscope
5. Bag and masks of varying sizes, preferably a bag that is also capable of maintaining a positive end expiratory pressure
6. Infant laryngoscope with nos. 0 and 1 blades (ideally equipped with an oxygen channel to minimize hypoxia during intubation) and spare batteries and bulb
7. Endotracheal tubes sizes 2.5, 3, 3.5, and 4 mm, with adapter
8. Malleable wire stylet with lubricant
9. Miscellaneous syringes and needles, gloves, umbilical clamps, and ties
10. Umbilical vessel catheter tray and infusion set (see Appendix B)
11. Doppler type of blood pressure apparatus with varying-size soft rubber cuffs, the width of which should be sufficient to cover at least one half the length of the upper arm

Note the list of drugs, their solution strength, and dosage needed at the top of p. 95.

VENTILATION FOR THE NONBREATHING INFANT

(For details and techniques of intubation and assisted ventilation, see Chapter 10.)

1. Place infant on a flat surface with shoulders slightly elevated.
2. Attach skin electrodes and connect to heart rate monitor.
3. Suction oropharynx if meconium was noted in amniotic fluid; view larynx with laryngoscope and suction trachea.
4. Ventilate with bag and mask attached to an oxygen source; intubate and ventilate with bag those infants not improving with mask ventilation alone and infants likely to need prolonged ventilation (i.e., infants of of less than 1,000 gm birth weight or severely depressed infants [Apgar score less than 3]).
5. Check air movement into lungs by observing chest wall movement, and auscultate for equality of breath sounds.
6. Apply 30 to 40 cm H_2O pressure initially, holding for 1 to 2 seconds, two or three times.
7. Continue ventilating at 15 cm H_2O pressure at a rate of at least 30 to 40 breaths per minute until respirations are sustained. (Higher rates and pressures occasionally may be required.)
8. Raise oxygen concentration if infant's color is not pink.
9. Transfer infant to appropriate nursery depending on responses and degree of risk of infant (Chapters 11 and 12).

CONTINUED APNEA WITH ASSISTED VENTILATION

1. If heart rate continues to be slow or is barely audible or inaudible, proceed directly to circulatory and metabolic support.
2. If heart rate and color improve but apnea persists, obtain blood gas measurements and consider the following:
   a. Narcotic depression—if narcotics have been given to mother, infuse Naloxone, 0.01 mg/kg, into infant.
   b. Perinatal asphyxia or central nervous system disease or injury

Such infants are likely to need mechanical ventilation and transfer to a regional center.

CIRCULATORY AND METABOLIC SUPPORT

1. Perform external cardiac massage if heart rate persists under 80 beats/min or heart sounds are weak. Depress chest wall at midsternum approximately 1 cm at a rate of about two per second with enough force to produce femoral pulsations; place hands around chest and use two thumbs to depress sternum.
2. For persisting or worsening bradycardia inject directly into the heart 0.1 to 0.5 ml/kg of 1:10,000 epinephrine. Inject the drug into the endotracheal tube if there is no time to place an umbilical vessel catheter first.
3. Have an associate catheterize an umbilical vessel and draw blood for pH and hematocrit. The pH of venous blood is .05 lower than that of arterial blood. Use this line for emergency medication and fluid support.
4. Infuse plasmanate, albumin 5%, or blood, 10 to 15 ml/kg, if infant gives an appearance of shock. Follow blood pressures serially.

Drugs and solution	Dose
1. 10% dextrose, sterile water, normal saline	2.5 ml D10W/kg (0.25 gm) slowly by IV push; then 3 to 4 ml/kg/hr
2. Plasmanate or albumin (5%)	10 ml/kg, repeated if needed
3. Sodium bicarbonate ($NaHCO_3$) (0.9 mEq/ml)	2 mEq/kg diluted 1:1 with H_2O slowly by IV repeated on basis of blood gas results
4. Naloxone (Narcan) (0.02 mg/ml)	0.01 mg/kg IV or IM
5. 10% calcium gluconate (0.45 mEq/ml)	1 to 2 ml/kg diluted 1:1 with H_2O given slowly IV
6. Epinephrine (1:10,000 or 0.1 mg/ml)	0.1 to 0.5 ml/kg, IV push or endotracheal tube
7. Ampicillin	100 mg/kg IV; then 50 mg/kg every 12 hours
8. Digoxin (0.1 mg/ml)	0.01 mg/kg to start digitalization
9. Heparin (1,000 units/ml)	0.1 ml in 20 ml syringe for taking blood from cord, fetal side of placenta, or O Rh-negative persons
10. Atropine	0.03 to 0.1 mg/kg IV
11. Isuprel 1:5,000 (0.4 mg/100 ml D10W)	2 μg/kg/min
12. Dopamine	5 to 10 μg/kg/min

For treatment of specific causes of shock, e.g., acute blood loss, sepsis, and abnormal cardiogenic problems, see Chapter 29.

5. Administer 2 to 3 mEq of sodium bicarbonate per kg of body weight diluted 1:1 with water at a rate of 1 mEq/min. Continue adequate ventilation to aid release of additional carbon dioxide from metabolization of sodium bicarbonate. Additional sodium bicarbonate should be given only on a basis of blood gas determinations (p. 258).
6. Start infusion of 10% glucose solution. Begin at a rate of 3 to 4 ml/kg/hr. This rate supplies 0.3 to 0.4 gm of glucose per hour, which is near the maximum rate for its metabolization by most preterm infants after birth. Infants of diabetic mothers, those who are asphyxiated, and babies small for gestational age may require more. Small preterm infants may tolerate only 0.2 to 0.3 gm/kg/hr.
7. Add 3 ml of calcium gluconate per 100 ml of glucose solution. Many depressed and most preterm infants develop hypocalcemia after birth.

PRECAUTIONS: Hyperosmolar solutions, which include sodium bicarbonate, calcium gluconate, and 15% or more glucose solutions, when injected too rapidly in too great a quantity or through an improperly placed catheter, can cause tissue and organ damage or intracerebral vessel rupture because of sudden fluid shifts in serum hyperosmolality.

CONTINUED RESPIRATORY DIFFICULTY FROM BIRTH

If, after intubation, the infant has only weak respirations and is unable to maintain color, suction and ventilate as follows:

1. Continue to ventilate infant, giving enough pressure with each inflation to ensure sufficient air exchange (determined by auscultation) without overexpansion of chest wall.
2. Supply oxygen in sufficient concentration to avoid cyanosis (if possible). Later regulate oxygen concentration on the basis of oxygen tension of the infant's blood.
3. Note scaphoid abdomen or displacement of cardiac impulse (usually to right) to indicate diaphragmatic hernia (Chapter 33).
4. Pass catheter to rule out esophageal atresia (Chapter 33).
5. Order emergency x-ray examination of chest to identify any abnormality (e.g., pneumothorax, pneumonia, congenital defects).
6. Consider sepsis (Chapter 25).

These serious events require transfer to a neonatal center. Respiratory distress syndrome (RDS), which develops gradually over 3 to 6 hours, is discussed in Chapter 27.

INCREASING CYANOSIS

Infants having increasing cyanosis may or may not have respiratory distress or apnea.

Oxygen is administered by a hood to achieve stable concentrations (Chapter 27). Conditions to be considered are as follows:
1. Congenital heart disease (usually not manifest at birth unless extremely serious) (Chapter 29)
2. Persistent pulmonary hypertension with right-to-left shunting of blood away from lungs (Chapter 29)
3. Metabolic disease caused by hypoglycemia and hypocalcemia
4. Polycythemia (Chapter 31)
5. Rarely congenital methemoglobinemia

Most of the conditions mentioned are of a serious nature and require transport to a regional neonatal center. Nevertheless, the early care and continued support of the infant by the local team until transfer is accomplished is vital to infant survival.

BIBLIOGRAPHY

Abramson, H., editor: Resuscitation of the newborn infant and related emergency procedures in the perinatal center special care nursery, ed. 3, St. Louis, 1973, The C.V. Mosby Co.

Behrman, R.E., James, L.S., Klaus, M., et al.: Treatment of the asphyxiated infant, J. Pediatr. **74:**981, 1969.

Carson, B.S., Losey, R.W., and Bowes, W.A., Jr.: Combined obstetric and pediatric approach to prevent meconium aspiration syndrome, Am. J. Obstet. Gynecol. **126:**712, 1976.

Gregory, G.A.: Resuscitation of the newborn, Anesthesiology **43:**255, 1975.

Hey, E.: Resuscitation at birth, Br. J. Anaesth. **49:**25, 1977.

Lees, M.H.: Cyanosis of the newborn infant, J. Pediatr. **77:**484, 1970.

National Conference on cardiopulmonary resuscitation and emergency cardiac care: standards and guidelines for cardiopulmonary resuscitation and emergency cardiac care, JAMA **244:**453, 1980.

Rogers, M.C.: New developments in cardiopulmonary resuscitation, Pediatrics **71:**655, 1983.

10

Techniques of resuscitation and stabilization

Up to 5% of infants require resuscitation in the birth room, and at least one fifth of these babies will continue to receive some form of mechanical ventilation for days and even weeks. In this chapter, along with detailed supplemental information in the Appendix, is presented an outline for initiation of laryngoscopy, intubation and endotracheal tube fixation, and assisted ventilation. These procedures should be practiced on anesthetized cats. Catheterization of umbilical vessels should also be practiced, using fresh umbilical cords.

LARYNGOSCOPY AND ENDOTRACHEAL INTUBATION
(Fig. 10-1)

(For a list of equipment and its preparation, see Appendix B.)
  1. Procedure
     If heart rate falls below 100 beats/min while you are attempting to intubate, stop and ventilate the infant with a mask and bag until the infant is pink and the heart rate is over 100 beats/min. If no favorable response occurs after several breaths, proceed to intubate. Problems such as bradycardia and cyanosis can be minimized by the use of laryngoscopes equipped with oxygen channels.
     a. Have equipment at hand, infant under radiant heat, and heart rate monitor attached.
     b. Elevate shoulders slightly with folded towel without extending or flexing the neck.
     c. Hold laryngoscope between thumb and index finger of left hand with third and fourth fingers firmly grasping the chin, decreasing the likelihood of laryngoscope slipping and injuring the infant.
     d. Insert laryngoscope slightly to right of midline and, while advancing it, move it toward the midline, gently deflecting the tongue.
     e. When base of tongue and epiglottis are in view, advance blade just short of epiglottis and raise blade gently obliquely upward and forward. The epiglottis will be moved anteriorly, revealing the larynx and vocal cords.
     f. Choose endotracheal tube size suitable for neonate's estimated weight as follows:

Birthweight (gm)	Size (mm)
<750	2.5
750-2,000	3
2,000-3,500	3.5
>3,500	4

     g. Have endotracheal tube marked for insertion distance on the basis of the following table:

Birthweight (gm)	Lip-to-tip distance (cm)
1,000	7
2,000	8
3,000	9
4,000	10

        This distance should place the tip midway between vocal cords and carina at T2.
     h. Lubricate stylet slightly and insert into endotracheal tube, making sure it does not protrude beyond tip of tube.

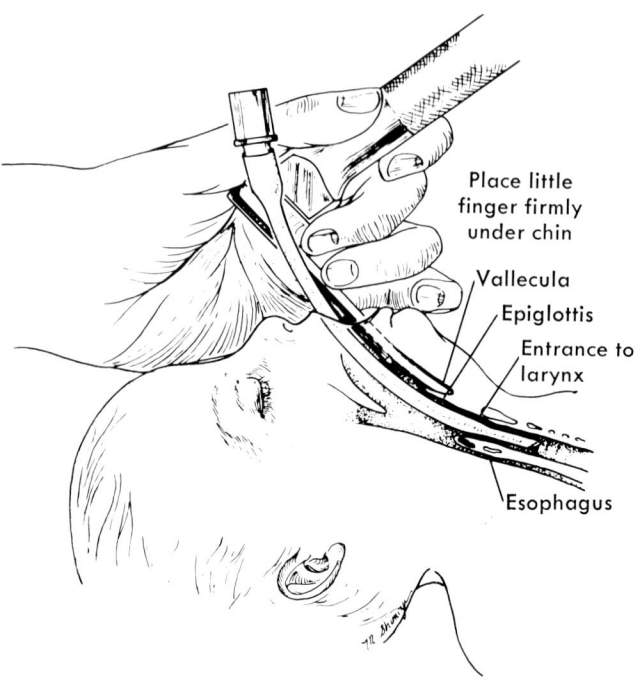

Fig. 10-1. Position of head, laryngoscope, and endotracheal tube during intubation of a newborn. (From Klaus, M.H., and Fanaroff, A.A.: Care of the high-risk neonate. Philadelphia, 1973, W.B. Saunders Co.)

    i. Holding endotracheal tube with adapter attached in your right hand, with bevel parallel to the cords, advance it from the right corner of the mouth and insert it while maintaining a direct view.

    j. Carefully withdraw laryngoscope blade and stylet while maintaining tube's position by holding your finger firmly over tube on roof of infant's mouth.

    k. Auscultate for equality of breath sounds while infant is ventilated and make sure that tube is inserted to previously measured length.

2. For prolonged intubation, secure tube in place as follows:
    a. Using applicators, paint with tincture of benzoin under nose and along cheek areas where tape is to be applied.
    b. When benzoin is dry, apply Elastoplast butterfly to fit snugly below infant's nose and approximately 3 to 5 cm onto cheeks.
    c. Suture endotracheal tube to Elastoplast on each side, being careful to place suture so that it will not obstruct passage of suction catheter (use 4-0 silk with taper needle).
    d. Tape endotracheal tube to Elastoplast and baby's cheeks with adhesive tape (approximately 10 cm long and 0.5 cm wide).
    e. Verify by x-ray examination placement of tip of endotracheal tube at T2.

3. Problems of intubation
Most problems result from failure to visualize the glottis when attempting to intubate. One can facilitate bringing the glottis into view by applying pressure over the larynx with the little finger of the left hand. The blade should never be used as a guide for introducing the endotracheal tube.
    a. Entry into esophagus is indicated by lack of chest movement, gastric distention, and absent breath sounds over lungs on auscultation.
    b. Entry into the right main bronchus is

suggested by diminished breath sounds over left side of chest.
c. Use of too small a tube impairs air exchange, interferes with suctioning, and promotes tube obstruction.
d. Injury to the cords or esophagus is the result of blind force or stylet protruding beyond endotracheal tube end.

METHODS OF ASSISTED VENTILATION

For the initial support of ventilation in apneic or poorly breathing infants, all perinatal personnel should be trained in the use of bag and mask. To learn the insufflation pressure required by finger squeeze on a bag one should practice with a pressure manometer. Chest wall movement and pressure of breath sounds on auscultation indicate adequacy of tidal volume.

I. Positive-pressure breathing devices

A number of manual positive-pressure breathing devices are on the market, (e.g., Laerdal, Penlon, Ambu, and Hope). Each has advantages as well as disadvantages. To perform satisfactorily, an infant bag should

A. Deliver up to 100% oxygen
B. Create variable pressures
C. Be equipped with masks of various sizes that fit comfortably over infant's nose and mouth
D. Connect to endotracheal tubes
E. Have a safety pop-off valve
F. Be connected by T-piece to a manometer to give operator better surveillance over inspiratory pressures used during ventilation

Technique of use

1. If infant is intubated, connect the endotracheal tube to a bag and ventilate the infant in this manner.
2. When applying bag-to-mask ventilation, cover infant's nose and mouth snugly with mask, and lift mandible upward to prevent airway obstruction.
3. Initially apply one or two inflations at pressures of 30 to 40 cm of water, holding pressure for 1 to 2 seconds to expand infant's lungs.
4. Continue to ventilate with lower pressures (10 to 20 cm of water) at a rate of 40 to 50 inflations/min.
5. Gastric distention may occur during mask ventilation; decompress stomach by placing orogastric tube.

II. Mouth-to-tube ventilation

A. To minimize danger of overexpansion of lung, use cheek muscles only when blowing into tube.
B. Deliver oxygen by placing a tube connected to an oxygen source into operator's mouth while operator is applying mouth-to-tube ventilation.

III. Mouth-to-mouth ventilation

This technique can be used by persons inexperienced with other methods and requires no equipment.

A. Place airway, if available, into infant's pharynx.
B. Place mouth firmly over infant's nose and mouth and inflate infant's lungs gently by blowing from cheeks.
C. Remove mouth from infant to let infant's lungs recoil.
D. Repeat maneuver at a rate of 30 to 40 inflations/min.
E. Oxygen can be given as above.

UMBILICAL VESSEL CATHETERIZATION

(For details of equipment and preparation, see Appendix B.)

Catheterization of an umbilical artery or vein for emergency use has become a standardized procedure in the birth room as well as the neonatal intensive care unit for the infant requiring intensive care. Although the hazards are of consequence (sepsis, emboli, thrombosis, necrosis), advantages are impressive and include the ability to monitor arterial or venous pressures, as well as the easy provision of parenteral medication, fluid and electrolytes, and nutrition during the period when serial arterial blood sampling is necessary for precise management. An important advantage for the small, weak infant is freedom from excess handling and skin puncture. Disturbing infants interferes with ventilation and gas exchange resulting in extended hypoxic periods not always recognized by skin color change. Although some infants can accept an arterial line in place for many weeks, the incidence of sepsis increases with time, as well as the chance of obstructive emboli formation. As soon as the infant becomes stable and has recovered from the acute phase of his disease, peripheral veins should be used for infusion sites.

Candidates for catheterization

1. Candidates for arterial catheterization include infants who:
   a. Are asphyxiated at birth or are in shock who may require blood volume expansion or metabolic support based on laboratory evaluation and pressure recording
   b. Continue to have or develop respiratory distress requiring over 30% ambient oxygen and serial blood gas determinations*
   c. Weigh less than 1,500 gm at birth
2. Candidates for umbilical vein catheterization include infants who:
   a. Need emergency replacement of blood or plasma
   b. Are in need of a central line when attempts at arterial catheterization are prolonged or unavailing
   c. Need infusions or intravenous medications when other avenues are impossible
   d. Require monitoring of central venous pressure

Placement of catheters

1. Place umbilical vein (UV) catheter tip in thoracic inferior vena cava about 5 to 7 cm through the umbilicus. A more precise figure is two thirds of the perpendicular distance from the shoulders to the umbilicus (S-U length).
2. Position† the umbilical artery (UA) catheter tip either above the diaphragm (110% of the S-U length) or just above the aortic bifurcation (60% of the S-U length).
3. Check position by x-ray film as follows:
   UV tip at T 6 = 9
   UA tip at T 7 = 10 or between L 3 and 4

Reasons for immediate removal

1. Arterial spasm with pale or pulseless leg
2. Discoloration or coolness of one leg in comparison to the other
3. Darkening tips of toes
4. Hypertension (systolic pressure of greater than 100 mm Hg) suggesting blockage of renal arteries
5. Signs of omphalitis (redness around umbilicus)
6. Clots visible in the catheter that cannot be aspirated

TECHNIQUES OF CATHETERIZATION
Umbilical artery

1. Take a radiopaque catheter (Fr 3½ for infant under 1,500 gm or Fr 5 for infant over 1,500 gm).
2. Cut off and discard the last 9 cm of the wide end of the catheter.
3. Insert a blunt no. 18 needle into this end to reduce dead space.
4. Attach a sterile stopcock, fill the system with heparinized solution (1 unit of heparin per ml of 5% glucose solution), free of air bubbles, and turn stopcock off toward the catheter.
5. Make a fresh cut across cord 0.5 cm from its base.
6. Use a small iris forceps for initial dilatation of the umbilical artery when inserting catheter into this vessel.
7. Overcome obstruction at level of abdominal wall by applying gentle traction on umbilicus.
8. Relieve obstruction at level of bladder by

---

*Capillary blood may be used when catheterization is impossible or conditions are less serious. However, results may be inaccurate in the first few hours of life, but obtaining blood by arterial puncture can be very helpful. For the technique of blood gas sampling, see Chapter 27.

†The best position for umbilical artery catheters has not been determined. For emergency use, the higher position may be better. For prolonged use, the lower position may be safer. The upper position tends to develop embolic extensions down the aorta, which may block important ostia producing ischemia or, in case of the renal vessels, hypertension. Lower settings are likely to block circulation to legs or toes. If close observation is maintained and catheter removed with onset of complication, permanent damage is infrequent.

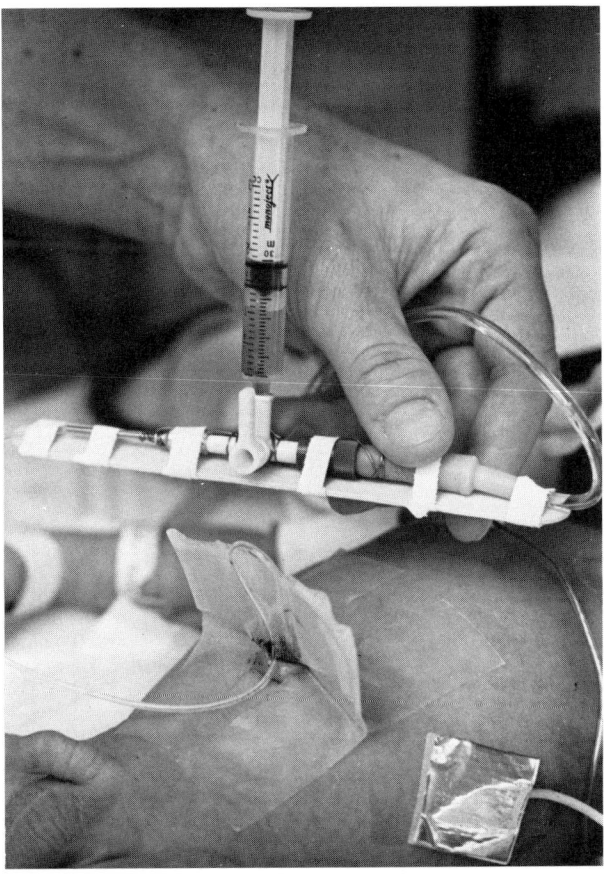

Fig. 10-2. Tape bridge for securing an umbilical vessel catheter and a method of fixating stopcock and tubing to tongue blade.

applying gentle steady pressure for 30 seconds. *Never use force.*
9. Advance to predesignated distance.
10. Observe lower extremities for blanching.
11. Check for return blood flow and flush with 5% dextrose containing 1 unit of heparin per ml.
12. Infuse any medications and attach catheter to intravenous line.
13. Start infusion pump *to prevent backflow and clotting.*
14. Use fused stopcocks with Luer-lok adapters *to prevent disconnection and loss of blood.*
15. Secure catheter with tape bridge as shown in Fig. 10-2.
16. Obtain x-ray film of abdomen and chest to ensure proper location. If catheter needs to be repositioned, do not advance it farther once the sterile field has been contaminated, but reinsert a new catheter using sterile technique. However, you may withdraw the catheter to a new position if necessary.
17. To minimize infection, apply 1.67% povidone-iodine solution daily to umbilical stump. Have stopcock and syringes changed every 12 hours, whenever they do not appear to be clean, or when they contain visible clots. If clots or debris are seen in a catheter and cannot be aspirated (never flush them into the infant), the catheter must be removed.
18. To prevent clotting of an umbilical catheter
    a. Use catheter for continuous infusion of parenteral fluids containing 20 U heparin per 100 ml.
    b. After obtaining blood samples, flush catheter with heparinized saline solution (1 unit of heparin per ml).

Umbilical vein

1. Grasp thin-walled vein with forceps; vein will be located anteriorly.
2. Gently insert Fr 5 or 8 fluid-filled radiopaque catheter while exerting traction on cord stump (helps to relieve obstruction at level of abdominal wall).
3. Withdraw tip several centimeters and rotate forward if obstruction is met in portal area.
4. Attempt to place catheter in inferior vena cava (avoids liver damage).
5. Check placement by x-ray examination for continued use for emergency infusions.
6. Observe *precautions* emphasized for umbilical artery techniques.

Securing catheter

1. Using 4-0 silk with a cutting needle, make a purse-string suture around cord.
2. Tie several knots around catheter, 2 to 3 cm from insertion site.
3. Clean Betadine off abdomen with alcohol, paint with tincture of benzoin, and tape catheter securely in place with bridge of clear plastic tape (Fig. 10-2).

Removal of umbilical vessel catheter

1. Obtain:
   No. 11 blade
   Sterile instrument set containing scissors and hemostat
   Package of sterile 4 × 4 inch gauze pads
2. Turn off intravascular infusion and wait 5 minutes.
3. Cut suture with no. 11 blade if necessary.
4. Remove catheter slowly, withdrawing it approximately 3 cm at a time. Procedure should take about 5 minutes.
5. Apply pressure to umbilicus with 4 × 4 inch gauze pad, or, if necessary, clamp vessel with hemostat.
6. Leave umbilicus uncovered and observe for hemorrhage.

BIBLIOGRAPHY

Boon, A.W., Milner, A.D., and Hopkin, I.E.: Lung expansion, tidal exchange, and formation of the functional residual capacity during resuscitation of asphyxiated neonates; J. Pediatr. **95**:1031, 1979.

Tochen, M.L.: Orotracheal intubation in the newborn infant: a method for determining depth of tube insertion, J. Pediatr. **95**:1050, 1979.

Zmora, E. and Merritt, T.A.: Control of peak inspiratory pressure during manual ventilation, Am. J. Dis. Child. **136**:46, 1982.

11

Classification into risk categories at birth

WHAT ARE THE RISK GROUPS?

Between 3% and 4% of newborn infants are at high risk, of whom the majority can be identified in the first hours of life. Most will require transfer to a regional center (Chapter 13) depending on the skills available in the hospital of birth. Mothers with serious problems in pregnancy will have been transferred to a perinatal center for delivery. The infants at greatest risk are those who:

1. Are very immature, weighing less than 1,500 gm (about 1% of infants born)
2. Remain depressed after resuscitation (about 0.5%)
3. Show increasing signs of respiratory distress (about 1%)
4. Have surgically correctable defects (about 0.5%)

Another group (0.5%) develops serious problems after birth (e.g., seizures or sepsis).

Between 70% and 80% of infants born are at low risk and well nourished. The remaining 15% to 25% are infants at medium risk most of whom can be cared for at a well-staffed community hospital. They may be at increased risk because of pregnancy history (e.g., prolonged rupture of membranes), stressful events during labor or delivery (indicated by FHR fluctuations or reduced Apgar score), or long or short gestations or disproportions in size and weight for gestational age. Specific care for these infants is outlined in Chapter 12.

Awareness at birth of all infants at medium risk is not always assured unless a physician for the infant is present or a nurse capable of careful observation and assessment has been assigned the task. To prevent a gap in continuity of medical care after resuscitation of the infant and the often delayed examination in the nursery, interim assessments should be performed by the perinatal nurse. In this way potential dangers may be anticipated.

ASSESSMENT BY WEIGHT AND GESTATION

The division of infants into term and premature on the basis of weight above and below 2,500 gm has little biologic significance. Many term infants (40% in some countries) weigh less than 2,500 gm, and in some areas, many preterm infants weigh over 2,500 gm.

Yet both weight and gestational age are important in classifying infants at birth so that morbidity and mortality risks can be anticipated to ensure optimal care. An accurate weight on admission to the nursery is necessary for statistical requirements, as well as for drug dosage. A careful menstrual history is an important method of estimating gestational age but should not supplant a clinical estimate of gestational age as part of the physical examination, particularly when the history is inexact or a discrepancy between birth weight and gestational age exists. Prenatal estimation of gestational age is discussed in Chapter 3. Table 11-1 presents a guide for the combined estimation of gestational age by measurement, appearance, neuromuscular behavior, and responses. More extensive criteria have been developed by Dubowitz et al. (Copies of a modification of the estimation of gestational age by Kempe, Silver, and O'Brien are supplied by the Mead Johnson Laboratories, Evansville, Indiana.)

Table 11-1. Postnatal estimation of fetal age on the basis of maturity (assuming normal growth)

	27 weeks	28 to 33 weeks	34 to 37 weeks	38 to 41 weeks	42 weeks or more
Anatomic maturity					
Sole creases	None	Minimal—one or two creases	Anterior third	Extend to heel	Deep creases over entire sole
Scrotum	Testes undescended	Testes high in scrotum; few rugae	Testes above raphe; more rugae	Testes bulge below raphe; rugae complete	Pendulous, deep rugae, well pigmented
Labia	Labia majora undeveloped	Minora prominent	Labia of equal prominence	Majora covers minora	Same
Ear cartilage	Pinna soft and folded	Still folded	Returns from folded position	Erect, with sharp ridges	Same
Breast tissue	None	None	Up to 4 mm (if not undergrown)	5 mm or more	Usually more than 10 mm; areolae very prominent
Skin	Translucent and edematous	Red	Pink to red	Pinkish white	Thicker and white; often desquamated
Nails	Visible; soft and small	Soft and extending to fingertips	Soft and extending to fingertips	Extending to just beyond fingertips; not as soft	Hard in consistency and extending well beyond fingertips
Eyes	Closed	Eyes opening	Wrinkles brows	Eyes will fixate	Good fixation; head will follow
Neuromuscular maturity					
Body flexion	None	Flexes legs—froglike	Flexes arms	Same	Same
Moro reflex	Aimless	Lateral extension	Knees under abdomen / Beginning embrace	Embrace	Same
Neck tone	Limp	Limp	Head control on arm flexion (36 to 37 weeks)	Raises head in prone position	Raises head in prone position; turns head from side to side
Sucking and deglutition	Not synchronized	Insufficient for total nipple feeding	Adequate for normal intake	Same	Perfect
Glabella tap (blink)	No response	Develops (32 to 33 weeks)	Good response	Same	Same
Pupil to light	No response	Gradual contraction	Good response	Same —begins to follow	Same
Measurements					
Weight (gm ± 1 SD)	1,000 ± 350	1,150-2,000 ± 450	2,200-2,950 ± 450	3,150-3,600 ± 500	3,300-4,100 ± 500
Length (cm ± 1 SD)	37 ± 1.5	38-44 ± 1.5	45-47.5 ± 1.5	48.5-53 ± 2	50-54 ± 2
Head circumference (cm ± 1 SD)	24.5 ± 1	25.5-30.5 ± 1	31.5-33.5 ± 1	34-36.5 ± 1.5	35-37.5 ± 1.5

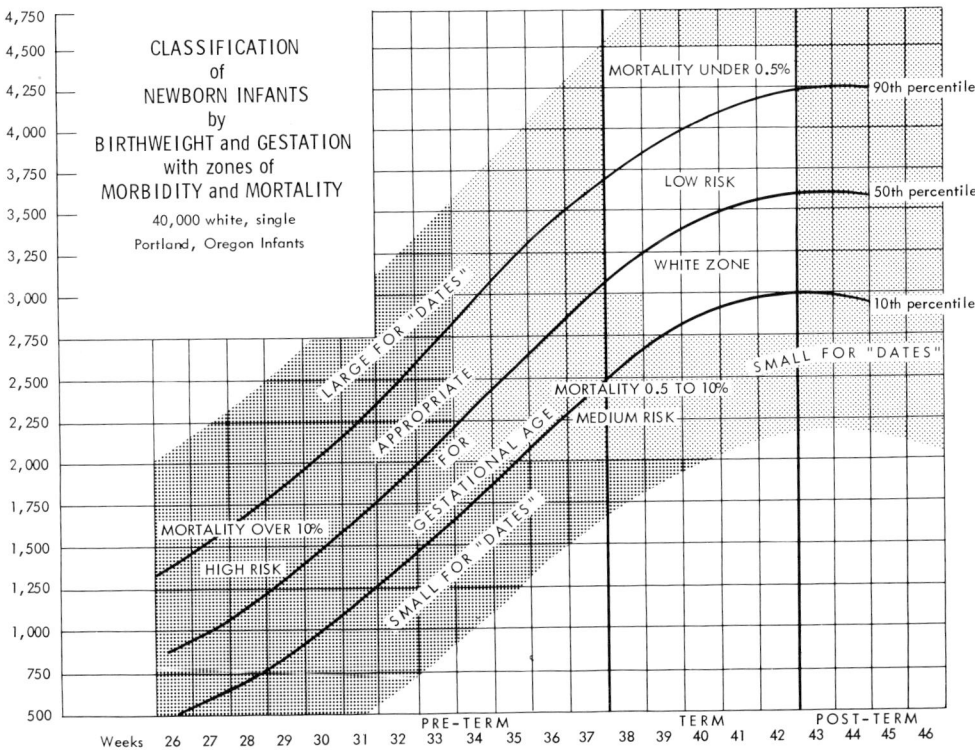

Fig. 11-1. Zones of mortality and morbidity in relation to both birth weight and gestation. Note changes in percentages that now apply as shown in text. (From Behrman, R.E., and Babson, S.G.: Am. J. Dis. Child. **121:**486, June 1971, Copyright 1971, American Medical Association.)

The classification by gestational age and growth pattern proposed by Battaglia and Lubchenco has been modified to conform with the expected mortality and pattern of fetal growth in 40,000 single, white infants born to a middle-class population in Portland, Oregon. These data are shown in Fig. 11-1, which presents zones of neonatal mortality and morbidity on the basis of weight and gestational age, and which may apply to many similar populations. The infants at high risk, with a mortality over 4%, are grouped together in the heavily shaded zone. They represent 1% to 3% of all infants, including those born before 33 weeks of gestational age and those weighing under 2,000 gm, regardless of gestation. Several times this number may be added to the high-risk group because of complications of pregnancy or delivery. Infants falling into the white zone have a neonatal mortality of less than 0.5%. They have a weight range from 2,750 to 4,500 gm (usually between the 10th and 90th percentiles) and a gestational age of 38 through 42 weeks and seldom present difficulty in the delivery room. All the remaining newborn infants, numbering about 15% to 25% of all deliveries, are placed in the medium-risk category (lightly shaded zone); they have a mortality of 0.3% to 4%. This zone of infants includes the postterm baby (often clinically dysmature), the undergrown infant with or without loss of subcutaneous tissue, and the otherwise normal large-for-dates infants, including a sizable group of preterm infants who weigh over 2,500 gm but are 33 weeks or more of gestational age. Thus small- and large-for-gestational-age infants (SGA and LGA) should be designated, as well as those who are preterm and postterm, so that they receive extra vigilance in the first days of life.

USE OF BODY MEASUREMENTS IN EVALUATION OF RISK GROUPS

In addition to a precise weight, best performed on an automatic beam scale (Toledo Babyweight), we recommend careful measurements

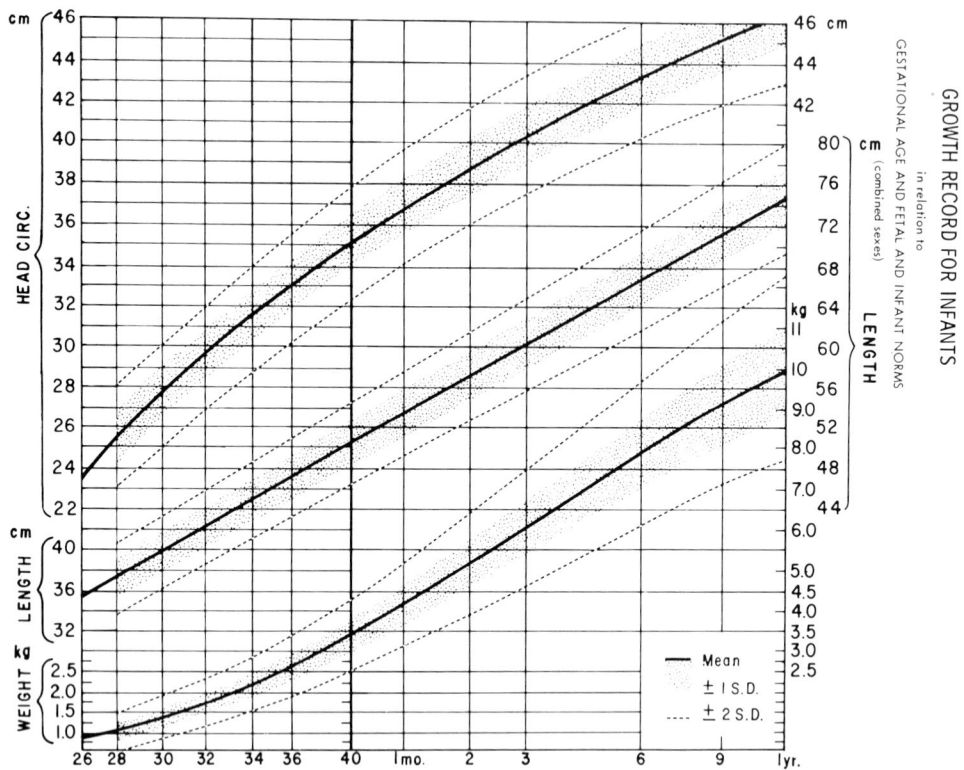

Fig. 11-2. Fetal infant growth graph, which shows growth curves of weight, length, and head circumference from 26 weeks of gestational age through 1 year of life after "term" has been reached. The curves have been smoothed through the usual transitional period of growth. Any disproportion among the three measurements, as well as deviations from the normal, can be easily recognized for evaluation. (From Babson, S.G., and Benda, G.I.: J. Pediatr. **89**:814, 1976.)

of head circumference and length. A disposable paper tape is placed snugly around the head over the forehead and occiput, and the greater circumference is recorded after two trials. Length is measured by placing the infant stretched out in a measuring tray with a movable footboard (Infa-Length, Olympic Surgical Co., Seattle, Washington). The head turned to the side will help extend the foot on the same side. (When an infant's condition is unstable, length can be measured in place. An extra hand increases the accuracy of both methods.) The measurements are then plotted on the growth graph (Fig. 11-2) according to the estimated gestational age. This additional screen will disclose any disproportion among the three measurements as well as variations from the fetal-infant norms.

Disproportionate head size in relation to length or a head-to-length ratio above 73 or below 65 may suggest hydrocephalus or microcephalus (see Fig. 30-1). Weight-length differences of more than 1 SD in which the infant is heavy or light for length deserve consideration. In the first instance it suggests an infant of a diabetic mother; in the other, it suggests dysmaturity or fetal wasting (Fig. 11-3). Such infants are not necessarily LGA or SGA. With carefully performed baseline measurements, later apparent aberrations in the plotting of growth will be more meaningful.

BIBLIOGRAPHY

American Academy of Pediatrics, Committee of Fetus and Newborn: Nomenclature for duration of gestation, birthweight and intrauterine growth, Pediatrics **39**:935, 1967.

American College of Obstetricians and Gynecologists, Committee on Terminology: Nomenclature—dissenting views, Pediatrics **39**:942, 1967.

Amiel-Tison, C.: Neurological evaluation of the maturity of newborn infants, Arch. Dis. Child. **43**:89, 1968.

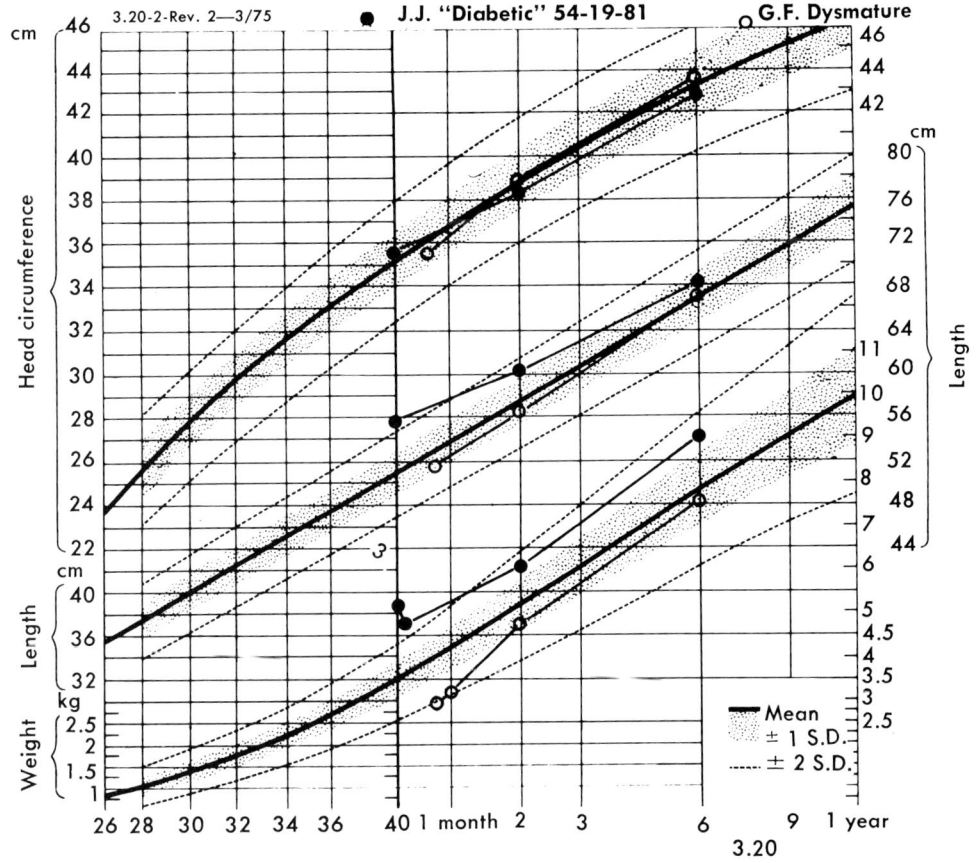

Fig. 11-3. J.J., ●, an infant of a diabetic mother who shows disproportionate overweight at birth in relation to other measurements. G.F., ○, a dysmature and postmature infant who is light in weight in relation to head and length. Note tendency to readjust toward the mean by 6 months of age.

Avery, M.E., and Fletcher, B.D.: The lung and its disorders in the newborn infant, ed. 3, Philadelphia, 1974, W.B. Saunders Co.

Babson, S.G., Osterud, H.T., and Thompson, H.: The congenitally malformed, Northwest Med. **65:**729, 1966.

Battaglia, F.C., and Lubchenco, L.O.: A practical classification of newborn infants by weight and gestational age, J. Pediatr. **71:**159, 1967.

Dubowitz, L.M.S., Dubowitz, V., and Goldberg, C.: Clinical assessment of gestational age in the newborn infant, J. Pediatr. **77:**1, 1970.

Engle, R., and Benson, R.C.: Estimate of conceptional age by evoked response activity, Biol. Neonate **12:**201, 1968.

Gruenwald, P.: Infants of low birth weight among 5,000 deliveries, Pediatrics **34:**157, 1964.

Koenigsberger, M.R.: Judgment of fetal age. I. Neurologic evaluation, Pediatr. Clin. North Am. **13:**823, 1966.

Lind, J.E., Tahti, E., and Hirvensalo, M.: Roentgenologic studies of the size of the lungs of the newborn baby before and after aeration, Ann. Paediatr. Finn. **12:**20, 1966.

Moss, A.J., and Monset-Couchard, M.: Placental transfusion: early versus late clamping of the umbilical cord, Pediatrics **40:**109, 1967.

North, A.F.: Nomenclature—dissenting views, Pediatrics **39:**941, 1967.

Oh, W., Wallgren, G., Hannson, J.S., et al.: The effects of placental transfusion on respiratory mechanics of normal term newborn infants, Pediatrics **40:**6, 1967.

Usher, R., McLean, F., and Scott K.E.: Judgment of fetal age. II. Clinical significance of gestational age and an objective method for its assessment. Pediatr. Clin. North Am. **13:**835, 1966.

World Health Organization, Expert Committee on Maternal and Child Health: Public health aspects of low birth weight, WHO Tech. Rep. Ser. **217,** Ch. 11, 1961.

12

Infants at medium risk and their specific care

Infants at low risk (70% to 80%) have been identified and either placed in the observation nursery* or kept with their mother in a combined recovery room, a preferable option. In either event, a modified form of medium-risk care is advised for a 3- to 6-hour period for all low-risk infants. When normal behavior and activity are apparent, vital signs are stable, and satisfactory feeding is noted, the baby may be discharged home or placed in the regular nursery. This period will allow sufficient time for recovery from the birth process, metabolization of any transferred analgesic or anesthetic agents, and the emergence of most serious problems not apparent at birth. Eye prophylaxis and vitamin K should have already been given. A Coombs' test must be negative; a peripheral hematocrit (taken after 3 hours) should be between 40% and 65% before discharge is authorized.

INFANTS WHO JUSTIFY MEDIUM-RISK CARE

1. Birth asphyxia (Apgar score usually below 6 at 1 minute) requiring resuscitation but stable at 30 minutes
2. Birth trauma (e.g., excessive bruising, paralyses)
3. Abnormal behavior (e.g., lethargy, irritability, poor feeding)
4. Early appearance of jaundice (within 24 hours) and requiring phototherapy (Chapter 28)
5. Anemia (Hct less than 35%) and polycythemia (venous Hct greater than 65%) (Chapter 31)
6. Increased respiratory rate without cyanosis or distress, (e.g., tachypnea of newborn) (Chapter 27)
7. Multiple births (Chapter 20)
8. Prolonged rupture of membranes (Chapter 18)
9. Major congenital anomalies not requiring immediate surgery or critical care (Chapter 33)
10. Preterm infant 33 to 36 weeks' gestation
11. Dysmature or malnourished infant
12. Small-for-gestational-age (SGA) and undergrown infant
13. Large-for-gestational-age (LGA) and infant of a diabetic mother (IDM)

See this chapter for discussion of points 10 to 13.

General care requirements for medium-risk infants

1. Temperature control
   Place the neonate undressed on side or stomach in a prewarmed incubator or under radiant heat to maintain skin or axillary temperature between 36.0° to 36.5° C (97° to 98° F). Check temperature every 30 to 60 minutes until stable and then every 4 to 8 hours.
2. Attach heart rate monitor or heart rate and apnea monitor, and set low alarm for heart rate between 80 and 100 beats/min. Set low alarm for apneic periods at 15 seconds if apnea monitor is used.

---

*In many hospitals, the observation nursery is combined with the special-care or medium-risk nursery where close nursing supervision can be maintained.

3. Record heart and respiratory rate every hour for six times or until stable and then every 2 to 4 hours.
4. Take blood pressure by transcutaneous Doppler method; report if systolic pressure is below 50 mm Hg (40 in the more immature) or above 90 mm Hg.
5. Be prepared to offer parenteral fluids (Chapter 15) when oral feeding is risky or unsatisfactory.
6. Order peripheral hematocrit.
7. Perform Dextrostix test at 2, 12, and 24 hours (more often in LGA infants, infants of diabetic mothers, and SGA babies, Fig. 12-1).
8. Offer a milk feeding by 3 hours, if active and responsive and if in no distress, and then every 3 hours or when hungry (Chapter 16). Instead of milk, some physicians prefer to start with sterile water for fear of aspiration. We do not do this but give feedings with caution after stomach contents have been emptied and when patency of esophagus is shown.
9. Treatments
Administer eye prophylaxis against gonococcal ophthalmia, such as ophthalmic ointment containing 0.5% erythromycin. Give intramuscularly 0.5 to 1 mg of vitamin K_1, for example, AquaMephyton.
10. Skin care
When condition and temperature are stable, wash off excess blood and mucus. Bathing is not necessary, and plain water to cleanse genital and buttock area is sufficient.
11. Cord care
Keep cord stump uncovered. Treatment with 1.67% povidone-iodine solution lessens chance of colonization with pathogenic

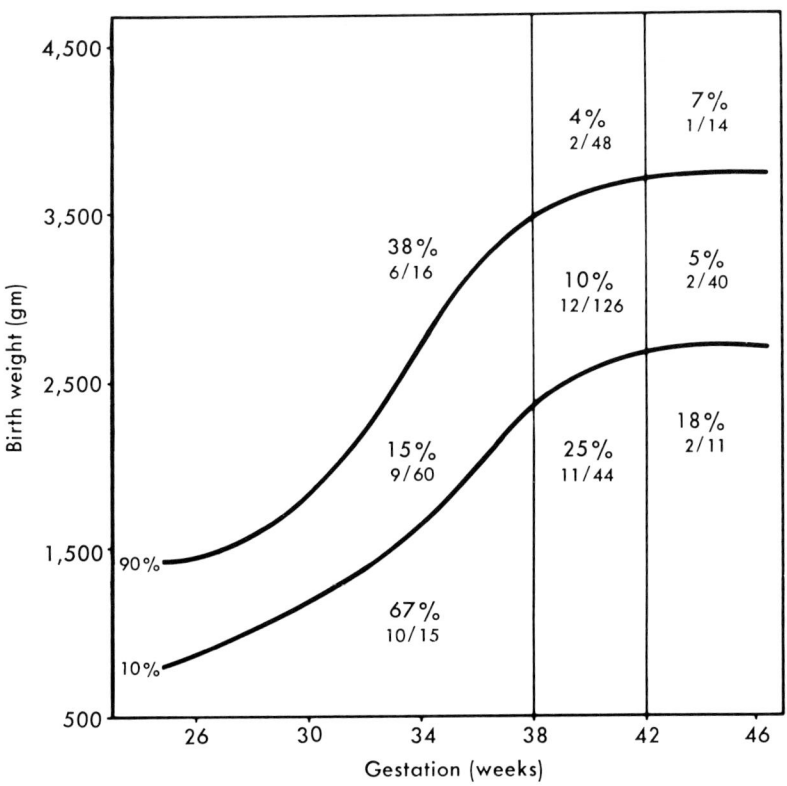

Fig. 12-1. Incidence of hypoglycemia (glucose levels less than 30 mg/100ml prior to first feeding) in newborn infants, classified by birth weight and gestational age. Numbers below percentages indicate number of hypoglycemic infants per total number of infants studied. (From Lubchenco, L.D., and Bard, H.: Pediatrics **47**:831, 1971. Copyright American Academy of Pediatrics, 1971.)

organisms. If stump is macerated or moist, apply 70% alcohol each shift. If infection is suspected, culture and consider parenteral antibiotics.

PRETERM INFANTS (33 TO 37 WEEKS OF GESTATIONAL AGE—1,500 TO 2,750 gm)

The preterm group is the largest at medium risk, accounting for 5% to 7% of all newborns with a mortality of 1% to 5%, depending on maturity. If not depressed at birth, they will usually accept the bottle, and the more vigorous will be able to nurse from their mothers. Infants of 32 weeks gestation or less, usually weighing under 1,600 gm and accounting for 1% of all babies born, should be cared for in a neonatal intensive care unit because of their high-risk status. The special problems of the small premature infant are discussed in Chapter 26.

Requirements of care

1. Offer medium-risk care as outlined above.
2. Increase level of care if:
   a. Respiratory rate rises above 60 per minute.
   b. Chest retractions or expiratory grunting develops.
   c. Bradycardia (less than 100 beats/min) is observed.
   d. Apnea (longer than 10 seconds) occurs.
   e. Cyanosis, pallor, or other changes in behavior develop.
3. Weigh daily. Loss in weight over 10% requires assessment of fluid and calorie intake.
4. Observe for jaundice every 6 hours and obtain bilirubin level at first sign of jaundice. See discussion on neonatal hyperbilirubinemia in Chapter 28.
5. Begin oral feedings with human milk or 20-calorie formula at 3 hours if infant is stable and active. For detailed instructions see Chapter 16.
6. Place infant to breast when able to nurse. Usually this act is unsatisfactory until infant is 35 weeks of postmenstrual age.
7. Discharge home when the following occur (Chapter 14):
   a. Infant has started to gain and feeds well. Weight is not important if infant is sufficiently mature (36 or more weeks of postmenstrual age) and vigorous.
   b. Jaundice is minimal or bilirubin level has fallen under 10 mg/100 ml.
   c. Axillary temperature is maintained in bassinette above 36° C (97° F).
   d. Mother and home are ready (a public health nurse report on home is acceptable).
   e. Arrangements for continuing care have been made, and a phone number is available for advice.

POSTTERM INFANTS (42 WEEKS OR MORE OF GESTATIONAL AGE)

(Prolonged pregnancy is discussed in Chapter 18.)

Postterm infants comprise about 3% of infants born. The slowing in growth as the fetus reaches term is accentuated as term is passed. With aging of the placenta, a decrease in the provision of nutrients to the fetus, including oxygen, occurs, resulting at times in loss of fetal weight with actual wasting of the subcutaneous tissues (dysmaturity) (Fig. 18-3). These infants are often asphyxiated and experience prolonged exposure to meconium-contaminated amniotic fluid. Special attention at birth with early provision of calories and glucose as outlines for SGA infants is indicated.

Some postterm fetuses have large placentas with efficient transport of nutrients and when labor does not ensue, growth and development may continue unabated until 45 weeks of gestational age. The larger size and increased calcification of their bones places them at risk for birth injury.

LARGE-FOR-GESTATIONAL-AGE INFANTS

(See discussion in Chapter 19.)

We restrict this group to the 5% of infants whose measurements at birth are near +2 SD on the growth chart (Fig. 11-2). When these babies are the products of large mothers no birth difficulty would normally occur, but when women gain weight excessively in pregnancy, they tend to oversupply nutrition to the fetus. Such infants may be injured from difficult labor because of cephalopelvic disproportion or shoulder dystocia.

Approximately 1% of all infants are oversized from frank or latent diabetes in the mother. They are big as well as heavy for length, as shown on Fig. 11-3. In addition to the chance of temporary hyperinsulinism (and hypoglycemia), these infants are often delivered early and are especially subject to respiratory distress syndrome, hyperbilirubinemia, and hypocalcemia.

Because of the risks faced by LGA infants, they should be given medium-risk care as follows:

1. Early feedings (when tolerated) at 1 hour of life of an isosmolar formula (20 kcal/30 ml) (Chapter 16)
2. Dextrostix testing on admission and every hour until glucose is stabilized between 50 and 90 mg/100 ml

    When blood glucose level falls below 40 mg/100 ml, an infusion of 10% dextrose at the rate of 5 microdrops/kg/min (5 ml/kg/hr) is started until feedings are begun and blood glucose is stable. Occasionally hypoglycemia persists, and solutions containing 15% glucose may be necessary.
3. Add 3 ml of 10% calcium gluconate to each 100 ml of infusion to maintain serum calcium levels above 8 mg/100 ml.

SMALL-FOR-GESTATIONAL-AGE INFANTS

A discussion of the growth-retarded fetus with etiology and management is found in Chapter 19. Anticipation at birth of an SGA infant or its prompt recognition is essential for the special care required. This includes any infant at birth who plots near the -2 SD line on Fig. 11-2 or is below the 10th percentile on the Colorado grid (Fig. 4-2). Differentiation of the undergrown infant from the preterm appropriate-for-gestational-age (AGA) infant of the same weight is outlined in Table 12-1. In addition to the search for genetic malformations and chromosomal defects (such as Down's syndrome), fetally contracted infections (such as rubella), and teratogenic insults (such as alcohol), support of the infant's undernutrition and avoidance of hypoglycemia is important. These babies, as well as those who show tissue wasting (dysmaturity), should be given medium-risk care as follows:

1. Start feedings as soon as infant is active and stable. Increase by 5 ml per feeding every 2 to 3 hours and continue up to easy tolerance; 24 or 27 calorie milk (0.8 or 0.9 kcal/ml) help to satisfy caloric requirements (Chapter 16).
2. Perform a Dextrostix test soon after birth and every 4 hours until blood glucose level stabilizes over 50 mg/100 ml.
3. Infuse 10% glucose if feedings are taken poorly or glucose level falls below 40 mg/100 ml.
4. Monitor glucose levels during glucose infusions and after discontinuation to avoid hyperglycemia and hypoglycemia, respectively.

HYPOGLYCEMIA (see also Chapter 32)

The increased frequency of hypoglycemia in the preterm infant and high incidence noted in all infants who are SGA as presented in Fig. 12-1 is compelling evidence for careful monitoring of blood glucose in all infants at any risk. Although there is usually no evidence of permanent damage in hypoglycemic infants short of convulsions, the risk of hypoglycemia is sufficiently great to avoid its occurrence.

PROBLEMS DEVELOPING THAT MAY REQUIRE TRANSFER TO REGIONAL CENTER

1. *Increasing tachypnea or breathing effort* (Chapter 27)
    a. Keep infant undressed in warmed environment.
    b. Maintain clear airway.
    c. Give sufficient oxygen to just relieve cyanosis of mucous membranes.
    d. Start glucose infusion of 10% concentration at a rate of 3 ml/kg/hr (Chapter 15).
    e. Obtain pH, blood gas measurements, and chest x-ray film.

    If infant's condition requires over 30% ambient oxygen, transfer to neonatal intensive care unit.
2. *Development of cyanosis* (Chapter 29). In addition to offering medium-risk care, check heart for activity and rate and maximum impulse, liver for enlargement, and femoral arteries for pulsations. Take blood pressure in arms and legs and obtain an ECG. If infant continues to have cyanosis that is unresponsive to oxygen or demonstrates any heart failure, he may have congenital heart disease and should be transferred to a tertiary center.
3. *Seizures* (Chapter 30). Any seizure in the first 48 hours of life is most likely caused by asphyxia at birth. Hypoglycemia, hypocalcemia, and infection must be considered, how-

Table 12-1. Comparison of clinical features of growth-retarded term infants with those of large premature babies, both approximately 2,250 gm (5 lb)

	Growth retarded (38+ weeks)	Large premature (34 weeks)
Body size	Reduced body size for gestation; weight in general reduced more than length or head circumference; head circumference usually reduced least	Body measurement proportional and appropriate for gestational age
Weight loss	Minimal weight loss, if any, after birth, usually under 5%	5% to 10% of birth weight
External appearance		
Skin	Minimal subcutaneous tissue, often loose and wrinkled; scaly and cracked in dysmaturity	May be edematous and shiny
	Milia often present	Milia not seen
Color	Whiter from thicker epidermis despite higher hematocrit	Pink
Vernix	Minimal to absent	Abundant
Lanugo	None	Moderate
Hair	Sparse, straight, and silky	Fine and fuzzy
Sole creases	Extend over whole sole	Anterior third only
Skull bones	Firm on palpation to edges—often suture separation without increase in spinal fluid pressure	Soft and pliable—skull bones overlap at sutures
Ear cartilage	Erect, with sharp ridges	Soft and pliable
Scrotum	Testes pendulous with well-developed rugae	Not completely descended, few rugae
Labia	Labia minora tend to be covered	Labia minora more prominent
Breast tissue	Nodule with or without gland swelling, depending on degree of fetal malnutrition	Nodule absent
Cord stump	Thin and often discolored; dries early	White and thickened
Behavior		
Activity	Active—eyes open with anxious appearance	Inactive, torpid, eyes closed
Feeding	Takes nipple eagerly, sucks fingers; gains rapidly	Takes nipple poorly; slow to regain birth weight
Neurologic signs		
Tone	Increased tone—holds head well on traction; raises head from mattress	Head lag on traction; cannot raise head
Moro reflex	Brisk, complete, but often restricted	Incomplete
Eye response	Fixes and follows with eye	No recognition
Transillumination	Under 2 cm of reflected light	2 to 4 cm
Electroencephalogram	Mature cerebral waves, short response to photic stimulation (157.4 ± 2 msec)	Mean peak latency of photic response (212.5 ± 20 msec)
Physiologic signs		
Oxygen consumption	Increased per kilogram of body weight over preterm infant	Slightly decreased compared to term infants
Temperature control	Better able to defend against heat loss (muscular activity, brown fat presence); however, heat conservation limited by reduced subcutaneous fat	Supplemental heat required to maintain body temperature
	Perspires and shivers	Neither perspires nor shivers
Organ systems	Regular respiration unless airway obstruction	Periodic breathing
	Concentrates urine well; minimal delay in bilirubin conjugation; decreased glycogen stores	Urine dilute; delay in conjugation of bilirubin; glycogen stores reduced, but usually adequate
Ossification centers		
Knee	Presence of both proximal tibial and distal femoral epiphyses—delay influenced by degree of fetal malnutrition	Absent

ever. A Dextrostix test should be performed immediately while an infusion of glucose is prepared. If the test shows less than 40 mg/100 ml, take a blood sample for glucose level and obtain blood for a calcium determination. Proceed with the infusion as outlined on p. 297.

4. *Early or intensifying jaundice* (Chapter 28). Any jaundice visible within the first 24 hours of life, or bilirubin levels above or around 10 mg/100 ml by 36 hours of age requires investigation.
5. *Pallor or anemia and plethora or polycythemia.* A hematocrit less than 40% at birth or less than 20% after 1 month of age are levels for which one considers transfusion. A peripheral hematocrit greater than 70% is an indication for screening to rule out hyperviscosity (Chapter 31).
6. *Bleeding diathesis.* If one is assured that vitamin K has been given, any acquired petechial hemorrhage after the birth process or easy bleeding on skin prick may be evidence of severe disease. Platelet counts are a most useful screening test because most neonates with serious bleeding problems are thrombocytopenic. Platelet counts may be estimated from a peripheral smear, that is, the average number of platelets per oil immersion field × 15,000. A more complete investigation of the infant's clotting factor is indicated.
7. *Apnea* (Chapter 28). All preterm infants must be monitored for apneic episodes. This can be accomplished in most instances by heart rate monitoring alone. Apnea leading to bradycardia and cyanosis not responding to simple stimulation requires investigation. Early apnea in the preterm and any apnea in the term infant could be a sign of sepsis or meningitis. Early apnea in the preterm may also indicate respiratory insufficiency.
8. *Lethargy and hypotonia.* Consider infection even before neurologic disease (Chapter 33).
9. *Feeding problems* (Chapter 16). Distention, regurgitation, and the presence of stomach residuals 3 hours after feeding on two successive occasions may mean overfeeding, but they also may be a sign of infection or necrotizing enterocolitis (Chapter 16). If such infants demonstrate lethargy, color change (increase in jaundice or pallor), or increase in apnea, a blood culture and a spinal tap should be performed and the infant should be given antibiotics (Chapter 25). Feedings should always be discontinued (nothing by mouth) and stomach kept empty until reassessment or recovery.

BIBLIOGRAPHY

Desmond, M.M., Rudolph, A.J., and Pineda, R.G.: Neonatal morbidity and nursery function, JAMA **212:**281, 1970.

Sjöstedt, S., Engleson, G., and Rooth, G.: Dysmaturity, Arch. Dis. Child. **33:**123, 1958.

13

Transport of the high-risk perinate

FETAL TRANSPORT

With careful evaluation of pregnant women and identification of the factors that significantly increase the risk of perinatal disaster, the development of special centers for the care of high-risk pregnancy has helped to reduce perinatal mortality. Some years ago an analysis of perinatal deaths in a Wisconsin study (Schneider, Sixty-sixth Ross Conference) indicated that two thirds of neonatal deaths and half of fetal deaths at that time were preventable. Further observation in that state showed that 80% to 90% of perinatal care in hospitals was given by nurses who in general had no special training.

These data strongly suggested that the 5% to 10% of women who contribute to the majority of perinatal mortality (Chapter 2) should be identified so that they can be referred for evaluation and perhaps delivery in a 24-hour perinatal team setting. This team may include house staff, but it should be emphasized that such personnel are in the learning process and should not have the prime responsibility for critical decisions. The more serious conditions requiring the support of a perinatal center are as follows:

1. Eclampsia and severe preeclampsia
2. Bleeding from placental separation
3. Multiple gestations
4. Significant maternal disease
5. Severe diabetes or isoimmunization
6. Hydramnios or oligohydramnios

Of more urgent nature is the fetus discovered to be at high risk when the pregnant mother demonstrates actual or threatened labor. Such women with fetuses of less than 34 weeks may be candidates for drug treatment that inhibits labor. Other complications are delineated in Chapter 2.

When these complications are identified in a community hospital, the physician may elect to consult with a perinatal center. The degree of progress toward birth is assessed and the time factor judged in relation to emergency transfer.

Transport is best not attempted under the following conditions:

1. When active labor is in progress with cervix dilated 4 cm or more, and the referral center is over 30 minutes away
2. When bleeding is brisk and transfusion capability is at hand
3. When fetal heart recordings show deceleration patterns and cesarean section can be effected promptly

NEONATAL TRANSPORT

The development of intensive care units for the severely ill infant during the last 15 years has been followed by the development of specialized transport systems in many areas of the country. Modern neonatal transport has become a necessary community and regional medical resource. The transfer of sick and small, preterm infants is not new, but the use of full intensive care during the trip, after any necessary stabilization—temperature, acid-base balance, and oxygen requirements—prior to the transport, has almost eliminated the hazards of travel. In fact, most jeopardized infants may arrive at a specialized center in better condition than they exhibited while they were in the referring hospital.

All regions should have coordinated programs of intercommunication and specialized teams for transport of neonates who are sick or at risk to specialized centers. For the type of infant problems suggesting need for transport from community hospital to a regional center, see Chapter 36.

High-risk infants
MODES OF TRANSPORT

1. Specially equipped ambulances or vans must be suitable for transport up to 100 miles from center, depending on traffic density, type of highway, and weather conditions. Equipment should include an AC power inverter, space for two transport incubators, an an adequate supply of compressed air and oxygen to operate a ventilator for 3 to 4 hours, suction, a transillumination light, and a resuscitation table with a source of heat for the infant.
2. Helicopters may be used for transports from 50 to 150 miles from center. Their use is advisable if road conditions are unfavorable and time of transport would be more than 2 hours by ground.
3. Twin-engined airplanes with all-weather capability can be used for transports 100 to 500 miles from center.

All transport vehicles should be capable of carrying three transport team members, a transport incubator with ventilator, equipment boxes, and at least two 80 cubic foot gas cylinders (air and oxygen).

TRANSPORT TEAM (IN ADDITION TO DRIVER, PILOT, AND AUXILIARY PERSONNEL BETWEEN HOSPITAL AND AIRPORT OR HELIPAD)

The transport team should be composed of a physician trained in neonatal care, a neonatal nurse, and a respiratory therapist, or a respiratory therapist and two neonatal nurses trained in providing the following specialized care:
1. Establishment of a peripheral or umbilical vessel infusion route
2. Endotracheal intubation and ventilatory support by bag and mask, constant positive airway pressure (CPAP), or ventilator
3. Fluid and metabolic support (e.g., prevention of hypoglycemia)
4. Special requirements as indicated by the baby's condition (e.g., treatment of possible sepsis, insertion of chest tubes)

ARRANGEMENTS TO BE MADE BY ADMITTING OR TRANSPORT OFFICER

1. Obtain pertinent clinical information (e.g., prolonged rupture of membranes, condition at birth) (Appendix D).
2. Give referring physician specific information on temporary care, including any specific treatment or laboratory aids.
3. Coordinate specific travel requirements and flight plans.
4. Obtain photocopies of referring hospital's chart forms (maternal and infant), collect x-ray films, obtain maternal blood (clotted and unclotted) and placenta, if possible.
5. Notify members of other services who might be involved (e.g., pediatric surgeon or cardiologist).
6. Obtain written consent for transport from parents.
7. Notify hospital admission and neonatal center personnel and provide appropriate information.

TRANSPORT TEAM ARRANGEMENTS

1. Check charge of all battery-powered equipment.
2. Check oxygen and compressed air supplies.
3. Make sure all equipment is assembled (Appendix C).

EQUIPMENT AND SUPPLIES FOR TRANSPORT (ASSEMBLED AND FUNCTIONING AT ALL TIMES)

1. Neonatal transport incubator with full temperature support—120-volt AC and 12-volt DC converters
2. Air cylinders: Oxygen and compressed air tanks with pressure regulating valves and tank-volume meter connected to air-oxygen blender with oxygen humidifier and sufficient supplies of each for length of trip and equipment to be used
3. Neonatal resuscitation bag with masks of various sizes (Laerdal or Penlon)
4. Heart rate monitor (battery powered) with skin electrodes (Squibb Vitatek, Inc., Hillsboro, Oregon, 97123)
5. Battery-powered infusion pump with complete intravenous administration set (IMED, Holter, Autosyringe)
6. Telethermometer and skin probe (Yellow Springs, Yellow Springs, Ohio)

7. Doppler blood pressure equipment, with sphygmomanometer (Parks Electronics, Beaverton, Oregon) and/or pressure transducer setup for direct pressure monitoring through arterial catheter
8. Bulb syringe, DeLee suction trap, or portable suction
9. Small plastic hood for oxygen administration with oxygen analyzer
10. Apparatus for delivering continuous positive airway pressure (CPAP) or intermittent positive-pressure breathing (IPPB) with positive end-expiratory pressure (PEEP)
11. Transcutaneous oxygen monitor
12. Tackle boxes containing additional equipment for the following purposes (Appendix C)
    a. Resuscitation
    b. Peripheral intravenous administration
    c. Umbilical artery catheterization
    d. Endotracheal suction
    e. Chest drainage
    f. Administration of emergency drugs
13. Clipboard with transport log, consent for transport form, and information booklets for parent

CARE AND STABILIZATION OF HIGH-RISK INFANTS, PARTICULARLY THOSE WITH RESPIRATORY DISTRESS

Before infants are transported between hospitals, sufficient stabilization and diagnostic procedures should be performed to avoid unnecessary emergencies en route and to ensure safe arrival.

I. Oxygenation/ventilation
   A. Determine patency of airway, color, respiratory efficiency, and need for assisted ventilation.
   B. If any respiratory distress or need for increased fraction of inspired oxygen ($F_{I_{O_2}}$) is present, obtain a chest x-ray film.
   C. Direct oxygen into plastic hood (Oxyhood), humidified with sterile water, to keep mucous membranes pink.
   D. If an $F_{I_{O_2}}$ of 0.35 or greater is needed, obtain arterial blood gas measurements.
   E. Consider starting CPAP if an $F_{I_{O_2}}$ of 0.5 or more is needed, there is clinical and x-ray evidence of hyaline membrane disease, the P_{CO_2} is less than 50, and there is no apnea.
   F. Intubation and artificial ventilation should be carried out if there is severe apnea, the P_{CO_2} is above 60, or an $F_{I_{O_2}}$ of 0.8 or greater is needed to maintain oxygenation. Clinical judgment may determine the need for intubation in unstable patients prior to transport.
   G. Rule out and treat pneumothorax prior to transport (p. 263).
II. Temperature control (p. 122)
   A. Attach skin probe of battery-powered telethermometer, and make sure temperature reading agrees with infant's axillary temperature.
   B. If infant is hypothermic (a temperature of less than 36°C or 97°F), increase the environmental temperature to warm infant gradually over 1 hour.
      If you are unable to maintain infant's temperature, use plastic coverings, heat lamps, or hot water bottles *with care*. Monitor blood pressure to detect any hypotension from too rapid rewarming. In cold weather, cover incubator with a blanket or aluminum foil to reduce radiant heat loss.
III. Metabolism, fluid, and glucose support
   A. Assess infant's blood glucose level with Chemstrip (Bio Dynamics Co., Indianapolis) test. If reading is below 25 to 40 mg/100 ml, give 5 ml/kg of D10W as intravenous push, and then follow with continuous infusion (3 ml/kg/hr).
   B. Place intravenous line for continuous infusion of fluid.
      1. Infuse D10W if Chemstrip reading is less than 125.
      2. Place an umbilical artery catheter for infants who are very tiny or very unstable or who require an $F_{I_{O_2}}$ above 0.35.

C. Correct acidosis (p. 256).
IV. Monitoring of vital signs
   A. Attach battery-powered heart rate monitor.
   B. Measure blood pressure (Doppler method) and repeat every 15 to 30 minutes if infant is hypotensive or tissue perfusion is poor.
   C. Check respiratory rate every 15 to 30 minutes.
V. Consider shock and be prepared to give blood, albumin, or Plasmanate (Cutter Biological, Berkeley, Calif. 94710) if
   A. Blood pressure is below normal (Chapter 29).
   B. Hematocrit is under 40.
   C. Infant has mottled or pallid skin suggesting poor tissue perfusion.
VI. Emptying stomach
   A. Aspirate stomach contents prior to transport to prevent vomiting and aspiration.
   B. If gastrointestinal obstruction is suspected, or if transport is by air, leave orogastric tube to gravity drainage.
VII. Suspected sepsis
   A. Obtain blood culture and gastric aspirate and, if possible, perform lumbar puncture and suprapubic bladder tap.
   B. Begin antibiotic therapy.
VIII. Pneumothorax
   A. Suspect if following signs occur: sudden worsening of infant's condition, onset of cyanosis, sudden onset of abdominal distention, falling blood pressure, increased anterior diameter of chest.
   B. Support infant with oxygen as needed.
   C. Confirm diagnosis by x-ray examination or transillumination of chest if possible.
   D. If baby is in severe distress, insert 18-gauge Angiocath into fourth intercostal space on midaxillary line, connect to three-way stopcock and large syringe, and aspirate air.
   E. A chest tube (Fr 10 or 12) for chest drainage during transport should be placed and connected to a Heimlich valve.
IX. Surgical problems
   A. *Intestinal obstruction.* Pass large-bore orogastric tube and leave to gravity drainage. Aspirate frequently.
   B. *Esophageal atresia.* Position baby on right side on an inclined plane (45 degrees) in head-up position. Pass a feeding tube into the upper pouch of the esophagus and aspirate frequently. Aspirate oropharynx with bulb syringe or DeLee trap frequently.
   C. *Omphalocele or gastroschisis.* Cover site with warm moist saline gauze, wrap with Kerlix, and cover with sterile plastic to prevent hypothermia. Avoid use of tape on abdomen. Pay special attention to temperature control.
   D. *Diaphragmatic hernia.* Insert orogastric tube and aspirate frequently. Attempt to maintain skin color with oxygen. Use no positive pressure unless there is increasing cyanosis, and then accomplish this by use of endotracheal tube only, with pressures under 30 cm H_2O, if possible.
   E. *Choanal atresia.* Tape oral airway in place.
   F. *Pierre Robin syndrome.* Position infant on abdomen. Tape airway in place or intubate, if necessary.
X. Parents
   A. Discuss infant's condition and explain need for special care.
   B. Obtain a brief history.
   C. Provide parents with information regarding the neonatal intensive care center, including telephone numbers, visiting policies, and names of key personnel.
   D. Obtain written consent for transport of infant.
   E. Before departing, wheel infant into mother's room to explain equipment, and lend support and en-

couragement to the parents and to have them touch their baby.
XI. Miscellaneous
  A. Consider regulations and sensitivities of referring hospital and staff.
  B. Administer vitamin K and eye prophylaxis if this has not been done.
  C. Record problems identified, vital signs, treatments, procedures, and medications given during transport on a transport log.

CARE OF INFANT DURING TRANSPORT

1. Observe color, respirations, and heart rate.
2. Maintain skin temperature at 36° to 36.5° C (97° to 98° F).
3. Adjust ventilatory support and oxygen as required.
4. In case of sudden worsening of infant's condition, consider:
   a. Respiratory tract obstruction by mucus or fluid
   b. Pneumothorax or pneumopericardium
   c. Endotracheal tube or left mainstem bronchus obstruction
   d. Extubation
   e. Oxygen equipment or ventilator malfunction
5. Notify parents and referring hospital of baby's arrival.
6. Reassemble and clean equipment in preparation for next transport.
7. For care of infant on admission to neonatal intensive care center, see p. 127.

SUMMARY

Neonatal transport for the infant in severe distress requires the prompt mobilization of a team not only trained in transport details but able to give emergency care aimed at the stabilization of the infant's physiologic state prior to transport. In most instances the infant will arrive at the neonatal center in better condition than he was in when first referred.

Infants at medium risk

Transport from a community or primary hospital to an intermediary hospital for infants at only moderate risk is a new concept in neonatal care. Such transfers should be restricted to one geographic area, preferably within a 50-mile radius, and should include babies with hyperbilirubinemia, moderate prematurity (over 32 weeks' gestation and weighing 1,500 gm), failure to thrive, and mild-to-moderate respiratory distress (see Chapter 12). Infants not responding to intermediary hospital care can in turn be sent to a tertiary neonatal center.

Requirements

1. Arrangements and equipment requirements are similar to those outlined on p. 115.
2. Personnel, equipment, and support, depending on the situation and condition of the baby, should include one or two nurses experienced in observation of the newborn, temperature control, suction, oxygen and full ventilatory support, and maintenance of parenteral infusion.

SUMMARY

There are two services to be performed in medium-risk transport:
1. Removal of infants at medium risk from primary hospitals (usually delivering fewer than 1,000 babies per year) to a designated intermediary hospital able to give continuing specialized care
2. Transfer of infants from a tertiary center to the intermediate care center for the continued growth and recovery of an infant who no longer requires intensive care

Because the parents will live closer to this unit, better parent-infant relations can be established.

Problems of transport

The effectiveness of neonatal transport in lowering morbidity and mortality depends on the efficiency of team care before and during transport. The following unsatisfactory situations have been repeatedly documented before and during transport services:
1. Inadequate resuscitation at birth
2. Failure to give basic support before transport team arrives
3. Cooling of infant as a result of failure of equipment or inexperience of personnel
4. Hypoventilation with or without airway obstruction; failure to intubate and offer sufficient oxygen and ventilatory support
5. Undetected pneumothorax or displacement of endotracheal tube

6. Failure to use essential monitoring equipment
7. Inadequate nursing observation of critically ill infant
8. Use of untrained personnel for transport responsibility
9. Inadequate physician communication between referring center and neonatal intensive care unit

TRAINING OF TRANSPORT NURSES

If nurses are used as leaders of a neonatal transport team, special training is required to familiarize them with equipment and emergency procedures. Telephone contact with a physician in the neonatal intensive care center is also desirable, along with a set of written guidelines. Training should include a combination of didactic and practice sessions as well as experience under supervision on actual transports.

1. Suggested didactic sessions
   a. Assessment of the infant and identification of problems
   b. Interpretation of x-ray films and laboratory values
   c. Treatment of conditions such as hypoglycemia, seizures, respiratory distress syndrome, sepsis, shock, and surgical problems
   d. Resuscitation of the neonate
   e. Use of transport equipment
   f. Obtainment of maternal history
2. Suggested practice sessions
   a. Peripheral intravenous insertion
   b. Umbilical artery and vein catheter insertion using model made with pieces of umbilical cord
   c. Endotracheal intubation of model and anesthetized cats
   d. Chest drainage—insertion of Angiocath and chest tubes in anesthetized rabbits

BIBLIOGRAPHY

Baker, G.L.: Design and operation of a van for the transport of sick infants, Am. J. Dis. Child. **118:**743, 1969.

Butterfield, J.: Denver newborn transport service manual, Denver, Colo., 1974, The Children's Hospital.

Chance, G.W., Mathew, J.D., Gash, J., et al.: Neonatal transport: a controlled study of skilled assistance, J. Pediatr. **93:**662, 1978.

Chance, G.W., O'Brien, M.J., and Swyer, P.B.: Transportation of sick neonates, 1972: an unsatisfactory aspect of medical care, Can. Med. Assoc. J. **109:**847, 1973.

Cunningham, M.D., and Smith, F.R.: Stabilization and transport of severely ill infants, Pediatr. Clin. North Am. **20:**359, 1973.

Ferrara, A., and Harin, A.: Emergency transfer of the high-risk neonate: a working manual for medical, nursing, and administrative personnel, St. Louis, 1980, The C.V. Mosby Co.

Jung, A.L., and Bose, G.L.: Backtransport of neonates: improved efficiency of teritiary nursery bed utilization, Pediatrics 7:918, 1983.

Pettett, G., Merenstein, G.B., Battaglia, F.C., et al.: An analysis of air transport results in the sick newborn infant: Part I. The transport team, Pediatrics **55:**774, 1975.

Segal, S., editor: Manual for the transport of high-risk newborn infants: principles, policies, equipment, techniques, Vancouver, British Columbia, 1972, Canadian Pediatric Society.

Shepard, K.S.: Air transportation of high-risk infants utilizing a flying intensive care nursery, J. Pediatr. **77:**148, 1970.

14

Intensive care of high-risk infants

NURSERY FACILITIES*

Improved knowledge and greater emphasis on protection of the fetus during labor and the infant at delivery have resulted in an increased number of living, immature infants who require nursery care. The larger general hospital is geared to intensive care for the severely ill and postoperative adult patients. Such an institution has a similar responsibility for ensuring optimal treatment for newborns with critical problems.

The very small, premature infants are too often recipients of substandard care in the expectation that they will die. They may be deposited in incubators of uncertain efficiency, and if they show signs of survival after a period of neglect, consultation may be sought. If they do live, the delay in metabolic and nutritional support may have impaired their chances for normal development.

The smaller premature infants, as well as infants with recognizable problems, should be transferred to a medical center if facilities and skills for appropriate care are not available. General nursery facilities for intensive newborn care should include the following:

1. Scrub facilities at the entrance with hot and cold water, knee or arm controls, orange sticks, and an organic iodine solution or chlorhexidine
2. Open radiant warmers or incubators with controlled-air environments and bacterial filters over the air intake vents for all high-risk neonates (Fig. 14-1 shows a current intensive care module.)
3. Accurate monitoring equipment for oxygen concentration, heart rate, respirations, and blood pressure
4. Facilities to provide phototherapy
5. An accurate scale, preferably of the automatic beam type, such as the Toledo Baby Weigh scale
6. Approximately 60 square feet for each infant (Critical care in an open warmer will require more space, whereas a recovering infant in an Isolette will need less.)
7. Effective illumination for vision (A daylight fluorescent light source, placed at 7 to 8 feet from the floor, will improve observation of the infant and should supply approximately 75 to 100 footcandles at the incubator level.)
8. Eight to 12 electrical outlets for each infant, with adequate grounding and half of the outlets on an emergency power circuit
9. Two oxygen outlets and at least one outlet each for vacuum and compressed air for each infant
10. Temperature of the nursery maintained at 24° C (75° F)
11. Air conditioning under positive-pressure ventilation (12 changes per hour), with neutral humidity in the range of 50%
12. Rooms for preparation of formula and intravenous solutions
13. Diaper and soiled linen receptacles in each nursery division, with foot-

---

*See also the discussion of regionalization of perinatal care and requirements for personnel and services in Chapter 36.

Intensive care of high-risk infants 121

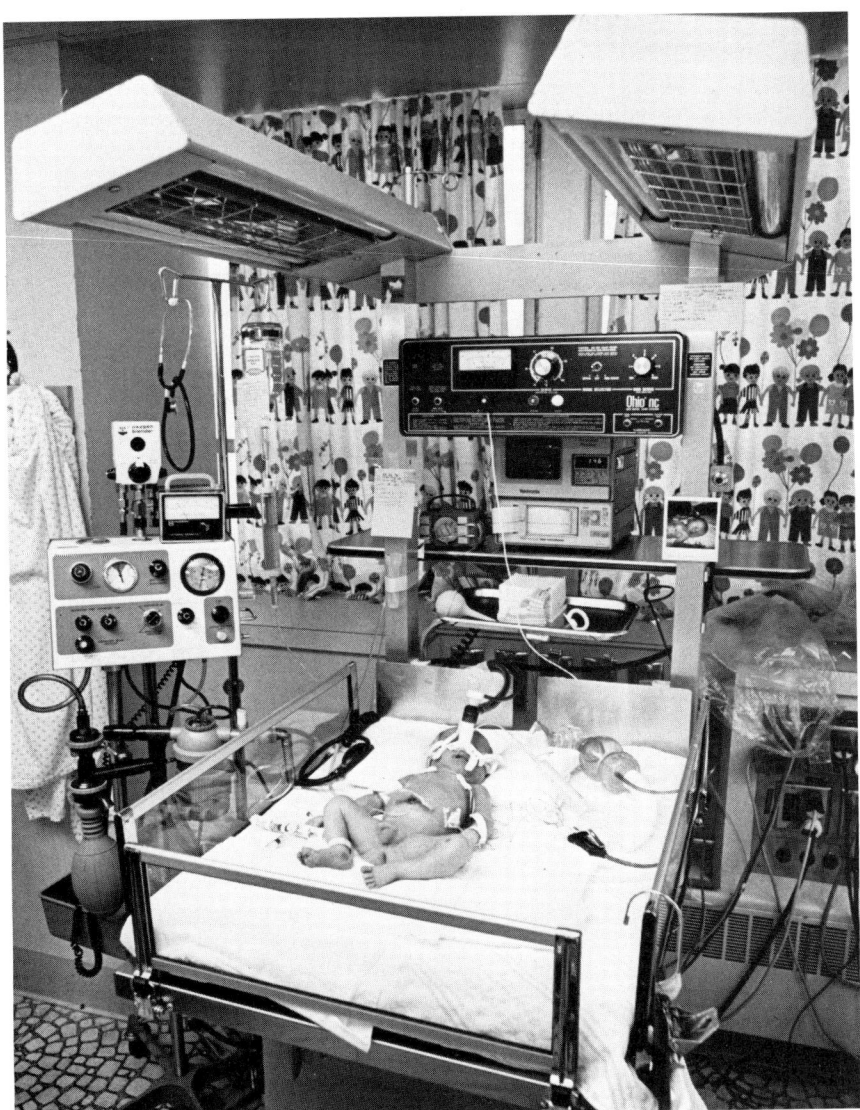

Fig. 14-1. Current intensive care module for use in care of a critically ill infant. Temperature of infant is monitored through sensor attached to his skin and connected to overhead radiant heating units. Surface electrodes attached to infant are connected to monitoring cable of neonatal monitor equipped to give digital, oscilloscope, and strip recorder readouts of heart and respiratory rate. Direct arterial blood pressure and temperature display is also possible with monitor (not in use in picture). Infant is receiving transpulmonary distending pressure with nasal prongs. A Laerdal resuscitation bag is positioned on mattress as backup in case of respirator failure. Umbilical artery catheter is placed for sampling of blood gases and administration of parenteral fluids, which are infused by pump (on shelf). (See also Fig. 10-2).

controlled covers (Disposable diapers are recommended.)
14. Demonstration room for instructing mothers in the care of their infants
15. Rocking chairs for the comfort of parents, nurse, and infant during feeding periods
16. Autoclave available for laundering soiled clothing separately from the regular hospital laundry
17. An area for special segregation of infants requiring isolation technique

NURSERY REGULATIONS FOR CONTROL OF INFECTIONS

Nursery infections are spread to healthy infants from other babies who are infected, from contaminated equipment and incubators, or from insufficient handwashing, poorly treated laundry, and infected personnel.

The head nurse of any nursery must have the responsibility of policing the nursery and firmly but gently enforcing the rules of cleanliness. Regulations have become less restrictive, and many nurseries now allow nurses to wear regular short-sleeved uniforms in the nursery, although they must cover with gowns to pick up infants. Caps and masks are considered unnecessary. Emphasis continues to be on handwashing. This easing of regulations has improved care of the patient and opened up off-limit areas to students and parents under supervision.

1. Technique to be used before entering the nursery
   a. Remove watch and ornamental rings, and wash hands.
   b. Scrub hands and arms to elbows for 1 minute with soap containing an organic iodine solution or chlorhexidine gluconate.
   c. Clean fingernails with an orange stick and repeat b.
   d. Dry hands with a paper towel.
   e. Physicians and visitors should don short-sleeved gowns if they handle infants.
2. Technique in nursery
   a. Wash hands just before and after handling any infant or touching one's own face, handkerchief, etc.
   b. Consider the incubator's tops, sides, controls, and handles as part of the baby's environment.
   c. Do not consider pencils, tape measures, thermometers, bulb syringes, etc., as interchangeable but as part of each baby's environment.
3. Responsibilities of charge nurse
   a. Limit entry to nursery to only those who are responsible for care, those who would benefit from observation of the infants, or parents.
   b. Exclude from nursery any person with infection, that is, open, draining skin lesions, or viral, bacterial, respiratory, or gastrointestinal infections.
   c. Orient and supervise all new personnel, students, and parents in the routines for infection control.
   d. Maintain strict protective techniques.
4. Equipment and cleaning
   a. Sterilize all equipment at the time of infant's discharge by autoclaving or gas sterilization, if possible; otherwise, use a quaternary ammonia solution.
   b. Clean humidity tanks if they are to be used, and replace sterile water daily.
   c. Wet-mop floors daily with a commercial antiseptic, for example, Microphene (1:1,000).
   d. Clean inside and outside surfaces of incubators and cribs with a quaternary ammonia solution.
   e. Wipe stethoscopes and other equipment between use with a similar antiseptic solution.

TEMPERATURE CONTROL*

Temperature homeostasis is impaired in the premature infant after birth because of his relatively large surface area, the paucity of subcutaneous tissues (including "brown fat"), lessened muscular activity, decreased metabolic response to cooling, and limited ability to sweat or shiver. A temperature that seems warm to adults is cool for babies.

To maintain the skin or axillary temperature of the unclothed, depressed, premature neonate at 36.5° C (98° F), and so to provide for minimal oxygen consumption by the infant, a surrounding temperature between 32° and 36° C (90° and 97° F) will be required, depending

---
*See conversion table for Fahrenheit to Celsius degrees inside the back cover.

on the infant's maturity, size, and metabolic activity (Table 14-1).

This neutral zone of temperature should be maintained from the period of birth, during transfer to the nursery, and throughout any procedure.

Hazards from excessive temperature

1. Obligatory increase in metabolic rate and oxygen requirement
2. Increase in apneic episodes
3. Danger of shock from vasodilation

Hazards from cooling

1. Obligatory increase in metabolic rate and oxygen requirement
2. Vasoconstriction with increase in acidosis with hypoxia
3. Rise in free fatty acid level of the blood, with reduction in glucose and interference with bilirubin binding

Table 14-1. Incubator air temperatures for the first 24 hours

Birth weight		Temperatures* (median ± range)	
gm	lb oz	°C	°F
	1' 0"	35.5 ± 0.5	96.0 ± 0.9
500		35.5 ± 0.5	96.0 ± 0.9
	2' 0"	35.0 ± 0.5	95.0 ± 0.9
1,000		34.9 ± 0.5	94.9 ± 0.9
	3' 0"	34.2 ± 0.5	93.6 ± 0.9
1,500		34.0 ± 0.5	93.2 ± 0.9
	4' 0"	33.7 ± 0.5	92.7 ± 0.9
2,000		33.5 ± 0.5	92.3 ± 0.9
	5' 0"	33.3 ± 0.7	92.0 ± 1.3
2,500		33.2 ± 0.8	91.8 ± 1.4
	6' 0"	33.1 ± 0.9	91.6 ± 1.6
3,000		33.0 ± 1.0	91.4 ± 1.8
	7' 0"	32.9 ± 1.1	91.2 ± 1.9
3,500		32.8 ± 1.2	91.0 ± 2.1
	8' 0"	32.8 ± 1.3	91.0 ± 2.3
4,000		32.6 ± 1.4	90.7 ± 2.5
	9' 0"	32.5 ± 1.4	90.5 ± 2.5

From Segal, S., editor: Manual for the transport of high-risk newborn infants: principles, policies, equipment, techniques, Vancouver, British Columbia, 1972, Canadian Paediatric Society; adapted from data published by Scopes and Ahmed (1966) and Oliver (1965).

*Temperatures given are recommended for use as an initial guide when relative humidity is approximately 50%. A lower humidity would require higher temperatures. Various other factors in the thermal environment and the individual infant's requirements will justify a temperature that is higher or lower than those given here. Some very immature infants require a somewhat higher ambient temperature.

4. Increase in apneic episodes
5. Increase in mortality (may intensify hyaline membrane disease)

Techniques of temperature regulation

I. A clinical thermometer capable of registering to 29° C (84° F) is needed.
   A. Hold thermometer firmly in infant's axilla* for 90 seconds.
   B. Take infant's temperature every hour until it is stabilized at 36.5° ± 0.5° C (98° ± 1° F) by adjustment of incubator control dial; then take and record temperature every 2 to 4 hours.
II. A closed incubator offers good visibility of infant, bacterial air filtering, and stable humidity, as well as a controlled environmental temperature. Incubator should be warmed to infant's neutral thermal environment before using (see Table 14-1). Axillary and incubator temperatures should be checked and recorded at least every 3 hours.
   A. Manual adjustment
      1. Take axillary temperature every 30 to 60 minutes until it is stabilized by adjustment of incubator temperature control dial.
      2. To avoid inadvertent wide temperature swings, adjust temperature control knob only slightly when necessary and check incubator and infant's temperature frequently until it is stable.
   B. Servo control—an automatic sensing device used in the modern incubator for maintaining the infant's temperature at a prescribed level through a thermistor attachment to the skin
      1. Attach thermistor with heat-reflecting patches or nonirritating plastic tape at infant's abdomen between navel and xiphoid process, while infant is kept on his back; attachment to side of abdomen allows baby to be on his abdomen as well as on his back.

---

*We do not recommend rectal temperature measurement because of hand contamination, possible injury to the infant, and delayed response of core temperature to sudden thermal changes.

2. When infant's temperature is low or high, check probe placement and contact with skin. Monitor axillary and incubator temperatures frequently until they are stable.
III. An open radiant warmer offers good accessibility to infant requiring frequent or prolonged procedures (i.e., umbilical artery catheterization, ventilator care) and controls infant's temperature automatically. Insensible water loss may be increased significantly in small infants.
   A. Use servo control as described under IIB.
   B. Check thermistor site frequently for good skin contact and make sure temperature alarm is turned on. Monitor and record infant's temperature at least every 3 hours.
   C. Place heat shield or piece of plastic over infant to reduce heat loss from air currents and water loss through skin.
IV. Additional techniques for the very low birth weight infant include the following:
   A. Place a plastic shield over the baby.
   B. Temporarily focus a 150-watt Sylvania or General Electric spotlamp on baby through incubator top from a distance of about 1 meter (3 feet).
   C. Line several walls of incubator with aluminum foil.
   D. Wrap infant in clear plastic.
   E. Carefully apply warm well-wrapped hot water bottles.
   F. Ensure that air-oxygen mixtures entering incubator or hood are warmed to required environmental temperature of infant.

Problems in temperature regulation

1. Check the infant's temperature if his body or extremities are cool to the touch.
2. Report a temperature drop of more than 1° to 2°. Suspect the following:
   a. An unadjusted or disconnected incubator
   b. Radiation loss to a cold window, wall, or cool environment (The use of a plastic shield placed over the infant will minimize this radiant heat loss.)
   c. Air-oxygen mixtures that have not been adjusted to the required environmental temperature of the infant entering incubator and thereby cooling or overwarming him
   d. Impending sepsis
3. Note and report infant's temperature if it is over 37° C (99° F). Identify:
   a. An overwarm incubator
   b. The heat effect of direct sunlight
   c. Abnormally high temperature of air-oxygen mixture entering plastic hood
   d. Developing illness

Gradual rewarming of the hypothermic infant (skin temperature less than 35.5° C [96° F]) may be achieved by keeping the Isolette temperature 1° C above his skin temperature. Intermittent readjustments of the incubator temperature may be necessary as the skin temperature reaches a normal level (36.5° C). Limiting the temperature difference between infant and environment ensures minimal metabolic demands.

Rapid rewarming should be tolerated as long as attention is paid to the possibility of vasodilation of the skin by the heat. Administration of volume expander may be necessary to prevent shock.

HUMIDIFICATION

Humidity* should be maintained in the neutral range of 40% to 60%, allowing no visible mist or moisture to form on incubator walls. This level usually is produced without adding water to humidity trays. Controlled studies have failed to demonstrate any favorable influence of high humidity, nebulized water, or detergent mist in the treatment or prevention of idiopathic respiratory distress. When high humidity is desired, ultrasonic nebulization may be preferable to standard techniques because of the smaller droplet size.

Increased humidity (nebulization) may be desirable in the following situations:
1. High-oxygen environments, since oxygen dries mucous membranes
2. Meconium aspiration syndromes with signs of respiratory obstruction
3. Excessive or thickened mucus secretions such as occur in tracheoesophageal fistulas, although humidity is no substitute for proper hydration

---

*A wet and dry bulb hygrometer is necessary for occasional checks of the nursery and incubators.

4. Prolonged intubation
5. Following extubation for about 24 hours

MONITORING HEART RATE AND RESPIRATION

Interruption of the usual respiratory pattern by apneic episodes or disorganized breathing resulting in hypoventilation are the most serious and frequently recurring problems in any intensive care unit caring for preterm and sick neonates. Causes are many but are usually related to lack of maturation of the respiratory center or pulmonary and airway complications.

Early detection and appropriate management of apnea are essential in avoiding death or damage to the central nervous system. Technical difficulties remain even today in the accurate detection of all apneic episodes. Methods of detection include use of respiration monitors that register chest wall movement, or heart rate monitors for the recognition of bradycardia, which typically occurs during apneic episodes (Chapter 27).

Types of monitoring

1. Routine heart rate monitoring is recommended for all babies at medium or high risk. A small battery-powered monitor is especially useful because it offers protection from severe electrical shock.
2. Use of cardiac monitors with oscilloscope and ECG strip recorder is recommended for infants experiencing frequent or severe apneic episodes or severe respiratory distress, and those with cardiac anomalies or arrhythmias. The oscilloscope is useful in distinguishing actual heart rate abnormalities from inaccurate pickup by the monitor and for determining optimal lead placement when difficulty in monitoring is encountered because of signal problems.
3. Respiration-apnea monitors measure impedance across the chest throughout respiratory movements. We have found them unreliable when used alone because of frequency of false alarms and inconsistency in detecting apneic spells.
4. Heart rate and respiration monitor combinations are desirable, nevertheless, for monitoring infants with frequent apneic episodes, especially those who become cyanotic with little or no drop in heart rate.

Use of heart rate monitors

I. Selection of electrodes
  A. Needle electrodes* provide good contact, take up little space, and require minimal amounts of tape to secure so that the insertion site may be easily observed. Possible complications in the use of needle electrodes are skin abscesses at the insertion site and breaking off of the needle under the skin.
  B. Surface adhesive electrodes are easy to apply and noninvasive. Skin breakdown may occur unnoticed under the electrodes if they are not changed regularly. Other disadvantages are faulty skin contact in some cases, impaired interpretation of x-ray films, impeded chest auscultation because of their relatively large size, and interference with intramuscular injections into the thigh.
II. Application of electrodes
  Most models require two electrodes placed over the anterior chest (right upper and left lower sternal area) and an additional electrode on each leg. Application of an electrode near each axilla is often most effective for respiration monitoring.
  A. Surface adhesive electrodes
  Apply to clean dry skin in previously mentioned areas and change site twice weekly.
  B. Needle electrodes
  Clean skin with organic iodine followed by alcohol; let dry. Insert needle parallel to skin surface just beneath skin; cover needle with clear tape to keep in place. Connect electrodes to monitor cables. Change electrodes twice weekly. Clean with acetone and gas autoclave before reusing.
III. Alarm settings
  A. Heart rate
  Set low alarm at 100 beats/min (higher for infants who become cyanotic with a minimal or delayed fall in heart rate); set high alarm at 200 beats/min.
  B. Respiration
  Set alarm for 10 to 20 seconds of apnea.

---

*Grass Instruments Co., Quincy, Mass. 02169.

IV. Use of oscilloscope and ECG recorder
   A. To improve accuracy of heart rate monitoring, place electrodes to produce maximum signal amplitude.
   B. If monitor is recording abnormal heart rate or rhythm, compare the QRS indicator light or audible QRS beep with the oscilloscope reading. If these are not synchronous, the problem is likely to be in the monitoring system rather than in the baby.
   C. Permanent readout of monitored data, a feature of some neonatal monitors, may be obtained as needed or automatically for 10 to 20 seconds each time monitor alarm sounds.
V. When alarm is sounded, proceed as follows:
   A. Rule out false alarm (infant shows respiration and usual color), caused by
      1. Lead failure—faulty placement, detached leads, etc.
      2. Monitor failure or wrong alarm settings
   B. If infant is apneic, treat as suggested on p. 268.

Blood pressure monitoring

Accurate blood pressure measurement is an important aspect of monitoring the premature or critically ill newborn. Shock, recognizable by pallor and hypotension (see Fig. 29-1) occurs frequently as a result of blood loss, sepsis, asphyxia, and pneumothorax. High-risk infants should have regular blood pressure monitoring and observation of capillary filling at least every 3 hours from birth (see Chapter 29).

METHODS OF MEASURING BLOOD PRESSURE

I. Transcutaneous Doppler method may be used to obtain accurate indirect systolic and, with automatic models, diastolic blood pressure measurements.
   A. Equipment
      Equipment needed includes Doppler scanner with transducer probe,* electrode gel, neonatal blood pressure cuff,† and sphygmomanometer.
   B. Procedure
      Place cuff around extremity and attach to manometer. Apply electrode gel to probe, turn on Doppler scanner, locate brachial or popliteal pulse with probe and adjust volume as necessary. Do not apply pressure to probe because this will occlude artery. Inflate manometer to between 100 and 150 mm Hg and slowly release pressure. The point at which the pulse is heard is recorded as systolic pressure.
   C. For use of automatic digital blood pressure monitors, follow manufacturer's instructions.
II. The flush method may be used if other equipment is not available. It is less accurate and generally not recommended for newborn infants.
   A. Equipment
      Equipment needed includes neonatal blood pressure cuff, an elastic bandage, and a sphygmomanometer.
   B. Procedure
      Place cuff around extremity, wrap extremity from distal end up to cuff with elastic bandage, and inflate manometer to between 100 and 150 mm Hg. Remove bandage and allow pressure to fall slowly. The point at which capillary filling occurs is recorded as flush pressure.
III. Direct intraarterial blood pressure measurement by means of a transducer is the most accurate way of obtaining values of systolic, diastolic, and mean blood pressures. It offers the option of continuous monitoring, and the pressure waveform is displayed. Direct monitoring of aortic blood pressure should be used on critically ill infants with umbilical artery catheters if equipment is available.
   A. Equipment
      Equipment needed includes blood pressure transducer and monitor, pressure tubing, three-way stopcocks, needle, 30 ml syringe filled with normal saline.
   B. Procedure
      1. Assemble system according to diagram (Fig. 14-2) making sure all connections are well secured to prevent accidental disconnection and hemorrhage from artery.

---

*Parks Medical, Beaverton, Oregon, 97006.
†Newborn BP Cuff, Dupaco Inc., San Marcos, Calif. '2069; part no. 22080.

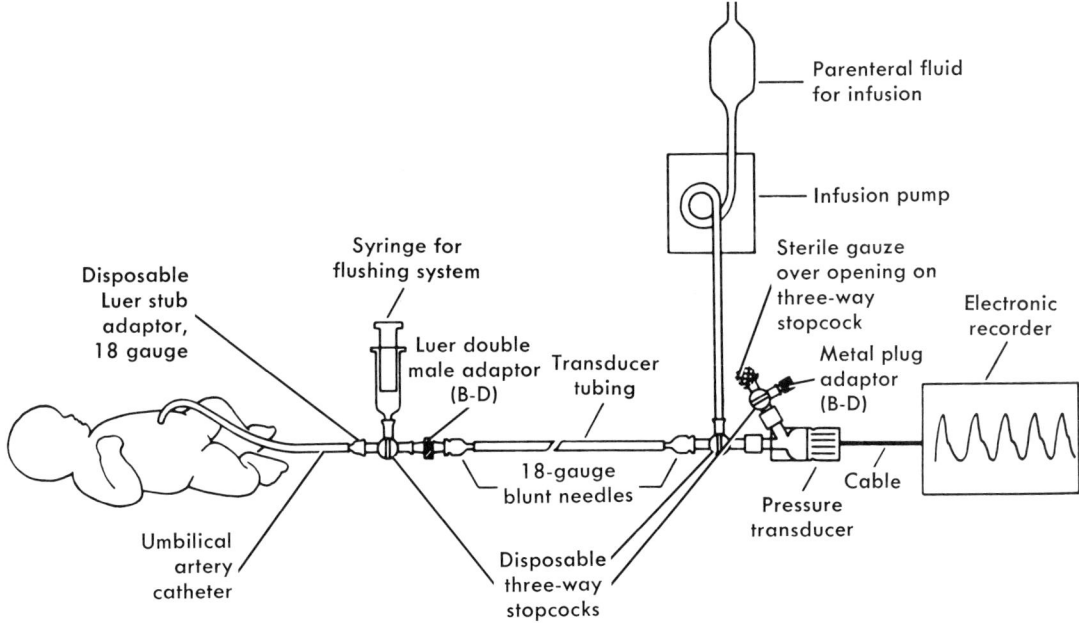

Fig. 14-2. System for direct measurement of arterial blood pressure in newborn infants. (From Kitterman, J.A., Phibbs, R.H., and Tooley, W.H.: Pediatrics **44**:959, 1969.)

2. Flush tubing with normal saline and keep it clear of air bubbles and blood at all times.
3. Calibrate transducer using a mercury-column or water-column manometer.
4. Position transducer at level of infant's heart. If infant is in radiant warmer, mount transducer outside of bed, or cover to protect it from radiant heat.
5. Allow temperature of transducer to stabilize for 30 minutes.
6. Obtain a zero-pressure baseline for the recording system according to instructions for monitor used.
7. Obtain pressure readings according to manufacturer's instructions.

DETAILS OF CARE
Admission care

1. Place infant in radiant warmer; attach thermistor to skin and switch on automatic temperature control mode.
2. Attach monitoring equipment.
3. Check identification and eye prophylaxis.
4. Check and record axillary temperature, heart rate, respiratory rate, and blood pressure.
5. Weigh infant and measure length and head circumference; these values are necessary for baseline observations, precise medication administration, and meaningful collection of vital statistics.
6. Note and record color of infant, rate and type of breathing, activity, state of nutrition, signs of bleeding or infection, and abnormality. Infants with purulent skin infections or watery diarrhea should be admitted only after consulting physician in charge.
7. Administer 0.5 to 1 mg of vitamin K_1 (e.g., AquaMephyton), if not given previously.
8. Obtain rectal and nasopharyngeal swabs for culture.
9. Label incubator with the name and sex of infant, date and hour of birth, birth weight, gestational age, age at admission (hours, if under 72 hours of age), and admission weight. The depressed and premature infant should be handled minimally. Cold exposure should be avoided and bathing postponed.

Positioning

1. Place infant in a position of comfort, such as on abdomen with head to the side, on side with a blanket roll at the back, or on back with some elevation of the shoulders (may be useful in respiratory distress).
2. Change infant's position every 2 to 3 hours.

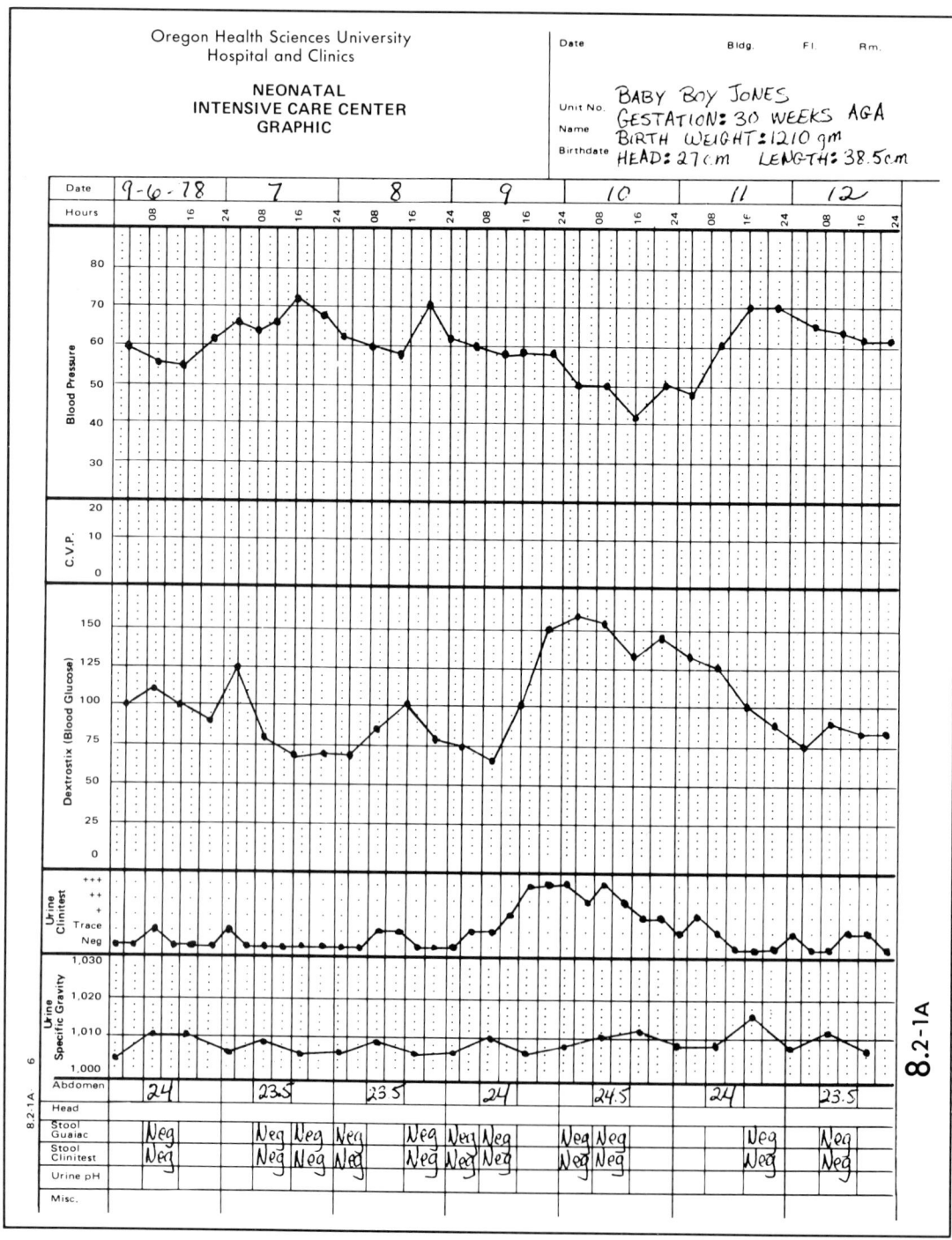

Fig. 14-3. Bedside graph for recording blood pressure and test results of Dextrostix and Clinitest, along with other important data. Note glycosuria, hyperglycemia, and falling blood pressure along with increased abdominal circumference (distension) of infant also described in Fig. 14-4. These data indicated the likely onset of sepsis, which was corroborated by a positive blood culture 24 hours after antibiotic therapy was started.

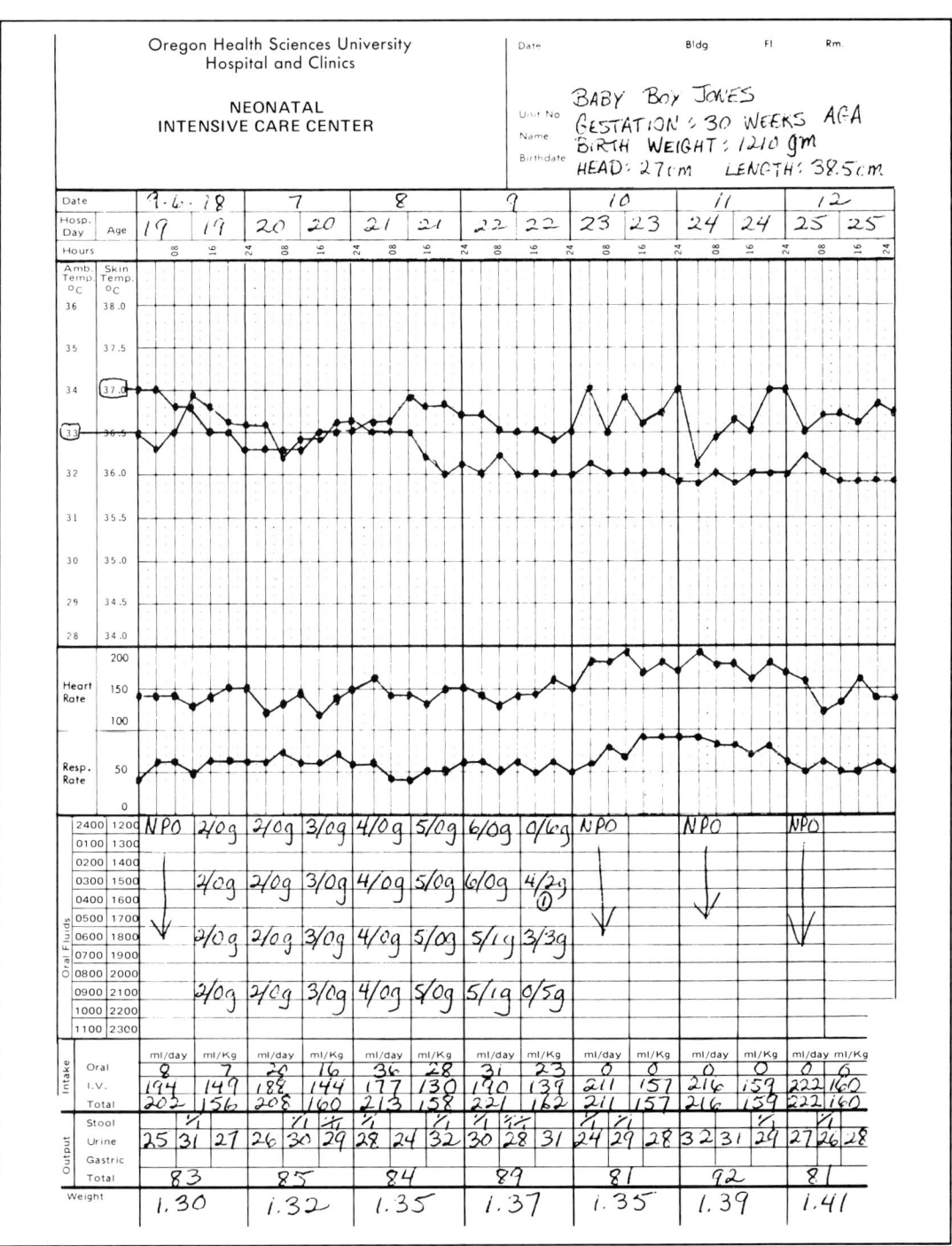

Fig. 14-4. Bedside graph for recording incubator temperature, infant's temperature, heart rate, respiratory rate, and feeding experience (see Chapter 16). Volumes of fluid and formula are calculated in ml/kg/day. Note increasing feeding residuals beginning on day 22, which preceded an illness, as indicated by physiologic alterations on day 23. Prompt discontinuance of feedings and substitution with intravenous fluids and calories followed during diagnostic workup and therapy until recovery of the infant. (See also Fig. 14-3.)

Clothing and crib transfer for the premature infant

1. Use no clothing on infants weighing under 1,500 gm during first week of life.
2. Diaper infants over 1,250 gm who are in good condition after first week.
3. Dress infants weighing around 1,800 gm and transfer to open cribs when they are sufficiently mature to maintain their own temperatures in a surrounding nursery environment of 24° C (75° F) and their conditions are stable.

Nursing notes and recording of data

Any variation in appearance or behavior may be extremely important and an early warning of disease or physiologic imbalance. Personnel on each nursery shift should record and report changes in color, activity, feeding, respirations, and so forth. The neonatal intensive care center graphic shown in Figs. 14-3 and 14-4 present a longitudinal record for the high-risk infant.

1. Graphically chart temperature of incubator, infant's temperature, heart rate, respiratory rate, arterial blood pressure, Dextrostix test, central venous pressure, urine Clinitest, and urine specific gravity (see Fig. 14-4).
2. Feedings
   Record volume of feeding in appropriate time slot.
   a. Signify mode of feeding by writing *n* (nipple) or *g* (gavage) after volume.
   b. Note gastric residuum as follows: milliliters of feeding given per milliliter of residuum.
   c. Record emesis by drawing a circle around estimated milliliters of regurgitation.
3. Intake
   a. Total and record oral and parenteral intake.
   b. Calculate and record milliliters per kilogram of weight daily.
4. Output
   a. Mark each stool individually.
   b. Check each voiding or record 8-hour urine totals.
   c. Total and record 24-hour output.
5. Record weight in kilograms (see conversion table inside front cover).
6. Record abdominal and head circumferences, stool guaiac and Clinitest, and urine pH in space provided. Nursing notes are minimized by use of this record, and basic information is easily interpreted by the physician and nurse from its inspection.

Miscellaneous care

1. Skin
   a. Sponge bathe infant with pH balanced soap twice weekly if condition permits; otherwise dry skin care is recommended, except for cleansing of contaminated areas, such as buttocks, with plain water. Bathing with dilute pHisoHex (less than 3%), followed by thorough rinsing of skin, may be indicated for infant with skin lesions culturing *Staphylococcus aureus* or for all cohorts of a nursery during a *Staphylococcus* epidemic. pHisoHex for routine use should be avoided because of the chance of neurotoxicity.
   b. Swab umbilical stump daily with small amount of povidone-iodine solution (1.67%).
   c. Place infant weighing less than 1,500 gm or those with limited mobility on sheepskin, waterbed, or air mattress to minimize apnea.
   d. Limit use of tape and Band-aids; remove tape using adhesive remover to lessen skin breakdown.
2. Nose, eyes, and mouth
   a. Aspirate any nasal secretions gently with a bulb syringe.
   b. Flush any eye debris or discharge with cotton dipped in sterile water (smear and culture recurring material).
   c. Inspect mouth daily for the white patches of thrush.
3. Urine and stool
   a. Expect urine to be passed in the first 24 hours. Time first voiding and note adequacy of stream (especially in males). Urine output may be measured by weighing diaper on a gram scale before and after voiding. The difference in grams equals milliliters of urine.
   b. Observe for time of first stool passage. There may be a delay of several days in the immature infant. Any distention should be reported to the physician. Ob-

serve and record color, consistency, and frequency of stools. Perform stool Clinitest and guaiac testing for premature infants, those with a history of perinatal asphyxia, and infants suffering from diarrhea, abdominal distention, or other feeding problems.

4. Weighing and measuring
   a. Weigh infant daily (sometimes more often) to gauge excessive weight changes. Any weight change of 2% or more daily after initial weight loss (usually 5% to 10% of body weight for the preterm infant) is an indication for clinical assessment.
   b. Measure head circumference and body length weekly to monitor infant's growth and for comparison of growth with fetus-infant norms (Fig. 11-2).
5. Intramuscular injections
   a. Use a tuberculin syringe with a 25-gauge needle attached.
   b. Pick up thigh tissues between thumb and forefinger.
   c. Place needle on skin surface and gently insert 1 to 1.5 cm.
   d. Aspirate and inject material at right angles into midanterolateral area. This technique avoids injury to the sciatic nerve and major leg vessels.

PARENT-INFANT RELATIONSHIPS

One very important yet easily neglected aspect of the care of a critically ill neonate, or even a "well" premature infant, is the role of parents. Their emotional shock over the premature birth or the delivery of an infant with a major cardiac or surgical problem may be magnified as the infant is admitted to an intensive care unit.

It is the responsibility of the medical team to minimize the emotional stress of parents and to encourage a mother-father-infant relationship in the following ways:

1. Prepare parents antenatally for the problems their baby might have and the type of care their infant will probably receive.
2. Explain the purpose of equipment used for the care of their infant.
3. Exhibit empathy and tact in outlining the prognosis.
4. Keep parents informed at regular intervals about the progress of their infant or call them promptly should the child's condition change drastically.
5. Encourage parents to see and touch their baby as soon and as often as possible, even if the infant is still critically ill or in an Isolette.
6. Provide parents with a Polaroid picture of their baby and footprints as soon as possible after birth.
7. Have parents share in the care of their baby whenever possible.
8. Let mother feed her baby as soon as the infant can suck adequately on a soft nipple.
9. Encourage breast feeding once the infant is vigorous enough.
10. Offer information the parents might desire about high-risk infants in general.
11. Be frank and honest with parents about their infant.
12. Refer parents to a parent support group, if available. Establishment of such groups for intensive care nurseries should be encouraged, since they are known to be helpful to parents with sick or immature infants.

By strengthening parent-infant ties during hospitalization of their infant, the confidence of parents in caring for their baby after discharge is supported and the emotional stability of that family unit fostered.

CRITERIA FOR DISCHARGE FROM THE INTENSIVE CARE UNIT

Discharge is not dependent on weight but on the maturity and general health of the infant and the efficiency of the mother. A thorough physical examination is required, with neurologic assessment and visualization of the retina. Response to auditory and visual stimuli should be ascertained. Measurements of head circumference and length are useful. The following are prerequisites to discharge from the nursery:

1. The assurance of at least 36 weeks of postmenstrual age, as determined by the infant's developmental state from longitudinal observations (growth and development, Chapter 36)
2. Maintenance of normal body tempera-

ture outside of incubator with ambient temperature of 25° C (76° F)
3. The conclusion of treatment for disease or congenital anomalies
4. Adequate oral intake and satisfactory gain in weight
5. Adequate oxygenation in room air
6. Absence of apnea or bradycardiac episodes for at least 7 days or evidence of a stable sleep polygraph (see also Chapter 27, "Apnea of prematurity")
7. A hematocrit over 25% (8 gm/100 ml of hemoglobin), or, if it is less, a reticulocyte count of 3% or more
8. An adequate home environment, as determined by the visiting public health nurse or the private physician, and freedom from infectious diseases in the home
9. Ability of the mother to care for her infant
10. The conclusion of thorough instruction and evaluation of the parents' capabilities in special nursing care procedures that may be required after discharge

RESPONSIBILITIES OF THE COMMUNITY HEALTH NURSE

A visit to the home by a community health nurse should be scheduled as soon as possible after the infant's admission to the neonatal intensive care unit (NICU) to ensure a smooth-functioning referral system between the NICU and the community. The nurse should make home visits for the following purposes:
1. Establishing a meaningful relationship with parents to be able to give effective help in getting the home ready for the baby and to provide on-going supervision if needed
2. Determining the capabilities of the mother and recognizing and working on special needs and problems
3. Reporting observations and plans to the physician and hospital staff
4. Supporting the family through the period of separation while the baby is hospitalized
5. Reassuring the parents as they become acquainted with parenthood and the new baby
6. Demonstrating procedures such as formula preparation, feeding, bathing, and dressing the baby
7. Supplying information that will increase parental understanding of the child's behavior
8. Observing the growth and development of the child
9. Emphasizing the need for good medical supervision
10. Providing emotional support and counseling to parents of a baby who has died
11. Informing and describing community resources that might provide help for families

Many emotionally immature parents are not ready to assume the responsibility of raising an infant. By design or through ignorance some infants are neglected. Recognition of this fact by the alert nurse or physician is important for the child's welfare.

Because of the circumstances surrounding the baby's birth, the mother has been identified as at high risk. An important aspect of the nursing visits is to ensure interpregnancy health supervision in an effort to prevent subsequent high-risk infants.

RESPONSIBILITIES OF THE SOCIAL WORKER

The hospital social worker is part of the ward team and participates in planning at discharge to be aware of the needs of the family and any special requirement deemed advisable by the physician. The social worker is a supportive person as well as a sympathetic listener; most high-risk infants are a source of anxiety to parents.

Social service does not duplicate the services of community health nursing or other disciplines. It implements team recommendations for optimum care and personal adjustment of the patient and family.

Discharge planning is a process that begins with the patient's admission to the hospital. The social worker's role is to (1) interview the family regarding social health, attitudes toward the infant's problems, and acceptance of the infant by both father and mother; (2) provide the health team with information on social, economic, or family problems; (3) contact resources in the community for the provision of health care needed by the family in total care of the infant; and (4) give support directly to the family by providing a relationship of trust and setting the stage for the alleviation of anxieties.

Information obtained by social service contact combined with that provided by the community nurse will contribute to appropriate medical planning and cooperation on the part of families.

SPECIAL ADVICE FOR THE MOTHER

When discharged, low birth weight infants may be as sturdy as full-term newborn infants. Therefore they should be handled in the same easy way and with the same loving attention.

I. General instructions
   A. Protection against illness
      All babies are susceptible to illness. We therefore recommend the following specific care:
      1. Wash hands before feeding or handling and after diapering baby.
      2. Keep everyone who has flu, a cold, sore throat, cough, diarrhea, or skin infection away from baby during first year.
      3. Restrict handling of infant by friends and relatives during first few months.
   B. Control of room temperature
      1. Maintain temperature at about 22° C (70° to 72° F) during the day.
      2. Prevent a drop in temperature below 16° C (60° F) at night until infant is 6 months of age.
   C. Clothing
      1. Clothe infant according to the temperature, always lightly enough to avoid perspiration or heat rash.
      2. Avoid rubber or plastic pants, which promote diaper rash.
      3. Do not dress infant in clothes that will restrict his activity.
   D. Bathing (two or three baths a week are sufficient)
      1. Use a warmer room, about 25° C (75° to 78° F). The water temperature should be comfortable to the elbow.
      2. Apply a mild antiseptic soap such as Dial, and use it sparingly. Oils and lotions are best avoided.
   E. First outing
      1. Delay outings until after first visits to physician or clinic.
      2. Avoid crowds during first year.
II. Feeding

Directions for making formula are given at time of discharge. The following points will be helpful to the mother in feeding her baby:

A. Hold baby in arms in a comfortable, relaxed way.
B. Tilt bottle so that milk fills nipple to help prevent the sucking of air.
C. Rest baby for a few minutes during feeding.
D. Burp baby by gently patting his back while holding him in an upright position. This should be done at least once during feeding and again at the end to allow air out that has been swallowed with the milk. Placing infant on his stomach will often help in the release of the air. Failure to burp baby well may cause discomfort later.
E. See that nipple holes are of adequate size.
   1. Holes should be large enough to permit milk, when cooled a little, to drop about as fast as it can without running in a stream.
   2. If holes are too small, the baby may get tired and stop before having enough to eat. *This is the most common feeding problem.*
   3. Holes may be enlarged by inserting the point of a red-hot needle held in a cork or raw vegetable, or with pliers.
F. Ignore the spitting up of small amounts of milk unless choking occurs.
G. Do not give baby more milk than he desires. The amount may vary from feeding to feeding. The baby is the best judge of the proper amount, provided the nipple hole is large enough.
H. Allow baby to set feeding intervals (between 3 and 5 hours). The night

feeding may be skipped if infant does not wake for it.
III. Special supplements
   A. Iron medication is to be given daily for the first year of life unless it is contained in the formula. It will be added to milk according to the physician's directions.
   B. Vitamin mixtures are to be given daily for at least the first year of life.
IV. Medical care for premature infants
   A. Have mother report any variation in behavior such as the following to physician or clinic responsible for infant's care:
      1. Repeated vomiting or diarrhea
      2. Difficulty with breathing
      3. Change in color
      4. Refusal of milk
      5. Overly quiet or extremely irritable behavior
   B. Suggest an appointment within the first week after discharge, depending on physician's decision.

RESPONSIBILITIES OF THE NEONATAL NURSE

As in other intensive care units, the neonatal nurse specialist works with the physician as a team member. Because such nurses have more contact with the infant, they are likely to be the first to recognize a significant change in an infant's clinical state and to offer appropriate care, often as an emergency. Therefore they must be trained and knowledgeable in the diagnosis and management of conditions encountered in neonates in an intensive care unit. Other responsibilities of the neonatal nurse in a specialized center include the following:
1. Maintaining parenteral infusions
2. Obtaining blood gas determinations and recognizing numerical deviations in blood gas measurements
3. Applying monitoring equipment
4. Administering oxygen appropriately on the basis of hypoxia
5. Performing Dextrostix and Clinistix tests and understanding their significance
6. Passing of orogastric tube, suctioning, and maintaining tube in situ when indicated
7. Understanding correct drug dosages and methods of intravenous and intramuscular administration
8. Measuring blood pressure and recognizing variations and abnormalities
9. Initiating rewarming and maintaining infant's thermoneutral environment
10. Skilled suctioning and positive-pressure ventilating with bag and mask during extended apnea
11. Reporting promptly all significant variations in patient behavior to physicians in charge
12. Encouraging and supporting parent-infant bonding

In the sophisticated center capable of offering continued assisted ventilation, in addition to the previous list, the specialized neonatal nurse should be trained in and capable of the following:
1. Recognizing respiratory failure and need for ventilatory support
2. Performing tracheal suction and pulmonary physiotherapy for infants on respirators
3. Recognizing failure in ventilator support because of the following:
   a. Mechanical failure of equipment
   b. Obstruction in or displacement of endotracheal tube
   c. Pneumothorax
   d. Shock and hypotension
4. Performing emergency intubation
5. Placing umbilical artery catheter

In the transport of high-risk infants to a regional intensive care center (Chapter 13), the specially trained neonatal nurse stands out as a key figure. The success of such a program is directly related to the degree of training and capability of the transporting team. The vast numbers of high-risk neonates requiring transport and specialized care lend importance to the development of training programs for such highly skilled nurses. The intact survival of neonates at high risk may well be more dependent on the alert and trained nurse who has elected to make a profession of neonatal nursing than on any other member of the neonatal team.

PROCEDURES

Any procedure performed on a distressed or small infant should be accomplished in an incubator or under radiant heat and appropriate supplemental oxygen. See Chapter 10 for umbilical vessel catheterization.

Peripheral vein infusion

1. Use a scalp vein set (23- to 25-gauge) suitable to the vein size.
2. Prepare skin with suitable antiseptic.
3. Fill set with flush solution (normal saline or D5W containing 1 unit of heparin per ml).
4. Insert needle, bevel up, into skin a short distance distal to selected site of venipuncture.
5. Introduce needle into center of vein and advance it until blood appears. If using intravascular over-the-needle catheter, advance catheter and withdraw stylet.
6. Flush carefully to clear blood and check patency of IV line.
7. Tape needle securely in place.
8. Attach needle and infusion tubing to infusion pump after clearing contained air.

Transillumination

The standard cuffed flashlight (technique below) has been superseded by more efficient transillumination methods, for example, fiberoptic light (Medgeneral Minilight). Transillumination can be used in subdued light and is helpful in detecting the following: major pneumothorax; fluid (clear) distended organs, such as the kidney and bladder; location of blood vessels for puncture; and size of abdominal organs in the presence of ascites.
   1. Technique
      Chest illumination is the method of choice in diagnosis of pneumothorax in the distressed and deteriorating infant. It is much less time consuming than a chest x-ray examination, and therefore allows the infant to be treated promptly, minimizing further worsening of his condition. Because of their increased skin thickness, this technique may not disclose pneumothorax in term or large preterm infants.
      a. Turn off ceiling light and lamps on warmers, phototherapy units, etc., to enhance visualization of pneumothorax with transilluminator.
      b. Apply tip of transilluminator directly to skin of chest wall and gradually move it over the area, maintaining contact with skin at all times. Examine both right and left sides of thorax to allow comparison and facilitate identification of pneumothorax (if unilateral air leak is suspected). In normal cases (i.e., absence of pneumothorax) a 1 cm ring of transmitted light can be seen. Pneumothorax will usually be detected by a much larger area of transmitted light visible around the probe, and the affected chest may "light up."

Spinal fluid tap

1. Technique
   a. Have infant held firmly in a sitting or side position, with his spine flexed but neck extended to prevent obstruction of airway.
   b. Use a 22-gauge short spinal needle or a 23-gauge disposable needle. The disposable L-P kit* has all needed equipment.
   c. Mark iliac crests with a skin pencil.
   d. Enter intervertebral space opposite crest marks.
   e. Slowly insert needle (0.5 to 1.5 cm), directed toward sternum. Remember that blood-colored fluid from trauma should become clear.
   f. Supply external heat to infant.
2. Usual findings
   a. Cells less than $10/mm^3$ (More than five polymorphonuclear leukocytes suggests meningitis.)
   b. Protein less than 100 mg/100 ml
   c. Glucose more than 20 mg/100 ml (Less than 50% of the blood glucose level supports a diagnosis of bacterial meningitis.)
   d. Xanthochromia (at 1 to 20 days of age)

Technique of retinal examination

1. Dilate pupils with 1 drop of tropicamide (Mydriacyl) or 1% phenylephrine (Neo-Synephrine) 1 hour before observation.
2. Darken room and hold lids away from pupils with the help of an assistant.
3. Keep a nipple in infant's mouth to relax him.

---

*Myelo-Nate L-P Kit, Gesco International, Inc. San Antonio, Tex.

Techniques of urine collection

Urine examinations for bacteria are of questionable value unless collection is critically supervised. Occasionally, unsuspected pyuria may be discovered during the nursery course. A carefully collected urine specimen is particularly important when illness is considered. A few pus cells per high-power field or the presence of one or more bacteria in a stained, concentrated smear under the oil immersion lens indicates the necessity for a culture and bacterial count of urine obtained by bladder tap.

1. Urethra or penis
   a. Wash genital area thoroughly with organic iodine solution.
   b. Apply plastic urine collector* to infant after diaper has remained dry for at least 1 hour.
   c. Observe closely for urination so that a clean, freshly voided specimen can be immediately processed.
2. Bladder tap
   When positive cultures are obtained by urine collection or sepsis is considered possible, urine specimens for smear and culture are best obtained by bladder tap.
   a. Wait at least 1 hour after urine passage.
   b. Obstruct urethra with a finger or fingers.
   c. Prepare suprapubic skin.
   d. Slowly insert a 3 cm, 22-gauge needle just above the symphysis pubis in the midline toward the vertebral column applying slight negative pressure to the syringe plunger.

Technique for blood glucose screening

Longitudinal qualitative blood glucose screening is necessary for oversized infants, infants of diabetic mothers, and all small-for-dates or malnourished infants. Infants demonstrating apnea, eye-rolling, tremors, or other signs of hypoglycemia are also screened.

1. The screening test using Chemstrip† is the preferred method. It is performed at the bedside. For precise technique follow manufacturer's instructions.
2. The Dextrostix test is the older method and although it is less accurate than the Chemstrip test it is more widely known. Follow manufacturer's instructions.
3. Obtain a quantitative laboratory confirmation in all screens under 30 mg/100 ml.

STOOL CLINITEST

1. Collect stool. If stool is liquid, collect with urine bag or place Saran Wrap inside diaper.
2. Mix 1 volume of stool with 2 volumes of water. Centrifuge for several minutes.
3. Transfer 15 drops of supernatant fluid to another tube.
4. Add Clinitest tablet. Wait for reaction to stop and read color exactly 15 minutes later.
5. Values up to 1+ may normally be seen with breast-fed infants.

STOOL GUAIAC

1. Spread small amount of stool on white piece of paper, using tongue blade.
2. Place 2 drops of each of the following solutions on stool specimen in this order: solution 1, glacial acetic acid; solution 2, guaiac solution; solution 3, hydrogen peroxide.
3. Occult blood is present if area of stool tested turns bright blue.

APT TEST

1. Mix meconium with equal parts of water.
2. Centrifuge to show pink supernatant fluid.
3. Mix 5 parts of supernatant fluid with 1 part of 0.25% sodium hydroxide.
4. If pink color persists over 2 minutes, fetal hemoglobin is present. A change to a yellow color indicates presence of adult hemoglobin.

Intubation

See p. 97.

Aspiration of tension pneumothorax

See p. 264.

---

*Two-chambered U-Bag (Hollister).
†Bio Dynamics Co., Indianapolis 46250.

BIBLIOGRAPHY

Baker, D.H., Berdon, W.E., and James, L.S.: Proper localization of umbilical arterial and venous catheters by lateral roentgenograms, Pediatrics **43**:34, 1969.

Buctow, K.C., and Klein, S.W.: Effect of maintenance of "normal" skin temperature on survival of infants of low birth weight, Pediatrics **34**:163, 1964.

Chernick, V., and Raber, M.B.: Electrical hazards in the newborn nursery, J. Pediatr. **77**:143, 1970.

Cochran, W.D., Davis, H.T., and Smith, C.A.: Advantages and complications of umbilical artery catheterization in the newborn, Pediatrics **42**:769, 1968.

Dunn, P.: Localization of the umbilical catheter by post mortem measurements, Arch. Dis. Child. **41**:69, 1966.

Fletcher, M.A., MacDonald, M.G., and Avery, G.B., editors: Atlas of procedures in neonatology, Philadelphia, 1983, J.B. Lippincott Co.

Guidelines for perinatal care, Evanston, Ill., American Academy of Pediatrics, Washington, D.C., 1983, American College of Obstetricians and Gynecologists.

Hey, E.N., and Mount, L.E.: Heat losses from babies in incubators, Arch. Dis. Child. **42**:75, 1967.

Klaus, M.H., and Kennell, J.H.: Maternal-infant bonding, ed. 2, St. Louis, 1982, The C.V. Mosby Co.

Krauss, A.N., and Stavis, R.L.: Complication of neonatal intensive care, Clin. Perinatol. **7**:107, 1980.

Kuhns, L.R., Bednarek, F.J., Wyman, M.L., et al.: Diagnosis of pneumothorax or pneumomediastinum in the neonate by transillumination, Pediatrics **56**:355, 1975.

Neal, W.A., Reynolds, J.W., Jarvis, C.W., et al.: Umbilical artery catheterization: demonstration of arterial thrombosis by aortography, Pediatrics **50**:6, 1972.

Schwartz, R.H., Hey, E.N., and Baum, J.D.: Management of the newborn's thermal environment. In Oliver, T.K., editor: Monographs in neonatology, New York, 1978, Grune & Stratton, Inc.

Silverman, W.A.: The effect of the atmospheric environment on the premature infants, J. Pediatr. **58**:581, 1961.

Silverman, W.A.: Diagnosis and treatment: use and misuse of temperature and humidity in care of the newborn infant, Pediatrics **33**:276, 1964.

Silverman, W.A.: Intensive care of the low birth weight and other at-risk infants, Clin. Obstet. Gynecol. **13**:87, 1970.

Silverman, W.A., Agate, F.J., Jr., and Fertif, J.W.: A sequential trial of the nonthermal effect of atmospheric humidity on survival of newborn infants of low birth weight, Pediatrics **31**:719, 1963.

Stein, B., Lucey, J.F., and Tooley, W.H.: Grounding and electrical leakage of phototherapy equipment, Pediatrics **44**:614, 1969.

Vapaavuori, E.K., and Raiha, N.C.R.: Intensive care of small premature infants, Acta Paediatr. Scand. **59**:353, 1970.

Wigger, H.J., Bransilner, B.R., and Blane, W.H.: Thromboses due to catheterization in infants and children, J. Pediatr. **76**:1, 1970.

15

Parenteral administration of fluid and electrolytes

Supplying water, electrolytes, and calories by parenteral means to neonates at risk has revolutionized their care. Not only have chances for survival been greatly improved, so also has the quality of survivors. Not long ago, starvation and dehydration were allowed because of fear of aspiration of milk feedings and lack of skills in fluid administration.

The preterm infant given water alone can live for only 5 to 10 days. Even with glucose additions, this survival time is merely doubled. Babies require 50 to 85 kcal/kg/day for maintenance support (basal, activity and cold stress), which without oral feedings or parenteral calories can be met only by their limited stores of glycogen, muscle, and fat. Growth, including brain cell division, must cease. The biochemical hazards of starvation include hypoglycemia, acidosis, hypernatremia, and hyperbilirubinemia. Although infusing glucose solutions limits protein losses secondary to catabolism of muscle tissue, the infant remains in negative nitrogen balance as long as oral feedings are delayed or parenteral alimentation (amino acids, glucose, and lipids) is not substituted (see Chapter 17).

The following are signs and symptoms in infants for whom parenteral fluids are to be considered in place of oral feedings:

At birth
1. Severe asphyxia—Apgar score under 4 at 1 minute or under 6 at 5 minutes
2. Weight of under 1,500 gm
3. Major surgically correctable defects
4. Stressed infant of a diabetic mother

Later
1. Signs of respiratory distress
2. Increasing apnea or cyanosis
3. Intolerance of oral feedings
4. Signs of infection

GLUCOSE, WATER, AND ELECTROLYTES FOR SHORT-TERM NEEDS*

Insensible water loss (IWL) in infants is increased with decreased maturity. This loss is reduced by higher relative humidity environments (mechanical ventilation) and any plastic material (heat shield, Saran Wrap) interposed between the infant and his environment (radiation and air circulation). However, with open incubation under radiant heating and use of phototherapy insensible water losses may be increased from approximately 1 ml to as much as 4 ml per hour. Basal water requirements, including urinary output, are approximately 60 to 80 ml/kg/day, but uncontrolled rates of loss and variability in preterm infants can easily double the amount that should be given. Assessment of fluid requirements is best determined by weighing the infant every 8 to 12 hours at the start and attempting to limit total weight

---

*For long-term needs, see Chapter 17 on parenteral nutrition; for introduction of oral feeds, see Chapter 16.

Table 15-1. Fluids (ml/kg/day) and electrolytes (mEq/kg/day)

Day	<1,000 gm 7.5% glucose	1,001-1,500 gm 10% glucose	>1,500 gm 10% glucose
1	90-100	80-100	70- 90
2	100-120	100-110	80-100
3	120-130	110-130	90-110
4	130-140	130-140	110-130
5	140-150	140-150	130-150
Na^+ (as chloride)	1-2	2	2
K^+ (as acetate)	2	2	2
Ca^{++} (gluconate 10%) (1 ml = 0.45 mEq)	1-2	1-2	1-2

Table 15-2. Laboratory monitoring for parenteral infusions

Parameter	Frequency	Acceptable range
Weight	Three times a day to once daily	Birth weight loss <12% (preterm); later ±2% daily
Glucose	Dextrostix* every 4 hours for 24 hours; then every 8 hours	50 to 125 mg/100 ml
Sodium Potassium Chloride	Daily for 3 days; then 3 times per week	130-145 mEq/L 4-6 mEq/L 95-105 mEq/L
Calcium pH	Daily for 3 days; then 2 times per week	8 to 10 mg/100 ml 7.30 to 7.42

*See p. 135, once stabilized, testing urine by Clinitest every 12 hours is sufficient; glucosuria over 1+ indicates possible hyperglycemia.

loss to 10% to 12%. Babies with respiratory distress or renal shutdown usually require more limited volumes of water. Table 15-1 outlines the recommendations for starting fluids and electrolytes according to weight.

Infants vary greatly in these requirements, and serial laboratory determinations are required for adjustment in biochemical control. Table 15-2 outlines recommended laboratory monitoring procedures and the range of acceptable determinations.

Urine volume and electrolytes should be measured in the very small infant. Values should be within the following ranges:

Urine volume	50 to 100 mg/kg/day
Osmolarity	75 to 300 mOsm/l
Specific gravity	1005 to 1012

ROUTES OF INFUSION

An umbilical vessel line, preferably arterial, is used for critically ill infants. When the infant is no longer in critical condition or a complication with the umbilical catheter demands its removal, a peripheral vein is used. A central venous catheter may be required in some larger infants who will need prolonged postsurgical alimentation.

HOMEOSTATIC IMBALANCE
(see also p. 141)
Water imbalances

Excessive weight loss (greater than 15% of birth weight) in the preterm infant accentuates bilirubin rise, hypernatremia, and metabolic acidosis from hyperchloremia.

Limiting weight loss to about 10% of birth weight may not be possible because of the high insensible water loss of the preterm infant, particularly when he is placed under radiant heat and phototherapy. Efforts to control water losses by increasing fluid volumes have created several problems: (1) hyponatremia from excessive sodium losses in the urine, (2) hyperglycemia from an excessive glucose load that may be offered, (3) edema with impaired respiratory gas exchange, and (4) possible opening of the ductus. Edema or early weight gain, however, may be the result of respiratory distress syndrome with oliguria or renal injury from asphyxia.

Sodium imbalances—hyponatremia and hypernatremia

The term infant fed human milk receives at most 200 ml/kg/day, which contains approximately 30 mg or 1.3 mEq of sodium. The preterm infant requires more than this to meet the needs of tissue growth and mandatory urinary losses and ensure a normal serum sodium level of 135 mEq/L. His reabsorption of sodium from the glomerular filtrate is inefficient, and an increased urine volume will lead to increased sodium loss. Thus hyponatremia (serum sodium less than 130 mEq/L) is common with the usually recommended sodium intake. Therefore, if serum sodium level is reduced, correction over a 24-hour period is advised. Chloride is usually reduced proportionately. Hyponatremia can be corrected by use of the following formula:

$$\text{mEq Na}^+ \text{ deficit} \times \text{Weight (kg)} \times 0.6 = \text{mEq Na}^+ \text{ needed for correction}$$

Example: 1.5 kg infant's sodium level is 121 mEq.
Formula: $135 - 121 \times 1.5 \times 0.6 = 12.6$ mEq Na^+ to be administered

This amount is added to the daily fluid volume, using a concentrated electrolyte solution of NaCl (1 ml = 2.5 mEq of NaCl).

Hypernatremia with a serum sodium level over 150 mEq/L is a common and potentially serious problem in the preterm infant. It is primarily the result of insensible losses of water from the extracellular fluid space without associated sodium losses. Early or excessive sodium additions as well as delays in fluid administration intensify the condition.

The resulting hyperosmolarity of the blood may lead to fluid shifts from brain cells. In this event, bridging vessels may be ruptured and hemorrhage may occur. Hypernatremia is treated by rehydration, for example, an infusion of 150 ml/kg/day of 5% glucose solution with 4 mEq/kg of NaCl over a 24-hour period. The increased volume will promote urine formation and sodium excretion.

Glucose imbalances—hypoglycemia and hyperglycemia

Carbohydrate is essential for the infant in distress, both to support his glucose needs for energy and to avoid hypoglycemia, so common in the asphyxiated infant and in those who are large or small for dates.

Of equal seriousness is hyperglycemia, an iatrogenic consequence of excessive administration of glucose beyond the ability of the infant to metabolize it. The smaller infants who require greater fluid loads to avoid dehydration are also those with limited means for glucose control.

The premature baby may only metabolize 0.3 to 0.4 gm/kg/hr with daily increases of approximately one tenth of this amount. If 10% glucose is given in the larger volumes mentioned, hyperglycemia will result. Not only does hyperglycemia increase osmolarity of the blood (18 mg/100 ml = 1 mOsm/L), but the resulting glucosuria also carries away additional body water (osmotic diuresis).

Hypocalcemia

Thirty percent of preterm infants have serum calcium levels below 7 mg/100 ml in the first 48 hours of life. Although this level is not dangerous, a low level in conjunction with low blood glucose levels or previous asphyxial insult may promote hyperactivity or seizures. To maintain serum calcium levels above 8 mg/100 ml, the small preterm and stressed infant requires at least 1 mg/kg/hr. This amount may be met by a dosage of 1.5 mEq/kg/day of calcium in the form of 3 ml of 10% calcium gluconate. Each milliliter of 10% calcium gluconate contains 9 mg of calcium or 0.45 mEq. This amount of calcium, although it can maintain serum levels, is by no means sufficient for growth and calcification of the skeleton.

BIBLIOGRAPHY

Bell, E.F., Neidich, G.A., Cashore, W.J., et al.: Combined effect of radiant warmer and phototherapy on insensible water loss in low-birth-weight infants, J. Pediatr. **94**:810, 1979.

Doyle, L.W., and Sinclair, J.C.: Insensible water loss in newborn infants, Clin. Perinatol. **9**:453, 1982.

Engelke, S.C., Shah, B.L., Vasan, U., et al.: Sodium balance in very-low-birth-weight infants, J. Pediatr. **93**:837, 1978.

Lorenz, J.M., Kleinman, L.I., Kotagal, U.R., et al.: Water balance in very low-birth-weight infants: relationship to water and sodium intake and effect on outcome, J. Pediatr. **101**:432, 1982.

Roy, R.N., and Sinclair, J.C.: Hydration of the low-birth-weight infant, Clin. Perinatol. **2**:393, 1975.

Tsang, R.C., Light, I.J., Sutherland, J.M., et al.: Possible pathogenic factors in neonatal hypocalcemia of prematurity, J. Pediatr. **82**:423, 1973.

Wu, P.Y.K., and Hodgman, J.E.: Insensible water loss in preterm infants, Pediatrics **54**:704, 1974.

16

Nutritional requirements and oral feeding of the low birth weight infant

WATER BALANCE AND CALORIES

Early and adequate provision of calories and water is now recognized as vital for the preterm, malnourished, or stressed infant who, in addition to exposure to asphyxia at birth, has been abruptly separated from the placental lifeline. Limited or depleted nutritional reserves, increased metabolic demands because of respiratory effort, evaporation losses under radiant heat and phototherapy, and gastrointestinal and renal immaturity, as well as the requirements for growth at a critical period, pose a challenge. Supplying thermoneutral environments for minimal caloric expenditure and giving attention to the nutritional and water requirements of infants are undoubtedly major factors contributing to the decrease in neonatal mortality and morbidity during the last 10 years.

Heird and associates have estimated that an infant weighing 1,000 gm, if supplied with water alone, can survive for 4 or 5 days with his calorie stores. The addition of 10% glucose (75 ml/kg/24 hr) can support his life for only 10 or 11 days. The hazards of thirsting and fasting include depression of blood glucose, nitrogen loss, acidosis, rise in plasma osmolarity,* and delay in meconium passage, which is likely to intensify bilirubinemia.

Weight loss

The large fluid component of the preterm infant (up to 85% of body weight, most of which is extracellular water) allows a greater percentage weight loss than occurs in infants born at term.

Other factors contributing to early weight loss include the following:
1. Insufficient fluid intake
2. Evaporation losses through the thin skin exposed directly to radiant heat (up to 4 ml/kg/hr)
3. Insensible water loss from lungs, increased by tachypnea and low humidity (15 ml/kg/24 hr)
4. Water loss from catabolism
5. Miscellaneous: osmotic diuresis, inhibition of antidiuretic hormone (ADH), passage of meconium

Acceptable weight loss limits are as follows:
1. Preterm—10% to 12%
2. Term—5% to 8%
3. Dysmature and undergrown—zero to 5%

After the first 3 days of life, weight loss or gain should not exceed 2% of the weight on the previous day. With ample calories and protein, the preterm infant should gain 15 gm/kg/24 hr, with an accretion of as much as 360 mg/kg/24 hr of nitrogen.

Renal solute load

In the first week after birth, the capacity of the kidney to concentrate urine is limited because of its low rate of excretion of urea, the shortness of the loop of Henle, and its diminished response to antidiuretic hormone (ADH). The kidney may concentrate up to 700 mOsm/L or, in the very premature, maximal urine concentration can be as low as 300 mOsm/L. Therefore an infant weighing 1,000 gm may not be able to excrete more than 18 mOsm in 60 ml of urine

---

*Plasma osmolarity should be maintained below 300 mOsm/L and can be estimated from this simple equation:

$$2 \times \text{Na(mEq/L)} + \frac{\text{Glucose (mg/100 ml)}}{18} + \frac{\text{BUN (mg/100 ml)}}{3}$$

(approximate volume with fluid intake of 150 mg/kg/24 hr). Some high-solute formulas offer more solute load than can be excreted in the available urine volume, particularly when extrarenal losses are high. Each gram of tissue accreted, however, requires 0.9 mOsm (Sinclair and colleagues), sparing the kidney from excretion of this solute in the growing infant.

A satisfactory estimate of potential renal solute load can be determined by the Ziegler-Fomon formula:

$$\left.\begin{array}{c} \text{gm/100 ml protein} \times 4 \\ + \\ \text{mEq of Na}^+, \text{K}^+, \text{Cl} \times 1 \end{array}\right\} \text{mOsm/100 ml of milk*}$$

With decreased capacity for net acid excretion in the preterm infant, development of oliguria in respiratory distress syndrome (RDS), and acute tubular necrosis (ATN) after perinatal asphyxia, frequent use of bicarbonate infusions and increased evaporation loss through the skin make diligent and careful attention to electrolyte balance vital. At times, a striking polyuria occurs, with a loss of Na^+, resulting in hyponatremia with hypotonicity of serum and increased urinary osmolarity. Inappropriate ADH secretion may be an important factor. The most effective therapy is the restriction of fluids. Administration of isotonic saline solution will cause a further loss of Na^+ in the urine.

Caloric expenditure

The energy metabolism of the low birth weight infant is at first less than that of the term infant, but metabolism gradually accelerates so that by 2 weeks of age it is considerably higher. The stressed or small-for-dates infant's oxygen consumption per kilogram is even greater than that of the average preterm infant. Table 16-1 presents the ranges in daily caloric expenditure of growing preterm infants.

Factors limiting efficiency of oral feedings

1. The weak sucking reflex and incoordination between sucking and swallowing make nipple feeding unsatisfactory until 33 to 34 weeks of gestational age has been reached.

---

*In Similac 24 given at 150 ml/kg 24 hr:
    3.3 gm protein × 4 = 13.2
  9.2 mEq of electrolyte × 1 =   9.2
                             22.4 mOsm/150 ml

Table 16-1. Caloric requirements for preterm infants

Item	kcal/kg/24 hr
Resting	40 to 50
Activity*	10 to 20
Cold stress	5 to 10
Specific dynamic action	8 to 10
Fecal loss†	2 to 20
Growth‡	25 to 40
TOTAL	90 to 150

*Influenced by crying, work of breathing.
†Parenteral feedings as opposed to underabsorption of nutrients (notably fats).
‡Undergrowth retardation increases caloric needs.

2. The relaxed cardiac sphincter and depressed intestinal mobility in low birth weight infants allow easy regurgitation and delay in stomach emptying.
3. Limited gastric capacity in the more immature infant, along with the above, permit overdistention and aspiration of feedings. Therefore caution in determining proper food volumes and appropriate rate of increase in feeding amounts is necessary to reduce these common hazards.
4. Physiologic malabsorption limits full use of calories. The delay in maturation of enzymes (e.g., lactase and lipase) affects the absorption of lactose and saturated fats.
5. The solute load of formulas high in protein and electrolyte content can exceed the concentrating ability of the kidney, thus raising the blood urea nitrogen (BUN) and serum osmolarity. Hyperaminoacidemia, hyperammonemia, and late metabolic acidosis can also occur. On the other hand, milks of low protein and electrolyte content can impede growth and allow hypoalbuminemia and mineral insufficiency (demineralization of bones).

NUTRITIONAL REQUIREMENTS

With interruption in the nutritional supply line to the fetus, a period of enforced starvation begins. Undue delay in the resumption of cell division and growth at this important period may have serious and lasting consequences. Ideally the very low birth weight infant should grow at the corresponding fetal rate that is at least 50% greater than that expected for term

Table 16-2. Range in daily feeding requirements of low birth weight infants per kilogram of body weight

Nutrient requirements		First week of life	Active growth period
Water (ml)		80-150*	130-200
Calories		50-100	110-150+
Protein	(gm)	2	3-4
Glucose		7-12	12-15
Fat		3-4	5-8
Sodium	(mEq)	1-2	3-4
Potassium		1-2	2-4
Chloride		1-2	2-4
Calcium	(mg)	20-50	210
Phosphorus		—	140
Magnesium		—	9

*Part or all of this volume is supplied by parenteral fluids in the risk infant.
+Calorie requirements of over 120 per kilogram apply to undergrown infants.

Table 16-3. Daily vitamin requirements

A	1,500	IU
Thiamine	0.2	mg
Riboflavin	0.4	mg
Pyridoxine	0.4	mg
B_{12}	1.5	µg
C	60	mg
D	600	IU
E	30	IU
Niacin	6	mg
Panthenol	300	µg
Folic acid	60	µg
K	15	µg

newborn. A further challenge is supplying sufficient minerals, since two thirds of the mineral content of the growing fetus is deposited during the last 2 months of gestation. If these goals are to be reached, formulas of similar composition to human milk are insufficient unless volumes given are large and possibly excessive. Yet overconcentrated feedings may jeopardize survival by surpassing the capabilities of the developing metabolic and excretory systems.

Daily feeding requirements

Table 16-2 presents the ranges in nutrients recommended for the preterm infant in consideration of their accumulation by the fetus and the absorptive and excretory capabilities of the infant.

1. Protein is accreted by the corresponding fetus at a rate of just over 2 gm/kg/day (320 to 350 mg of nitrogen). In view of nitrogen losses in the urine and stool (about 150 mg/kg/day), one can make a case for offering the preterm infant 3 to 4 gm/kg/day or 10% to 12% of the total calories given. Essential amino acids such as cystine should be present in sufficient amounts.
2. Carbohydrate should make up about 40% to 45% of total caloric intake. Because of the difficulty of the small premature infant to digest lactose, sucrose, or other sugars, glucose should probably make up 50% or more of this amount.
3. Fat in the diet, 3% of which should be in the form of essential linoleic acid, should supply 45% to 50% of total calories. By increasing medium-chain triglycerides and limiting the percentage of saturated fats, both fat and calcium absorption are enhanced.
4. Improved bone mineralization is achieved in the very low birth weight infant when calcium and phosphorus intakes are raised sufficiently to allow retention resembling the amount accreted in utero by the fetus of a similar gestational age.
5. Caloric density refers to the number of calories per volume of milk. Standard formulas of 20 kcal/oz (67 kcal/100 ml) are recommended for term infants, whereas 24 kcal/oz (81 kcal/100 ml) is recommended for more premature infants. Occasionally 90 or even 100 kcal/100 ml is given to the undergrown or chronically stressed infant who has higher caloric requirements. Increased protein and electrolyte content raises the renal solute load; thus one must supply sufficient total water (150 mg/kg/day) and avoid excessive water losses (mainly diarrhea and exposure to dry heat) to prevent azotemia.

Vitamins and iron

Table 16-3 presents vitamin requirements that are tentative because of the uncertainty regarding the preterm infant's needs.

1. Administer vitamin K_1 (AquaMephyton), 0.5 to 1 mg or equivalent, on the first day of life.

Table 16-4. Contents of various milks (per 100 ml)

	Human milk	SMA Premie	Similac Special Care	Enfamil Premature
Protein (gm)	1.1*	2.0	2.2	2.4
Casein:whey ratio	40:60	40:60	40:60	40:60
Fat (gm)	4.5	4.4	4.4†	4.1†
Carbohydrate (gm)	7.2	8.6‡	8.6‡	8.9‡
Minerals (mg)				
Calcium	34	75	144	95
Phosphorus	14	40	72	48
Sodium	16	32	35	32
Potassium	51	75	100	90
Chloride	42	53	65	69
Iron	0.02	0.3	0.3	0.13
Vitamins				
A (IU)	280	320	550	254
D (IU)	5	51	120	51
E (IU)	0.5	1.5	3	1.6
K (µg)	1.5	0.007	0.01	0.008
C (mg)	5	7	30	7
Calories (kcal)	74	81	81	81
Osmolality (mOsm/kg)	300	270	300	300
Potential renal solute load (mOsm)	8	18	21	22

*Protein in human milk varies from 0.8 to 1.3 gm/100 ml.
†Approximately 50% MCT (medium-chain triglycerides) oil.
‡Approximately 50% lactose and 50% polycose.

2. Add multivitamin mixtures, including pyridoxine and vitamin E, daily to the formula by the third day of life. Vitamin E is poorly absorbed by the preterm infant, and 30 IU of the water-soluble form is recommended daily. This increased amount is supported by the knowledge that polyunsaturated fats in the diet and iron supplementations interfere with vitamin E absorption and its protection of erythrocyte hemolysis.
3. Supply parenteral vitamin mixtures when oral feedings are delayed (see Chapter 17).
4. Add 10 to 15 mg of elemental iron (e.g., Ferro drops) daily by the age of 6 to 8 weeks. Milk products containing iron supplements are sufficient for iron requirements when a formula intake of approximately 1 L per 24 hours is achieved.

Formulas

Nutrient compositions of human milk and formulas at 810 kcal/L designed for the preterm infant are presented in Table 16-4. These higher density formulas should be diluted one third with water until 125 ml/kg/day are taken, unless parenteral fluids are given. This additional water allows sufficient urinary water for solute excretion.

Recent reports have associated the recent increase in lactobezoar with the use of 24 kcal/oz formulas designed for the low birth weight infant. Stomach distention because of the accumulation of milk curd can be confirmed by x-ray examination. Delay in enteral feeding of the asphyxiated preterm infant and limiting volume increases may reduce lactobezoar incidence.

Criteria for assessment of adequacy of feeding

1. Plot daily growth in weight and weekly length and head circumference on fetal-infant growth chart (Fig. 11-2). Growth lines tend to parallel standard growth curves after the first week or two of life.
2. A blood urea nitrogen (BUN) level between 10 and 25 mg/100 ml will ensure an ample but not excessive protein intake.
3. Aim at a serum albumin level of over 3 gm/100 ml to avoid edema.
4. Observe for metabolic acidosis and keep base deficit under -5.
5. Check electrolytes triweekly. Maintain urine

specific gravity at 1.012 or less and osmolarity under 300 mOsm/L.

Breast milk controversy

An examination of the mineral and protein content of human milk (Table 16-4) shows that it is unable to meet the growth needs of the preterm infant (Table 16-2) even at 200 ml/kg/day. Studies disagree regarding the adequacy of human milk in promoting growth in the premature in comparison to modified cow's milk formulas. Although the protein content of human milk decreases with postnatal age, higher levels have been found in milk from mothers of preterm infants. One must weigh the possible nonnutritive advantages of using human milk (for example, protection against infection, favorable gut flora, and improved iron absorption), against the theoretical disadvantage of using it and not providing sufficient nutrients to allow growth as it would be if the infant had remained in utero.

Unfortunately, heat treatment and freezing of human milk for milk bank use destroys much of its nonnutritive advantages, particularly its antibody and cellular immunity protection. Although storage of expressed breast milk at 4° C protects its immunologic advantage, dangers from bacterial contamination (streptococci and staphylococci) in transporting and handling remain.

Commercial breast milk additives are a newer approach to adapting human milk for use by the preterm infant. Additives can improve protein, calcium, phosphorus, vitamin, and calorie contents.

Modifications of commercial formulas designed specifically for the preterm infant (Table 16-4) have included the use of types of proteins similar to that found in human milk, predominantly whey protein.

Long-term studies must give the final answers, but there is general agreement that when breast feeding must be postponed women who wish to nurse later must be helped to maintain their milk supplies.

FEEDING PLANS
When to start oral feedings

The infant at risk requires water, glucose, and certain electrolytes from the time of birth. Early feedings by mouth may be tolerated by undergrown, dysmature, and many preterm infants sufficient to prevent hypoglycemia and further catabolic stress, but parenteral infusions are usually necessary to provide initial requirements. When gastric feedings must be delayed for days, and certainly when they are delayed beyond a week, parenteral alimentation—preferably through a peripheral vein line—should be given and can maintain most infants in positive nitrogen balance for many weeks until oral feedings can be offered safely. Some infants can accept and will benefit from indwelling catheters placed through the pylorus. We do not recommend any feedings until the following conditions are met:

1. Stable respirations, with little or no respiratory distress
2. Absence of distention, with adequate bowel sounds
3. Acceptance of feedings with minimal residual and apneic episodes

When beginning enteral feedings, refer to Table 16-5 for guidance. Because of the prematurity of the infant, initial feeding volumes are kept small and increases are made gradually, as outlined in the table, being especially conservative with very small infants. Feeding volumes in Table 16-5 are given in total daily amounts, to be divided into hourly, or two or three hourly aliquots, depending on the feeding method used.

Very small infants (unable to suck, usually weighing under 1,300 gm but otherwise in fair condition)

1. Start 10% glucose infusion (7.5% for infants weighing less than 800 gm) in the first few hours of life at a rate of 100 ml/kg/24 hr.
2. Add 3 ml of 10% calcium gluconate* (1 ml = 0.45 mEq Ca^{++}) per 100 ml of solution and 1 to 2 mEq of Na^+, K^+, and Cl^-. See also Chapter 15.
3. Increase rate of infusion by 10 to 20 ml/kg/24 hr to a total of approximately 150 ml/kg/24 hr, depending on weight loss (Fig. 16-1).

---

*Intravenous calcium prevents acute hypocalcemia common in low birth weight infants after interruption of the placental lifeline.

Table 16-5. Enteral feeding schedule for preterm infants

Day of enteral feeding	<1,000 gm birth weight		1,001-1,500 gm birth weight		>1,500 gm birth weight	
	Amount of feeding (ml/kg/day)	Parenteral fluids	Amount of feeding (ml/kg/day)	Parenteral fluids	Amount of feeding (ml/kg/day)	Parenteral fluids
1	12	yes	16	yes	24	yes
2	24	yes	24	yes	40	yes
3	36	yes	32	yes	64	yes
4	48	yes	48	yes	88	yes
5	60	yes	64	yes	112	yes
6	72	yes	80	yes	136	no
7	84	yes	104	yes	152	no
8	96	yes	128	no		
9	120	yes	152	no		
10	144	no				
11	156	no				

4. Check urine every 3 hours with Clinistix and if 1+ or more or if Dextrostix shows over 130 mg/100 ml, obtain blood glucose value. If above 150 mg/100 ml, reduce glucose concentration or rate of infusion. When sufficient urine is collected, the use of Clinitest tablets is a more accurate method of assessing glucosuria.
5. Begin oral feedings of 2 ml/kg of formula by gavage every 3 hours when the condition has definitely stabilized (see Table 16-5).
6. Increase feeding by approximately 1 ml/kg/12 hr.
7. Clinitest stool daily for sugar—over 2+ signifies possible malabsorption. (See p. 136 for method.)
8. Reduce volume of infused fluids as oral feedings are increased, keeping total volume at approximately 150 ml/kg/24 hr.
9. Do not discontinue intravenous fluid until oral feedings have reached 100 ml/kg/24 hr.
10. Limit gavage feedings to 150 ml/kg/24 hr, and calories to 120/kg/24 hr when using a 24 kcal/oz formula. Increases above 150 ml/kg/24 hr should continue gradually when using a 20 kcal/oz milk or human milk until intakes of approximately 180 ml/kg/day are reached.
11. Begin multivitamins, 0.3 ml daily, with first milk feeding.
12. Discontinue oral feedings if there is abdominal distention,* regurgitation, repeated residual over 2 ml, or an increase in apneic periods. Reinstate parenteral fluids and consider intravenous alimentation (see Chapter 17).

Larger premature infants in good condition

1. Start with 4 to 10 ml of human milk or 20 kcal/oz formula by 3 hours of age if condition has stabilized and offer every 2 to 3 hours if infant accepts formula by nipple.
2. Increase by 3 to 5 ml every 12 hours if accepted, to achieve an intake of 100 to 150 ml/kg of body weight by 1 week of age, and 150 to 180 ml/kg by 2 weeks. Generally, bottle-fed infants may choose their volume.
3. Gradually strengthen calorie concentration to 24 kcal/oz in small-for-dates infants or infants who act hungry.
4. Discontinue or reduce feeding if distention, regurgitation, diarrhea, or cyanosis occurs and supplement or substitute parenteral nutrition.
5. Give multivitamins, 0.3 ml, by the third day.
6. Breast feeding may begin at 35 to 36 weeks of postmenstrual age if the infant is vigorous.

---

*Distention and ileus are serious signs that may indicate infection or overfeeding, or presage necrotizing enterocolitis or lactobezoar. Daily measurement of circumference of abdomen will signify possible pathosis.

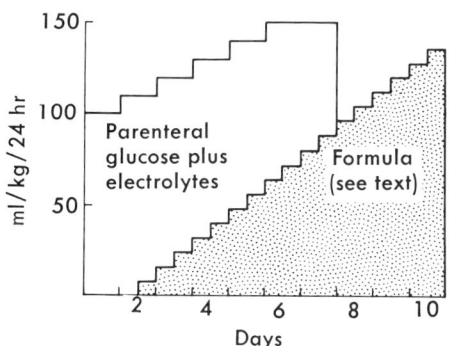

Fig. 16-1. Example of combined parenteral and oral feeding in milliliters per kilogram per day for a newborn infant weighing less than 1,500 gm at birth who is unable to suck. Increases of 2 ml/kg/24 hr of oral feeding from an initial intake of 2 to 3 ml achieve an intake of approximately 100 ml/kg/24 hr by 7 days of age. Many infants will not tolerate this volume of intake without abdominal distention, regurgitation, and risk of aspiration; continuation of parenteral fluids is advisable for these infants. (Modified from Babson, S.G.: J. Pediatr. 79:694, 1971.)

Undersized and undernourished (small-for-dates and dysmature) infants

1. Feed 20 kcal/oz formula, if tolerated, to active and stable infants at 2-hour intervals, starting soon after birth.
2. Change to a formula of 24 kcal/oz after a day or two.
3. Perform Dextrostix* test every 4 to 6 hours for 48 hours until blood glucose is stabilized over 50 mg/100 ml.
4. Infuse 10% glucose if oral intake is not satisfactory, there is evidence of hypoglycemia, or weight loss exceeds 5%.
5. Continue to monitor blood glucose even after starting intravenous glucose and a few hours after its discontinuation to avoid rebound hypoglycemia.
6. Wash stomach with 5 to 10 ml of water or saline solution if there is evidence of mucus vomiting (common in the dysmature).

---

*The use of Dextrostix (Ames) offers a qualitative test for blood glucose and tends to underestimate the true level at the low end of the color range. If the test paper shows an absence of easily recognizable pale blue color, a blood level below 30 mg/100 ml is likely, and an accurate quantitative determination is necessary.

General precautions in oral feedings

1. Consult infant's physician regarding volume increases.
2. Encourage prompt discontinuation and reporting of feeding difficulties.
3. Spitting up is a sign of excessive or too early feedings.
4. Note change in feeding habits such as disinterest in sucking, delayed emptying, or distention, which may indicate sepsis or necrotizing enterocolitis.
5. Do not give gastric feedings when there is tachypnea or respiratory distress (particularly with assisted ventilation). Use parenteral feedings, followed by transpyloric feedings when extended ventilatory support is required.

FEEDING TECHNIQUES

No method of feeding the neonate at risk can be satisfactory to the exclusion of other methods. Frequently, indications justify a combination of methods as well as a progression in methods, beginning with parenteral fluid infusions, moving to gavage or transpyloric feedings, and ending with the nipple. None of the described feeding methods has been evaluated in sufficient depth to warrant its recommendation as the best way to feed low birth weight infants. Percentage of weight loss, time needed to regain birth weight, and time needed to reach discharge weight are all useful measures of success in feeding. More important are the neurologic and intellectual end points that will eventually determine the success of any method or combination of methods currently in use.

Intermittent gavage

Intermittent gavage is preferred for the smaller preterm infant in no distress until sucking is established because it is safe, simple, quick, and easily taught.

1. Place the infant either on his side or his back. No restraint or handling of infant is necessary.
2. Insert a soft Fr 8 catheter through the mouth, for a distance equal to that from the bridge of the nose to the xiphoid process.
3. Observe for choking or gasping, indicative of possible tracheal entry.

4. Attach a syringe to feeding tube and aspirate gently. If there is a feeding residual of 1 to 2 ml prior to next feeding, amount of feeding should be decreased by amount of residual. Do not discard residual—refeed it to infant with the new formula. Report residual of more than 2 ml and skip that feeding.
5. Pour formula through barrel of syringe, allowing milk to run slowly, with no pressure and with minimal elevation of syringe.
6. Pinch to close tube, and withdraw it quickly.
7. Place infant on right side or abdomen to promote emptying of stomach.
8. Elevate upper part of body slightly.

Bottle feeding

Bottle-feeding technique requires a good sucking and swallowing reflex and should be tried when the infant sucks the gavage tube (32 to 33 weeks of postmenstrual age). The time of feeding should not exceed 15 minutes. The procedure is accomplished by the following:
1. Use a soft, medium-sized nipple with an adequate opening.
2. Apply gentle pressure on infant's chin and touch his lip with the nipple to help him open his mouth.
3. Hold infant semierect to facilitate nursing and burping when he is kept in incubator during feeding.
4. Turn infant on his side or abdomen when feeding is finished. When infant is dressed, he is removed from the incubator or bassinet and held by the nurse in a rocking chair for all feedings.

Precautions

1. Do not urge infant to accept more than is easily taken. Be prepared to remove nipple if he is getting milk too fast.
2. Assess clinically any infant showing reluctance to eat on two successive occasions.
3. Stop feeding if baby vomits or becomes cyanotic, if abdomen becomes distended, or stools become liquid or frequent.
4. Do not prop bottle.

Any change in feeding habits may be the first sign of illness.

Nasogastric feeding

Smaller plastic catheters, Fr 3½ to 5, have an advantage over larger catheters for indwelling tube feedings. Many centers successfully use this method for intermittent or continuous feeding of the immature infant. The catheter is replaced every 3 days through alternate nostrils. We believe that nasogastric feeding is less safe for the small healthy preterm infant than intermittent gavage feeding for the following reasons:
1. The tube acts as a foreign body, producing mucus, and both tube and mucus may block the airway of the weak premature infant.
2. Purulent rhinitis may develop.
3. The catheter may disturb some infants, and stabilizing tape may irritate skin.

Nevertheless, for the infant who has apneic attacks with gavage feeding, but who has adequate gastrointestinal motility, nasogastric feeding either intermittently or by continuous infusion with a pump is useful. Frequent checks for excessive feeding residuals and prompt identification of any distention are necessary. Volumes are started at 0.5-1 ml/kg/hr and are increased somewhat more slowly than they are with transpyloric feeding.

Transpyloric feeding

Transpyloric feeding of infants is accomplished by an indwelling tube placed through the pylorus and formula administered by a constant-infusion pump. The infants who may benefit from this method are those who:
1. Exhibit repeated apnea with gavage feedings (from tube insertion as well as stomach distention)
2. Show continued gastric residuals without ileus
3. Require prolonged assisted ventilation

Technique*

1. Pass a French 8 feeding tube through mouth and into stomach and instill 10 ml/kg of air.
2. Take a 36-inch radiopaque tube Fr 5 (3½ for very small infants) and mark the distance

---

*Modified from Shaff-Blass, E., Kuhns, L.R., and Wyman, M.L.: Gastric air insufflation as an aid to placement of oroduodenal tubes, J. Pediatr. **89**:954, 1976.

from the nose to the xiphoid plus 8 to 10 cm.
3. Lubricate tip and pass through nose, with infant held upright and slightly to right.
4. Secure catheter and intermittently aspirate until presumed duodenal contents are obtained. Check for bile-stained color or a pH reading over 7.
5. Remove gastric tube after removing air.
6. Attach infusion pump and give milk or formula at a rate of 0.5-1 ml/kg/hr. Increase by 0.5-1 ml/kg/hr each 12 to 24 hours if feeding is tolerated until approximately 150 to 180 ml/kg/day is reached, depending on caloric density.
7. Check for reflux by orogastric aspiration every 3 to 6 hours. Distention or reflux of over 3 ml demands caution and possible discontinuation.
8. Change catheter every 3 days to prevent small bowel perforation from hardening of the catheter material.

Types of feedings. The possible association of hyperosmolar and excessive volume feedings with necrotizing enterocolitis demands caution by physicians in feeding infants, particularly those who weigh under 1,500 gm at birth.
1. Start with an isosmolar feeding—5% dextrose for 12 hours—and then switch to 20 kcal/oz (later 24 kcal/oz) of formula or human milk.
2. Consider addition of medium-chain triglycerides (MCT oil, 8.3 kcal/gm, or safflower oil at 1 to 3 ml/24 hr), which does not increase osmolarity but adds to caloric intake.

Precautions. Sufficient experience is not yet available to assess the role of transpyloric feeding in the neonate, but evidence so far suggests a definite role, particularly after, or along with, parenteral infusions. Nasojejunal placements may interfere with enzymatic digestion and nutrient absorption. The following hazards and warning signals should be anticipated:
1. Reflux into stomach of volume over 2 ml indicates the need to reduce feedings or extend the placement of the feeding tube. Aspirate stomach contents every 3 to 6 hours until the amount aspirated remains under 2 ml.
2. Distention may indicate ileus, an early sign of necrotizing enterocolitis.
3. Bradycardic episodes justify further dependence on parenteral feedings.
4. Diarrhea may indicate excessive feedings or insufficient absorption of nutrients.
5. Airway obstruction may indicate rhinitis or use of too large a tube.
6. Polyvinyl catheters harden when left in place for several days and may perforate the intestine.

NECROTIZING ENTEROCOLITIS

Necrotizing enterocolitis (NEC) is a disease of the gastrointestinal tract and is reported to occur in 1% to 9% of admissions to neonatal centers, with a mortality of 20% to 30%. Fluctuating incidence (up to 25%) in infants under 1,300 gm birth weight suggests invasion of bacteria as an important complicating factor. NEC is occassionally seen in the term and small-for-dates infant.

Major factors

1. Bowel ischemia secondary to patent ductus arteriosus, hyperviscosity of blood, perinatal asphyxia, or umbilical catheterization
2. Feedings of milk, which encourage bacterial growth.
   Excessive volumes of milk feeding and hyperosmolar formulas particularly have been indicated, but cases have been reported to occur with human milk feedings.
3. Invasion of enteric bacteria, particularly *Klebsiella* and *Enterobacter*, into the bowel wall producing mucosal ulceration and intramural gas (H^+) formation, often leading to perforation
   NEC has also occurred with invasion of other bacteria (i.e., *Clostridium* species) and with rotavirus infection.

Warning signs

1. Increased apneic episodes with lethargy
2. Abdominal distention with decreased motility and increasing gastric residuals
3. Guaiac-positive stools containing mucus

More ominous signs

1. Vomiting of bile-stained material
2. Palpable loops of bowel
3. Bloody diarrhea

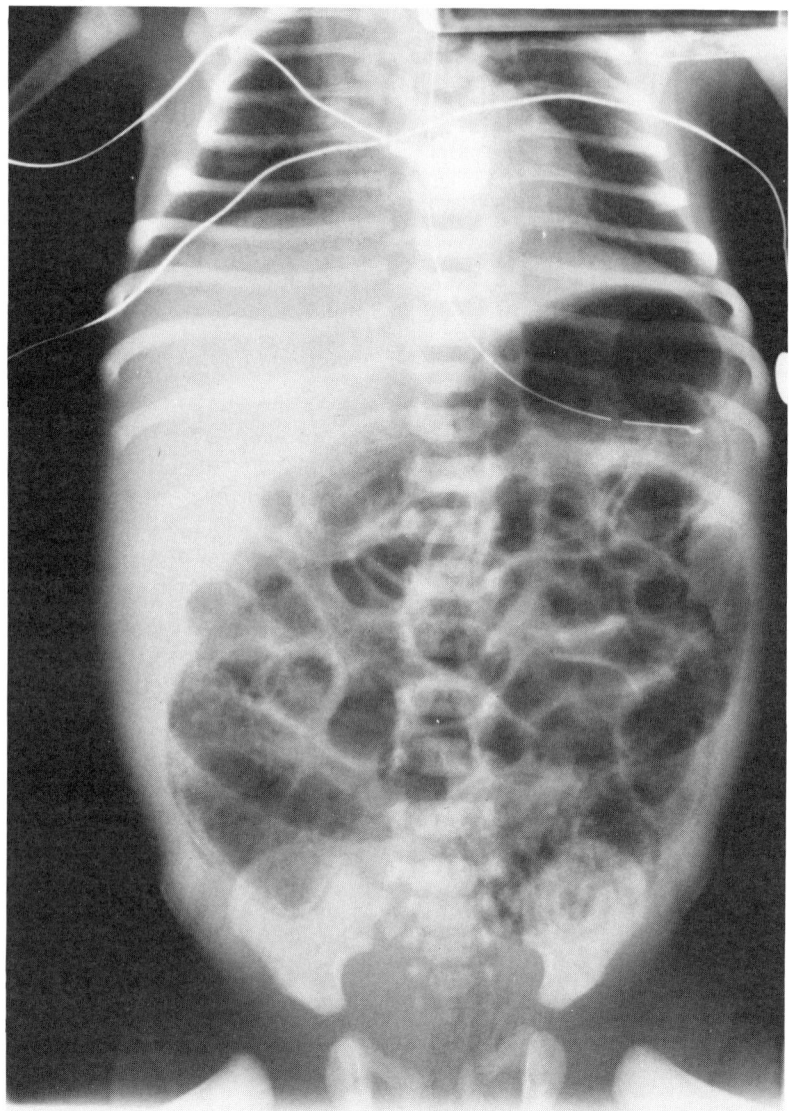

Fig. 16-2. Necrotizing enterocolitis. Small bowel is markedly dilated. Bowel wall contains small bubbles of gas, signifying pneumatosis intestinalis.

Confirmatory findings by x-ray examination (Figs. 16-2 and 16-3)

1. Dilated loops of bowel with thickened walls
2. Streaks of intramural air (pneumatosis intestinalis)
3. Air in hepatic vein or air in peritoneal cavity

Management

1. Correct acidosis (pH less than 7.30), hypotension, and anemia (Hct less than 40%).
2. Keep stomach empty by gentle continuous suction, for example, use of Stedman pump or intermittent gastric emptying with a feed-

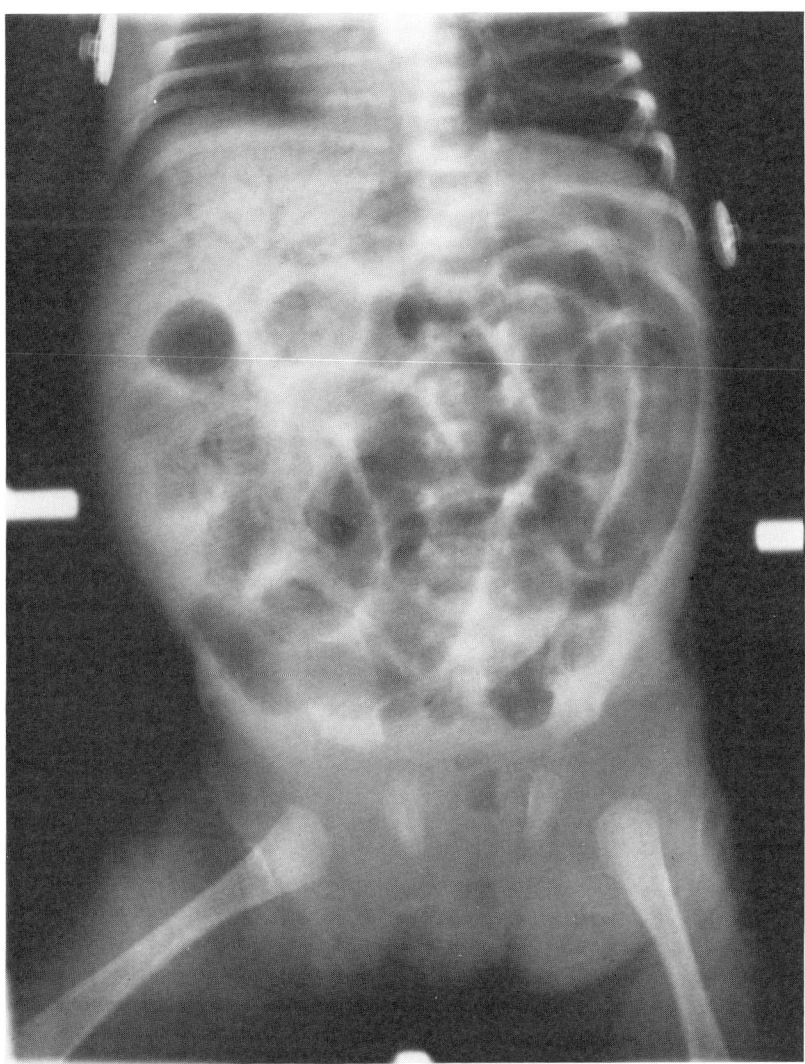

Fig. 16-3. Necrotizing enterocolitis. Small bowel is dilated and aligned in ropelike fashion. Linear lucencies are distributed throughout liver indicating gas in the portal system.

ing catheter. Feedings are not restarted until normal function is restored, usually after 7 to 10 days.
3. Culture blood and stool and give antibiotics (aminoglycosides and ampicillin).
4. Initiate parenteral nutrition.
5. Take series of x-ray films of abdomen.
6. Prepare for surgical intervention when there is intestinal perforation, evidence of abscess formation, or deteriorating clinical condition of infant. Resection of perforated or nonviable segment of intestine and placement of a temporary colostomy are the usual procedures in such cases.

Mortality with NEC is high when there is intestinal perforation or evidence of shock, but most infants will survive short of these events. Malabsorption may follow surgical treatment after removal of necrotic segments of bowel, leaving insufficient absorptive surface. Partial obstruction of intestinal tract may develop from healing contractures.

Prevention

We have been of the opinion for many years that the introduction of any oral feedings to the small, weak infant in too forceful a manner may encourage the development of NEC. Brown and Sweet have confirmed this impression. Therefore we advise:

1. Delay oral feedings of unstable preterm infants.
2. Give small volumes, increasing them very gradually.
3. Avoid hyperosmolar elemental feedings.
4. Discontinue feedings for distention, residual of 2 ml or more of milk, and guaiac-positive stools.
5. Administer antibiotics with any warning sign.

BIBLIOGRAPHY

American Academy of Pediatrics, Committee on Nutrition: Nutritional needs of low-birth-weight infants, Pediatrics **75**:976, 1985.

Atkinson, S.A., Anderson, G.H., and Bryan, M.H.: Human milk comparison of the nitrogen composition in milk from mothers of premature and full-term infants, Am. J. Clin. Nutr. **33**:811, 1980.

Atkinson, S.A., Radde, I.C., and Anderson, G.H.: Macromineral balances in premature infants fed their own mother's milk or formula, J. Pediatr. **102**:99, 1983.

Babson, S.F.: Feeding the low-birth-weight infant, J. Pediatr. **79**:694, 1971.

Books, L.S., Overall, J.C., Jr., Herbst, J.J., et al.: Clustering of necrotizing enterocolitis, N. Engl. J. Med. **297**:984, 1977.

Brown, E.G., and Sweet, A.Y.: Preventing entercolitis in neonates, JAMA **249**:2452, 1978.

Brown, E.G., and Sweet, A.Y., editors: Neonatal necrotizing enterocolitis, Monographs in neonatology, New York, 1980, Grune & Stratton, Inc.

Cheek, J.A., and Staub, G.F.: Nasojejunal alimentation for premature and full-term newborn infants, J. Pediatr. **82**:955, 1973.

Davies, P.G.: Adequacy of expressed breast milk for early growth of preterm infants, Arch. Dis. Child. **52**:296, 1977.

Erenberg, A., Shaw, R.D., and Youzefzadeh, O.: Lactobezoar in the low-birth-weight infant, Pediatrics **63**:642, 1979.

Fomon, S., Ziegler, E., and Vasquez, H.: Human milk and the small preterm infant, Am. J. Dis. Child **131**:463, 1977.

Greer, F.R., Steichen, J.J., and Tsang, R.C.: Effects of increased calcium, phosphorus, and vitamin D intake on bone mineralization in very low-birth-weight infants fed formulas with polycose and medium-chain triglycerides, J. Pediatr. **100**:951, 1982.

Gross, S.J., David, R.J., Bauman, L., et al.: Nutritional composition of milk produced by mothers delivering preterm, J. Pediatr. **96**:641, 1980.

Heird, W.C.: Nasojejunal feeding: a commentary, J. Pediatr. **85**:111, 1974.

Kliegman, R.M., and Fanaroff, A.A.: Neonatal necrotizing enterocolitis: a nine-year experience. I. Epidemiology and uncommon observations, Am. J. Dis. Child. **135**:603, 1981.

Kliegman, R.M., and Fanaroff, A.A.: Neonatal necrotizing enterocolitis: a nine-year experience. II. Outcome assessment, Am. J. Dis. Child. **135**:608, 1981.

Lundstrom, V., Sūmes, M.A., and Dallman, P.R.: Iron supplementation of low-birth-weight infants, J. Pediatr. **91**:878, 1977.

Rhea, J.W., Ahmed, M.S., and Menge, M.S.: Nasojejunal (transpyloric) feeding, J. Pediatr. **86**:451, 1975.

Rönnholm, K.A.R., Sipilä, I., and Siimes, M.H.: Human milk protein supplementation for the prevention of hypoproteinemia without metabolic imbalance in breast milk-fed very low-birth-weight infants, J. Pediatr. **101**:243, 1982.

Saigal, S., and Sinclair, J.C.: Urine solute excretion in growing low birth weight infants, J. Pediatr. **934**, 1977.

Santulli, T.V., Shullinger, J.N., Heird, W.C., et al.: Acute necrotizing enterocolitis in infancy: a review of 64 cases, Pediatrics **55**:376, 1975.

Shenai, J.P., Reynolds, J.W., and Babson, S.G.: Nutritional balance studies in very-low-birthweight infants: enhanced nutrient rates by an experimental formula, Pediatrics **66**:233, 1980.

Sinclair, J.C., Driscoll, J.M., Jr., Heird, W.C., et al.: Supportive management of the sick neonate: parenteral calories, water, and electrolytes, Pediatr. Clin. North Am. **17**:863, 1970.

Tomarelli, R.M.: Osmolality, osmolarity and renal solute load of infant formulas, J. Pediatr. **88**:454, 1976.

Ziegler, E.E., and Fomon, S.J.: Fluid intake, renal solute load and water balance in infancy, J. Pediatr. **78**:561, 1971.

17

Total parenteral nutrition

CANDIDATES FOR PARENTERAL NUTRITION

Parenteral nutritional support is indicated when conventional feeding methods are either impossible or hazardous for the infant and the likelihood of sufficient oral feedings will be unduly delayed. Candidates for total parenteral nutrition (TPN) are those who:

1. Have undergone complicated surgical procedures especially involving the gastrointestinal tract
2. Are in critical condition because of extended and severe respiratory distress
3. Experience complications with oral feedings, which are as follows:
    a. Recurrent or increasing apneic episodes
    b. Abdominal distention
    c. Vomiting or continued feeding residuals
    d. Abnormal stools containing blood or reducing sugars (Clinitest less than 2^+).*
    These positive findings are often associated with necrotizing enterocolitis.
4. Are very immature, particularly those less than 28 weeks of gestational age or weighing under 900 gm at birth

If one is able to provide by parenteral means 80 to 100 calories and 2 to 3 gm of protein per kilogram daily, positive nitrogen balance can be ensured and tissue catabolism prevented in most cases. In addition, continued growth and organ development will occur, and tissue healing as well as resistance to infection, should be enhanced.

A further advantage of established parenteral nutrition is the allowance of very gradual increments in oral feedings (see Fig. 16-1). This approach reduces numbers of those who must be placed on "nothing by mouth" and incidence of necrotizing enterocolitis.

SOURCES OF MAJOR NUTRIENTS
Protein

Proteins available for parenteral use are hydrolysates of casein or fibrin, which contain free amino acids and peptides, or free amino acid mixtures, such as TrophAmine,* which contain synthetic amino acids only and are used more commonly because of their higher amount of usable nitrogen (approximately 310 mg/100 ml in a 2% amino acid solution). Because cysteine is considered to be an essential amino acid in infants its addition as cysteine hydrochloride 1mM/kg/24 hr is recommended.

Carbohydrate

Dextrose is the carbohydrate of choice even though the sick and immature infant has difficulty with its metabolization. Hyperglycemia (less than 150 mg/100 ml) and glucosuria (greater than 1^+ by Clinitest) with possible dehydration from osmotic diuresis must be avoided. Therefore initial glucose infusion

---

*See p. 136 for techniques of Clinitest and guaiac testing.

*American McGaw, Irvine, Calif. 92714.

Table 17-1. Solutions for parenteral nutrition

Item	Al* 8	Al 10	Al 13	Al 18
Amino acids†	1.0	2.0	2.0	2.0
Carbohydrate (hydrous dextrose) (gm/100 ml)	8	10	13	18
Calories (per 100 ml)	27	34	44	61
Na^+ (mEq/100 ml)‡	2.6	2.7	2.7	2.7
K^+ (mEq/100 ml)	2.1	2.1	2.1	2.1
Ca^{++} (mEq/100 ml)	2.0	2.0	2.0	2.0
Mg^{++} (mEq/100 ml)	0.4	0.4	0.4	0.4
P (mM/100 ml)	0.9	0.9	0.9	0.9
Cl^- (mEq/100 ml)	2.5	2.5	2.5	2.5
Gluconate (mEq/100 ml)	2.0	2.0	2.0	2.0
SO_4 (mEq/100 ml)	0.4	0.4	0.4	0.4
Acetate (mEq/100 ml)	0.8	0.8	0.8	0.8

*"Al" stands for alimentation solution; the numbers following indicate gm/100 ml of dextrose present.
†TrophAmine (6%).
‡Sodium contribution from TrophAmine is included.

should not exceed 10 gm/kg/day (7.5 gm/kg/day in infants weighing under 1 kg).

Fortunately, tolerance is gained when the amount of carbohydrate is gradually increased. Increases must be supervised by frequent monitoring. Solutions containing up to 13% dextrose can be infused through peripheral veins, provided the infusion rate does not exceed 20 to 25 ml per hour.

Fat

Fat is an excellent calorie source and essential for prevention of fatty acid deficiency. Intralipid* is a 10% soybean emulsion offering 1.1 kcal/ml. Tolerance is limited to the range of 2 to 4 gm/kg/day (20 to 40 ml/kg/day). Amounts above tolerance level will cause hyperlipemia, and possibly deteriorating pulmonary function. Because of these potential dangers overadministration of parenteral lipids must be avoided. For the immature infant and those with significant pulmonary disease, 2 gm/kg/day of parenteral fat should probably not be exceeded.

Tolerance of lipids will improve with extension of the infusion period to 24 hours. Lipids cannot be mixed with TPN solutions and need to be infused separately by adding piggyback distally to the infusion set. Accurate infusion pumps are required.

Water, electrolytes, and trace elements

Water and electrolyte requirements are similar to those specified in Chapter 15. Additional calcium and phosphorus are essential to parenteral nutrition. Amounts indicated in Table 17-1, however, are significantly below those required by the low birth weight infant to avoid their precipitation in the solution. For prolonged use of TPN, 1.5 ml/kg/24 hr of a trace element mixture containing (per ml) 200 µg zinc, 13 µg copper, 0.1 µg chromium, 3.5 µg manganese, and 1 µg selenium should be added.

Vitamins

A multivitamin preparation, MVI-Pediatric* is added in the amounts listed below:

Weight	Amount
< 1 kg	1.5 ml/24 hr
1-3 kg	3.25 ml/24 hr
> 3 kg	5.0 ml/24 hr

This recently released preparation includes vitamins B_{12}, K, and E.

---

*Cutter Laboratories, Inc., Berkeley, Calif. 94710.

*Armour Pharmaceutical Co., Kankakee, Ill. 60901.

Table 17-2. Metabolic assessment for infants receiving TPN

Factor	Initially	After stabilized
Weight	Twice daily	Daily
Blood glucose	2 to 6 hours	Twice daily
Serum electrolytes	Daily	Thrice weekly
Serum turbidity (when infusing fats)	Twice daily	Daily
Base deficit	Daily	Thrice weekly
BUN		
SGOT		
Bilirubin		
Albumin	Weekly or as indicated	
Cholesterol		
Triglycerides		
Free fatty acids		
Ammonia		
Urine glucose (Clinitest)	4 to 6 hours	Twice daily
Urine electrolytes		
pH	Daily	Thrice weekly
Specific gravity		

TECHNIQUES OF CARE AND USE
Preparation

Scrupulous care by a trained team is necessary in the mixing of these solutions, which is performed, ideally, in the pharmacy. Extreme accuracy, cleanliness, and the use of closed mixing systems and laminar flow hoods are recommended. Solutions should be mixed in 12-hour aliquots (greater volumes can be prepared but must be kept refrigerated until used.)

The solutions we use for parenteral nutrition are shown in Table 17-1.

Administration

1. Regular infusion sets are attached to the bottle containing the amino acid solution and connected to the catheter or peripheral infusion site.
2. Intralipid (in a separate infusion set) is connected piggyback (using a Y-connector) to the amino acid infusion set, as close to the infusion site as possible, and infused with a pump. Because of the possibility of free fatty acids displacing bilirubin from albumin-binding sites, bilirubin levels should be below the range requiring phototherapy before Intralipid infusion begins. Other considerations in giving Intralipid are as follows:
   a. Begin with 1 gm/kg/24 hr and increase by 0.5 gm/kg daily.
   b. Infuse Intralipid over 24 hours to improve tolerance. The use of accurate infusion pumps is essential.
   c. Avoid serum turbidity by checking a spin-down hematocrit tube twice daily. Persisting marginal turbidity, increases in jaundice, or levels of serum cholesterol, triglycerides, and SGOT require consideration of the discontinuation of Intralipid infusion.
   d. Do not use microfilters for Intralipid infusion.
3. In-line filters (0.22-micron pore size) should be used for the amino acid solution, but placed proximally to the Intralipid entry site.

Infusion sites

1. *Peripheral veins.* We prefer this approach for most infants and have been successful in supporting growth for as long as 3 months and up to 3 kg in weight with this route as the sole source of calories.
2. *Central vein.* We use this method only in infants who require a greater caloric load than can be given by the peripheral route or when peripheral veins have been "used up."
3. *Umbilical artery.* We offer nutrition by way of the aorta only as long as a catheter is required for obtaining blood for serial blood gas measurements.
4. *Umbilical vein.* TPN is administered by this route if the catheter is in position for central venous pressure monitoring.

Metabolic assessment for infants receiving TPN

This information is given in Table 17-2.

Suggested use of parenteral nutrition solutions

Tables 17-3 and 17-4 offer a plan for a total parenteral nutrition program intended for immature infants and larger preterm or term

Table 17-3. Example of TPN program for a small preterm infant whose tolerance to glucose and fat is somewhat limited

Day*	Solution	Rate (ml/kg/day)	Lipid (ml/kg/day)	Total (ml/kg/day)	Calories (kcal/kg/day)
1	Al 8	100	—	100	27
2	Al 8	110	—	110	30
3	Al 8	130	—	130	35
4	Al 10	140	—	140	48
5	Al 10	140	10	150	59
6	Al 13	135	15	150	77
7	Al 13	130	20	150	79
8	Al 13	125	25	150	83

*If parenteral alimentation is started later than day 1 of life, the amounts of glucose infused can be higher, although caution is advised and careful monitoring of blood glucose levels by Dextrostix is necessary. Fluid amounts and electrolyte dosages have to be adjusted according to the infant's needs. Lipid infusion may be started if hyperbilirubinemia is not present, but it should be delayed as long as serum bilirubin levels remain high.

Table 17-4. Example of a TPN program for a larger preterm infant or term infant

Day	Solution	Rate (ml/kg/day)	Lipid (ml/kg/day)	Total (ml/kg/day)	Calories (kcal/kg/day)
1	Al 10	80	—	80	27
2	Al 13	90	10	100	51
3	Al 13	95	15	110	59
4	Al 13	110	20	130	70
5	Al 13	115	25	140	79
6	Al 13	120	30	150	86
7	Al 13	125	35	160	94

Table 17-5. Example of combined enteral and parenteral feedings

| Day | Parenteral fluids | | | Enteral feeding (24 kcal/30 ml) | Total (ml/kg/day) | Calories (kcal/kg/day) |
	Solution	Rate (ml/kg/day)	Lipid (ml/kg/day)	(ml/kg/day)		
1	Al 10	80	—	—	80	27
2	Al 10	90	10	—	100	42
3	Al 13	90	15	16	121	70
4	Al 13	90	20	24	134	81
5	Al 13	90	25	32	147	94
6	Al 13	80	20	48	148	96
7	Al 13	80	10	64	154	98
8	Al 13	70	10	80	160	107
9	Al 13	50	10	96	156	111
10	Al 13	50	—	112	162	113
11	—	—	—	128	128	104
12	—	—	—	144	144	117
13	—	—	—	160	160	130

infants. These are guidelines only, and use of such a program depends on individual patient needs and tolerance.

Supplemental parenteral nutrition

Small preterm infants started on enteral feedings usually need 1 to 2 weeks of cautious increases of these feedings. Supplementing their nutrition by parenteral means therefore allows an improved calorie intake during that time. Similarly, infants recovering from major surgery of the gastrointestinal tract will benefit from parenteral alimentation while enteral feedings are gradually increased. Attention must be paid to total volumes of fluid, electrolytes, and so forth, that are given. Table 17-5 gives examples of combined enteral and parenteral feedings. Larger and more mature infants will metabolize glucose more easily and can accept higher concentrations of it.

HAZARDS IN USE OF PARENTERAL NUTRITION
Infection

The use of peripheral veins can significantly reduce the incidence of sepsis caused by contaminated central catheters. Nevertheless, these are necessary at times for the provision of nutrition when sufficient calories cannot safely be given through peripheral veins or when these have been "used up."

Aseptic technique in the use of central catheters and in preparation and handling of infusates will keep the incidence of major infections to a minimum.

Hyperglycemia and hypoglycemia

Maintenance of normoglycemia is important because elevated serum glucose levels (greater than 150 mg/100 ml) and subsequent hyperosmolality and osmotic diuresis, or hypoglycemia (less than 40 mg/100 ml), are dangerous for the infant.

Main factors causing abnormal serum glucose levels are as follows:
1. Limitation in glucose tolerance because of immaturity
2. Sudden changes in tolerance to glucose because of stress (e.g., sepsis)
3. Inaccuracy of infusion pumps
4. Interruptions of infusion (with rebound hypoglycemia) and subsequent increase in infusion rate (with hyperglycemia) after infiltration of infusion sites

Tissue necrosis

One may encounter sloughs when using peripheral veins if significant infiltration of tissues at infusion site is allowed to occur before infusion is discontinued. The increased osmolarity of the infusate is very irritating to tissues. Careful observation of infusion sites, minimal taping of an extremity to prevent restriction of venous return, as well as to allow visibility, and prompt discontinuation of infusion at the earliest sign of infiltration or skin irritation all help to keep this complication at a minimum.

Cholestasis

Significant elevations of direct bilirubin and liver function tests indicating cholestasis are observed occasionally after several weeks of parenteral nutrition with or without the use of lipids. Although most infants recover after several weeks, progressive deterioration and death have been observed in some cases.

Therefore monitoring of liver functions and discontinuation of parenteral nutrition in symptomatic infants is advised.

Miscellaneous observations

Metabolic acidosis, hyperammonemia, and elevations of plasma amino acids have been observed with parenteral nutritional support. Reduction in amounts of protein infused (to less than 4 gm/kg/day) will usually limit these derangements, and also minimize chances for imbalance of plasma amino acids levels.

BIBLIOGRAPHY

Benda, G.I.M., and Babson, S.G.: Peripheral alimentation of the small premature infant, J. Pediatr. **79**:494, 1971.

Brans, Y.W.: Parenteral nutrition of the very low birth weight neonate: a critical view, Clin. Perinatol. **4**:367, 1977.

Bryan, M.H., Wei, P., Hamilton, J.R., et al.: Supplemental intravenous alimentation in low birth weight infants, J. Pediatr. **82**:940, 1973.

Committee on Nutrition, American Academy of Pediatrics: Commentary on parenteral nutrition, Pediatrics **71**:547, 1983.

Dweck, H.S., and Cassady, G.: Hyperglycemia and very low birth weight, Pediatrics **53**:189, 1974.

Heird, W.C., and Winters, R.W.: Total parenteral nutrition, J. Pediatr. **86**:2, 1975.

Oh, W.: Fluid and electrolyte therapy and parenteral nutrition in low-birth-weight infants, Clin. Perinatol. **9:**637, 1982.

Pildes, R.S., Ramamurthy, R.S., Cordero, G.V., et al.: Intravenous supplementation of L-amino acids and dextrose in low-birth-weight infants, J. Pediatr. **82:**945, 1973.

Rigo, J., and Senterre, J.: Parenteral nutrition in the very low-birth-weight infant. In Kretchmer, N., and Minkowski, A., editors: Nutritional adaptability of the gastrointestinal tract, New York, 1983, Raven Press.

Shaw, J.C.L.: Parenteral nutrition in the management of sick low birth weight infants, Pediatr. Clin. North Am. **20:**333, 1973.

Sinclair, J.C., Driscoll, J.M., Jr., Heird, W.C., et al.: Supportive management of the sick neonate: parenteral calories, water and electrolytes, Pediatr. Clin. North Am. **17:**863, 1970.

18

Untimely termination of pregnancy

PREMATURE LABOR

Labor is the process by which the products of conception are normally expelled. It is subject to a variety of complications, but one of the more frequent is premature termination of pregnancy.

Premature labor has been defined as labor that occurs earlier in pregnancy than normal. It is generally recognized as the presence of two or three uterine contractions at 10-minute intervals, with or without cervical changes. Other useful criteria for defining premature labor include the following:

1. Gestational age of less than 36 weeks
2. Observation for at least 30 minutes of regular, painful uterine contractions that occur at least twice every 10 minutes, or uterine contractions with demonstrated cervical effacement or dilatation
3. Intact membranes (although labor may be premature with ruptured membranes, those cases are considered premature rupture of membranes)

By this definition premature labor occurs in over 10% of all pregnancies* and accounts for nearly two thirds of infant deaths (approximately 25,000 infants annually in the United States).

The exact etiology of premature labor may be difficult to determine. However, there are strong clinical correlates that allow identification of many of the pregnancies at risk before the complication develops so that appropriate preventive measures may be taken. Additionally, both indirect supportive measures and direct approaches aimed at the extension of pregnancy are now available for the patient with established premature labor. Thus much of the perinatal mortality and morbidity experienced in the past with this pregnancy complication may be prevented.

Chapter 37 attempts to focus on the social, economic, and educational factors that so often relate to early birth as well as to low birth weight. No doubt these influences have much to do with the fact that the incidence of liveborn infants weighing less than 1,500 gm in Sweden is one third that of infants in this category in the United States (Table 34-2).

Iatrogenic prematurity

Prematurity can be prevented in the 1% to 3% of those infants who are premature because the physician misjudged fetal maturity and performed an untimely elective cesarean section or induction of labor. This continuing tragedy can be sharply curtailed or entirely eliminated if all elective deliveries are screened for maturity by use of the simple rapid surfactant ("bubble") test (p. 40), lecithin/sphingomyelin ratio determinations, or phosphatidylglycerol tests on the amniotic fluid.

Although size of fetal head is not precisely related to gestational age, a biparietal diameter of 9.5 cm or more, measured by ultrasonography, ensures that the fetus is of adequate size for delivery when determination of maturity by amniocentesis is not desirable.

---

*Another 3% of pregnancies result in mature low birth weight infants (less than 2,500 gm).

Diagnosis of premature labor
I. Clinical correlates of premature labor
   A. Previous obstetric history
      1. Premature or low birth weight babies
      2. Complications listed in B to F
   B. General medical complications
      1. Hypertension (primarily chronic hypertensive vascular disease)
      2. Renal disease
      3. Heart disease
      4. Pyelonephritis
      5. Acute systemic infections
      6. Heavy cigarette smoking
      7. Alcoholism or drug addiction
      8. Severe anemia
      9. Malnutrition (excessive or inadequate nutrition) and inadequate or excessive weight gain with pregnancy
   C. Obstetric complication
      1. Severe hypertensive states of pregnancy
      2. Abruptio placentae
      3. Placenta previa
      4. Circumvallate placenta
      5. Placental insufficiency
      6. Premature rupture of membranes
      7. Multiple gestation
      8. Polyhydramnios
      9. Pregnancy occurring less than 3 months after previous pregnancy's termination
   D. Genital tract anomalies
      1. Uterus
         a. Bicornuate
         b. Subseptate
         c. Unicornuate
      2. Cervical incompetence
         a. Congenital
         b. Acquired
            (1) Surgical (conization, abortion)
            (2) Obstetric (lacerations)
      3. Uterine leiomyomas
   E. Infection
      1. Maternal urinary tract infections
      2. Maternal genital tract infections (e.g., genital mycoplasma, Neisseria gonorrhoeae, herpes simplex)
      3. Specific fetotoxic maternal infections (e.g., cytomegalovirus, toxoplasmosis, listeriosis)
      4. General sequelae of massive maternal systemic infections (e.g., pneumonia, influenza, malaria)
      5. Maternal intraabdominal sepsis (e.g., appendicitis, cholecystitis, diverticulitis)
      6. Maternal intraabdominal aseptic irritation (e.g., leaking benign cystic teratoma, perforation of gastric or duodenal ulcer, adnexal torsion)
   F. Miscellaneous
      1. Maternal trauma or burns
      2. Surgical procedures (particularly intraabdominal)
      3. Low socioeconomic status
II. Presenting symptoms and signs
   A. Labor contractions
      In majority of cases, strong premature contractions initiate labor.
   B. Premature rupture of membranes
      The membranes rupture prematurely in approximately 20% to 25% of all premature deliveries and may be the first abnormal sign. The etiology of premature rupture of membranes is unknown. However, it has been shown that membranes that rupture prematurely have a lower bursting tension than do membranes that do not rupture prematurely.
   C. Vaginal bleeding
      Second-trimester vaginal bleeding may be caused by a circumvallate placenta, abruptio placentae, or placenta previa. Each of these creates relative placental insufficiency and gestational instability. They are discussed in greater detail in Chapter 22.
   D. Increased vaginal discharge and vaginal pressure
      Incompetent cervix is usually seen with discharge and pressure.
III. Examination in premature labor
   A. Fetal size
      Special care should be taken to determine fetal size (ultrasonography) and well-being (electronic fetal monitoring).
   B. Presenting part
      The presenting part should be noted. An increased incidence of breech presentation occurs with early labor
   C. Contractions
      The duration and frequency of contrac-

tions must be determined. This is usually best accomplished by external electronic fetal monitoring.
D. Cervix
Cervical dilatation, cervical effacement, status of membranes, presence or absence of mucous plug, evidence of infection, fetal presenting part, and fetal station all are important in evaluation of labor.
E. Laboratory
Obtain same laboratory information as for premature rupture of membranes (see p. 168).

Exclusions to treatment of labor

It would seem at first glance that one should attempt to suppress every instance of premature labor because of the devastatingly high perinatal mortality and morbidity that accompanies prematurity. This is illogical, however, because many cases of premature delivery and perinatal death are related to a serious disorder that cannot be diagnosed ante partum. Moreover, it may be best to actually encourage early birth in some conditions to spare the mother or her fetus. Nonetheless, one must identify instances in which the only threat to the offspring appears to be premature labor. Thus labor should be permitted to continue in the following:

1. Maternal conditions that jeopardize the intrauterine environment or make birth the lesser risk
   a. Severe hypertensive disease (e.g., acute exacerbation of chronic hypertension, eclampsia, severe preeclampsia)
   b. Cardiac or pulmonary disease (e.g., valvular disease, tachyarrhythmias, pulmonary edema)
   c. Hemorrhage or extraordinary potential for hemorrhage (e.g., abruptio placentae, disseminated intravascular coagulation)
   d. Hyperthyroidism
   e. Other states that might be adversely affected by therapy
2. Fetal disorders that tend either to precipitate early delivery or to make attempts to stop premature labor profitless
   a. Fetal death
   b. Fetal distress
   c. Intrauterine infection
   d. Polyhydramnios
   e. Therapy adversely affecting the fetus
   f. Other critical fetal problems where the fetus is safer if delivered than left in utero (e.g., erythroblastosis fetalis, severe intrauterine growth retardation)
3. Clinical conditions in which it is obvious that attempts to check premature labor will be futile
   a. Ruptured membranes
   b. Cervix dilated more than 4 cm
   c. Cervical effacement greater than 80%
4. Mature (as determined by physiologic maturity testing) fetuses

If one excludes all patients for whom attempts at arrest of labor are either contraindicated or likely to be unsuccessful, only about 25% of the total low birth weight fetuses remain as candidates for labor-suppression drug therapy. Also, the excellent prognosis for neonates when lecithin/sphingomyelin ratios, presence of PG, or rapid surfactant tests indicate maturity obviates any reasonable attempt to delay their delivery.

Pharmacologic control of labor

After observation and analysis, therapeutic decisions usually depend on the variables of uterine contractions and cervical change (Table 18-1).

I. General measures
   A. Bed rest
   B. Initial pelvic examination only
II. Hydration and sedation
   Because of demonstrated success in several centers, hydration and sedation are increasingly used as first treatment or as "pretherapy" for premature labor.
   A. Criteria for admission to protocol
      1. Confirmation of premature labor
      2. Pregnancy beyond 20 weeks (this level is variably set by different institutions)
      3. Cervical dilatation of 4 cm or less
      4. Cervical effacement of 80% or less
      5. No contraindications to therapy
   B. Protocol
      1. Thirty min observation with electronic fetal monitoring to ascertain uterine activity
      2. One hour observation with the following:
         a. Continuous electronic fetal monitoring

Table 18-1. Therapy for premature labor based on various combinations of uterine contractions and cervical change.*

Group	Diagnosis	Usual therapy
I (No uterine contractions; no cervical change)	No labor	None
II (Uterine contractions but no cervical change)	Premature labor	Hydration/sedation protocol
III (Cervical change but no uterine contractions)	Incompetent cervix	Bed rest, consider cerclage
IV (Uterine contractions and cervical change)	Labor	Tocolytic protocol

*For purposes here uterine contractions are considered present when there are more than two contractions every 10 minutes and cervical change when effacement is greater than 80%, or dilatation is greater than finger tip, or there is change in either effacement or dilatation with observation.

    b. Hydration with 500 ml 5% dextrose/0.5% normal saline (or 5% dextrose/lactated Ringer's solution) given intravenously over 30 min
    c. Morphine sulfate 8 to 12 mg IM (provided no allergy exists, delivery is not imminent, and naloxone is available should delivery occur and fetal respiration be depressed)
3. At the end of 1 hour assess progress of labor and proceed as follows:
    a. With progressive cervical change proceed to use of tocolytics or other appropriate therapy.
    b. With no cervical change but continued uterine activity proceed to use of tocolytics.
    c. With no cervical change and cessation of uterine activity continue observation for risk of premature labor.

It may be anticipated that those in group *a* will represent only a small percentage, those in group *b* less than half, and those in group *c* the majority of patients. Moreover, both groups *b* and *c* are at risk for subsequent premature delivery.

III. Tocolysis

The decision to use a tocolytic drug must be carefully considered and once that decision is reached, the choice of which tocolytic drug to use must be carefully weighed. Many drugs potentially dangerous to the fetus, including barbiturates, anesthetics, progesterone, epinephrine, chlordiazepoxide (Librium), and diazepam (Valium), have been abandoned as effective agents against premature labor. Clearly the standard that other drugs are now judged by is ritodrine.* Although each of the drugs listed below (in descending order of effectiveness) has certain contraindications, they may be effective for the suppression of uterine contractility in threatened premature labor.

  A. Ritodrine - *p* - hydroxyphenylethyl - *p* - hydroxy - norepinephrine, administered intravenously
  B. Ethanol, administered intravenously
  C. Magnesium sulfate, administered intravenously

IV. Tocolytic regimens
  A. Ritodrine administered intravenously
    1. Determinations to be made before beginning ritodrine therapy:
      a. All criteria for premature labor are met.
      b. Fetus is (or is very likely to be) premature but is over 20 weeks' gestation. In emergencies or when it seems certain that fetus is premature, therapy may be initiated before physiologic maturity studies are obtained.
      c. No reason for allowing labor to continue exists.
    2. General contraindications to ritodrine therapy

---

*Information on ritodrine from Astra Pharmaceutical Products, Inc.: YUTOPAR Solution and Tablets (ritodrine hydrochloride), 1982, (AST-2613) Worcester, Massachusetts.

a. Pregnancy that is near term or of less than 20 weeks
   b. Maternal condition making continuation of pregnancy hazardous
   c. Fetal condition making continuation of pregnancy hazardous
3. Specific contraindications to ritodrine therapy
   a. Antepartum hemorrhage that demands immediate delivery
   b. Eclampsia and severe preeclampsia
   c. Intrauterine fetal death
   d. Chorioamnionitis
   e. Maternal cardiac disease
   f. Pulmonary hypertension
   g. Maternal hyperthyroidism
   h. Uncontrolled maternal diabetes mellitus
   i. Preexisting maternal medical conditions that would be seriously affected by the known pharmacologic properties of beta-mimetic drugs, such as hypovolemia, cardiac arrhythmias associated with tachycardia or digitalis intoxication, uncontrolled hypertension, pheochromocytoma, bronchial asthma already treated with beta-mimetics or steroids
   j. Known hypersensitivity to any component of the product
4. Precautions to be observed with intravenous ritodrine therapy
   a. Patient must be hospitalized.
   b. Administration must be closely monitored. Attendants must know pharmacology of ritodrine and be qualified to identify and manage complications of drug administration and pregnancy.
   c. Cardiovascular responses (including maternal pulse, maternal blood pressure, and FHR) must be closely monitored. Danger signs (because of propensity for cardiovascular response or unmasking of occult cardiac disease) include:
      (1) Persistent high tachycardia (greater than 140 beats/min)
      (2) Tachypnea
         Either or both of the above may be signs of impending pulmonary edema.
      (3) Chest pain or tightness of chest
         Temporarily discontinue medication and obtain an ECG as soon as possible.
   d. Avoidance of maternal pulmonary edema
      Development of serious and even fatal maternal pulmonary edema during ritodrine therapy has been reported both ante partum and post partum and appears to occur more frequently with concomitant corticosteroid usage.
      (1) Avoid fluid overload.
      (2) Carefully monitor patient's hydration state.
      (3) Discontinue the drug immediately if signs of pulmonary edema develop.
   e. Laboratory parameters for monitoring ritodrine administration
      Monitoring the following is particularly important with prolonged intravenous administration of ritodrine because the drug elevates plasma insulin and glucose and decreases plasma potassium concentrations. Assessment of hydration state is also important and may be assisted by the hemogram.
      (1) Plasma glucose
      (2) Serum electrolytes
      (3) Hemogram
5. Adverse effects of ritodrine related to beta-mimetic activity
   Effects noted below pertain to intravenous therapy. The only adverse effects of oral therapy are small increases in maternal heart rate (maternal blood pressure and

FHR are unaffected), palpitation, tremor, nausea, jitteriness, rash, and cardiac arrhythmias (about 1%).
  a. Usual effects (80% to 100% of patients will experience one or more of these effects)
     (1) Increased maternal heart rate (to average of 130 beats/min)
     (2) Increased systolic blood pressure (average increase of 12 mm Hg) and decreased diastolic blood pressure (average decrease of 23 mm Hg)
     (3) Increased FHR (to average of 160 beats/min)
  b. Frequent effects (10% to 50% incidence)
     (1) Tremor
     (2) Nausea
     (3) Vomiting
     (4) Headache
     (5) Erythema
  c. Occasional effects (5% to 10% incidence)
     (1) Nervousness
     (2) Jitteriness
     (3) Restlessness
     (4) Emotional upset or anxiety
     (5) Malaise
  d. Infrequent effects (1% to 3% incidence)
     (1) Chest pain or tightness (rarely associated with ECG abnormalities)
  e. Other reported adverse effects
     Anaphylactic shock
     Heart murmur
     Ileus
     Constipation
     Dyspnea
     Hemolytic icterus
     Lactic acidosis
     Drowsiness
     Rash
     Epigastric distress
     Bloating
     Diarrhea
     Hyperventilation
     Glycosuria
     Sweating
     Weakness
6. Reported neonatal symptoms
  a. Infrequent effects
     (1) With no other maternal beta-mimetic agent used
        (a) Hypoglycemia
        (b) Ileus
     (2) With other maternal beta-mimetic agent used
        (a) Hypocalcemia
        (b) Hypotension
7. Symptoms of overdose
   The amount of ritodrine required to produce symptoms of overdose is individually variable. No deaths caused by overdose have been reported. Symptoms of overdosage are those of excessive beta-adrenergic stimulation.
   a. Tachycardia (maternal and fetal)
   b. Palpitation
   c. Cardiac arrhythmia
   d. Hypotension
   e. Dyspnea
   f. Nervousness
   g. Tremor
   h. Nausea
   i. Vomiting
8. Method of administration
   In management of preterm labor, initial intravenous treatment should usually be followed by oral administration. The optimum dose of ritodrine is determined by a clinical balance of uterine response and unwanted effects.
   a. Intravenous therapy
      Do not use intravenous ritodrine if solution is discolored or contains any precipitate or particulate matter. Solution should be used promptly after preparation, never later than 48 hours after preparation.
      (1) Maintain patient in left lateral position.
      (2) Pay careful attention to hydration. Fluid overload must be avoided.

(3) Use a controlled infusion device to adjust rate of flow in drops/min. An IV microdrip chamber (60 drops/ml) can provide a convenient range of infusion rates within recommended dose range.
(4) Use recommended dilution of 150 mg ritodrine (3 ampuls) in 500 ml fluid, which yields a final concentration of 0.3 mg/ml. Ritodrine for intravenous infusion should be diluted with one of the following:
   (a) 0.9% sodium chloride solution
   (b) 5% dextrose solution
   (c) 10% dextran 40 in 0.9% sodium chloride solution
   (d) 10% invert sugar solution
   (e) Compound sodium chloride solution (Ringer's solution)
   (f) Hartmann's solution
(5) Start intravenous therapy as soon as possible after diagnosis. The usual initial dose is 0.1 mg/min (0.33 ml/min or 20 drops/min using a microdrip chamber at recommended dilution), to be gradually increased according to results by 0.05 mg/min (0.17 ml/min or 10 drops/min using a microdrip chamber at recommended dilution) every 10 minutes until desired result is attained. Effective dosage usually lies between 0.15 and 0.35 mg/min (0.50 to 1.17 ml/min, 30 to 70 drops/min using a microdrip chamber at recommended dilution).
(6) Monitor maternal uterine contractions, heart rate, and blood pressure, and FHR frequently, titrating dosage according to response. If other drugs need to be given intravenously, use piggyback method or other site of intravenous administration to maintain independent control of rate of infusion.
(7) Continue infusion for at least 12 hours after uterine contractions cease. With recommended dilution, the maximum volume of fluid that might be administered after 12 hours at the highest dose (0.35 mg/min) is approximately 840 ml.
(8) Monitor amount of IV fluids administered and rate of administration to avoid circulatory fluid overload (overhydration).

b. Oral administration

Oral maintenance begins with 1 tablet (10 mg) given approximately 30 minutes before termination of intravenous therapy. The usual dosage schedule for the first 24 hours of oral administration is one tablet every 2 hours. Thereafter, usual maintenance is one or two tablets (10 to 20 mg) every 4 to 6 hours, the dose depending on uterine activity and unwanted effects. The total daily dose of oral ritodrine should not exceed 120 mg. Treatment may be continued as long as desired to prolong pregnancy. Recurrence of unwanted preterm labor may be treated with repeated infusion of ritodrine.

B. Ethanol, administered intravenously
1. Infuse 100 ml 95% ethanol with

900 ml D5W to equal 1,000 ml 9.5% ethanol (75.4 gm/L).
   2. Give loading dose of 15 ml/kg body weight over 2 hours.
   3. Give maintenance dose of 1.5 ml/kg body weight/hr.
   4. If treatment has been discontinued less than 10 hr earlier calculate dose to reload patient as follows (Fuchs and colleagues):

   $$\text{Loading dose} \times \frac{\text{No. of hours}}{10}$$

C. Magnesium sulfate, administered intravenously
   1. Determine that all criteria for premature labor are met.
   2. Determine that maternal or fetal contraindications to therapy exist.
   3. Infuse 4 gm of $MgSO_4$ (40 ml of 10% solution) slowly enough to prevent flushing and vomiting.
   4. Continue constant infusion of 2% maintenance solution (200 ml 10% $MgSO_4$ to 800 ml D5W) at 100 ml/hr until labor subsides or progresses to an irreversible stage (spontaneous rupture of membranes or cervical dilatation of 5 cm).
   5. Reduce rate of $MgSO_4$ infusion if magnesium toxicity is observed.
   6. Repeat procedure if contractions reappear after discontinuation of infusion.
V. Glucocorticoid therapy
   Glucocortocoid therapy, as demonstrated by Liggins and others (Table 18-2), can reduce the incidence of respiratory distress syndrome, particularly in infants under 32 weeks of gestational age. Ballard's work indicates that this is brought about by an increased production of pulmonary surface-active material. Evidence is accumulating (Taeusch et al., Papageorgiou et al.) in support of steroid therapy.

We have chosen to use steroid therapy in selected circumstances, with patients carefully monitored and studied. The dosage and type usually administered is betamethasone (Celestone) 12 mg IM with the dose repeated once in 12 hours and then once weekly. Other circumstances to be considered are noted in the next section (premature rupture of membranes).

Management of preterm delivery

See Chapter 7.

PREMATURE RUPTURE OF MEMBRANES

Spontaneous rupture of membranes may happen at any time during pregnancy. When it occurs prior to the onset of labor, the condition is termed premature rupture of membranes (PROM). By this definition approximately 10.7% of all pregnancies suffer this "complication." However, there is a vast difference between potential maternal and perinatal morbidity and mortality when this occurs with a mature fetus and when it happens at 27 weeks' gestation. Thus, "premature" rupture of membranes is unfortunate terminology. It is more accurate to term the event "prelabor" rupture of membranes if a mature fetus is involved and "preterm" rupture if a less than mature fetus is involved. When more than 24 hours elapses

Table 18-2. Respiratory distress syndrome (RDS) related to gestational age in live-born infants of unplanned deliveries 24 hours to 7 days after entry into trial

Gestational age at delivery	Betamethasone			Control			Statistical significance p
	No RDS	RDS	%RDS	No RDS	RDS	%RDS	
28 to 30 weeks	36	10	27.8	26	15	57.7	0.04
30 and 31 weeks	23	2	8.7	25	14	56.0	0.001
32 and 33 weeks	50	0	0.0	31	4	12.9	0.04
34 weeks or more	73	4	5.5	74	4	5.4	NS

between rupture of membranes and onset of labor, the problem is one of prolonged premature rupture of membranes. Amniotic fluid may gush through the cervix, denoting a wide rent in the membranes; in other cases a persistent trickle suggests a small tear or perforation. With considerable loss of fluid, the onset of labor usually occurs within a few days, but it is not inevitable and is clearly related to the size of the fetus when there is no intervention (Table 18-3).

Periodic discharge of amniotic fluid may also occur, but occasionally the presenting part will prevent great loss, or the perforation may seal off. In these instances the mother and fetus usually are unaffected, and the pregnancy will continue. However, this condition remains an extremely serious cause of morbidity and mortality in the preterm fetus.

I. Associations
Recognized relationships to premature rupture of membranes include the following:
A. Maternal urinary tract infections
B. Lower genital tract infection
C. Intrauterine infection
D. Cervical incompetence
E. Multiple pregnancy
F. Hydramnios
G. Gonorrheal infections
Gonorrheal infections predispose pregnancy to a 2.5-fold increase in rupture of membranes, even if infection is asymptomatic.
H. Nutritional
1. Ascorbic acid deficiency
2. Copper deficiency
I. Decreased membrane tensile strength
Although not all causes of decreased membrane strength are known, it is associated with the nutritional deficiencies noted above.
J. Familial
If a woman is the product of a pregnancy complicated by PROM, she is at a five-fold greater risk of having PROM as a pregnancy complication. The exact reasons for this remain unclear.

There are a number of factors previously thought to be correlated with membrane rupture that have subsequently been disproved including maternal age, maternal parity, fetal weight, fetal position, and trauma.

II. Pathologic physiology
A. Premature rupture of membranes is an important cause of premature labor, prolapse of the cord, and intrauterine infection.
B. So-called dry labor, which eventually occurs after gross loss of amniotic fluid, may be desultory or prolonged if
1. Patient is not at term
2. Uterus in not "sensitized" to labor
3. Malpresentation exists
4. Intrauterine infection is present
C. The fetus may appear similar to one with Potter's syndrome, with extraordinary flexion, drying of the skin, etc. It has been reported, but not confirmed, that various anomalies may result from chronic absence of amniotic fluid caused by rupture of membranes.

III. Diagnosis
A. Symptoms
1. Persistent or recurrent loss of fluid, often including flecks of vernix
2. Reduction in size of uterus
3. Increased prominence of fetus to palpation
B. Sterile speculum exam
A most important step is accurate diagnosis of premature rupture of membranes and accurate assessment of fetal maturity. On admission the

Table 18-3. Occurrence of onset of labor after rupture of membranes related to fetal weight

Weight group	% PROM resulting in onset of labor	% prolonged membrane rupture resulting in onset of labor
>2,500 gm	94.3	19
1,000-2,500 gm	5.3	49
<1,000 gm	0.4	74

following procedure has proved useful:
1. Examine abdomen carefully.
2. Culture cervix mucus.
3. If vaginal pool exists, collect fluid for
   a. KOH and wet mount examinations
   b. Nitrazine and fern tests
4. Observe for leakage of fluid from os with
   a. Valsalva maneuver
   b. Cough
   c. Fundal pressure
5. Collect fluid from posterior lip of speculum (if uncontaminated) for L/S ratio, phosphatidylglycerol (PG), or bubble test.
6. Determine cervical status.
7. Check for cord prolapse.

C. Examination of fluid
The following tests are useful in the identification of rupture of membranes:
1. pH
   Amniotic fluid is clear or milky, slightly alkaline (pH greater than 7; nitrazine test paper deep blue), and has a seminiferous odor.
2. Arborization test (when fluid is uncontaminated with gross blood or meconium)
   a. Obtain fluid from vagina as close to cervix as possible, or from posterior lip of a Graves' speculum.
   b. Spread fluid on a clean glass slide and allow to dry.
   c. Observe for a distinct pattern of crystallization resembling a palm or fern design, which indicates amniotic fluid.
   d. Also observe another sample of fluid microscopically for lanugo hair.
3. Dye test
   a. Aspirate 5 ml of amniotic fluid transabdominally.
   b. Inject 5 ml of dilute Evans blue solution.
   c. Insert vaginal speculum after 15 to 20 minutes.
   d. Blue-colored fluid in vagina indicates ruptured membranes.

The dye test should only rarely be necessary. Use of the other tests mentioned, including a careful history within 2 hours of the presumed rupture of membranes, will allow an accurate diagnosis.

IV. Evaluation on admission
   A. Physical examination
      1. Search for signs of infection.
         a. Urinary tract (i.e., pyelonephritis)
         b. Amnionitis
         c. Other possibly treatable foci of infection
      2. Perform a careful abdominal examination.
      3. Search for signs of other infection.
   B. Laboratory tests
      1. Complete blood count with differential
      2. Catheter urine for analysis, culture, and antibiotic sensitivity
      3. Ultrasonography for fetal size
      4. If diagnosis is equivocal, amniocentesis may be done, with fluid withdrawn for fetal-maturity studies and culture, and dilute indigo carmine injected; a tampon in the vagina will reveal PROM by its blue color
   C. Amnionitis
      1. Seek to diagnose early by frequent monitoring for
         a. Fever—check temperature every 4 hours
         b. Maternal leukocytosis—obtain leukocyte count and differential daily, or more frequently if elevated
         c. Fetal tachycarida—auscultate fetal heart tones every 4 hours
         d. Uterine tenderness—check every 4 hours
      2. Difficulties in diagnosis of amnionitis
         a. Frequent fundal examinations may cause uterine tenderness.
         b. Steroid administration may cause mild leukocytosis.

c. Labor is associated with leukocytosis.
  3. If diagnosis of amnionitis is equivocal, amniocentesis should be performed to look for bona fide evidence of amnionitis:
     a. Bacteria on Gram's stain
     b. Bacterial growth on culture
     c. Numerous leukocytes in amniotic fluid
V. Differential diagnosis
  A. Vaginal fluid is mucoid and acid and will not crystallize, nor does it contain exfoliated fetal cells or lanugo hair.
  B. The incontinent patient may have vaginal fluid that has the odor of urine and contains urate crystals but does not reveal fetal elements and does not dry to form fernlike crystal patterns.
  C. Hydrorrhea gravidarum fluid is periodic, but it may also be profuse. It is most frequently found as part of a triad consisting of circumvallate placenta, abruptio placentae, and hidrorrhea gravidarum. The fluid is thought to be a serum transudate. It does not contain fetal cells or lanugo hair and does not form the fern pattern.
  D. Vaginitis of a pronounced degree may be confused with ruptured membranes. A microscopic examination should aid in the diagnosis of the infection's etiology.
VI. Prevention
  A. Treat vaginitis and cervicitis before and during pregnancy.
  B. Repair incompetent cervix when indicated.
  C. Provide prolonged bed rest for patients with multiple pregnancy or hydramnios.
  D. Screen patients for and treat urinary tract infections.
  E. Screen patients for and treat gonorrheal and chlamydial infections.
VII. Treatment
  At present there is controversy concerning management of premature rupture of membranes. One school of thought holds that nonintervention (no vaginal manipulation or attempts at delivery) may have greater benefit to the preterm fetus than attempts to deliver. The second school of thought holds that delivery should be induced within a reasonable interval for all fetuses over 33 weeks' gestation. Both groups present good data supporting these opposing views.
  It has been suggested that differences in populations studied may account for these disparate results. That is, for populations where puerperal febrile morbidity is low, nonintervention may be appropriate, but for populations with common puerperal febrile morbidity, the mother and perinate may benefit from delivery within 24 hours.
  If nonintervention is selected, care should be exercised to determine that amnionitis has not occurred (see C., Amnionitis, above). If intervention is selected, proceed as follows:
  A. Prepare patient for impending labor.
  B. Check for evidence of multiple pregnancy, malpresentation, fetal anomaly, or prolapsed cord.
  C. Avoid frequent vaginal or rectal examinations to minimize chance of introducing intrauterine infection.
  D. Manage preterm delivery as discussed in Chapter 7.
  E. Determine whether delivery or induction or inhibition of labor is indicated.
    1. 36 weeks or greater—induce labor if it does not occur within 2 hours of rupture of membranes.
    2. 32 to 36 weeks—determine physiologic maturity status. Inhibit labor for 24 to 48 hours in absence of amnionitis, if needed for possible enhancement in pulmonary maturation.
    3. Less than 32 weeks
       a. If amniotic fluid for bubble test, and L/S ratio and PG determinations can be obtained and indicate fetal maturity, deliver at once.
       b. In absence of amnionitis, fol-

low until 32 weeks, after glucocorticoid therapy, observing for amnionitis. In patients for whom bed rest has been prescribed, miniheparin and foot boards should be used. Limited ambulation may be allowed. Deliver at 32 to 36 weeks or when physiologic maturity testing is at least intermediate.
F. Use glucocorticoid therapy when indicated (restricted to fetuses of 27 to 32 weeks' gestation with immature physiologic maturity statuses)—betamethasone (Celestone) 12 mg IM, to be repeated in 12 hours.
G. Inhibit labor if indicated.
1. In absence of amnionitis, inhibit labor as needed with tocolytics.
2. Presence of bleeding may indicate abruption, in which case inhibitors of labor usually are not successful or indicated (see Chapter 22).

Amnionitis

Intrauterine infection after rupture of membranes shows an almost linear progression beginning after a lag period of 12 to 18 hours. As time passes after rupture of membranes from any cause, exposure of the fetus to infected fluid leads to intrauterine pneumonia; omphalitis and septicemia usually are secondary to placentitis but may occur after amnionitis.
1. Fetal risk is much greater for the premature than for the term fetus because
    a. Resistance to infection is much less for the immature fetus and is directly related to the degree of maturity.
    b. The lag period prior to spontaneous or even induced labor is longer for the woman who is not at term than for one who is close to the expected date of confinement.
    c. Many premature infants present in breech position, and trauma during vaginal delivery may cause injury.
2. Antibiotics of the broad-spectrum type, even in large doses, do little to protect the fetus from intrauterine infection.
3. Presence of amnionitis is indicated by the following signs:
    a. Fever in mother (often accompanied by a tender uterus)
    b. Maternal polymorphonuclear leukocytosis
    c. Fetid odor of amniotic fluid
    d. Placental membranes and cord showing "smoky" or "steamy" translucence (A frozen section of these structures will show abnormal collections of neutrophils with infection.)
    e. Polymorphonuclear leukocytes found on a smear of the chorionic surface of the amnion
    f. Polymorphonuclear leukocytes found on a smear of a gastric aspirate from the infant
4. Treat mother
    a. Administer appropriate broad-spectrum antibiotics.
    b. Deliver infant rapidly.

Management of neonate (see also Chapter 25)

Every infant born after prolonged rupture of membranes or obvious signs of amnionitis in the mother (fever, leukocytosis, tender uterus, foul-smelling amniotic fluid) should have gastric aspiration (a swab from the external ear canal also can be used). Gram stain is applied to the material for microscopic examination. An unmixed collection of morphologically similar bacteria is more significant than a multiplicity of forms. The presence of more than five polymorphonuclear neutrophils (PMNs) per high-power field indicates exposure to infection but not necessarily active infection (approximately 10% to 15% of such infants develop sepsis); thus treatment is not mandatory. For infants with a positive gastric aspirate, obtain a blood culture (not from an umbilical vessel) and consider antibiotic treatment with gentamicin and penicillin or ampicillin when:
1. Gram-positive cocci (likely to represent group B streptococci) are observed on the smear
2. Infant is delivered with low Apgar score (under 7)
3. Infant is preterm
4. Evidence of respiratory distress, especially with an x-ray film demonstrating pneumonia, is observed
5. There is abnormal behavior or change in behavior of the infant compatible with infection

6. Neutrophils fall under 4000/mm³ or platelet count is under 100,000/mm³

Duration of antibiotic treatment must be individualized depending on results of cultures and infant's clinical behavior. We generally discontinue antibiotic treatment if blood culture remains negative for over 48 hours and the infant does not appear to be ill. For infants with obvious infection treat as described in Chapter 25.

INCOMPETENT CERVIX

Cervical incompetence, premature painless dilatation and effacement of cervix, is caused in most cases by damage sustained during previous cervicouterine surgery or delivery, although it may be a congenital condition. Repeated second trimester abortion or premature birth may be caused by cervical incompetence, which is found approximately once in every 500 to 600 pregnancies. Two percent of premature births are ascribed to cervical incompetence. No particular age or race is prone to this disorder.

I. Pathogenesis
   A. Forcible dilatation of the cervix in the nongravid patient and traumatic labor, delivery, or induced abortion lead to cervical damage. Lacerations may or may not be apparent, but as pregnancy progresses, containment of the products of conception becomes more and more difficult.
   B. Congenital shortness or weakness or abnormal function is assumed in the occasional primigravida with cervical incompetence.
II. Pathosis
   A. Note lacerations, even a site of rupture of cervix into lower uterine segment.
   B. Concealed damage—perhaps multiple tears—may be present.
III. Pathologic physiology
   A. Cervix (and perhaps lower uterine segment) cannot hold products of conception within uterus.
   B. With painless thinning and widening of cervix, membranes usually rupture; this will be followed by untimely delivery.
IV. Clinical findings
   A. Progressive insensitive dilatation and effacement of cervix after first trimester, premature rupture of membranes, and premature labor and delivery are typical of cervical incompetence.
   B. Neither laboratory findings nor x-ray studies are diagnostic during pregnancy.
   C. Repeated, gentle sterile-glove vaginal examinations may disclose abnormal progressive opening of cervix. Although examination is usually recommended on a weekly basis, it is not uncommon for cervical change to occur in a lesser interval.
V. Differential diagnosis of second trimester abortion
   A. Consider lower genital tract infection, severe isoimmunization, active maternal syphilis, premature separation of placenta, placenta previa, extrachorial placenta.
   B. Congenital uterine deformity reduces uterine capacity, in midtrimester abortion and premature labor and delivery.
VI. Complications and sequelae
   A. Incompetent cervix will usually result in repeated midpregnancy termination.
   B. Offspring usually is considerably undersized; prematurity rate for cervical incompetence is increased eight or nine times over average.
VII. Treatment
   A. Emergency measures
      Cervical cerclage may be successful if the os is not more than 9 cm dilated or 50% effaced, assuming pregnancy is otherwise normal and viable.
   B. Specific measures
      1. Bed rest and avoidance of stress
      2. Laxatives when needed
      3. Avoidance of hormone therapy
      4. Only mild sedation for mother to avoid narcotizing immature fetus if early delivery follows despite therapy
   C. Surgical measures
      1. Cervical cerclage may be
         a. Temporary, in which case

there are two major types. One is the McDonald method, in which a heavy permanent suture is passed alternately submucosally and extramucosally to encircle the cervix. The second is the Würm procedure, in which two heavy nonabsorbable mattress sutures are placed through the cervix at right angles to each other.
  b. Semipermanent, in which a ribbon of inert material is passed around the cervix just over the fascia with tightening and securing of the strand followed by closure of the mucosa with additional absorbable sutures (Fig. 18-1). This procedure may also be accomplished in the nonpregnant state.
  c. Permanent, in which a cervical cerclage is accomplished abdominally using inert material to encircle the cervix at the level of the internal os. In this circumstance the material may not be removed vaginally and all deliveries must be by cesarean section. There are relatively few indications for this procedure (cervix too short or too scarred or lacerations of too great an extent to perform a vaginal procedure, and possibly subacute cervicitis), and it is quite difficult to perform after week 17 or 18. However, it may provide for better isthmic support and decreased slippage, and it possibly prevents premature cervical ripening. It may be used for more than one pregnancy per cerclage and be useful in cases that are not amenable to a vaginal approach.

Determining which of these various approaches is attempted must be an individualized surgical decision

2. When labor ensues
  a. Würm sutures must be cut for vaginal delivery.
  b. If a buried cerclage has been inserted, it may be severed for vaginal delivery, or a transverse lower-segment cesarean section may be elected.
  c. Cervicouterine infection, fetal death, or severe bleeding will require removal of cerclage followed by emptying of uterus.
  d. With abdominal cerclage cesarean section must be performed. In the very early ges-

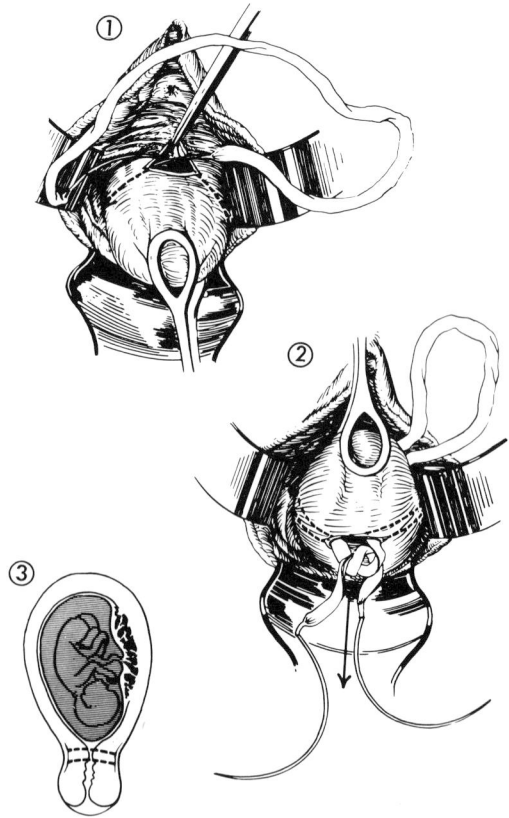

Fig. 18-1. Cerclage of cervix (Shirodkar) with incompetent os in pregnant patient. (From Benson, R.C.: Handbook of obstetrics and gynecology, ed. 5, Los Altos, Calif., 1974, Lange Medical Publications.)

tation loss, a small suction curette may be used to evacuate aborted products of conception.

VIII. Prevention
   A. Avoid trauma to cervix in obstetric or gynecologic operations.
   B. Correct cervical lacerations or close abnormally patulous cervix before pregnancy.

IX. Prognosis
   A. Repeated late abortions or premature deliveries will occur if cervix is incompetent. Most fetuses are lost before the thirty-second week. A 25% to 75% perinatal mortality was usual prior to use of cerclage.
   B. In otherwise uncomplicated cases, two thirds to three fourths of offspring in cases where cervical cerclage is used will now go well beyond viability (28 weeks), with a perinatal mortality of 10% to 15%.

PROLONGED PREGNANCY
(see also Chapter 12)

The majority of fetuses whose gestation is prolonged or who have reached 42 weeks of completed gestation from the last menstrual period will show the effects of impairment of nutritional supply, perhaps from an aging process of the placenta. Many of these infants will have suffered an actual loss of weight in utero, with evidence of reduced subcutaneous tissue, scaling, and parchmentlike skin—a condition usually referred to as dysmaturity. This common event in the postterm stage has led to the use of the term "postmaturity" to mean placental insufficiency, even in infants who are not in the postterm stage. Since many postterm babies do not suffer placental inadequacy but continue to grow and gain weight (Fig. 18-2), the term "postmaturity" should be abandoned as a term for fetal wasting. In contrast to the infant shown in Fig. 18-2, Fig. 18-3 shows a postmature infant who has suffered chronic fetal distress (dysmaturity).

At least 3% of infants are born after 42 completed weeks of gestation. Because of the potential risk of perinatal asphyxia or injury it is recommended that studies designed to ascertain fetal well-being be initiated and repeated weekly when a patient's pregnancy continues past her confirmed due date. If pregnancy is followed past 42 weeks, consideration should be given to performing these tests no less than twice a week. Should any evidence of placental insufficiency appear, hospitalization is mandatory. Moreover, consideration should be given to elective cesarean section for those with proven fetopelvic disproportion. Additionally, at 42 weeks the following plan is suggested:

1. Recalculate expected date of delivery.
2. Consider amniocentesis for pulmonary maturity testing and to determine whether there has been meconium staining.

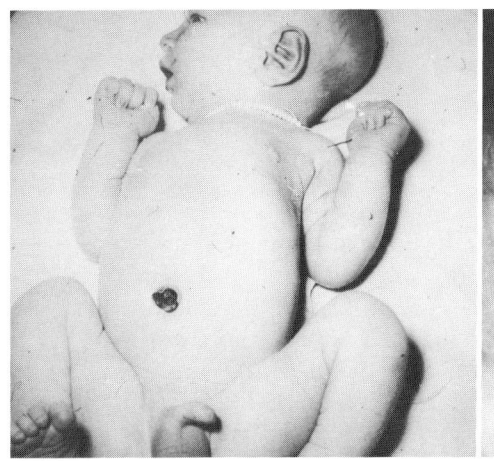 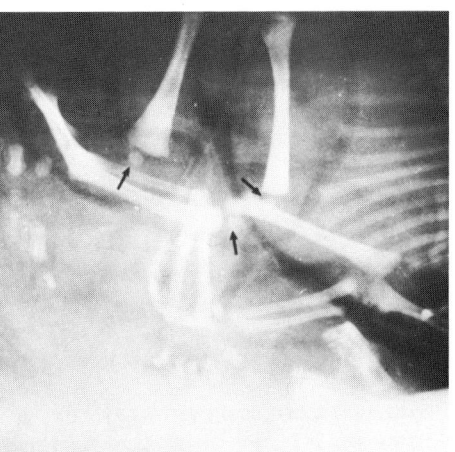

Fig. 18-2. A, An oversized (4,400 gm) postmature (44 weeks' gestation) newborn. **B,** Fetogram of infant in **A,** with large distal femoral and proximal tibial epiphyses.

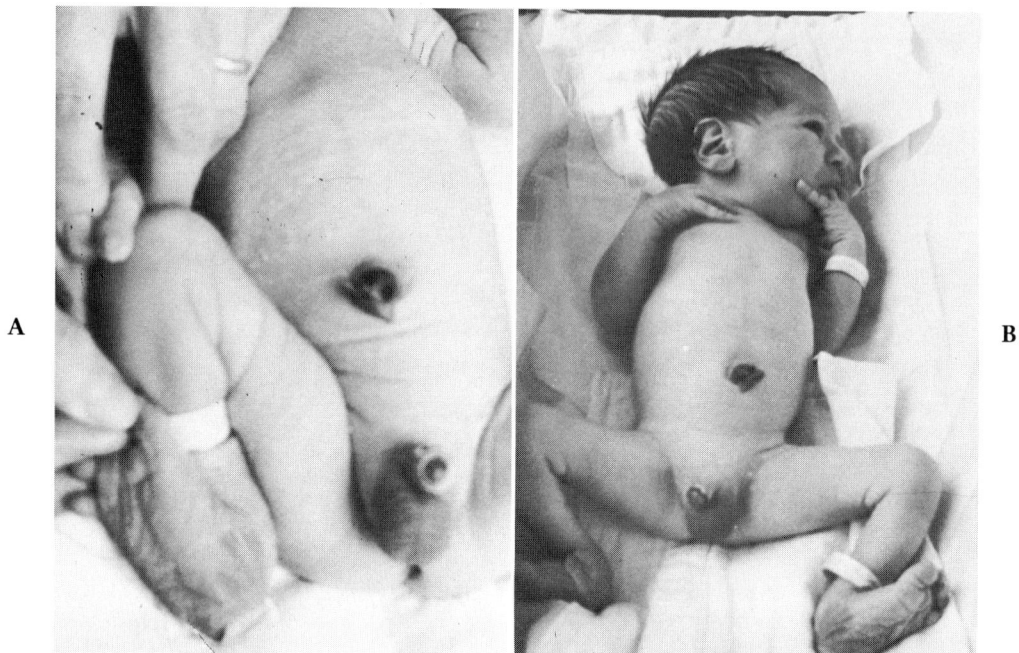

Fig. 18-3. A, This 2,600 gm infant was delivered after term and shows severe dysmaturity with scaling of the skin and loss of subcutaneous tissue. **B,** The open eye, hunger, wrinkled soles of the feet, and excessive fingernail length support a diagnosis of postmaturity.

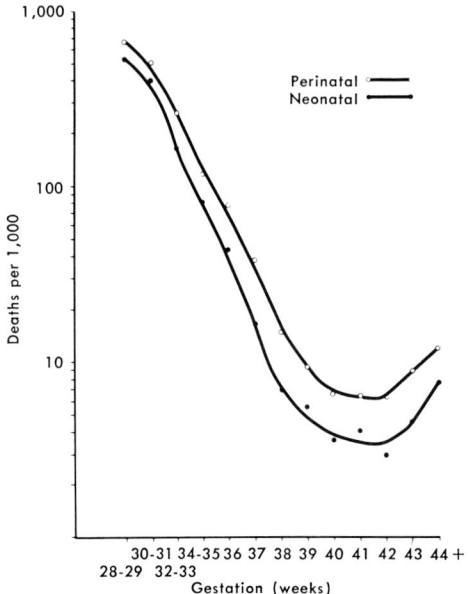

Fig. 18-4. Perinatal and neonatal mortality by weeks of gestation from over 40,000 births. (From Behrman, R.E., Babson, S.G., and Lessel, R.: Am. J. Dis. Child. **121:**486, 1971.)

3. Identify oversized fetus or fetopelvic disproportion by ultrasonography.
4. Identify fetal distress (biophysical profile, nonstress test, or contraction stress test).
5. If there is no evidence of fetopelvic disproportion or fetal distress, induce labor while employing continuous fetal monitoring.
6. Perform cesarean section if fetus is in abnormal position, if there is evidence of fetopelvic disproportion, or if fetal distress is evident.

Complications

1. Fetal or neonatal death
   There is a sharp rise in perinatal mortality after 42 weeks' gestation (Fig. 18-4).
2. Fetal injury from fetopelvic disproportion
3. Asphyxial damage from fetal distress, which is particularly hazardous in the primigravida

These complications in the survivors increase the chance of mental subnormality and neurologic sequelae.

MECONIUM IN THE AMNIOTIC FLUID

The passage of meconium into the amniotic fluid is thought to indicate fetal stress and perhaps even distress. Although there is some controversy regarding the associated perinatal morbidity and mortality, there is unanimity that if the perinate takes gasping respirations sufficient to carry meconium-laden amniotic fluid into the small airways or alveoli, and proper therapy is not instituted, meconium aspiration syndrome will complicate extrauterine respiration. An effective management plan for this problem follows:

1. The nares and pharynx should be suctioned with a catheter as soon as the head is delivered and prior to delivery of the chest.
2. As soon as the infant is delivered the trachea should be visualized with a laryngoscope, and if any meconium is present the trachea should be suctioned thoroughly. Suctioning may need to be performed directly through an endotracheal tube when meconium is extremely viscous.
3. Occasionally saline washing of the tracheobronchial tree will be necessary.
4. Proper ventilatory support must be immediately and meticulously applied.

BIBLIOGRAPHY

Andreyko, J.L., Chen, C.P., Shennan, A.T., et al.: Results of conservative management of premature rupture of the membranes, Am. J. Obstet. Gynecol. **148:**600, 1984.

Ballard, P., Benson, A., and Brehier, A.: Glucocorticoid effects in fetal lung, Am. Rev. Respir. Dis. **115:**29, 1976.

Barden, T.P., Bieniarz, J., Cibils, L.A., et al.: Premature labor: its management and therapy, J. Reprod. Med. **9:**93, 1972.

Barford, D.A.G., and Rosen, M.G.: Cervical incompetence: diagnosis and outcome, Obstet. Gynecol. **64:**159, 1984.

Bartolucci, L., Hill, W.C., Katz, M., et al.: Ultrasonography in preterm labor, Am. J. Obstet. Gynecol. **149:**52, 1984.

Berkowitz, R.L., Bonta, B.W., and Warshaw, J.E.: The relationship between premature rupture of the membranes and the respiratory distress syndrome, Am. J. Obstet. Gynecol. **124:**712, 1976.

Bieniarz, J., Motew, M., and Scommegna, A.: Uterine and cardiovascular effects of ritodrine in premature labor, Obstet. Gynecol. **40:**65, 1972.

Bolognese, R.J.: Ampicillin: transfer into fetus and amnionic fluid, Rocky Mt. Med. J. **65:**72, 1968.

Clark, D.M., and Anderson, G.V.: Perinatal mortality and amnionitis in a general hospital population, Obstet. Gynecol. **31:**714, 1968.

Cotton, D.B., Hill, L.M., Strassner, H.T., et al.: Use of amniocentesis in preterm gestation with ruptured membranes, Obstet. Gynecol. **63:**38, 1984.

Crombleholme, W.R., Minkoff, H.L., Delke, I., et al.: Cervical cerclage: an aggressive approach to threatened or recurrent pregnancy wastage, Am. J. Obstet. Gynecol. **146:**168, 1983.

Curet, L.B., Rao, A.V., Zachman, R.D., et al.: Association between ruptured membranes, tocolytic therapy, and respiratory distress syndrome, Am. J. Obstet. Gynecol. **148:**263, 1984.

Garite, T.J.: Premature rupture of the membranes: the enigma of the obstetrician, Am. J. Obstet. Gynecol. **151:**1001, 1985.

Hameed, C., Tejani, N., Verma, U.L., et al.: Silent chorioamnionitis as a cause of preterm labor refractory to tocolytic therapy, Am. J. Obstet. Gynecol. **149:**726, 1984.

Hatjis, C.G., Nelson, L.H., Meis, P.J., et al.: Addition of magnesium sulfate improves effectiveness of ritodrine in preventing premature delivery, Am. J. Obstet. Gynecol. **150:**142, 1984.

Huddleston, J.F.: Preterm labor, Clin. Obstet. Gynecol. **25:**123, 1982.

Hummer, W.K., and Sheldon, R.S.: Prolonged gestation, Minn. Med. **52:**333, 1969.

Iams, J.D., Talbert, M.L., Barrows, H., et al.: Management of preterm prematurely ruptured membranes: a prospective randomized comparison of observation versus use of steroids and timed delivery, Am. J. Obstet. Gynecol. **151:**32, 1985.

Lauersen, N.H., Merkatz, I.R., Tejani, N., et al: Inhibition of premature labor: a multicenter comparison of ritodrine and ethanol, Am. J. Obstet. Gynecol. **127:**837, 1977.

Lauersen, N.H., and Fuchs, F.: Experience with Shirodkar's operation and postoperative alcohol treatment, Acta Obstet. Gynecol. Scand. **52:**77, 1973.

Liggins, G.C.: Lung maturation and the prevention of hyaline membrane disease, Proceedings of 70th Ross Conference on Pediatric Research, Columbus, Ohio, 1977, Ross Laboratories.

Liggins, G.C., and Howie, R.N.: Prevention of respiratory distress with corticoids, Pediatrics **50:**515, 1972.

Minkoff, H.: Prematurity: infection as an etiologic factor, Obstet. Gynecol. **62:**137, 1983.

Minkoff, H., Grunebaum, A.N., Schwarz, R.H., et al.: Risk factors for prematurity and premature rupture of membranes: a prospective study of the vaginal flora in pregnancy, Am. J. Obstet. Gynecol. **150:**965, 1984.

Moberg, L.J., Garite, T.J., and Freeman, R.K.: Fetal heart rate patterns and fetal distress in patients with preterm premature rupture of membranes, Obstet. Gynecol. **64:**60, 1984.

Naver, E.: The incompetent cervix and its treatment in habitual abortion and premature labour, Acta Obstet. Gynecol. Scand. **47:**314, 1968.

Nimrod, C., Varela-Gittings, F., Machin, G., et al.: The effect of very prolonged membrane rupture on fetal development, Am. J. Obstet. Gynecol. **148:**540, 1984.

Papageorgiou, A.N., Desgranges, M.F., Masson, M., et al.:

The antenatal use of betamethasone in the prevention of respiratory distress syndrome: a controlled double-blind study, Pediatrics **63**:73, 1979.

Richardson, C.J., Pomerance, J.J., Cunningham, M.D., et al.: Acceleration of fetal lung maturation following prolonged rupture of the membranes, Am. J. Obstet. Gynecol. **118**:1115, 1974.

Sampson, M.B., Lastres, O., Tomasi, A.M., et al.: Tocolysis with terbutaline sulfate in patients with placenta previa complicated by premature labor, J. Reprod. Med. **29**:248, 1984.

Scanlon, J.: The early detection of neonatal sepsis by examination of liquid obtained from the external ear canal, J. Pediatr. **79**:247, 1971.

Socol, M.L., Dooley, S.L., Tamura, R.K., et al.: Perinatal outcome following prior delivery in the late second or early third trimester, Obstet. Gynecol. **150**:228, 1984.

Taeusch, H.W., Jr., Frigoletto, F., Kitzmiller, J., et al.: Risk of respiratory distress syndrome after prenatal dexamethasone treatment, Pediatrics **63**:64, 1979.

Tamura, R.K., Sabbagha, R.E., Depp, R., et al.: Diminished growth in fetuses born preterm after spontaneous labor or rupture of membranes, Am. J. Obstet. Gynecol. **148**:1105, 1984.

Taylor, J., and Garite, T.J.: Premature rupture of membranes before fetal viability, Obstet. Gynecol. **64**:615, 1984.

Zwerdling, M.A.: Factors pertaining to prolonged pregnancy and its outcome, Pediatrics **40**:202, 1967.

19

Disproportionate fetouterine growth

GROWTH-RETARDED FETUS

A perinate below the 10th percentile (Fig. 4-1) indicates moderate growth retardation. One below 2 standard deviations from the mean (approximately 3rd percentile) indicates severe growth retardation. Thus incidence depends on the criteria used. Fig. 19-1 illustrates the linearity of normal growth and the more common variations from it.

Growth impairment during the first half of pregnancy is most likely attributable to embryonic injury, genetic defect, or viral invasion of the fetus. Such fetuses often die in utero. Slowing of growth during the last half of pregnancy is usually related to a reduction in the flow of nutrients or oxygen to the fetus. There is often decreased uterine blood flow in such cases and sometimes uterine contractions. Severe impairment of maternal-fetal transfer may cause arrest in cell division or even hypoxic damage to the brain. Therefore the added asphyxial effects of labor further jeopardize the fetus. Early identification of the slowly growing fetus and intensive team management are imperative to ensure intact survival.

I. Associations of intrauterine growth retardation
  A. Maternal (Fig. 4-1)
    Small women married to small men usually have small babies. This is fortunate, for these women often have limited pelvic capacities. There is little evidence that this deviation from the norm of a heterogeneous population is true intrauterine growth retardation. Thus consideration of offspring size should be related to parental size, currently only a rudimentary practice at best.

Pathophysiologic changes that interfere with fetal gaseous exchange or nutritional supply include limitation of uterine blood flow, reduction in area of placental exchange, lowered maternal arterial concentration of essential gases (oxygen) and nutrients, impairment of diffusion across placental membrane, and possibly diversion of fetal blood flow from the umbilical circulation. Factors to be considered are as follows:
1. Insufficiency of growth substrate because of
   a. Maternal undernutrition
   b. Close spacing of pregnancies, and infants born after four pregnancies
   c. Limited maternal weight gain, or weight loss in the last trimester
2. Vascular disease, including:
   a. Chronic hypertension
   b. Atherosclerosis
   c. Collagen diseases with superimposed hypertensive states of pregnancy
3. Chronic decreased function of vital organ, including:
   a. Chronic renal disease
   b. Severe heart disease
   c. Pulmonary diseases causing decreased maternal-fetal gaseous exchange

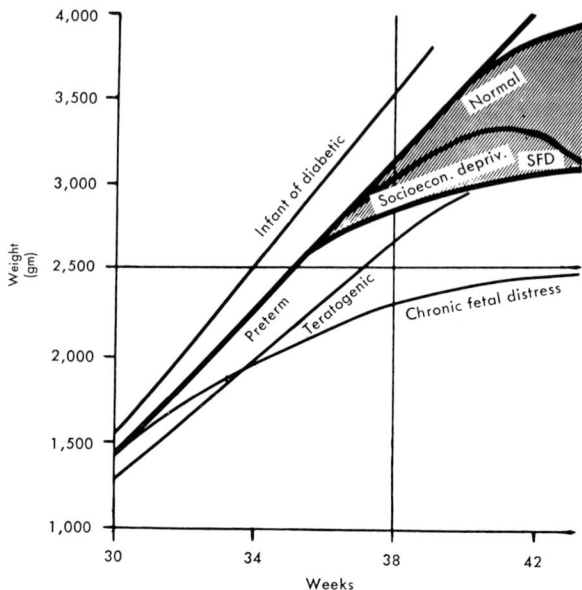

Fig. 19-1. Birth weight curves of population *(shaded area)* and several abnormal groups. Subacute fetal distress *(SFD)* is indicated by the only curve representing a weight loss. *Heavy line* continuing straight above the normal range is the extrapolated curve. (From Gruenwald, P., and Babson, S.G. In Davis' gynecology and obstetrics, Hagerstown, Md., 1972, Harper & Row, Inc.)

  4. Chronic hypoxia, including:
    a. Gravida living at high altitude
    b. Severe maternal anemia
  5. Substance abuse, including:
    a. Smoking
    b. Alcoholism
    c. Use of narcotics
  6. Previous growth-retarded infant
    Tendency to have growth-retarded infant is likely to be caused by a recessive gene. Moreover, women whose sisters' pregnancies have been complicated with intrauterine growth retardation are at higher risk for this process.
 B. Placental and related to cord
  1. Chronic placental abruption or infarction
  2. Chorioangioma
  3. Placenta previa
  4. Circumvallate placenta
  5. Placental aging or postmaturity
  6. Two-vessel cord
  7. Velamentous cord insertion
  8. Marginal cord insertion
 C. Fetal
  1. Multiple gestation (Chapter 20)
  2. Infections (e.g., syphilis, toxoplasmosis, rubella, or cytomegalovirus)
  3. Fetal genetic defects (particularly chromosomal abnormalities)
  4. Fetal malformations (particularly cardiovascular)
  5. Prolonged pregnancy
    Fetus may have to metabolize its energy stores.
  6. Extrauterine pregnancy
    Impaired vascular supply is possible cause of growth retardation.
  7. Inherited family trait to be small neonate
II. Clinical identification
 A. Previous undergrown infant
 B. Slowly increasing fundal measurements (under 1 cm/wk)
 C. Slowly increasing, stable, or decreasing maternal weight
 D. Girth measurements steady or decreasing
 E. Presence of maternal disease, addic-

tive habits, or other associations noted above
III. Diagnosis by ultrasonographic measurements
   A. Growth under 2 mm/wk (biparietal diameter) from thirtieth to thirty-fourth week
   B. Growth under 1 mm/wk (biparietal diameter) from thirty-fifth week to term
   C. Disparity from other expected growth
IV. Management
   A. Rule out fetal distress by initiation of biometric testing
   B. Determine readiness for delivery by performing amniocentesis for rapid surfactant test, lecithin/sphingomyelin ratio, and/or phosphatidylglycerol (Chapter 4).
   C. Correct any maternal nutritive or substance abuse problems.
   D. Treat any disease process amenable to modern therapy.
   E. Place patient in lateral recumbent position to increase uterine blood flow.
   F. Offer full team care during labor and delivery, with continuous monitoring (Chapters 6 and 7) to accomplish atraumatic delivery.

SMALL-FOR-DATES NEONATES
(see also Chapters 4 and 12)

Infants who are below the 10th percentile on the Denver weight grid (Fig. 4-2) are suspect for fetal undergrowth. Only 5% of babies born at sea level with good health conditions are below the 10th percentile on this grid. Some of these infants are small because of family patterns, but these can be differentiated from undergrown infants by the presence of adequate subcutaneous tissue and proportionate body measurements. A substantial number of infants are adequate in size for gestational age but show signs of late fetal wasting and should be managed similarly to those with chronic fetal distress.

Undersized infants are classified into two groups: (1) those who are hypoplastic because of an intrinsic impairment of fetal cell division through injury or genetic influence, and (2) those who suffered fetal undergrowth or weight loss imposed by chronic nutritional limitation.

Hypoplastic infant

Hypoplastic infants usually, but not always, exhibit malformation.
   1. Etiologic factors
      a. Genetic defects and chromosomal disarrangements (e.g., trisomy syndromes, Down's syndrome)
      b. Placental transfer of infection (e.g., rubella)
      c. Exposure to teratogenic drugs, such as thalidomide
      d. Exposure to ionizing radiation, such as from x-ray studies or therapy
   2. Identification
      a. Careful inspection at birth of placenta and cord and volume of amniotic fluid may reveal placental abnormalities, hydramnios, oligohydramnios, amnion nodosum, or a single artery in the cord. Such findings vastly increase chances of malformation.
      b. Infant should be examined for signs of anomaly (Chapter 8).

Nutritional impairment

The perinate tolerates the anoxia and nutritional deprivation that accompany chronic placental impairment surprisingly well. An acceptable theory indicates that to conserve limited oxygen supplies for the most vital organs (heart and brain), much of the circulation to the viscera and limbs is reduced. This reduction of oxygenation to the skin may account for the parchmentlike scaling (less noticeable on the face) and absence of vernix in the moderately dysmature infant. Release of meconium and its staining of the skin suggest a more severely affected fetus.

CHRONIC FETAL DEPRIVATION (CHRONIC FETAL DISTRESS) (Fig. 19-2)

Chronically decreased maternal-fetal exchange usually occurs after midpregnancy. Gradual restriction in growth results in a proportionately small infant in all growth parameters (under the 3rd percentile). Brain weight is least affected, but if nutritional restriction is severe enough, brain cell division may cease.

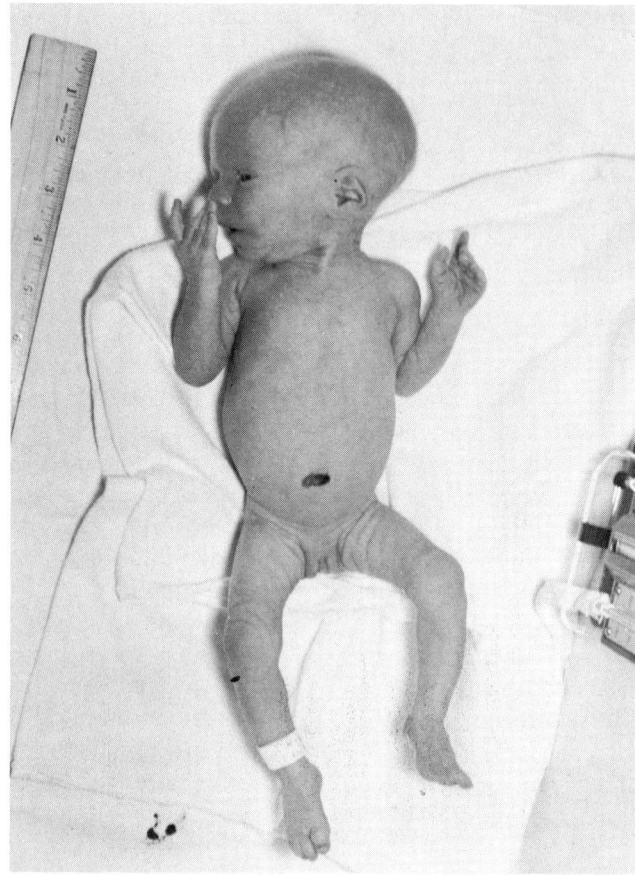

Fig. 19-2. Proportionately undergrown infant, 1,600 gm, who is 40 weeks of gestational age. Note observation of hand. She apparently contracted rubella in the second trimester without evidence of teratogenic effect.

SUBACUTE FETAL DEPRIVATION OF DYSMATURITY (Fig. 18-3)

Subacute fetal deprivation of dysmaturity is a common condition that affects the fetus near the end of pregnancy and is identified at birth by loss in body weight and generalized wasting, with reduction in fat and muscle. These tissues have been consumed to support the metabolism necessary for survival. The skin is often cracked and dry, and there is a loss of vernix. Length and head size may be within the normal range but are proportionately greater than they should be for weight. On the ponderal index—a weight/length ratio—the infant may be under 2 standard deviations of the mean, or under 2.20 (weight in grams $\times$ 100 $\div$ cm^3); yet the weight for gestation may be appropriate and over the 10th percentile. In other words, the infant is light for length but not necessarily small for dates. Nonetheless, metabolic jeopardy is often serious.

ACUTE FETAL DISTRESS

Acute fetal distress indicates relatively sudden and uncompensated hypoxic insult, which is an added hazard for the fetus with growth retardation. The combination of growth retardation and asphyxia, the latter intensified by labor, is a leading cause of perinatal morbidity and death. In this event rescue by immediate delivery is justified.

RECOGNITION OF UNDERGROWN MATURE INFANT

The special problems and requirements of undergrown mature infants are such that they need to be differentiated from preterm infants. Table 12-1 compares their clinical characteristics.

MANAGEMENT OF INFANTS WITH NUTRITIONAL IMPAIRMENT
See p. 145.

COMPLICATIONS
The following complications are sufficiently common and serious that they are discussed in other sections of this book. Term gestation infants whose sizes are under 2 standard deviations of the mean have eight times the perinatal mortality of infants of similar gestational age who are appropriate in size.

1. Asphyxia neonatorum, often with meconium aspiration (Chapter 27)
2. Hypoglycemia (Chapter 32)
3. Pulmonary hemorrhage (Chapter 27)
4. Congenital anomalies (incidence approximately 10 to 20 times that found in large mature infants) (Chapter 33)
5. Asphyxial convulsions (Chapter 30)

LATE DEVELOPMENT
1. Neurologic deficit

    The neurologic damage of symptomatic hypoglycemia and perinatal asphyxia is well known. Brain weight and size are less affected than are other organs in fetal undernutrition; yet limitation in brain cell division and numbers is possible, and so this potential handicap to future development must be faced. Although animal studies indicate a clear relationship between fetal growth retardation and suppression of both brain development and the learning process, evidence that intrauterine nutritional deprivation results in slowing of neurologic maturation and intellectual development in humans remains circumstantial.

    In studies of monozygotic twins who were discrepant in size by 25% or more at birth, the larger twin maintained a relatively small advantage over his smaller twin in IQ.

    Minkowski and associates have been impressed by the degree to which brain development during fetal life progresses independently of unfavorable gestational circumstances that may affect physical growth. Even if neurologic maturation of small-for-dates infants is appropriate for gestational age, cell multiplication may be suppressed. Drillien has shown that children who were small-for-dates infants did as well on IQ tests at 10 to 12 years of age when reared in better-than-average homes (but not when reared in poorer homes) as did those of the same age group who were much larger at birth. If the severely undergrown infant is free of disease and unhampered by significant asphyxia, normal school progress can be expected.

2. Growth retardation

    Physical growth in undersized term newborns, after a temporary acceleration in growth, continues at a reduced level during the early part of the growth period. Fig. 35-1, C, shows the longitudinal growth measurements of 12 severely undergrown term infants through the first year of life. Growth curves in weight and length are parallel to but much reduced compared to curves for normal infants. Head circumference is usually less reduced at birth and increases at a faster rate than other measurements in that the curve approaches curves for infants of normal size at 1 year of age. Studies of twins demonstrate that the smaller of monozygotic twins seldom attains the physical size of his twin, even after growth is completed. Head circumference in twins is the least affected, although significant difference in this measurement still remains.

OVERGROWN, OR LARGE FETUS
(see also Chapter 12)

During the past decade, especially, an increase in the weight of newborn infants has been recorded. Almost 2% of neonates at our institution weigh 4,500 gm (9 lb 15 oz) or more at birth, and 10% weigh over 4,000 gm. Body length and other measurements have increased concomitantly with weight. Although racial differences and better nutrition are major reasons for heavier babies, women's pelvic dimensions have not increased proportionately. The vast number of excessive-sized babies are born of multiparous mothers, a number of whom have gestational diabetes or diabetes mellitus or are obese.

The large infant is often exposed to serious birth trauma, which is most critical in breech presentation. Currently, the cesarean section rate for the excessive-sized fetus is about twice that for those of average weight. In addition, the baby of the diabetic mother is metabolically stressed.

It is well known that successive progeny are heavier and that excessive weight gain (over 24 lb) during pregnancy is associated with larger offspring. Moreover, if a woman produces a large baby, there is a very good chance that a later baby will be large, or even larger. About 35% of large babies are delivered after 293 days and are postmature.

Estimation of fetal size in utero is difficult. Nonetheless, the physician should try to determine whether an infant will be small (2,500 gm or less), average (2,500 to 4,000 gm), or large (4,000 gm or more).

Prolonged, difficult labor is usual with the oversized fetus. Instrumental delivery is the rule. Shoulder dystocia is common because of greater chest circumference, and posterior or transverse arrest is frequent.

I. Associations (Fig. 4-1)
   A. Infants delivered of women who are more than 25% overweight or who had a prepregnant weight/height ratio (cm/kg) of over 2.4
   B. Infants of women who gain more than 35 lb in weight during pregnancy
   C. Infants of diabetic or gestational diabetic mothers
   D. Infants with transposition of great vessels
II. Clues to excessive fetal development
   A. Past maternal history of large babies
   B. Large stature, multiparity, diabetes, or obesity
   C. Weight gain of over 35 lb in pregnancy
   D. Postmature pregnancy (294 days or more)
   E. Prolonged, dystotic labor
III. Diagnosis
   A. Biparietal head diameter (ultrasonography) over 10 cm
   B. Fundal measurement over 42 cm
   C. Fetal cephalometry combined with x-ray pelvimetry
IV. Management
   A. Consider fetal overgrowth in relation to size and structure of mother's pelvis.
   B. Be prepared for cesarean section because of malposition and dystocia.
   C. Reevaluate all pregnancies that approach 42 weeks of gestational age.
   D. Monitor electronically in any trial of labor.
   E. Prepare for shoulder-girdle dystocia.
V. Clinical features of infant
   A. Weight, head, and length are all proportionately large.
   B. Initial activity and hunger are usually reduced.
   C. Weight loss is nearly double that of normal-sized infants.
   D. Hyperbilirubinemia, hypocalcemia, and hypoglycemia are not uncommon in infants born before term.
VI. Complications (when delivered vaginally)
   A. Fetal asphyxia or trauma with dystocia or malpresentation
   B. Injury during birth
      1. Broken clavicle
      2. Brachial plexus injury
   C. Mental subnormality
      The increase in incidence of mental subnormality reported may reflect excessive fetal stress. This potential tragedy should be prevented by liberal use of cesarean section.

The large-for-dates perinate is defined as being over the 90th percentile in weight for gestational age. At term this percentile for middle-class, white infants peaks at approximately 4,250 gm (Fig. 11-1). This may be an excessive size for successful delivery. In a study of 70 infants who were over the 95th percentile for weight at birth, we found that at least 50% of the mothers were obese and had gained over 35 lb during pregnancy. Only about one third of these babies were born after 42 weeks of gestation. Additionally improved nutrition of many areas of the world has apparently resulted in increasingly larger fetuses, although pelvic capacities have not increased proportionately. This discrepancy (fetopelvic disproportion) also places many fetuses of lesser size at increased jeopardy. North European parents produce the largest infants (nearly 2% are over 4,500 gm at birth). In contrast to the multitude of factors that slow fetal growth, maternal diabetes or its tendency is the only known pathophysiologic correlate to accelerated fetal growth (Fig. 19-1).

HYDRAMNIOS AND OLIGOHYDRAMNIOS

Both excessive accumulation and paucity of amniotic fluid are associated with great hazard to the perinate. Hydramnios (polyhydramnios) is an increase over the normally expected 800 to 1,200 ml of amniotic fluid near term gestation and usually is not detectable until 2,000 to 3,000 ml is present. It may occur either acutely (2% of cases) or chronically (98% of cases), and although the exact causes are unknown, there are certain clinical correlates:

1. Diabetes (25% of cases)
2. Congenital malformation (20% of cases)
3. Erythroblastosis fetalis (12% of cases)
4. Multiple gestation (8% of cases)

Despite these correlates, the largest group (33%) is still idiopathic. It complicates 0.4% of all pregnancies, and nearly 40% of pregnancies so complicated result in perinatal demise. It is therefore imperative that any pregnancy with this complication be investigated by glucose tolerance test, repeat antibody screening, and ultrasonography, and be considered for amniography. Many modes of treatment have been attempted, and bed rest with diuretics may assist slightly. Ultimately, in the severe case, multiple amniocenteses may be necessary. This aggressive management, however, is indicated only for maternal indications (relief of dyspnea).

1. Possible causes of hydramnios
   a. Increased production of amniotic fluid
   b. Decreased clearance of amniotic fluid
   c. Fetal urine excess or reduced swallowing of amniotic fluid
   d. Gross transudate
2. Pronounced congenital abnormalities associated with hydramnios (approximately 50% of cases)
   a. Central nervous system anomalies such as anencephaly or spina bifida
   b. Gastrointestinal anomalies—esophageal atresia
3. Maternal problems related to hydramnios
   a. Eclamptogenic toxemia
   b. Multiple pregnancy
   c. Cardiac or renal diseases with edema
   d. Diabetes mellitus
   e. Syphilis (tertiary) of the viscera
   f. Isoimmunization of maternal blood resulting in erythroblastosis fetalis

Oligohydramnios is the rare condition in which there is a significant paucity of amniotic fluid (usually under 500 ml at term). It is difficult to diagnose because of the decreasing amount of amniotic fluid with lengthening gestation; however, diagnosis is suggested when the uterus is tightly apposed about the fetus and any form of ballottement is impossible. With ultrasonography the diagnosis is usually readily apparent, although it is more an observation than an exact quantification. During labor there is a much higher incidence of variable decelerations as a reflection of cord compromise. Comprehensive antepartum evaluation and careful electronic fetal monitoring with labor are mandatory.

There appears to be a multiplicity of causes of oligohydramnios; however, an exact etiology is undetermined. Clinical correlates are fetal renal agenesis and obstruction to the urinary tract. There is little disagreement that when pregnancy is complicated by oligohydramnios the fetus is at high risk; however, there is no known therapy.

Conditions associated with oligohydramnios include the following:

1. Pregnancy with placental insufficiency
2. Fetus with serious urinary tract abnormality—little or no urine excreted
3. Fetal death and absorption of amniotic fluid
4. Persistent, slight loss of fluid through a small membrane defect

Maternal diagnostic studies and observations in hydramnios and oligohydramnios

1. Obtain ultrasound scans or radiographs for discernment of
   a. Skeletal defects (e.g., anencephaly or hydrocephaly)
   b. Twinning and hydrops fetalis
   c. Signs of fetal death (e.g., overlapping of cranial bones and presence of fetal gas)
   d. Skeletal age; observation of presence and size of distal femoral epiphyses (Table 4-2)
2. Perform biometric monitoring (Chapter 4).

3. Screen mother for known associations.
4. Record appearance of abnormal amniotic fluid, (e.g., meconium or bile contamination)
Pigment is increased in hemolytic disease.

Treatment

I. Hydramnios
   A. Treat maternal disease appropriately: digitalize for cardiac failure; give diuretics for stasis edema.
   B. Accomplish amniocentesis when
      1. No gross fetal anomaly can be identified and maternal distension is extreme and refractory to other therapy
      2. Serious fetal or maternal disease is diagnosed and premature termination of pregnancy is necessary

II. Oligohydramnios
   A. Recalculate and reestimate duration of pregnancy. A smaller uterus may indicate a later expected date of confinement, not placental dysfunction.
      1. Avoid intervention if fetal or maternal jeopardy is uncertain.
      2. Terminate pregnancy if fetal anomaly is recognized or fetal death has occurred or when placental insufficiency is likely.
   B. Measure fetal growth by ultrasonography.

BIBLIOGRAPHY

Adamson, A.R., and Benster, B.: Renal agenesis, oligohydramnios, and diabetes mellitus, Postgrad. Med. J. **45**:189, 1969.

Babson, S.G., and Henderson, N.B.: Fetal undergrowth: relation of head growth to later intellectual performance, Pediatrics **53**:890, 1974.

Babson, S.G., Henderson, N.B., and Clark, W.M.: The preschool intelligence of oversized newborns, Pediatrics **44**:536, 1969.

Babson, S.G., and Kangas, J.: Preschool intelligence of undersized term infants, Am. J. Dis. Child. **117**:553, 1969.

Babson, S.G., and Phillips, D.S.: Growth and development of twins dissimilar in size at birth, N. Engl. J. Med. **289**:937, 1973.

Baxi, L., Barad, D., Reece, E.A., et al.: Use of glycosylated hemoglobin as a screen for macrosomia in gestational diabetes, Obstet. Gynecol. **64**:347, 1984.

Bolton, R.N.: Some considerations of excessive fetal development, Am. J. Obstet. Gynecol. **77**:118, 1959.

Boyd, M.E., Usher, R.H., and McLean, F.H.: Fetal macrosomia: prediction, risks, proposed management, Obstet. Gynecol. **61**:715, 1983.

Chamberlain, P.F., Manning, F.A., Morrison, I., et al.: Ultrasound evaluation of amniotic fluid volume: the relationship of increased amniotic fluid volume to perinatal outcome, Am. J. Obstet. Gynecol. **150**:250, 1984.

Chantler, C., and Baum, J.D.: Dextrostix in the diagnosis of neonatal hypoglycemia, Lancet **2**:1395, 1967.

Coustan, D.R., and Imarah, J.: Prophylactic insulin treatment of gestational diabetes reduces the incidence of macrosomia, operative delivery, and birth trauma, Am. J. Obstet. Gynecol. **150**:836, 1984.

Dor, N., Mosberg, H., Stern, W., et al.: Complications in fetal macrosomia, N.Y. State J. Med. **84**:302, 1984.

Drillien, C.M.: The small-for-dates: etiology and prognosis, Pediatr. Clin. North Am. **17**:9, 1970.

Fitzhardinge, P.M., and Stevens, E.M.: The small-for-date infant. II. Neurologic and intellectual sequelae, Pediatrics **50**:50, 1972.

Fleischer, A., Schulman, H., Farmakides, G., et al.: Umbilical artery velocity waveforms and intrauterine growth retardation, Am. J. Obstet. Gynecol. **151**:502, 1985.

Hill, L.M., Breckle, R., Wolfgram, K.R., et al.: Oligohydramnios: ultrasonically detected incidence and subsequent fetal outcome, Am. J. Obstet. Gynecol. **147**:407, 1983.

Jaschevatzky, O.E., Mor, G., Miller, M., et al.: Risk in the vaginal delivery of the large fetus, Aust. N.Z. J. Obstet. Gynaecol. **24**:178, 1984.

Miller, H.C., and Hassanein, K.: Fetal malnutrition in white newborn infants: maternal factors, Pediatrics **52**:504, 1973.

Naeye, R.L., Blanc, W., and Cheryl, P.: Maternal nutrition and the fetus, Pediatrics **52**:494, 1973.

Nelson, L.W., Horne, M.K., and Bradford, W.D.: Polyhydramnios: an infrequent etiology, South, Med. J. **65**:188, 1972.

Ott, W.J.: Fetal femur length, neonatal crown-heel length, and screening for intrauterine growth retardation, Obstet. Gynecol. **65**:460, 1985.

Ounsted, M., and Taylor, M.E.: The postnatal growth of children who were small-for-dates or large-for-dates at birth, Dev. Med. Child. Neurol. **13**:421, 1971.

Philip, A.G.S.: Fetal growth retardation: femurs, fontanels, and follow-up, Pediatrics **62**:446, 1978.

Queenan, J.T., and Gadaw, E.C.: Polyhydramnios: chronic versus acute, Am. J. Obstet. Gynecol. **108**:349, 1970.

Sack, R.A.: The large infant, Am. J. Obstet. Gynecol. **104**:195, 1969.

Scott, K.E., and Usher, R.: Fetal malnutrition: its incidence, causes, and effects, Am. J. Obstet. Gynecol. **94**:951, 1966.

Usher, R.H.: Clinical and therapeutic aspects of fetal malnutrition, Pediatr. Clin. North Am. **17**:9, 1970.

Weiner, C.P., Sabbagha, R.E., Vaisrub, N., et al.: A hypothetical model suggesting suboptimal intrauterine growth in infants delivered preterm, Obstet. Gynecol. **65**:323, 1985.

Westergaard, J.G., Teisner, B., Hau, J., et al.: Placental function studies in low birth weight infants with and without dysmaturity, Obstet. Gynecol. **65**:316, 1985.

Whitfield, C.R.: Effect of amniotic fluid volume on prediction, Clin. Obstet. Gynecol. **14**:537, 1971.

20
Multiple pregnancy

Multiple pregnancies are directly or indirectly responsible for approximately 15% of all premature births and 9% of all perinatal deaths, a rate seven times that of single perinate pregnancies. Wastage is largely caused by the increased chance of early birth and attendant physiologic immaturity with associated asphyxia neonatorium and respiratory distress syndrome. Indeed, 55% of twins weigh less than 2,501 gm at birth, 80% of mortality in twin pregnancies occurs in those under 31 weeks of gestational age, and 93% of twin pregnancy deaths are of infants with birth weights of less than 1,500 gm.

However, wastage for multiple gestation infants is not confined to the sequelae of prematurity. Multiple pregnancy also contributes approximately 17% of all growth-retarded infants. There is delayed mental and physical development of surviving twins and a higher incidence of cerebral palsy than occurs with singletons. One fetus is sometimes aborted or absorbed or becomes a fetus papyraceus. There is suggestion of a higher risk of both fetuses being aborted (compared with singletons), but quantification of this is lacking.

There is also increased maternal risk from the hypertensive states of pregnancy, uterine rupture, hemorrhage, and other complications. Thus the approximate 1% of pregnancies with multiple fetuses (2% of infants born) place both mother and offspring at extreme high risk. Reduction in the untoward sequelae of multiple gestation could significantly decrease overall maternal and perinatal morbidity and mortality.

Diagnosis of multiple birth early in gestation is vital. Unfortunately, only around 75% are currently diagnosed prior to delivery. Indeed, the majority of immature twin pairs (which, as noted, account for most problems) referred to neonatal centers have been undiagnosed prior to delivery. Multiple gestations cannot be taken lightly by either patients or professionals and must be treated as high-risk pregnancies if satisfactory results are to be achieved.

INCIDENCE AND ASSOCIATIONS

Weinberg's formula is often applied to express the natural frequency of multiple gestation: twins, 1:90; triplets, $1:90^2$; quadruplets, $1:90^3$, etc. However, the true frequency for a given population may vary considerably from these estimates. Monozygotic twinning occurs at a constant rate of approximately 2.3 to 4 per 1,000 pregnancies in all populations, has no known predispositions, and accounts for approximately 30% of plural pregnancies. The inherent risk of twin gestation resulting from a single ovum is considerably influenced by the timing of the separation, as shown in Table 20-1.

Multiple monozygotic fetuses are at a 2½ times greater risk of death than are dizygotic twins. The majority of multiple gestations result from separate ova, so that up to 70% of twins may be the result of dizygotic gestations. In contrast to monozygotic twins, the incidence of dizygotic twinning is influenced by a variety of factors:

Previous birth of dizygotic twins (tenfold increase of subsequent multiple pregnancy)
Race (1.3:1,000 in Japan, 12:1,000 in the United States, 40:1,000 in western Nigeria)

Table 20-1. Monozygotic twinning

Division timing	Results
Prior to 4 days* (before morula stage)	Separate or fused placentas Two chorions (dichorionic) Two amnions (diamniotic)
4-8 days (after trophoblast differentiation, before amnion differentiation)	Single placenta Common chorion (monochorionic) Two amnions (diamniotic)
8-14 days (after amnion differentiation)	Single placenta Monochorionic Monoamniotic
8-14 days (incomplete)	Conjoined or "Siamese" twins
Later than 14 days	Incomplete twinning

*Division on or prior to day 5 accounts for approximately one third of monozygotic twins, and after day 5 for the other two thirds.

Table 20-2. Parental influence on the incidence of twins

Parent	Incidence of twins (total births)
Mother dizygotic twin	1.7% to 4.0%
Father dizygotic twin	0.8% to 1.7%

Table 20-3. Incidence of males in pregnancies of increasing fetal number

Fetal number	Males (%)
1	51.59
2	50.85
3	49.54
4	46.48

Heredity (probably an autosomal recessive trait passed on via female descendants with the father's genetic contribution having little or no impact on multiple gestation) (Table 20-2)

Maternal age (peak occurrence between 35 and 45 years of age)

Maternal parity (up to para seven, the higher the parity the higher the rate, with rate doubled by para four)

Maternal height and weight (higher incidence of twinning among taller and heavier women)

Among whites, blood groups O and A (more multiple births—cause unknown)

Pregnancy that occurs in the first menstrual cycle after cessation of long-term oral contraceptive therapy

Maternal polyovulation (possible resulting from excessive production of pituitary gonadotropins)

Artificial polyovulation (from induction of ovulation with human pituitary gonadotropins or clomiphene citrate, the latter increasing the incidence of twins to 7% and triplets to 0.3%)

Approximately 75% of all twin gestations result in twins of the same sex, with 45% being male pairs and 30% being female pairs. When both twins are male there is an unexplained enhancement of premature delivery (as opposed to female-male and female-female pairs) and the resulting infants are smaller and lighter (correct for gestational age). However, numbers of male fetuses decrease as numbers of fetuses in multiple pregnancies increase (Table 20-3). Although there are various speculations regarding the cause of this phenomenon, the etiology remains obscure.

IDENTIFICATION BY CLINICAL ASSOCIATIONS AND OBSERVATION

Approximately 25% of twin gestations are undiagnosed until labor or delivery, partly because of failure of patients to avail themselves of prenatal care. However, to influence outcomes beneficially diagnosis must be made early, and proper care must be instituted in every case. Screening patients for the associations noted above allows identification of certain patients who are at risk. Physicians should retain a high index of suspicion and consider all pregnancies as possible multiple gestations until it can be determined that only a single fetus exists. Specific physical findings suggesting multiple gestation include:

Larger uterine size than expected (greater than 4 cm over expected measurement according to gestational age estimate)

Greater maternal weight gain than expected (especially during first trimester)

Greater quantity of and more persistent fetal movements (usually useful in multiparous women only)

Manual abdominal examination can detect or confirm the diagnosis of twinning in over 75%

of cases. The most common findings noted are:
- Outline or ballottement of more than one fetus
- Palpation of a multiplicity of small parts
- Palpation of three or more large parts

Auscultation of more than one fetal heart is the usual clinical tool used to confirm the suspicion of multiple pregnancy. To confirm multiple pregnancy, fetal hearts must be auscultated simultaneously and should vary at least 8 beats/min from each other and from the maternal pulse.

Certain pregnancy complications merit investigation because of their association with multiple gestation. These include:
- Polyhydramnios (10 times more frequent in multiple gestation)
- Maternal anemia (hypochromic normocytic)
- Preeclampsia-eclampsia
- Maternal complaints of increased visceral pressures
- Lutein cysts and ascites
- Glucose intolerance

DIAGNOSIS BY LABORATORY PROCEDURES

The laboratory modality currently most often used to confirm the clinical suspicion of multiple gestation is ultrasonic scan. It is possible to use ultrasonography, even early in pregnancy (from 8 to 10 weeks separate gestational sacs may be visualized). Consistently correct diagnoses can be expected after 12 to 14 weeks. It is imperative to determine placental placement, and, as early as possible, to determine biparietal diameters, abdominal circumferences, femur lengths, and other measurements useful for following fetal growth patterns. These parameters should be obtained serially to ensure continued normal growth of all fetuses, since 25% of twins (and increasing percentages for perinates from pregnancies with a greater number of fetuses) suffer fetal growth retardation. Moreover, ultrasonography is the most viable method of discovering the effects of anastomotic circulations (twin-to-twin transfusion syndrome) in monozygotic multiple pregnancies.

Ultrasonography also allows discernment of the positional relationships of fetuses prior to delivery, discovery of malpositions, and detailing of anomalies such as incomplete twinning. Ultrasonography may also be used antenatally to accurately assess amniotic and chorionic features. Sonographic features to consider when assessing the latter include number of placental sites, whether a membrane separates fetuses, fetal position, and amount of amniotic fluid. Interpretations are as follows:

- Two placental sites—dichorionic, therefore diamniotic pregnancy
- Membrane separating fetuses—diamniotic pregnancy
- Disparate fetal position and movement (one fetus may move freely and the other appears to be restricted)—suggests diamniotic pregnancy
- Entanglement or intermingling of fetal parts or umbilical cords—suggests monoamniotic pregnancy

When ultrasonography is not available radiography of the uterus after the twentieth week usually reveals the number of fetuses and their presentations. However, fetal movement that occurs during radiography may obscure the true number of fetuses. Moreover, the accuracy of diagnosis and of critical mensuration by both ultrasonography and radiography decreases as the number of fetuses increases. Therefore extreme care must be taken in proper investigation of fetal number in multiple gestations.

Other laboratory modalities used to confirm multiple gestations include use of fetal electrocardiography, which will reveal multiple heartbeats, but unfortunately is usually accurate only in the latter stages of pregnancy. It has also been reported that a human placental lactogen assay above 3 µg/ml before 25 weeks' gestation, above 4 µg/ml at 25 to 30 weeks' gestation, or above 8 µg/ml after 30 weeks probably indicates multiple gestation.

Other studies significantly altered by multiple pregnancy include increases in chorionic gonadotropin, estriol, pregnanediol, cystine, leucine aminopeptidase, and alkaline phosphatase. However, none of these latter determinations are specific enough to be helpful in routine screening or clinical diagnosis.

Differential diagnosis

Differential diagnoses of multiple pregnancy include the following:
- Singleton pregnancy with inaccurate dates
- Singleton pregnancy with polyhydramnios
- Hydatidiform mole
- Singleton pregnancy with macrosomia
- Abnormal twin gestations such as conjoined twins or fetus papyraceous

Elevation of pregnant uterus by distended bladder or full rectum

Pelvic tumors

Abdominal tumors complicating pregnancy (most common are uterine fibroid tumors; however, ovarian tumors or diverse abdominal tumors may also be present)

Ultrasonic examination should identify most differential diagnoses.

SPECIAL CARE DURING PREGNANCY
Benefits of early detection

Early detection of multiple gestation will:
1. Enhance parents' concern for the pregnancy and fetal health
2. Allow augmentation of nutrition at an earlier date
3. Offer opportunity for earlier institution of a rest schedule
4. Allow earlier detection of premature labor
5. Encourage prompt introduction of therapy for threatened premature labor
6. Encourage better use of testing modalities for detection of fetal abnormalities and prompt initiation of appropriate therapy
7. Allow delivery to be planned in advance with sufficient perinatal facilities and personnel available

Indeed, early detection offers critical benefits of sufficient magnitude to perhaps warrant ultrasonic scans* of all pregnancies (between 16 and 20 weeks' gestation) as a means of screening.

Additional rest

It may be useful to curtail exercise during plural pregnancy and to initiate a program of additional rest from the time of diagnosis until 34 weeks' gestation has passed. The value (as measured by prolongation of gestation) of absolute bed rest for a week at the time of diagnosis (if under 30 weeks) and again at 32 weeks has

---

*The expense of ultrasonography is now a deterrent to its routine use in pregnancy care. Yet the possibility of achieving a delay of 6 weeks in the delivery of one set of surviving twins born at 27 weeks could result in savings of approximately $100,000. This could pay for approximately 1,500 ultrasonic scans, which should identify at least 30 multiple gestation fetuses. Other abnormalities such as uterine and fetal anomalies, placental aberrations, and ectopic and molar gestations could also be identified by such a screening program.

---

been questioned. However, increased uterine blood flow effected by decreased competition for cardiac output from skeletal muscle and enhanced by recumbent position certainly minimizes risk. Moreover, institutionalized bed rest is certainly warranted when serious problems threaten (such as toxemia, spontaneous labor, or cervical dilatation) or proper daily rest is impossible in the home environment.

Optimal antepartum care

Proper prenatal care has been demonstrated to lower perinatal mortality and morbidity.
1. Schedule a prenatal visit every 2 weeks during second trimester and weekly during third trimester. In addition to routine prenatal care, perform vaginal examinations for cervical effacement or dilatation. Ultrasonic scan may be advisable as frequently as every 2 weeks.
2. Follow carefully assessing for fetal growth retardation as often as every 2 weeks (ultrasonography). If biparietal diameters do not increase by more than 1 mm/wk, intrauterine growth retardation may be present.
3. Emphasize importance of abstinence from smoking and alcohol use.
4. Screen for complications seen more commonly with multiple gestations and initiate early therapy.

Nutrition

Maternal nutritional intake, including protein, iron, and calcium, should be increased. With multiple gestation maternal caloric needs exceed those of gravidas with singleton gestations by at least another 300 kcal/day. The overall goal should be to gain at least the weight that will be lost with delivery. Iron (60 to 100 mg/day) should be added to the diet, and folic acid addition should be considered.

Premature labor

Treat premature labor as detailed in Chapter 18.

SPECIAL CONSIDERATIONS FOR DELIVERY
General considerations

1. Multiple pregnancy is a high-risk category. If possible, deliver perinates in a maternity center with a physician-nurse team for each

infant in the delivery room, as well as full obstetric and anesthesia teams attending.
2. Obtain frequent maternal pulse and blood pressure measurements (also temperature and respiration, if indicated).
3. Employ electronic fetal monitoring for both first and second twins for detection of fetal distress. Should fetal distress occur in the second twin (even if the first is already delivered), it is safer to deliver the baby by cesarean section than to attempt a traumatic vaginal delivery.
4. Have an intravenous catheter (18 gauge or larger) in place and working. Consider hemodynamic monitoring (Swan-Ganz catheter or central venous pressure line) if there is greater than usual possibility of hemorrhage or shock.
5. Avoid or treat maternal hypotension.
   a. Increase intravenous fluids (administer blood if indicated).
   b. Try positional changes to move uterus from inferior vena cava. Maintain lateral recumbent position.
   c. Push uterus off inferior vena cava.
   d. Elevate (Trendelenburg) or wrap legs with elastic supports.
   e. Consider alternative positions (e.g., Sims) for delivery if supine hypotensive syndrome is severe.
6. Administer maternal oxygen if there is any evidence of fetal compromise.
7. Have type-specific blood available for both mother (also blood products, if necessary) and babies.
8. In addition, scrub abdomen with appropriate antiseptic in preparation for possible cesarean section.
9. Have a retention catheter and prep set ready for immediate insertion should cesarean section become necessary.
10. Develop a team plan for the most atraumatic delivery possible.

Analgesia

The use of analgesia and anesthesia for multiple gestation, especially in premature labor, poses very special problems. Medication poorly chosen or too liberally administered will be seriously depressing, particularly for the fetus that is not mature or is otherwise jeopardized. All procedures and agents used to relieve the discomforts of labor and delivery have some advantage or desirable characteristic, but none is perfect. Each case must be individualized with minimal amounts of analgesia and anesthesia employed and administered by experienced and qualified personnel only. It has been suggested that low doses of meperidine may be safely used for analgesia. A restricted segmental epidural block or nitrous oxide–oxygen has also been suggested as satisfactory for analgesia and delivery anesthesia.

Mode of delivery

1. Twins
   The mode of delivery for twin gestation is usually determined during intrapartum management. A protocol for intrapartum management and delivery based on the two crucial variables of fetal presentation and sonographically determined estimated fetal weight (EFW) is presented in Fig. 20-1. External version of the second twin when the first is vertex is a clearly emerging trend.
2. Three or more fetuses
   It is commonly agreed that a pregnancy with more than two fetuses, with few exceptions, indicates cesarean delivery.

CESAREAN SECTION

Cesarean section is increasingly being used when either twin is in a position other than vertex. An abnormal presentation is much more likely with twins (and other plural pregnancies) than singletons. The relative frequency of various twin presentation combinations is shown in Table 20-4. The first twin, in 70% of cases, and the second twin, in 50% of cases, may be expected to be in the vertex position.

Recent evidence has dispelled the notion that the second twin will be the smaller; indeed, it is usually the larger. Thus delivery may be complicated by a second twin who is in malposition and may be larger than the first. Additionally, the second twin is more subject to hypoxia. All monoamniotic twins should be delivered by cesarean section. Should the first twin be in breech and the second in vertex position, the hazard of the twins interlocking is so great that cesarean section is usually indicated.

The type of cesarean section to be used (low transverse cervical or low vertical) must be carefully considered and individualized on a

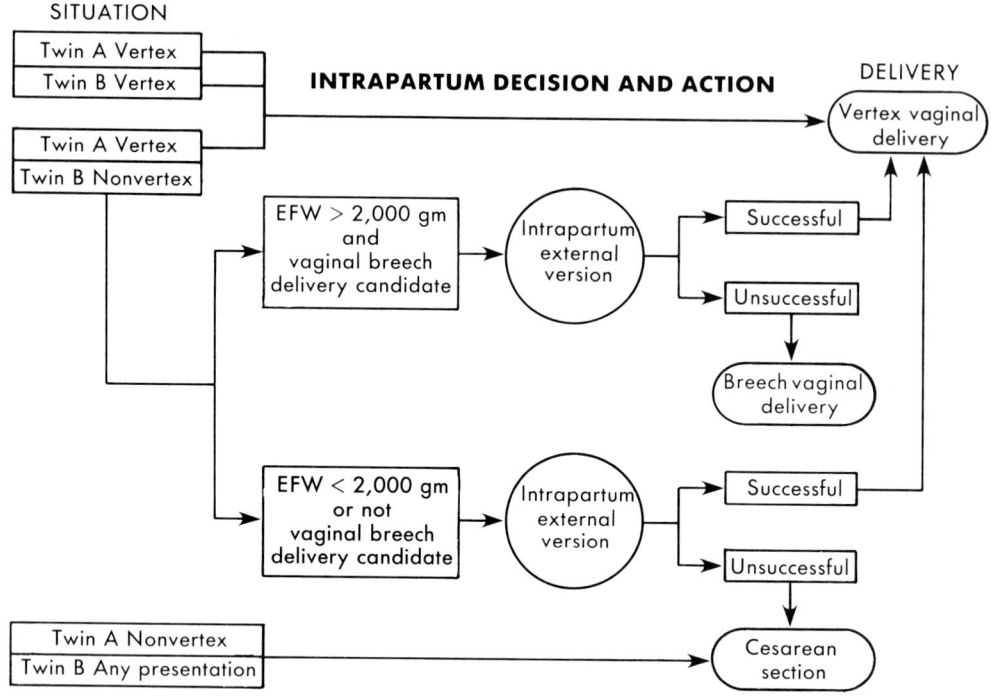

Fig. 20-1. Management of twin gestation, intrapartum protocol. (Modified from Chervenak, F.A., et al.: Intrapartum management of twin gestation, Obstet. Gynecol. 65:120, 1985.)

Table 20-4. Combinations of presentations in twins at labor

Twin A	Twin B	Percent
Cephalic	Cephalic	42.5
Cephalic	Breech	26.0
Cephalic	Transverse	11.3
Breech	Cephalic	6.9
Breech	Breech	6.1
Breech	Transverse	4.7
Cephalic	Oblique	1.1
Transverse	Cephalic	0.6
Transverse	Transverse	0.6
Breech	Oblique	0.3

From Chervenak, F.A., et al.: Intrapartum management of twin gestation, Obstet. Gynecol. 65:120, 1985.

case-by-case basis. The determining consideration in this choice is ease of delivery through the incision. Indications for cesarean section in twin gestation include, but are not limited to:
Accepted obstetric indications for singletons
Breech/vertex presentation.
Conjoined twins
Monoamniotic twins
Fetus-to-fetus transfusion syndrome

VAGINAL DELIVERY

1. A deep episiotomy is often recommended to shorten the second stage of labor and decrease compression of the fetal head, particularly when delivery is premature. Indeed, in this case use of forceps to cradle and protect the head should be considered. The umbilical cord should be cut immediately after delivery. However, in no circumstance should a cord around the neck of the first perinate be cut; it should be manipulated over the head. In numerous circumstances it has been found to be the cord of the second monoamniotic twin. When cut, the cord should be clearly identified with a marking clamp.
2. A vaginal examination must be performed immediately after delivery of the first child to ascertain the presentation of the second child. Do not administer oxytocin or ergot after delivery of the first child.
3. If the membranes are to be ruptured, this should be accomplished in the interval between contractions.
4. Use of oxytocin will infrequently be neces-

sary because of ineffectual uterine contractions. In light of the overdistended uterus and possible uteroplacental insufficiency, its use must be clearly indicated, and great care must be taken in administration.

5. Internal version and extraction should be performed only for known fetal deaths.
6. Although it has been stated that operative delivery for the second twin is indicated when the interval between delivery of the first and second twins exceeds 15 minutes, this is not necessarily the case if electronic fetal monitoring is available. However, the safest interval may still lie between 10 and 20 minutes.
7. Because of frequent postpartum hemorrhage, oxytocin should be administered (5 U IV and then 15 to 20 U/1,000 ml IV solution) after delivery of the second child. Other steps such as uterine elevation, use of ergots, and use of prostaglandins may be necessary.

SPECIAL PERINATAL CONSIDERATIONS

1. Fetus-to-fetus transfusion (twin-to-twin transfusion) is rarely if ever encountered in dizygotic multiple gestations. Although artery-to-artery and vein-to-vein communications are described, the most serious is the artery-to-vein connection where a pressure differential causes blood to be pumped out of one fetus into the other. As a result of the ensuing intrauterine deprivation, one twin may be essentially growth retarded and the other plethoric and relatively macrosomic. The smaller is likely to have oligohydramnios and the larger polyhydramnios.

In the extreme form this complication may lead to intrauterine death of one or more fetuses. Although maternal administration of digitalis has been reported to assist in fetal cardiac failure, there is little that can be done to alter the course of fetus-to-fetus transfusions.

An uncommon variant of this problem is the development of an acardiac amorphous fetus, in which the heart of one fetus is not functional and the acardiac fetus therefore exists as a parasite on the other fetus. Usually minimal cephalic development and numerous other anomalies are also apparent.

Labor may pose special and quite disparate hazards to fetuses unfortunate enough to be attached to an acardiac amorphous fetus, and each must be carefully and completely monitored. Cesarean section must be used quite liberally to prevent birth complications.

At birth there is likely to be a great differential in hemoglobin concentration between babies. Smaller infants will usually have anemia, hypovolemia, hypotension, microcardia, and other stigmata of intrauterine growth retardation. Larger infants are likely to have hypertension, cardiac hypertrophy, polycythemia, and hyperviscosity, which carries a 70% perinatal mortality. A partial exchange transfusion with equal volumes of plasma for the plethoric infant may be necessary when the venous hematocrit reading surpasses 65%. Packed cells may be necessary for anemic infants if the hematocrit reading is less than 35%. In an emergency, blood may be taken from the polycythemic infant and given to the anemic one via the umbilical vein.

2. Resuscitation and stabilization procedures are similar to those used for singletons. Important requirements are sufficient physician-nurse teams and equipment for each infant.
3. Discrepancy in size at birth and in fetal undergrowth is more likely in monozygotic pairs. In addition to twin-to-twin transfusion, this may be the result of a shrunken umbilical cord or a velamentous insertion at the cord's attachment to the placenta causing fetuses to receive unequal shares of placental blood (and nutrients). Discrepancy in birth size of twins may be marked (e.g., a recent pair weighed 800 and 2,650 gm respectively at birth). The nutritional bankruptcy in the smaller may end tragically unless care is taken to prevent hypoglycemia by early and frequent high-calorie feedings. If proper nutrition is utilized, some catch-up growth and favorable intellectual outcome may be anticipated.
4. Postnatal high-calorie feedings are necessary to assist in preventing further sequelae of growth retardation.
5. The death of one fetus may occur at any time. Indeed, ultrasonic evidence suggests this is much more common than was pre-

viously thought in very early gestation. When death occurs early, it is usual for complete absorption of the dead fetus to occur. At a later stage the dead fetus and its placenta and membranes may be compressed with loss of fluid and soft tissue and growth of the remaining fetus to form a fetus papyraceus.

An additional concern is the possibility (although rare) of either disseminated intravascular coagulation or consumption coagulopathy in the mother and/or the other fetus. Careful monitoring of maternal fibrinogen and fibrin degradation products should assist in detection of this very unusual complication.

6. Although amniocentesis for antenatal diagnosis may be safely accomplished with multiple gestation, great care must be taken to sample each sac. There are numerous reports of dizygotic gestations in which one fetus(es) is affected and the other fetus(es) is normal.

7. Other tests of fetal maturity and well-being (pulmonary maturity studies, nonstress tests, contraction stress tests, and probably biophysical profiles) may be used with relative assurance of results comparable to those obtained with singleton gestation.

COMPLICATIONS AND SEQUELAE
Maternal

Maternal morbidity with multiple pregnancy (excluding the commonly encountered anemia previously mentioned) is eight times that reported for singleton vaginal delivery. Common complications are noted below.

1. Preeclampsia-eclampsia
   This complication is three times more frequent in women bearing twins than those bearing singletons.
2. Abnormal labor
   a. Premature
      Premature labor (often after spontaneous rupture of membranes) and premature delivery are seven times more likely in multiple than in singleton pregnancy. The cause of this tendency toward early labor remains unclear, but crowding with uterine overdistention, preeclampsia, and the relatively diminished blood flow to the uterus per fetus are all likely factors. Treatment of premature labor includes bed rest, sedation, hydration, and use of betamimetics.
      Pulmonary maturity must be evaluated carefully. It may occur earlier in multiple gestation fetuses than it does in the singleton. Use of progesterone, cervical cerclage, and other agents demands further study.
   b. Abnormal labor patterns
      An abnormal and often ineffective labor pattern (most frequently desultory) is more common with multiple gestation, presumably because of uterine overdistention.
3. Maternal distress
   a. Anemia
      Dilution anemia is two to three times more common with multiple gestations.
   b. Sensation of breathlessness
      Even though respiratory tidal volume is greater than it is in a singleton gestation, the gravida with a multiple gestation often complains of being unable to "catch her breath."
   c. Visceral pressures
      Visceral pressures are usually enhanced in multiple gestation, especially in women with shorter abdominal lengths.
   d. Lutein cysts
      Lutein cysts, often with accompanying ascites, are much more common in multiple gestation.
   e. Hypotension
      Usual maternal propensity for peripheral venous pooling and vena caval obstruction is enhanced with multiple gestation.
   f. Glucose intolerance
      Incidence of both gestational diabetes mellitus and gestational hypoglycemia is increased with multiple gestation. Glucose tolerance testing may be indicated in all multiple pregnancies.
4. Urinary tract complications
   Infection of the urinary tract is at least twice as common with multiple gestation, and occasionally the uterus reaches a size sufficient to cause obstructive uropathy.
5. Postpartum hemorrhage
   Postpartum hemorrhage occurs five times

more often because of uterine atony after overdistention.
6. Operative intervention
Need for operative intervention is greater in multiple than in singleton gestations.
7. Morbid partum or postpartum course
Multiple gestation carries a five times greater chance of morbidity caused by infectious or other complications.

Table 20-5. Average duration of gestation and perinatal deaths related to number of fetuses

Fetal number	Weeks completed	Perinatal deaths (per 1,000 births)
1	39	39
2	35	152
3	33	309
4	29	509

Fetal

As could be expected, the earlier the termination of gestation and the smaller the fetuses, the more perinatal morbidity and mortality occurs. Twice as many triplets die in the perinatal interval as do twins (Table 20-5). Double ova twins generally fare better than single ovum twins. Other fetal complications and sequelae include the following:

I. Abortion (Chapter 3)
II. Malformations
Serious congenital anomalies occur with nearly two-fold greater incidence in multiple than in singleton gestations. Abnormalities are more frequent in monozygotic twins. Most commonly affected are the central nervous, musculoskeletal, respiratory, and cardiovascular systems. Extreme examples include conjoined twins and the acardiac amorphous fetus (a parasitic fetus without a heart and with distorted and rudimentary development).
III. Low birth weight
  A. Prematurity (Chapter 18)
  B. Intrauterine growth retardation
  Fetal undergrowth, which affects 25% of twins, contributes to the higher proportion of multiple gestation fetal deaths. Indeed, most twins demonstrate some degree of limitation after 34 weeks' gestation. Triplets and quadruplets are affected earlier. Restrictions in nutritional supply are added if traditional pregnancy weight gain limits are applied to women with plural pregnancies.
IV. Twin-to-twin transfusion
V. Polyhydramnios
Polyhydramnios in multiple gestation is sometimes associated with twin-to-twin transfusion syndrome or fetal anomalies. However, hydramnios may also occur when these complications are not present and poses the same but even more vexing problems than it does with the singleton. Indeed, hydramnios is five times more common in multiple than in singleton pregnancy.
VI. Perinatal death
  A. Fetal death occurs three times as often with twins (compared with singletons) because of:
    1. Abnormal fetal or placental development
    2. Circulatory competition
    3. Cord compression or other accidents
    Incidence of death of one fetus with monoamniotic twins is 50%
  B. Neonatal death is a sequelae of the events noted above and below.
VII. Central nervous system injury and other trauma may follow intervention and operative delivery. Thus the incidence of cerebral palsy and mental retardation is increased in multiple gestation. Examples of hazardous situations include:
  A. Manipulation at delivery (e.g., internal podalic version)
  B. Cervical "trapping" of the aftercoming head
  C. Delay in delivery of second twin
  D. Cord compression
  E. Malposition
  All of these increase chances of asphyxia as well as traumatic damage to tissues including the brachial nerves. Cesarean section is being used increasingly to avoid these hazards.

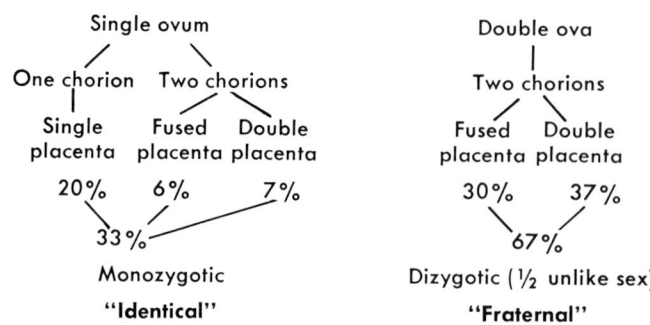

Fig. 20-2. Twin zygosity and placental form. (Based on data from Potter, E.L.: Am. J. Obstet. Gynecol. **87**:566, 1963.)

Placental and related to cord

1. Placenta previa
   Incidence of placenta previa is increased because of increased placental size.
2. Abruptio placentae
   Incidence of abruptio placentae is increased and is especially common after delivery of the first twin.
3. Single umbilical arteries
   Single umbilical artery occurs three times more often in twins than in singletons.
4. Velamentous cord insertion
   Velamentous insertion of the cord occurs seven times more frequently with multiple pregnancy.
5. Premature rupture of membranes
   PROM is often the cause of premature labor. It occurs in about 25% of twin, 50% of triplet, and 75% of quadruplet pregnancies.
6. Cord prolapse
   Incidence of cord prolapse is increased fivefold because of prematurity, polyhydramnios, unstable lie, and malposition.
7. Cord entanglement
   If monochorionic, monoamniotic twins are present (1% of twin pregnancies) the cords may become entangled. This complication poses special hazard for death before and particularly during labor.

Placental examination

Careful examination of cords and placenta(s) in multiple births offers immediate opportunity to determine with good accuracy whether fetuses are monozygotic. This simple observation can be of great clinical significance. Steps to be taken for precise observation are as follows:

1. With each delivery, identify that infant's cord by a particular clamp etc.
2. After delivery of placenta(s), place it on a flat surface and approximate the original configuration.
3. Study that portion of the membranes dividing the fetal cavities, even if two chorionic plates are found. Take a section of this area for microscopy.

Monoamniotic twins are always monozygotic. When two sacs are present, the area studied will consist of two amnions but only one chorion (indicating monozygotic fetus) or two amnions and two chorions (usually indicating dizygotic fetuses). (Fig. 20-2). All those of unlike sex are dizygotic. Only those left (diamniotic, dichorionic of like sex) will require extensive hematology and/or genetic study to determine zygosity. Accurate determinations of zygosity may be obtained by sophisticated studies of blood groups, serum proteins, red blood cell enzymes, red cell antigens, HLA typing, and chromosome markers.

BIBLIOGRAPHY

Babson, S.G., and Philips, D.S.: Growth and development of twins dissimilar in size at birth, N. Engl. J. Med. **289**:937, 1973.

Blake, G.D., Knuppel, R.A., Ingardia, C.J., et al.: Evaluation of nonstress fetal heart rate testing in multiple gestations, Obstet. Gynecol. **63**:528, 1984.

Chervenak, F.A., Johnson, R.E., Youcha, S., et al.: Intrapartum management of twin gestation, Obstet. Gynecol. **65**:119, 1985.

DeGeorge, F.V.: Maternal and fetal disorders in pregnancies of mothers of twins, Am. J. Obstet. Gynecol. **108**:975, 1970.

Dobbie, H.G., Whittle, M.J., Wilson, A.I., et al.: Amniotic fluid phospholipid profile in multiple pregnancy and the effect of zygosity, Br. J. Obstet. Gynaecol. **90**:1001, 1983.

Hanna, J.H., and Hill, J.M.: Single intrauterine fetal demise in multiple gestation, Obstet. Gynecol. **63**:126, 1984.

Jeffrey, R.L., Bowes, W.A., and Delaney, J.J.: Role of bedrest in twin gestation, Obstet. Gynecol. **43**:822, 1974.

Jonas, E.G.: The value of prenatal bed rest in multiple pregnancy, J. Obstet. Gynaec. Brit. Comm. **70**:461, 1974.

Knuppel, R.A., Rattan, P.K., Scerbo, J.C., et al.: Intrauterine fetal death in twins after 32 weeks of gestation, Obstet. Gynecol. **65**:172, 1985.

Leveno, K., Santos-Ramos, R., Duenhoelter, J.H., et al.: Sonar cephalometry in twins: a table of biparietal diameters for normal twin fetuses and a comparison with singletons, Am. J. Obstet. Gynecol. **135**:727, 1979.

Leveno, K.J., Quirk, G., Whalley, P.J., et al.: Fetal lung maturation in twin gestation, Am. J. Obstet. Gynecol. **148**:405, 1984.

MacGillivray, I.: Twin pregnancies, Obstet. Gynecol. Annu. **7**:135, 1978.

Mahony, B.S., Filly, R.A., and Callen, P.W.: Amnionicity and chorionicity in twin pregnancies: prediction using ultrasound, Radiology **155**:205, 1985.

Manlan, G., and Scott, K.E.: Contribution of twin pregnancy to perinatal mortality and fetal growth retardation: reversal of growth retardation after birth, Can. Med. Assoc. J. **118**:365, 1978.

Nance, W.E., editor: Twin research: proceedings, International Congress on Twin Studies, New York, 1978, Alan R. Liss, Inc.

Newton, W., Keith, L., and Keith, D.: The Northwestern University multihospital twin study, Am. J. Obstet. Gynecol. **149**:655, 1984.

Norman, R.J., Joubert, S.M., and Marivate, M.: Amniotic fluid phospholipids and glucocorticoids in multiple pregnancy, Br. J. Obstet. Gynaecol. **90**:51, 1983.

Pernoll, M.L., and Carnes, R.W.: Electronic fetal monitoring of twin gestations, Am. J. Obstet. Gynecol. **116**:583, 1973.

Rayburn, W.F., Lavin, J.P., Jr., Miodovnik, M., et al.: Multiple gestation: time interval between delivery of the first and second twins, Obstet. Gynecol. **63**:502, 1984.

Socol, M.L., Tamura, R.K., Sabbagha, R.E., et al.: Diminished biparietal diameter and abdominal circumference growth in twins, Obstet. Gynecol. **64**:235, 1984.

21

Hypertensive states in pregnancy

The hypertensive disease states of pregnancy are certain vascular derangements (usually vasopastic) that either antedate pregnancy or arise during pregnancy or the early puerperium. Synonyms include toxemia of pregnancy, eclamptogenic toxemia, edema-proteinuria-hypertension complex, and gestoses. These disorders are of unknown etiology and involve multiple metabolic aberrations, often involving low protein intake. In addition to vasospasm, sodium and water retention occurs, and there is depletion of serum albumin and globulin because of proteinuria. Primigravidas and women who have chronic hypertensive or renal disease are predisposed. The lower socioeconomic groups of all races are especially prone to eclamptogenic toxemia.

In the United States between 3% and 10% of pregnant women develop preeclampsia, but the incidence is as high as 20% in areas where poor medical care prevails. Eclampsia affects about 5% of toxemic patients in the United States.

Maternal mortality with preeclampsia is exceptional, but with eclampsia it may reach 15%. Perinatal mortality is two or three times the average in preeclampsia, whereas with eclampsia it may reach 20%, with most infants being of low birth weight.

DIAGNOSTIC CRITERIA
Hypertension

Hypertension is a rise in systolic pressure of 30 mm Hg or more; a rise in diastolic pressure of 15 mm Hg or more; or the presence of a blood pressure reading of 140/90 mm Hg or higher. Hypertension may also be determined by a mean arterial pressure of 105 mm Hg or higher or by a rise of 20 mm Hg or more. The level cited must be manifest on at least two occasions at least 6 hours apart and should be based on previously known blood pressure levels.

GESTATIONAL HYPERTENSION

Gestational hypertension is the development of hypertension during pregnancy or within the first 24 hours post partum in a previously normotensive woman. No other evidence of preeclampsia or hypertensive vascular disease persists or develops. Blood pressure returns to normal levels within 10 days after parturition. Some patients with gestational hypertension may develop preeclampsia or hypertensive vascular disease, but they do not initially satisfy the criteria for either of these diagnoses (e.g., lack of proteinuria or generalized edema) to substantiate preeclampsia.

Gestational edema

Gestational edema is a general accumulation of fluid in the tissues greater than 1+ pitting edema *after* 12 hours' rest in bed, or a weight gain of at least 2.3 kg in 1 week because of the influence of pregnancy.

Gestational proteinuria

Gestational proteinuria is the presence of proteinuria during (or under the influence of) pregnancy in the absence of hypertension, edema, urinary tract infection, or known intrinsic renovascular disease. Protein must occur in concentrations greater than 0.3 gm/L in a 24-hour urine collection, or greater than 1 gm/L (1+ to 2+ by standard turbidimetric methods) in a random urine collection on two or more occasions at least 6 hours apart. Specimens must be clean voided, midstream, or obtained by catheterization.

CLASSIFICATION

The hypertensive disorders of pregnancy have been classified by the American Committee on Maternal Welfare as follows:
 I. Preeclampsia-eclampsia (pregnancy-induced hypertension, toxemia, edema-proteinuria-hypertension complex, gestosis)
 II. Chronic hypertension
  A. Primary (essential, idiopathic)
  B. Secondary (to some known cause)
   1. Renal
    a. Parenchymal — glomerulonephritis, chronic pyelonephritis, interstitial nephritis, polycystic kidney disease
    b. Renovascular
   2. Adrenal
    a. Cortical — Cushing's disease, hyperaldosteronism
    b. Medullary — pheochromocytoma
   3. Other causes (e.g., coarctation of the aorta, thyrotoxicosis)
 III. Chronic hypertension with superimposed preeclampsia
 IV. Transient hypertension (a nebulous group of patients who develop hypertension during labor or immediately post partum)

CLINICAL STATES

A vigorous screening program is necessary for detection of the various degrees of the hypertensive states of pregnancy. Certain *predispositions* warrant especially rigorous scrutiny:
1. Primigravida
2. Multiple gestation
3. Hydramnios or fetal hydrops
4. Hydatidiform mole
5. Obesity
6. Diabetes mellitus
7. Renal disease (especially chronic hypertension)
8. Positive family history
9. Pheochromocytoma
10. Lupus erythematosus

Preeclampsia

Preeclampsia is the development of hypertension with proteinuria, edema, or both because of pregnancy or the influence of a recent pregnancy. It may occur anytime after 20 weeks of gestation, but most commonly occurs after 32 weeks. Should it develop before 20 weeks of pregnancy, the possibility of hydatidiform mole, choriocarcinoma, or chronic hypertension must be considered. Preeclampsia is predominantly a disorder of primigravidas and occurs in 7% to 8% of pregnancies.

Preeclampsia is a "disease of theories," its etiology unknown. Sodium and water retention and increased blood volume are normal concomitants of pregnancy. Considerable evidence suggests that plasma volume is contracted in preeclampsia, but whether this is a cause or a consequence of preeclampsia is debated. Assali believes that preeclampsia is a vasospastic process and that the slightly smaller blood volume is merely fitting a contracted vascular bed. This correlates with Swan-Ganz catheter data showing normal wedge pressures and normal or elevated cardiac outputs in preeclampsia.

Using the placental clearance of dehydroepiandrosterone sulfate (DHEA-S) as a measure of placental perfusion, Gant et al. found a decrease in DHEA-S clearance before the development of preeclampsia. Studies of angiotensin sensitivity indicate that the normal refractoriness to angiotensin II (A-II) is lost at 18 to 21 weeks' gestation in women destined to develop preeclampsia. Normal pregnant women lose their refractoriness to A-II after treatment with prostaglandin synthetase inhibitors such as aspirin or indomethacin, suggesting that prostaglandin is involved in mediating vascular reactivity to A-II in pregnancy. Furthermore, A-II refractoriness can be restored to patients with preeclampsia by administration of theophylline, a phosphodiesterase inhibitor that increases levels of cyclic AMP. Gant hypothesizes that prostaglandin synthesized in the arteriole may modulate vascular reactivity to A-II by altering the intracellular level of cyclic AMP in vascular smooth muscle.

Other studies relate preeclampsia to an imbalance between prostacyclin (PGI_2), a vasodilator and inhibitor of platelet aggregation, and thromboxane (TXA_2), a vasoconstrictor and platelet aggregator. Beer has noted that the renal histology in preeclampsia is similar to glomerulonephritis. Beer has also noted that the placental vascular changes of preeclampsia are similar to vascular changes that occur in transplanted organs when they are rejected and has marshalled other evidence to support an immunologic pathogenesis.

The characteristic renal lesion, glomerular capillary endotheliosis, features swelling of the glomerular capillary endothelium with narrowing of the capillary lumina. Subendothelial fibrinoid deposition is also seen. These changes have been shown on serial biopsy to be totally reversible by 6 weeks post partum.

Preeclampsia is divided into mild and severe forms.

I. Mild preeclampsia
   A. Hypertension: blood pressure greater than 140/90 mm Hg or a 30/15 mm Hg rise on two occasions 6 hours apart
   B. Weight gain: more than 5 lb/wk (2.3 kg)
   C. Edema: 15% to 50% of pregnant women have slight generalized edema, but only 4% have mildly elevated blood pressure and proteinuria
   D. Proteinuria: 0.3 gm/L or more on a random specimen on two occasions at least 6 hours apart
II. Severe preeclampsia (in addition to the above)
   A. Hypertension: blood pressure 160/110 mm Hg or higher on two separate occasions at least 6 hours apart with the patient resting in bed
   B. Proteinuria: 5 gm/24 hr or more
   C. Oliguria: 500 ml/24 hr or less
   D. Thrombocytopenia (less than 100,000 cells/mm^3)
   E. Other symptoms (noted primarily if the condition is worsening):
     1. Headache: violent, persistent, and generalized
     2. Ocular abnormalities
       a. Symptoms: visual disturbances, blurred vision, or scintillating scotoma
       b. Sign: retinal arteriolar spasm on funduscopic examination
     3. Epigastric pain
     4. Nausea or vomiting
     5. Nervousness and irritability
     6. Pulmonary edema or cyanosis
III. Differential diagnosis
   A. Essential hypertension
   B. Adrenal hyperplasia
   C. Coarctation of the aorta
   D. Unilateral or bilateral renal arterial disease
   E. Hyperaldosteronism
   F. Glomerulonephritis
   G. Nephrotic syndrome
   H. Pyelonephritis
   I. Pheochromocytoma

Eclampsia

1. Diagnosis
The diagnosis of eclampsia is based on the presence of the signs listed previously for severe preeclampsia, plus one or more of the following:
   a. Convulsions (tonic and clonic) or coma (often after an unobserved seizure) not attributable to other central nervous system disorders such as epilepsy or cerebral hemorrhage
   b. Hypertensive crisis or shock
2. Differential diagnosis
   a. Grand mal epilepsy
   b. Water intoxication
   c. Toxic reaction to local anesthetic agents
   d. Hysteria
   e. Cerebral tumor
   f. Hypoparathyroidism
   g. Acute porphyria
   h. Hypoglycemia
   i. Subarachnoid hemorrhage
   j. Alkalotic tetany
   k. Meningitis
   l. Systemic lupus erythematosus
   m. Strychnine poisoning

Chronic hypertension

1. Diagnosis
The criteria for diagnosis of chronic hypertension are:
   a. Blood pressure of 140/90 mm Hg or higher at 20 or more weeks' gestation
   b. Blood pressure of 140/90 mm Hg or higher before pregnancy or for longer than 6 weeks after pregnancy
Chronic hypertension antedates pregnancy

and includes both essential and secondary forms. Indeed, perinatal mortality and morbidity are related more to duration and severity of hypertension than to its underlying cause.

It is often difficult to distinguish chronic hypertension from chronic hypertension with superimposed preeclampsia. With the development of superimposed preeclampsia, hypertension worsens and edema, proteinuria, and hyperuricemia usually develop. Additionally, it is difficult to distinguish chronic hypertension from preeclampsia. Renal biopsy is the most definitive method of doing this; however, renal biopsy during pregnancy carries a significant risk of renal injury. In patients undergoing biopsy, 25% of patients with classic signs and symptoms of pure eclampsia had underlying renal disease and 21% of patients with a clinical diagnosis of chronic hypertension with superimposed preeclampsia had renal disease.

2. Incidence
The incidence of chronic hypertension in pregnancy is approximately 1.5%.

3. Associations
Patients with chronic hypertension in pregnancy tend to be older and multiparous. Obesity is common. Diabetes and other medical problems are frequently associated (see classification on p. 197).

4. Clinical course
Pregnant patients with chronic hypertension may deteriorate rapidly. After initially seeming to stabilize on admission to the hospital oliguria, thrombocytopenia, serious retinal detachment, or abruptio placentae may develop. Indeed, incidence of abruptio placentae increases from 0.5% to 2% in the general population to 9% to 15% in the chronic hypertensive group.

Superimposed preeclampsia or eclampsia

One of the most difficult complications in patients with chronic hypertension is superimposed preeclampsia or eclampsia.

1. Diagnosis
Superimposed preeclampsia or eclampsia is the development of preeclampsia or eclampsia in a patient with chronic hypertensive vascular or renal disease. When hypertension antedates pregnancy (as established by previous blood pressure recordings) a rise in the diastolic pressure of 15 mm Hg and the development of proteinuria and/or edema are required to establish the diagnosis. Additionally, hyperuricemia usually worsens. Nevertheless, it is still often difficult to distinguish chronic hypertension from chronic hypertension with superimposed preeclampsia.

2. Incidence
Unlike pure preeclampsia, which most frequently occurs after 35 weeks' gestation, chronic hypertension with superimposed preeclampsia often occurs at 30 to 33 weeks. The fetus is at risk for the complications of prematurity as well as those of intrauterine growth retardation. If the pregnant patient with chronic hypertension has normal renal function, the incidence of superimposed preeclampsia is 15% to 30%. Superimposed preeclampsia develops in virtually all chronic hypertensive patients when there is renal insufficiency.

3. Clinical course
The conditions of patients with this complication tend to be very unstable and must be carefully monitored (as outlined in the sections under severe preeclampsia on p. 200, and chronic hypertension on p. 204). Careful fetal evaluation and expeditious delivery must be considered.

Unclassified hypertensive disorders

Unclassified hypertensive disorders are those in which information is insufficient for classification. They should compose a minority of the hypertensive disorders in pregnancy.

LABORATORY STUDIES

The following laboratory studies should be obtained for every patient who is affected by the hypertensive states of pregnancy seriously enough to require hospitalization.

1. Hematocrit, hemoglobin
2. White blood count
3. Urinalysis
4. Culture and sensitivity of urine
5. Serum protein with albumin/globulin ratio
6. Serum electrolytes
7. Blood urea nitrogen

8. Uric acid
9. Twenty-four-hour urine collection for
   a. Creatinine clearance
   b. Protein
   c. Vanillylmandelic acid (if there are wide blood pressure fluctuations)
10. Coagulation series to include:
    a. Platelets
    b. Fibrinogen
    c. Prothrombin time
    d. Partial thromboplastin time
11. Additionally, depending on stage of gestation, maternal status, and acuity of the situation, it may be desirable to obtain the following:
    a. Ultrasonic scanning (to determine whether intrauterine growth retardation is present)
    b. Fetal physiologic maturity testing
    c. Studies of fetal well-being
    d. Chest radiograph (in any patient who has suffered a seizure or is chronically hypertensive and has not been evaluated previously)
    e. Electrocardiogram

Pregnant patients with chronic hypertension must be evaluated as early in pregnancy as possible with the following baseline laboratory studies (in addition to the usual prenatal laboratory work):

1. Hematocrit, hemoglobin, and white blood count
2. SMA-6, SMA-12
3. Urinalysis, culture and sensitivity
4. Twenty-four-hour urine collection for creatinine clearance and total protein
5. Chest radiograph
6. Electrocardiogram

A 3-hour glucose tolerance test is indicated after 20 weeks' gestation and a 24-hour urine vanillylmandelic acid test is necessary if the patient has hyperglycemia or wide blood pressure fluctuations.

TREATMENT

The objectives of all treatment for the hypertensive diseases of pregnancy are (1) to prevent or control convulsions, (2) to ensure survival of the mother with minimal morbidity, and (3) to deliver a surviving infant with minimal trauma.

I. General measures
   A. Diet
      1. General diet without sodium restriction
      2. Fluid intake not restricted but intake and output carefully monitored
   B. Diuretics
      Diuretics are not necessary or desirable. Most patients respond to bed rest in the lateral recumbent position (which increases renal blood flow and aids in alleviation of edema).
   C. Provision of high-risk prenatal care, as outlined in Chapter 14, with acute care for any complications that may develop

II. Mild preeclampsia
    A. Hospitalize gravida without delay and prescribe bed rest.
    B. Discharge to home with bed rest after obtaining the following favorable responses:
       1. Reduction in blood pressure to below 120/80 mm Hg
       2. Proteinuria of less than 150 mg/24hr
       3. Normal renal function
       4. No evidence of central nervous system irritability
    C. Rehospitalize for bed rest and possible delivery if any exacerbation occurs.
    D. Deliver when fetal maturity is sufficient to ensure neonatal survival.

III. Severe preeclampsia (in addition to treatment for mild preeclampsia)
     A. Ensure patient is cared for in fully capable prenatal centers only.
     B. Determine fetal pulmonary maturity and repeat testing at frequent intervals so that delivery can be effected as soon as the fetus is sufficiently mature for likely survival.
     C. Deliver fetus if condition worsens. Some useful criteria for delivery include:
        1. Diastolic blood pressure that is
           a. Consistently greater than 100 mm Hg in a 24-hour period
           b. 110 mm Hg or higher and confirmed at least once

2. Proteninuria greater than 1 gm/24 hr
3. An elevated creatinine level that continues to rise
4. Severe epigastric pain
5. Persistent, severe headaches
6. Abnormal liver function tests
7. Thrombocytopenia
8. Eclampsia
9. Pulmonary edema
10. Heart failure
11. Fetal distress

Attempt induction of labor if cervix and other conditions are favorable. Perform cesarean section immediately if maternal or fetal distress develop or if induction is unsuccessful.

D. Consider use of additional medication.
   1. Magnesium sulfate may be given to a blood level of 7 mg/100 ml. In addition to controlling irritability and hyperreflexia, magnesium sulfate prevents seizures. The usual dose is 4 gm IV loading dose followed by 1.5 gm/hr constant infusion.

   The patient must be examined every 4 hours for respiratory rate over 12 respirations/min, patellar or biceps reflexes, and urine output of at least 100 ml/hr.

   The drug is excreted by the kidney and dose adjustment is required with oliguria or renal insufficiency. While magnesium sulfate does decrease acetylcholine release at the neuromuscular junction and causes paralysis at a serum level of approximately 15 mg/100 ml, its chief mechanism of action is on the central nervous system. Magnesium sulfate potentiates both the depolarizing and nondepolarizing muscle relaxants.

   Calcium chloride or calcium gluconate (10 ml of a 10% solution) is the antidote for magnesium sulfate overdose.

   2. Phenobarbital 15 to 30 mg may be given four times a day intravenously, if delivery is not imminent.
   3. Antihypertensives may be necessary for control of hypertension.

   The critical blood pressure at which antihypertensive treatment should begin has not been established. There is fairly uniform agreement that a diastolic blood pressure exceeding 110 mm Hg requires therapy to prevent maternal stroke and heart failure. Whether milder degrees of hypertension require therapy is much debated. Some studies have shown a decrease in the incidence of superimposed preeclampsia with therapy for mild hypertension, but evidence of improved fetal outcome is not impressive. The central question is whether uterine blood flow is autoregulated. If it is, antihypertensive therapy will not decrease uterine blood flow. If the uterine vessels are maximally dilated at all times and flow is not autoregulated, as some evidence suggests, lowering maternal blood pressure will decrease uterine blood flow. Studies in various animals (with and without use of anesthesia) have given conflicting results, and accurate studies in humans have not been done. Therefore the use and benefit of these agents must be carefully weighed against the risks.

   To affect uterine perfusion minimally, one should lower blood pressure no more than 20% to 30% and use antihypertensives only if diastolic blood pressure exceeds 110 mm Hg.

a. Hydralazine
Hydralazine is the antihypertensive medication used most frequently with preeclampsia. The usual dose is 10 to 20 mg IV. The onset of action is in 15 to 20 minutes with a 4- to 6-hour duration of action. If diastolic pressure does not decrease to the therapeutic goal of between 90 and 100 mm Hg within 20 minutes the dose is repeated. Other methods of administration include 25 mg IM or 20 to 50 mg IV in 500 ml D5W given slowly. When stabilized, the patient may be weaned from the IV dose while the drug is administered orally (25 to 50 mg every 6 hours).
Hydralazine causes direct relaxation of arteriolar smooth muscle. There is a secondary baroreceptor-mediated sympathetic discharge that increases heart rate, stroke volume, and cardiac output. The drug is acetylated in the liver.
Side effects of hydralazine therapy include flushing, headache, dizziness, palpations, and angina. There are conflicting reports concerning its effect on uteroplacental blood flow.
Aldomet, 500 mg twice daily, may be used to prevent the reflex tachycardia seen with hydralazine. Hydralazine should not be given to patients with collagen diseases.
b. Diazoxide
Diazoxide is a direct arteriolar vasodilator that acts more rapidly than hydralazine. It causes a secondary baroreceptor-mediated sympathetic discharge as well. There is little change in uterine blood flow unless the patient becomes hypotensive. It is usually administered as a 300 mg bolus. Onset of action occurs within seconds and duration of action lasts 3 to 12 hours. "Overshoot" or hypotension is the biggest problem with use of this drug, particularly when it is given after 20 to 40 mg of hydralazine has failed to lower the blood pressure to a safe level. There are also patients who do not respond to diazoxide. Hyperglycemia and salt and water retention are usually not problems in obstetric usage of the drug, since one or two doses are usually all that is given. However, late decelerations, a sign of uteroplacental insufficiency, frequently develop with administration of the drug during labor, and it also stops labor in about half of patients. Diazoxide causes minimal change in the fetal cardiovascular system.
c. Sodium nitroprusside
Sodium nitroprusside may be the most potent agent yet used for hypertensive emergencies. It is often effective where other agents have failed and has been particularly useful in malignant hypertension accompanied by severe congestive heart failure. It reduces preload and afterload by dilating both resistance and capacitance vessels. It has no maternal autonomic or central nervous system effect and causes no change

in uterine blood flow. It is rapid-acting and ideally should be given with an arterial line in an intensive care setting. It is administered in a solution of 100 mg/L D5W at 0.5 to 8 µg/kg/min. The dose is titrated to pressure. Accumulation of blood thiocyanate may lead to toxicity that is particularly detrimental to the fetus. If nitroprusside is necessary to control maternal hypertension, expeditious delivery is probably indicated.

   d. Methyldopa

Methyldopa is the most popular oral antihypertensive drug used in the United States during pregnancy. It is well tolerated, drowsiness and orthostatic hypotension being the commonest problems with its usage. Concurrent use of diuretics is controversial, primarily because of lack of data. It is not known whether a patient receiving chronic diuretic therapy before pregnancy has a normal physiologic volume expansion if drug therapy is continued during pregnancy. The acute antihypertensive effect of thiazide diuretics is the result of volume depletion, but after 4 to 8 weeks of therapy plasma volume returns nearly to normal. The chronic antihypertensive effect is thought to involve sodium depletion from the arteriolar wall decreasing vascular sensitivity to endogenous catechols. However, the association of contracted blood volume with preeclampsia and chronic hypertension raises doubts regarding the safety of diuretic therapy during pregnancy.

   e. Beta-blockers

Beta-blockers have been popular for over a decade in the treatment of hypertension in the nonpregnant state because of the low incidence of side effects. Despite widespread use by obstetricians in Great Britain and Australia, they are not popular for obstetric use in the United States. Bradycardia, hypoglycemia, respiratory depression, intrauterine growth retardation, and blockade of the tachycardic response to hypoxia have been reported in newborns of mothers taking beta-blockers. Since most cases are isolated, the frequency with which these effects occur is unknown.

4. Heparin* may be added if disseminated intravascular coagulation is present.

5. With severe oliguria Lasix* may be helpful, although diuretics are best reserved for cases with cardiac failure, pulmonary edema, or acute renal failure.

6. Heart failure may be treated with digitalis* and oxygen. Indeed, oxygen should be used if there is tachycardia, cyanosis, pulmonary edema, or reduced blood pressure.

7. Corticosteroid administration is another controversial area. In Liggins's original study, perinatal mortality was higher for infants of steroid-treated

---

*Exact type and dosage are not given because therapy is best individualized for each of these critically ill patients. Interdisciplinary consultation is also a key feature of successful management.

than those of placebo-treated hypertensive mothers. Several small studies have recently supported the use of steroids; however, it is recommended that continuous fetal monitoring be employed while the obstetrician awaits enhancement of lung maturity. The obstetrician must also be ready to effect delivery before the requisite 48 hours after the first dose of steroids (to achieve the desired effect on fetal pulmonary maturity) if the maternal condition deteriorates.
  E. Consider placement of a central venous pressure monitor or Swan-Ganz catheter to accurately manage the patient who is in critical condition.
IV. Eclampsia
  Eclampsia is a medical emergency and requires the following:
  A. Airway maintenance (A plastic airway will usually suffice.)
  B. Place padded tongue blade or plastic airway to prevent patient from biting tongue.
  C. Suction as necessary to remove regurgitated stomach contents and thus prevent aspiration.
  D. Administer nasal oxygen at 6 L/min.
  E. One of the following may be used for control of the convulsion:
    1. Diazepam (Valium), 10 mg IV by slow push (5 mg/min)
    2. Magnesium sulfate, 4 gm IV over 5 to 10 minutes (usually given in a 20% solution) and then 1 gm/hr (1 gm/100 ml D5W) by intravenous drip if urine output is satisfactory
  F. Place bladder catheter for recording urine output per hour.
  G. Obtain chest x-ray film to rule out aspiration.
  H. When mother is stable, maturity status of fetus should be determined and delivery projected.
V. Chronic hypertension
  Mild hypertension may be followed closely and treated symptomatically; however, the following are key features in successful management of moderate to severe chronic hypertension:
  A. Consider abortion and sterilization only if pregnancy is threat to mother's life. Permit pregnancy to continue if patient responds to hospitalization, as outlined under treatment for severe preeclampsia.
  B. Prescribe a general diet without salt restriction and follow patient's condition every 2 weeks until 30 weeks, then weekly thereafter. Some investigators suggest admission to hospital for initial evaluation. Hospitalization is indicated if diastolic pressure exceeds 100 mm Hg.
  C. Evaluate fetal condition carefully. To ascertain gestational age and assist in detection of intrauterine growth retardation, two ultrasonic examinations, a month apart, should be obtained between 16 and 28 weeks. NST, CST, or other biometric evaluations should be performed weekly starting at 30 to 34 weeks' gestation or whenever superimposed preeclampsia develops.
  D. Deliver perinate immediately if
    1. Blood pressure rises above 200/120 mm Hg
    2. Retinal exudates or hemorrhages occur
    3. Congestive heart failure develops
    4. Renal insufficiency ensues
  E. Consider early delivery for patients with superimposed preeclampsia, severe hypertension requiring propranolol, or underlying medical problems such as diabetes or renal insufficiency, or when abnormal antepartum fetal well-being assessments, or intrauterine growth retardation are present. A patient beginning an accelerated phase of hypertension may be given steroids to accelerate fetal pulmonary maturity if the delivery can be delayed for 48 to 72 hours.

F. Antihypertensives should be used if diastolic blood pressure exceeds 90 mm Hg; the goal of therapy is to keep diastolic pressure below 90 mm Hg. If patient is already taking thiazide diuretics, these may be continued at the same dosage. If patient is taking no antihypertensive medication, methyldopa (750 to 2,000 mg daily) should be the first drug used. If blood pressure cannot be controlled with methyldopa, propranolol 40 to 240 mg per day is the next drug of choice.

VI. Control of acute hypertension
Although magnesium sulfate remains the drug of choice, it has poor antihypertensive action, and occasionally patients will have acute hypertensive problems, which may be a serious threat to life, and effective management of hypertension is mandatory. Such circumstances may include diastolic blood pressure of more than 120 mm Hg, rapidly accelerating hypertension, neurologic manifestations, and progressive papilledema. In these critical cases it may be necessary to initiate vigorous antihypertensive therapy (more than hydralazine). It should be stressed that *little is known about the effects of some antihypertensive medications (e.g., diazoxide and nitroprusside) on the fetus and their use should be undertaken only when, in the attending physician's opinion, jeopardy warrants their use and lesser agents have failed.* (See previous section for discussion of antihypertensive therapy.)

VII. Decision for delivery
The decision for delivery is based on the severity of the disease and fetal maturation. Mode of delivery is dictated by a total assessment of both patients.

VIII. Analgesia and anesthesia (Chapter 7)
Analgesia should be avoided in prematurity and used very cautiously in all pregnancies with this complication because of the already compromised fetoplacental exchange.

General anesthesia (i.e., epidural, caudal, or local blocks supplemented with nitrous oxide and oxygen) may be effectively used for delivery or cesarean section. However, regional anesthetic blocks (usually of the subarachnoid type) often create severe hypotension that may be difficult to control.

GENERAL CHARTING AND LABORATORY STUDIES

For appropriate treatment of severely affected patients the following is useful:

I. Laboratory studies
A. Every 6 hours obtain
1. Hematocrit
A rising hematocrit indicates a worsening of the disease process.
2. Urinary protein
Increasing urinary protein indicates a worsening of the process.
B. Every 24 hours obtain
1. Serum electrolytes
2. Creatinine or BUN
3. Uric acid
In the absence of underlying renal disease or a recent convulsion, greater than 4.5 mg/100 ml is virtually diagnostic. Additionally severity may be judged from the level before initiation of therapy. Above 5.5 mg/100 ml indicates severe toxemia.
4. Twenty-four-hour urine protein and creatinine
C. As needed, obtain
1. Studies of fetal well-being (e.g., NST)
2. Pulmonary maturity studies (e.g., L/S ratio, PG)
3. Serum proteins with albumin/globulin ratio

II. Vital sign monitoring
A. Every 15 minutes, depending on patient's condition, obtain
1. Blood pressure, pulse, respiratory rate
2. FHR
3. Fluid intake and output
4. Quality of deep tendon reflexes
B. Daily
1. Funduscopic examination for retinal arteriolar spasm
2. Weight

COMPLICATIONS

1. Maternal complications
   a. Development of preeclampsia into eclampsia when metabolic derangement cannot be controlled
   b. Blindness from retinal detachment or retinal involvement
   c. Abruptio placentae (with antepartum bleeding) and postpartum hemorrhage (more common in hypertensive states)
   d. Cerebral hemorrhage (resulting from hypertension and vascular fragility)
   e. Coma, delirium, and confusion (manifestations of toxicity, central nervous system abnormalities, or oversedation, usually after convulsions of eclampsia)
   f. Aspiration pneumonia, injuries accompanying convulsions (e.g., vertebral fractures, laceration of lips or tongue)
   g. Clotting alterations (chiefly thrombocytopenia)
   h. Microangiopathic hemolytic anemia
   i. Pulmonary edema
   j. Hepatocellular damage (chronic passive congestion, subcapsular hemorrhage and rupture)
   k. Renal lesions (glomerular capillary endotheliosis)
   l. Protein depletion (rare)
   m. Renal failure
   n. Death
2. Factors apparently increasing the chance of development of chronic hypertension
   a. Age of patient (older patients having a greater chance)
   b. High blood pressure during early pregnancy
   c. Higher blood pressure during the acute episode
   d. Duration of elevated blood pressure
   e. Degree and duration of proteinuria
   f. Persistence of hypertension in the puerperium
   g. Degree of obesity (greater incidence with greater obesity)
3. Fetal complications
   a. Fetal distress
      1. Decreased uterine blood flow
      2. Abruptio placentae
   b. Intrauterine growth retardation
   c. Premature labor or premature delivery
   d. Stillbirth or intrapartum death
4. Complications of treatment
   a. Magnesium sulfate overdosage (the therapeutic range is 7 mg/100 ml, and the LD_{50} is approximately 15 mg/100 ml) may create hyporeflexia, respiratory depression, and cardiac asystole. The antidote is calcium. It is our policy to have 10% of calcium gluconate in a syringe at the bedside whenever magnesium sulfate is being administered, so that the toxic effects of magnesium sulfate overdosage can be vitiated by direct intravenous injection of the calcium.
   b. If diuretic therapy is used, one must be extremely careful not to deplete the intravascular space and thus cause development of an extravascular low-salt syndrome.
   c. Injudicious use of antihypertensives may lead to hypotension or relative hypotension with a uterine blood flow decrease sufficient to compromise the fetus.

PROGNOSIS

Hippocrates accurately stated the prognosis for inadequately or poorly managed hypertensive states of pregnancy: "In pregnancy, drowsiness with headache accompanied by heaviness and convulsions is generally bad." This prognosis could well apply to both mother and fetus, for toxemia continues to be one of the three leading causes of maternal death each year in the United States (along with hemorrhage and infection) and remains a leading cause of perinatal mortality.

Mother

The outlook for the toxemia patient is good unless convulsions ensue, whereupon about one woman in 15 dies of an intracranial accident, hemorrhage, shock, or renal failure caused by premature separation of the placenta, aspiration pneumonia, cardiac or renal cortical necrosis, or lower nephron nephrosis. It is also probable that chronic hypertension is increased in patients affected by the hypertensive states of pregnancy.

Perinate

Perinatal mortality in eclampsia can be reduced from at least 20% to less than 10% by current intensive therapy. The necessity for early delivery diminishes with improved maternal management.

PREVENTION

1. Toxemia of pregnancy is avoidable in most instances.
2. Early, adequate antenatal care and proper nutrition often will protect patients against toxemia.
3. Key to prevention is recognition that a rise in blood pressure greater than 20 mm Hg systolic or 10 mm Hg diastolic during pregnancy is significant and that the development of proteinuria during pregnancy is always an indication for further investigation and treatment.
4. Prompt, vigorous treatment of preeclampsia will limit incidence of eclampsia drastically.
5. Definitive therapy for patients in the convulsive state will reduce maternal and perinatal mortality considerably.

NEONATAL CARE

1. Major problems
   a. Prematurity
   b. Undergrowth
   c. Combination of prematurity and undergrowth
   d. Perinatal asphyxia
   e. Hypotonia resulting from hypermagnesemia (because of magnesium sulfate therapy to mother) (see Chapter 32)
2. Management
   a. Deliver infant in a maternity center equipped with neonatal intensive care unit.
   b. Resuscitate infant immediately (Chapter 9).
   c. Assess infant for growth retardation and manage accordingly (e.g., hypoglycemia) (Chapter 12).
   d. Obtain magnesium level if indicated. Over 5 mEq/L requires special care (Chapter 32).
3. Other problems of the neonate in toxemia of pregnancy
   a. Paralytic ileus—caused by antepartum blocking agents given to mother
   b. Nasal stuffiness with respiratory obstruction—caused by antepartum therapy with reserpine
   c. Thrombocytopenia—caused by antepartum administration of thiazides
   d. Neonatal depression—caused by antepartum administration of tranquilizers and sedatives
   e. Methemoglobinemia—caused by antepartum administration of nitrites

BIBLIOGRAPHY

Arias, F.: Expansion of intravascular volume and fetal outcome in patients with chronic hypertension and pregnancy, Am. J. Obstet. Gynecol. **123**:610, 1975.

Assali, N.S., and Vaughn, D.L.: Blood volume in preeclampsia: fantasy and reality, Am. J. Obstet. Gynecol. **129**:355, 1977.

Beer, A.E.: Possible immunologic bases of preeclampsia/eclampsia, Semin. Perinatol. **2**:39, 1978.

Berkowitz, R.L.: Antihypertensive drugs in the pregnant patient, Obstet. Gynecol. Surv. **35**:191, 1980.

Brazy, J.E., Grimm, J.K., and Little, V.A.: Neonatal manifestations of severe maternal hypertension occurring before the thirty-sixth week of pregnancy, J. Pediatr. **100**:265, 1982.

Chesley, L.C.: Hypertensive disorders in pregnancy, New York, 1978, Appleton-Century-Crofts.

Cockburn, J., Ounsted, M., Moar, V.A., et al.: Final report of study on hypertension during pregnancy: the effects of specific treatment on the growth and development of children, Lancet **1**:647, 1982.

Gant, N.F., and Worley, R.J.: Hypertension in pregnancy: concepts and management, New York, 1980, Appleton-Century-Crofts.

Goodlin, R.C.: Severe pre-eclampsia: another great imitation, Am. J. Obstet. Gyecol. **125**:747, 1976.

Pritchard, J.A., Cunningham, F.G., and Mason, R.A.: Coagulation changes in eclampsia: their frequency and pathogenesis, Am. J. Obstet. Gynecol. **124**:855, 1976.

Pritchard, J.A., and Pritchard, S.A.: Standardized treatment of 154 consecutive cases of eclampsia, Am. J. Obstet. Gynecol. **123**:543, 1975.

Redman, C.W.G., Beilin, L.J., Bonvar, J., et al.: Fetal outcome in trial of antihypertensive treatment in pregnancy, Lancet **753**:956, 1976.

Ricke, P.S., Elliot, J.P., and Freeman, R.K.: Use of corticosteroids in pregnancy-induced hypertension, Obstet. Gynecol. **55**:206, 1980.

Rubin, P.C.: Beta-blockers in pregnancy, N. Engl. J. Med. **305**:1323, 1981.

Sibai, B.M., McCubbin, J.H., Anderson, G.D., et al.: Eclampsia 1: Observation from 67 recent cases, Obstet. Gynecol. **58**:609, 1981.

Zuspan, F.P., and O'Shaughnessy, R.: Chronic hypertension in pregnancy. In Pitkin, R.M., editor: Yearbook of obstetrics and gynecology, Chicago, 1979, Yearbook Medical Publishers, Inc.

Zuspan, F.P.: Problems encountered in the treatment of pregnancy-induced hypertension, Am. J. Obstet. Gynecol. **131**:591, 1978.

22

Late pregnancy hemorrhage

Third trimester bleeding sufficient to require investigation occurs in 5% to 10% of all gravidas. Bleeding may originate from several sites in the engorged pelvis. Nonobstetric causes of bleeding, save invasive carcinoma of the cervix, usually produce relatively small amounts of bleeding and are not a threat to either mother or baby. The most common obstetric cause, extrusion of the cervical mucus (bloody show), may be accompanied by enough bleeding to cause patient concern but is rarely if ever a problem. Nevertheless hemorrhage remains the major cause of obstetric deaths and a principal cause of maternal morbidity.

CERVICAL AND VAGINAL LESIONS

Bleeding during the third trimester may be caused by cervical or vaginal lesions. Conditions include:
1. Cervicitis
2. Cervical eversions
3. Cervical polyps
4. Cervical or vaginal benign neoplasias
5. Cervical cancer
6. Vaginal lacerations
7. Vaginal varices

These conditions usually cause only spotting that does not increase with activity. There are no uterine contractions, and definitive diagnosis can be made by speculum examination, Pap smear, cultures, or colposcopy.

Treatment and prognosis

Most cervical and vaginal conditions will require some treatment. Lacerations and varices may require repair and most neoplasias and eversions may require simple treatment, but prognosis for all of these is good. Likewise, for infections treated with proper agents prognosis is good. If cancer is not invasive, prognosis is good after therapeutic intervention has been employed. Maternal prognosis is poor when cancer is advanced.

COAGULOPATHIES

Bleeding in late pregnancy or the puerperium caused by coagulopathies, most commonly disseminated intravascular coagulation or hyperfibrinogenemia, is uncommon but is associated with abruptio placentae, intrauterine demise, amniotic fluid embolus, sepsis, and the hypertensive states of pregnancy. Signs and symptoms include easy bruising and spontaneous bleeding from mucous membranes, the bladder, rectum, or needle puncture sites. Diagnosis can be confirmed by abnormal findings in laboratory studies, including the following:
1. Low fibrinogen level (normal—350 mg/100 ml; critical—less than 100 mg/100 ml)
2. Increased prothrombin time (PT)
3. Prolonged partial thromboplastin time (PTT)
4. Detection of fibrin split products

Treatment and prognosis

Treatment for coagulopathies during pregnancy or puerperium is as follows:
1. Maintain maternal blood volume.
2. Correct coagulopathy. Use whole blood. If whole blood is not available, use packed red blood cells, platelets, and fresh frozen plasma.
3. Expedite delivery of fetus.

4. Treat patient for sepsis if present.
5. Administer life support measures if necessary.

Prognosis for associated disorders is grave, and overall, late pregnancy or puerperium coagulopathy is an extremely serious maternal and perinatal complication.

PLACENTAL AND UTERINE BLEEDING

The majority of serious hemorrhages (2% to 3% of all cases) are placental in origin, caused by abruptio placentae or placenta previa (Table 22-1). These two conditions continue to be vexing problems even in modern obstetric and neonatal practice. The full extent of fetal jeopardy caused by anoxia or even fetal hemorrhage is not known, but it must be considerable, since these conditions also contribute greatly to perinatal morbidity and mortality.

Uterine rupture is rarely (approximately 1:2000 cases) the cause for late pregnancy hemorrhage. Vasa previa is even more uncommonly a cause for the bleeding. Both of these uncommon occurrences markedly jeopardize the fetus and, in the case of uterine rupture, seriously threaten maternal life.

Other causes of obstetric hemorrhage during late pregnancy include bleeding from the peripheral portion of the intervillous space (ruptured marginal sinus) and placental hemorrhage associated with circumvallate placenta. The former is usually self-limiting and the latter, although not common during late pregnancy, is a major cause of hemorrhage during the second trimester. Thus, although both of these conditions may be associated with or contribute to abruptio placentae and premature delivery, they are more likely to be diagnostic problems, rarely presenting the critical maternal and perinatal emergencies posed by placenta previa, abruptio placentae, or uterine rupture.

Fortunately, the majority of patients suffering third trimester bleeding have a blood loss of less than hemorrhagic proportions (500 ml). However, even minor blood loss may indicate life-threatening conditions. Therefore prudent management requires following the obstetric principle that *all patients with third trimester hemorrhage be hospitalized immediately with definitive evaluations performed to detail the cause of bleeding.* A second principle requires that *no*

Table 22-1. Major causes of third trimester hemorrhage

Condition	Incidence	Associations	Signs and symptoms	Diagnostic aids	Management priorities
Abruptio placentae	Mild 1:150 Severe 1:500	Hypertension; high parity; past abruption	Abdominal or back pain; dark red vaginal bleeding; tender, irritable uterus (possible hypertonus)	Ultrasonography Hematology	Maintain blood volume Treat coagulopathy Deliver viable infant
Placenta previa	1:200	Advanced age or parity; previous placenta previa; uterine operations	Bright red vaginal bleeding; no pain and soft uterus; unengaged fetal presenting part with possible malpresentation	Ultrasonography	Maintain blood volume Allow fetal maturity
Uterine rupture	1:2,000	Previous uterine trauma or operations; difficult delivery; uterine manipulations	Abdominal pain; shock; cessation of labor	None	Maintain blood volume Perform laparotomy immediately

rectal or vaginal examinations be performed until placenta previa is ruled out, the health care team is prepared to deal with severe hemorrhage, and preparations to deal with any maternal or perinatal complications are completed.

GENERAL CONSIDERATIONS

The obstetric patient with third trimester bleeding must be observed carefully for signs and symptoms of acute blood loss. These include the following:
1. Pallor
2. Cool, moist (sweating) skin
3. Syncope
4. Thirst
5. Air hunger (dyspnea)
6. Restlessness, agitation, anxiety, confusion
7. Falling blood pressure
8. Increased, thready pulse (tachycardia)
9. Oliguria (or anuria)

The general laboratory evaluations listed below must be obtained for the patient with late pregnancy or puerperium bleeding.
1. Hemoglobin and hematocrit
2. White blood count with differential
3. Blood type and cross match
4. Fibrinogen
5. Prothrombin time
6. Partial thromboplastin time
7. Platelet count
8. Peripheral smear for morphology

The general action plan for third trimester hemorrhage is as follows:
1. Obtain patient history including:
    a. Information pertaining to acute episode
    b. Obstetric information
2. Obtain vital signs assessments.
3. Perform abdominal examination.
    a. Mark top of uterus and measure uterine length in centimeters to determine approximate gestation duration.
    b. Perform Leopold's maneuvers to determine fetal size, presentation, position, and engagement.
    c. Palpate for uterine contractions, tone, or tenderness.
    d. Determine whether palpations evoke contractions.
    e. Obtain FHR and initiate appropriate monitoring.
4. Start intravenous infusion with large-gauge catheter.
5. Initiate laboratory workup.
6. Initiate urinary output monitoring (possibly Foley catheterization).
7. Prepare for determination of placental placement and fetal maturity evaluation by
    a. Ultrasonography
    b. Amniocentesis
8. Prepare for either expectant management or delivery.

Indeed, management of third trimester bleeding prior to delivery varies primarily with the severity of bleeding. If bleeding is life threatening to the mother a true emergency exists, and plans for delivery (often by cesarean section) must imediately follow implementation of the life support measures listed below. For many of these critically ill patients etiology may be determined only on the operating table.

Life support measures that must be implemented when a patient has serious third trimester bleeding include the following:
1. Act quickly!
2. Employ general antishock measures.
    a. Place patient in Trendelenburg position (not so extreme as to interfere with breathing).
    b. Establish adequate airway.
    c. Keep patient warm.
3. Initiate fluid replacement (taking care not to create cardiac overload) using the following, as indicated:
    a. Blood (whole or packed red blood cells)
    b. Plasmanate
    c. Plasma expanders
    d. Saline, dextrose, mannitol
    Fluid replacement considerations should include correction of bicarbonate deficits and adjustment of electrolyte imbalances.
4. Administer vasoactive drugs when indicated.
    Vasoactive drugs should be used only when specific pharmacologic effects are desired (e.g., increasing myocardial contractility), when volume expanders are not available, or when volume expansion and other measures are ineffective. Even in these cases efficacy may be questioned. Therefore these agents should be used only when their benefits clearly outweigh potential risk.
    a. Dopamine (a mixed alpha- and beta-adrenergic stimulant), 200 mg in 500

ml sodium chloride injection USP, should be started at 2 to 5 gm/kg/min and increased to 20 gm/kg/min.

b. Other drugs to consider using include levarterenol bitartrate, isoproterenol, metaraminol bitartrate, and phenylephrine.

Occasionally patients will be in hemorrhagic shock but will exhibit no evidence of external bleeding (approximately 5% of patients with third trimester bleeding). In these patients an occult hemorrhage has usually occurred. The most common causes of this are abruptio placentae, with the hemorrhage entirely concealed behind the placenta, and ruptured uterus. All of the measures employed for patients with external bleeding must be employed for those with concealed hemorrhage.

When the mother's life is not in immediate jeopardy management variables to consider include cause and extent of bleeding, fetal gestational age, fetal maturational status, indications of fetal well-being, and presence of labor. The diagnostic workup usually includes ultrasonography to ascertain placental location, determine whether there is a retroplacental blood clot, obtain an estimate of fetal gestational age, determine fetal position, and ascertain whether gross detectable anomalies exist or fetal death has occurred. Laboratory studies are essential to determine maternal status and whether coagulopathy is present.

Fetal physiologic maturity is best ascertained by consideration of gestational history, ultrasonic findings, and possibly by amniocentesis for rapid surfactant test, lecithin/sphingomyelin ratio, or phosphytidylglycerol. *If the fetus is premature, or if complexity of the maternal or fetal patient's condition exceeds the care capability of the facility where the patient is originally seen, it is essential to attempt stabilization and to arrange for transport to a center with full high risk care capability.*

Although blood loss is usually maternal, this is not always the case, for fetal blood loss may result from either trauma to the placenta or vasa previa. (Vasa previa is discussed in some detail later in this chapter.) Trauma to the placenta most commonly occurs with low placental implantation or abruptio placentae with retroplacental clot formation. Several laboratory tests are available for detection of fetal hemoglobin including the Apt test and the Kleihauer-Betke test. Hemoglobin electrophoresis is possible but is so time consuming that it is usually of little value.

After these general considerations have been met efforts must then be directed toward diagnosis and treatment of the specific cause of hemorrhage.

Generally, the sequence detailed in the action plan (p. 210) is employed and individualized to evaluate the several variables. Close monitoring of maternal vital signs and preparation for maternal life support during this interval will assist in ensuring continued maternal well-being. Fetal well-being may be assessed by FHR monitoring, ultrasonography, and amniocentesis. The importance of ultrasonography in evaluation of third trimester bleeding originating from the placenta cannot be overstressed.

Labor creates a more pressing need for cervical evaluation. Adequate vaginal examination includes both a speculum and a manual examination. These need not be delayed if ultrasonic scan rules out placenta previa and preparations to deal definitively with hemorrhage have been made. Indeed, with labor total placenta previa may be largely dismissed if the presenting part is fully engaged. However, there are many factors confounding the use of engagement as a criterion to exclude placenta previa, for example, inadequate examination (because of obesity, enhanced abdominal muscle tone, increased uterine tone) and partial placenta previa. Certainly the patient with an unengaged presenting part must not have vaginal or rectal examinations until placenta previa is ruled out.

Slight premature placental separation

Slight premature placental separation may occur and is usually more a diagnostic than a therapeutic problem. Even minimal uterine bleeding during the last half of pregnancy causes anxiety concerning hemorrhage and the possibility of premature delivery. Minor degrees of premature separation of the normally implanted placenta may be responsible for such blood loss. Other known causes are cervicitis and bleeding from the decidua. Pain, fetal distress, and early labor are unlikely unless the area of separation is large or retroplacental. In the mild form of the process strict bed rest and mild sedation for several days will usually arrest the bleeding, and the pregnancy may continue.

After ultrasonic scanning has dismissed placenta previa, if there is doubt about the diagnosis of mild placental separation visualization of the vagina and cervix to rule out nonplacental bleeding is necessary. However, palpation through the cervical canal is both unnecessary and unwise. The "double setup" examination so frequently employed in the past for diagnosis has a high false-negative rate and is hazardous. Therefore it is rarely used today.

Reassurance, increased bed rest, and close observation are necessary.

I. Pathogenesis
   A. Predisposition to early separation of the placenta occurs with
      1. Advanced age and multiparity (highly significant)
      2. Uterine distention (in multiple pregnancy or hydramnios)
      3. Previous abruptio placentae
      4. Hypertensive states of pregnancy
      5. Cigarette smoking
         Discontinuing smoking during pregnancy may reduce the vasoconstrictive effect of nicotine throught to produce decidual necrosis at the placental margin and may prevent the associated decreased placental perfusion as well.
   B. Precipitating causes of premature separation of the placenta
      1. Circumvallate placenta
      2. Sudden reduction in volume of uterus—rapid loss of amniotic fluid or delivery of first twin
      3. Trauma
         a. External or internal version
         b. Use of automobile lap belt restraints
            Although there is an increase in abruptio placentae with use of lap belts in collisions, this adverse effect is probably more than offset by the lower incidence of maternal deaths with the use of restraints.
      4. Abnormally short cord
      5. Uterine anomaly or tumor
      6. Abrupt or extreme vascular congestion, shock, and supine hypertensive syndrome (vena cava syndrome)
      7. Vascular deficiency, deterioration—toxemia, diabetes mellitus, or chronic renal disease complicating pregnancy
      8. Possible predisposition occurring in mothers with type O blood

II. Types
Two types of premature separation of the placenta are recognized:
   A. Marginal separation of placenta, with leakage of blood behind the membranes through the cervix (This external bleeding may be painless.)
   B. Central separation of placenta, with blood trapped behind the placenta and minimal external evidence of bleeding (This is painful, concealed bleeding—abruptio placentae. Failure of blood coagulation occurs in about 5% to 8% of serious cases of concealed hemorrhage.)
      1. Bleeding, with disruption of the vascular bed behind the placenta, results in extensive localized clotting and necrosis of the decidua basalis.
      2. Depletion of fibrinogen from the general circulation follows "fixation" of fibrinogen in retroplacental clotting.
      3. If peripheral blood fibrinogen falls to less than 100 mg/100 ml, generalized ecchymosis, free bleeding from all mucosal surfaces, and extravasation into the myometrium (Couvelaire uterus) often ensue.
         a. Couvelaire uterus is ligneous, agonizingly painful and tender.
         b. Dysrhythmic or arrested labor occurs. (Indeed, some 20% of these cases are complicated by uterine inertia that is resistant to amniotomy or oxytocin stimulation. It is thought that high

concentrations of fibrin degradation products inhibit myometrial contractility.)
　　　c. Maternal shock out of proportion to the estimated blood loss is the rule.
　　　d. Fetal death is nearly certain.
　　　e. Aminocaproic acid an antifibrinolitic agent, may be effective in some of these cases.
III. Clinical findings
　A. Symptoms
　　1. Painless vaginal hemorrhage may indicate unrestricted bleeding from the margin or a segment of the placenta.
　　2. Suspect concealed hemorrhage and perhaps premature separation of most of the placenta when severe pain, backache, unremittent uterine tenderness, an increased uterine tonus, enlargement of the uterus, or fetal distress develops prior to or during labor. Shock, bleeding from the nose, mouth, or needle puncture site, and loss of fetal heart tones indicate severe abruptio placentae and hypofibrinogenemia (consumption coagulopathy).
　B. Laboratory studies
　　1. Hemoconcentration and anemia.
　　2. Hypofibrinogenemia in association with abruptio placentae is confirmed by the following tests:
　　　a. Failure of clotting or fragile clot after 1 hour in Lee-White tube at 37° to 38° C
　　　b. Poor coagulation or no clot with Fibrindex test after 1 minute (reconstituted human thrombin added to 1 drop of patient's plasma)
　　　c. Fibrinogen determination (gravimetric test) less than 100 mg/100 ml
　　　d. Plasma protamine paracoagulation test
　　　　Disseminated intravascular coagulation is indicated if test is positive.
　C. Ultrasonic scan
　　Ultrasonography may reveal the retroplacental blood clot and assist in determination of placental location. Criteria for sonographic diagnosis of abruptio placentae include:
　　1. Retroplacental anechoic areas
　　2. Intraplacental anechoic areas not confined to superficial subchorionic areas
　　3. Separation and rounding of placental edge
　　4. Thickening of placenta (Although some controversy exists, if placenta is 5.5 cm or more thick, in absence of diabetes mellitus or Rh isoimmunization, the diagnosis must be entertained.)
IV. Differential diagnosis
　A. Nonplacental causes of bleeding—consider hemorrhagic lesions of cervix or vagina, "show" of cervical dilatation and effacement, and rupture of uterus.
　B. Placental bleeding from placenta previa usually will be ascertained by ultrasonography.
　C. Vasa previa can be diagnosed before delivery only by amnioscopy.
V. Complications
　A. Mother—hemorrhage, shock, hypovolemia, hypofibrinogenemia, small pulmonary emboli, renal cortical and lower nephron nephrosis, and fibrinolysis may occur, especially with abruptio placentae
　B. Fetus—hypoxia with resultant fetal distress may cause damage to fetal central nervous system with later cerebral palsy, mental retardation, or actual death of fetus. Additionally, fetus may suffer loss of blood from placental vessel interruption. Premature birth is also frequently seen with abruptio placentae.
VI. Treatment
　A. Emergency measures
　　1. Institute antishock measures.
　　2. *Rupture the membranes* (regard-

less of the likely method of delivery) to permit drainage, reduce the risk of consumption coagulopathy, and speed labor.
3. Obtain appropriate laboratory studies—complete blood count, type and cross match (3 to 6 units), fibrinogen, clot for observation, and appropriate studies as indicated by hematologic consultation.
4. *Restore blood clotting mechanism,* if deficient, before attempting any type of delivery.
5. Mark upper limit of fundus to monitor uterine expansion from intrauterine bleeding.
6. Institute direct electronic fetal monitoring.
7. Institute central venous pressure monitoring if indicated. (This or Swan-Ganz monitoring may be a very important guide to colloid and crystalloid replacement.)
8. Measure urinary output hourly.
9. Administer mannitol, 12.5 gm IV (supplied as 25% solution in 50 ml ampules), to protect against lower nephron nephrosis after shock, if severely oliguric or anuric.

B. Specific measures
1. Premature separation of placenta accompanied by external bleeding will probably require no operative intervention, unless hemorrhage or prolonged labor develops. Type, match, and hold blood for possible transfusion or cesarean section.
2. Treat lesser degrees of abruptio placentae in same manner. In severe abruptio placentae, if vaginal delivery is likely to occur within a reasonable time (less than 6 hours), plan on delivery from below; if a longer labor is likely, perform cesarean section strictly on maternal indication. Cesarean section is also indicated for any fetal distress.

C. General measures
1. Give oxygen by face mask for fetal distress.
2. Begin transfusion if gravida is in shock or is anemic.
3. If rapid labor or hasty delivery transpires, deny excessive analgesia, despite severe pain, to minimize fetal central nervous system depression.
4. Monitor FHR and record maternal pulse and blood pressure every 5 minutes.

D. Surgical measures
1. Use low forceps to expedite delivery. (Dührssen incisions are rarely if ever justified, even for fetal distress in a multipara, because of the danger of further hemorrhage and shock.)
2. Employ cesarean section when
   a. Desultory labor does not respond to amniotomy and cautious oxytocic stimulation. Although the use of aminocaproic acid (an antifibrinolitic agent) should be considered to improve labor, this is an extraordinary measure and must be undertaken with great care.
   b. Fetopelvic disproportion is recognized.
   c. Hemorrhage cannot be checked by amniotomy or restoration of the coagulation mechanism.
   d. Fetal distress occurs.
3. Hysterectomy may be necessary (although rarely) in abruptio placentae if normal blood coagulation cannot be achieved.

E. Treatment of complications
1. Coagulopathy and blood loss—treat with fresh whole blood, platelet packs, and cryoprecipitate.
2. Renal cortical necrosis—administer hydralazine, 25 to 40 mg diluted, by slow intravenous drip to possibly increase renal blood flow and thereby prevent

or reverse renal ischemia; obtain nephrology consultation for possible dialysis.
3. Cor pulmonale—give oxygen by mask or tent. Limit intravenous fluids. Administer digitalis.
4. Lower nephron nephrosis—balance fluid intake and output. Deny potassium-containing materials. Initiate dialysis or begin peritoneal lavage when serum potassium approaches 7 mg/100 ml.

VII. Prevention
A. Avoid trauma and toxemia.
B. Diagnose and treat promptly, especially by artificial rupture of membranes.
C. Have patient discontinue cigarette smoking.

VIII. Prognosis
A. Maternal mortality after premature separation of the placenta is 0.5% to 5% throughout the world. Hemorrhage and renal failure are major causes of maternal death.
B. Perinatal mortality is 30% to 50%. Almost half of these perinates have shortened gestations. In approximately a fifth of cases, fetus is dead at time of parturient's entry into hospital. Hypoxia, birth trauma, and prematurity are the principal causes of perinatal death.
C. The recurrence rate is between 5.6% and 17% for one previous placental abruption and up to 25% for two previous episodes. Proper counseling regarding recurrence is indicated.

IX. Care of neonate (Chapter 9)

Pathophysiology of concealed hemorrhage

In abruptio placentae, gross clotting occurs behind the placenta, and considerable damage is done to decidua and endometrium. With this tissue decomposition, clotting then occurs in small vessels in the uterus and elsewhere. Plasminogen is converted to plasmin, and secondary fibrinolysis starts. This process may be so extensive and rapid that many clotting factors may be expended in a very short time. Additionally, the secondary fibrinolysis dissolves fibrinogen into smaller molecules that exert a heparin-like anticoagulant action. In such instances the patient will begin to bleed from the uterus, sites of needle puncture, mucous membranes, and so forth. Bleeding time will be prolonged secondary to thrombocytopenia, and although a small, fragile clot may form, it will soon disintegrate by lysis. This coagulation disorder is termed "consumption coagulopathy" or "defibrination syndrome."

Shock often develops, and although the patient may remain normotensive for a time before becoming hypotensive from hypovolemia, the microcirculation particularly becomes constricted. Erythrocytes become damaged by being forced through a contracted vasculature partially blocked by clots. As a result, many broken, misshaped red blood cells ("helmet cells," schistocytes) appear in the peripheral blood smear as evidence of the microangiopathic hemolytic anemia.

LABORATORY INDICES OF CONSUMPTION COAGULOPATHY

1. Thrombocytopenia (notable even in smear of peripheral blood)
2. Consumption of coagulation factors I, II, V, and VII (prothrombin and partial thromboplastin)
3. Demonstration of fibrin monomer or fibrin degradation products (FDP) in plasma
4. Prolonged thrombin time

TREATMENT FOR ABRUPTIO PLACENTAE WITH CONSUMPTION COAGULOPATHY

1. Do not attempt vaginal delivery or cesarean section until coagulation problem is corrected.
2. Treat for shock with transfusion of *fresh* blood. If serious bleeding persists:
   a. Give cryoprecipitate in amounts sufficient to restore coagulation mechanisms. Cryoprecipitate contains both fibrinogen and factor VIII and is therefore more effective in restoring normal coagulation than the previously used lyophilized fibrinogen. Additionally, it has the advantage of minimizing transmission of serum hepatitis (between 10% and 30% of patients undergoing fibrinogen therapy acquire homologous serum jaundice).

b. In some cases, fresh frozen plasma or platelet administration, or both, will be necessary.
c. Rarely, when the uterus cannot be emptied or when there is continued disseminated intravascular coagulation, administration of heparin or aminocaproic acid will be necessary. It should be administered only after appropriate investigative studies and usually in consultation with a hematologist. If used, it is proper to administer heparin, 75 to 150 U/kg of body weight every 6 hours IV to maintain coagulation time at about 20 minutes. If the uterus remains well contracted post partum, persistent or delayed bleeding is unlikely. (Protamine sulfate will counteract heparin if unusual bleeding ensues.) Heparin has an antithrombin effect and blocks intrinsic activation of prothrombinase as well. Because consumption of coagulation factors is secondary to the proteolytic effect on thrombin, which increases the induction of a release phenomenon of platelet components, heparin corrects the problem.
3. When bleeding is checked and the coagulation defect is corrected, empty the uterus in the most expeditious way.

PLACENTA PREVIA

Placenta previa is the implantation of the placenta in the lower uterine segment. In this abnormality the placenta covers all or a portion of the internal os and precedes the fetus in vaginal delivery. Reduced vascularity in the fundus probably is of etiologic significance, but the cause in most cases cannot be determined.

I. Associations
   A. Older maternal age
   B. Multiparity
   C. Previous uterine surgery (particularly cesarean section)
   D. Multiple gestation
   E. Congenital abnormalities
   F. Cigarette smoking
   G. Male infant
II. Incidence
   A. Approximately 1:200 pregnancies
   B. Complete placenta previa—approximately one third of cases
   C. Marginal (or partial) placenta previa—approximately 50%
      Remaining cases are the result of low-lying placentas.
III. Pathogenesis, pathology, pathologic physiology
   A. Tumors and scarring in fundus encourage placentation low in uterus.
   B. Placenta covers a one-third greater area to obtain adequate circulation.
   C. Antepartum or intrapartum bleeding occurs with the following:
      1. Spontaneous dilatation and effacement of cervix
      2. Rectal or vaginal examination
   D. Low situation of placenta causes delay in or failure of engagement of presenting part. Breech (11%) and transverse (17%) presentations frequently occur. Moreover, placenta accreta is also related to placenta previa.
   E. If more than a small portion of placenta covers the os, vaginal delivery may not occur, even after rupture of membranes and full dilatation of cervix. This usually results in disruption of a portion of the placenta and hemorrhage and the need for operative assistance.
   F. Laceration of the edge of the placenta may result in fetal as well as maternal blood loss. Fetal hemorrhage may be severe when placenta previa is greater than 20% coverage of the internal os. Maternal hemorrhage may be extreme when placenta previa is greater than 30%.
IV. Degree of previa
   Attempts to designate placenta previa as marginal, partial, or complete, depending on the amount of placenta covering the cervical os, do not aid in prognosis or therapy. Unfortunately, neither does the classification of placenta previa based on estimation of the percentage of the placenta covering the fully dilated cervix. The literature of the last decade is marked by two approaches: individualization of therapy and increasing uses of cesarean section.

Individualization of therapy is based on maternal status, bleeding, and fetal status, not on the amount of the placenta covering the os.

The increasing cesarean delivery rate is based on several factors. Cesarean delivery has an excellent correlation with perinatal survival. Perinatal mortality is also lower with cesarean delivery for all degrees of placenta previa (especially for lesser degrees in which the physician is tempted to deliver the baby vaginally). In addition, cesarean section is the most important variable in decreasing both the perinatal and maternal mortality (other factors as important as blood transfusions and better neonatal care being considered). Thus many believe that vaginal delivery is contraindicated for patients with any degree of placenta previa whose babies are viable and of reasonable gestational age. Therefore estimation of degree of placenta previa appears to be of limited if any value.

V. Clinical findings
 A. Symptoms
  1. Uterine bleeding with placenta previa is painless unless the patient is in labor or has other complications (infection, tumor, etc.).
  2. Bleeding may be continuous or intermittent and is usually brighter red than that seen with abruptio placentae.
 B. Ultrasonography
  The diagnostic method of choice for determining placental location is ultrasonic scanning. The only other procedure that has sufficient reliability to warrant mention is angiography. However, because of the obvious associated risks, angiography is seldom if ever used for this purpose.
 C. Special management procedures
  1. Hospitalize patient with definite bleeding.
  2. Maintain adequate maternal blood volume.
  3. Attempt to maintain pregnancy until fetus achieves physiologic maturity.
  4. Prepare for cesarean section.
VI. Differential diagnosis
 A. Rule out nonplacental causes for vaginal bleeding: carcinoma, tuberculosis of the cervix or vagina, polyps, ruptured vaginal varices, lower genital tract infections, blood dyscrasias.
 B. Rule out other major placental cause for bleeding: premature separation of normally implanted placenta (often with painful uterine bleeding).
VII. Complications
 A. Fetus
  1. Delivery of a premature neonate occurs in one third to one half of cases.
  2. Early delivery accounts for 60% of perinatal deaths in placenta previa.
  3. Prolapse of cord may occur when membranes rupture and presenting part is unengaged.
  4. Hypoxia, birth injury, and transplacental hemorrhage exact an extremely high morbidity.
  5. When placenta is torn during cesarean section, the fetus may bleed.
 B. Mother
  1. Hemorrhage and hypovolemic shock may develop.
  2. Operative trauma, especially cervical laceration and uterine rupture, may occur.
  3. Vascular thrombosis and embolism often develop post partum.
  4. Placenta previa accreta may account for lack of separation of forelying placenta.
VIII. Treatment
 A. Emergency measures
  1. Hospitalize patient at once.
  2. Treat patient for hemorrhage and shock.
 B. Specific and supportive measures

1. Type and match blood, and have blood available for transfusion.
2. Postpone delivery until 36 weeks' gestation, if possible.
3. Avoid use of oxytocics and enemas.
4. Monitor FHR continuously during times of bleeding. During intervals use biometric testing (ultrasonography, fetal activity-acceleration determinations) to ascertain fetal well-being.
5. Deliver baby in manner least hazardous to both gavida and offspring.

Perform a cesarean section (preferably low cervical under general anesthesia, unless placenta is anterior, in which case a classic entry may allow avoidance of placenta and serious hemorrhage). Suture bleeding sinuses within the uterus for control of placental site.

Placenta previa accreta may require cesarean total hysterectomy.

IX. Prevention: none
X. Prognosis
   A. Maternal mortality is now less than 0.8% in major medical centers.
   B. Perinatal mortality is still 6% to 10%, even in large hospitals, despite improved methods.
   C. Approximately 10 times more offspring die when placenta previa complicates pregnancy than when pregnancy is uncomplicated.
   D. Perinatal mortality can be reduced to less than 10% with optimal treatment, including avoidance of reckless intervention at delivery of the undersized fetus.
   E. Cesarean section increases the likelihood of placenta previa in a subsequent pregnancy by about 5%.
   F. Multiparity and infection raise the incidence of placenta previa.
XI. Care of the neonate

The high perinatal mortality with placental bleeding suggests that labor and delivery should occur in a maternity center in which an experienced team can be present for both mother and infant. A neonatal intensive care unit should be part of the center.
   A. Special problems to be anticipated at birth include the following:
      1. Prematurity (labor usually ensues before term is reached)
      2. Asphyxia (result of disruption of fetal-placental circulation)
      3. Hypovolemia (loss of blood* from fetal side of placenta)
      4. Hyaline membrane disease (intensified by asphyxia, which reduces surfactant production in the preterm infant)
   B. Management
      1. Resuscitate infant immediately.
      2. Offer Plasmanate for shock unless forewarned by knowledge of fetal blood loss with appropriate blood available.
      3. Perform serial hematocrits three times per hour—a falling hematocrit indicates acute blood loss.
      4. Transfuse if hematocrit is less than 45.
      5. Support respiratory failure (Chapter 27).

CIRCUMVALLATE OR CIRCUMMARGINATE PLACENTA (EXTRACHORIAL PLACENTA)

Extrachorial placenta (circumvallate or circummarginate) is associated with increased rates of slight or moderate antepartum bleeding, early delivery (which is a major cause of second trimester losses), and perinatal death. Older multigravidas have a much greater predisposition. Nevertheless, circumvallate placenta and circummarginate placenta together represent only about 6% of all deliveries in which there has been prelabor bleeding. Despite well-documented obstetric-pediatric complications, extrachorial placenta is an uncommon, rarely

---

*Check vaginal blood before delivery for fetal bleeding by the Kleihauer technique (resistance to acid elution). Fixed blood smear is immersed in a citrate-phosphate buffer of acid pH (3.3 to 3.4). Hemoglobin A is eluted from erythrocytes, but hemoglobin F (fetal) is not.

serious clinical obstetric problem. Nevertheless, our experience demonstrates a high incidence of low birth weight infants of white mothers who had extrachorial placentas.

VASA PREVIA

Vasa previa occurs when the umbilical cord is not inserted on the chorionic plate, but at some point on the membranes. The fetal vessels course across the membranes from the cord site to the placental plate. Thus the vessels may lie over the cervix where fetal descent and rupture of the membranes will lead to their disruption and result in fetal hemorrhage. Unfortunately, the only detectable fetal response to this event may be tachycardia.

BIBLIOGRAPHY

Barret, J.M., Boehm, F.H., and Killam, A.P.: Induced abortion: a risk factor for placenta previa, Am. J. Obstet. Gynecol. **141**:764, 1981.

Brenner, W.E., Edelman, D.A., and Hendricks, C.H.: Characteristics of patients with placenta previa and results of "expectant management", Am. J. Obstet. Gynecol. **132**:180, 1978.

Carp, H.J.A., Maschiach, S., and Sher, D.M.: Vasa previa: a major complication and its management, Obstet. Gynecol. **53**:273, 1979.

Crenshaw, C., Jr., Darnell, J., and Parker, R.T.: Placenta previa: a survey of twenty years experience with improved perinatal survival of expectant therapy and cesarean section, Obstet. Gynecol. Surv. **28**:461, 1973.

Crosby, W.M., and Costiloe, J.: Safety of lap-belt restraint for pregnant victims of automobile collisions, N. Engl. J. Med. **284**:632, 1971.

DeValera, E.: Abruptio placentae, Am. J. Obstet. Gynecol. **100**:599, 1968.

Dunster, G.A., Davieser, Ross, F.G.M., et al.: Placental localization: a comparison of isotopic and ultrasonic placentography, Br. J. Radiol. **49**:940, 1976.

Golsemberg, B.B.: The identification of placenta previa, Radiology **128**:255, 1978.

Goujard, J., Rureau, C., and Schwartz, D.: Smoking during pregnancy: stillbirth and abruptio placentae, Biomedicine **23**:20, 1975.

Hertig, A.T., and Rock, J.: On the development of the early human ovum with special reference to the throphoblast of the previous stage: a description of 7 normal and 5 pathologic human ova, Am. J. Obstet. Gynecol. **47**:149, 1944.

Jaffe, M.H., Schoen, W.C., Silver, T.M., et al.: Sonography of abruptio placentae, AJR **137**:1049, 1981.

Jeffrey, R.B., and Laing, F.C.: Sonography of the low lying placenta: value of Trendelenburg and traction scans, AJR **137**:547, 1981.

Kohler, H.G., and Jenkins, D.M.: Chorionic haemangiomata and abruptio placentae, Br. J. Obstet. Gynaecol. **83**:667, 1976.

Naeje, R.L., Harkness, W.L., and Utts, J.: Abruptio placentae and perinatal death: a prospective study, Am. J. Obstet. Gynecol. **128**:740, 1977.

Naeje, R.L.: Abruptio placentae and placenta previa: frequency, perinatal mortality, and cigarette smoking, Obstet. Gynecol. **55**:701, 1980.

Paterson, M.E.L.: The aetiology and outcome of abruptio placentae, Acta Obstet. Gynecol. Scand. **58**:31, 1979.

Pritchard, J.A., Mason, R., Corley, M., et al.: Genesis of severe placental abruption, Am. J. Obstet. Gynecol. **108**:22, 1970.

Ricos, N., Doran, T.A., Miskin, M., et al.: Natural history of placenta previa ascertained by diagnostic ultrasound, Am. J. Obstet. Gynecol. **133**:287, 1979.

Sher, G.: Pathogenesis and management of uterine inertia complicating abruptio placentae with consumption coagulopathy, Am. J. Obstet. Gynecol. **129**:164, 1977.

Smith, J.J., Schinfeld, J., and Schulman, H.: Placenta previa: reappraisal and new therapeutic classification, NY State J. Med. **82**:1037, 1982.

Wexler, P., and Gottesfeld, K.R.: Early diagnosis of placenta previa, Obstet. Gynecol. **54**:231, 1979.

Section II SERIOUS OBSTETRIC PROBLEMS
AND THE PERINATE

23

Malpresentation and cord accidents

BREECH

Breech is a longitudinal presentation in which the cephalic pole of the fetus occupies the fundal segment, and the caudal or podalic pole lies in the lower segment of the uterine cavity or within the birth canal. There are three major types of breech presentation:

Frank breech: hips flexed, knees extended, buttocks presenting (approximately 65% of total)

Complete breech: hips partially extended, knees partially flexed, buttocks or feet, or both presenting (approximately 10% of total)

Incomplete breech: hips extended, knees extended, foot or feet presenting (approximately 25% of total)

Single footling if one leg is completely extended and the other flexed

Double footling if both legs are extended below the level of the buttocks

The incidence of term breech presentations is 3% to 4%. Previous or habitual breech presentation is found in approximately 20% of cases. The incidence of breech presentation is higher with decreasing gestational age.

Correlations predisposing to breech presentation

As the fetus grows, it occupies a greater volume in the uterine cavity and tends to adapt to the shape of the corpus. The etiology of breech presentation may be an aberration of this adaptation process or of the fetal attitude. For example, in premature infants, when the head is larger than the buttocks, the head is more likely to be in the fundus than it is at term. In other cases the site of placental implantation may encourage breech presentation. Although 80% of breech presentations have no discernible causation or associations, the following factors are thought to be correlates of breech presentation:

Maternal
  Previous breech presentation
  Congenital uterine abnormalities (e.g., septate or bicornuate uterus)
  Contracted pelvis (not confirmed in several recent studies)
  Multiparity
  Tumors of the uterus, cervix, vagina, or ovaries
  Uterine scars

Placental
  Placenta previa or cornual-fundal placentation

Fetal
  Fetal anomalies (primarily anencephaly, hydrocephaly, macrosomia, or other conditions that prevent normal fetal attitude of flexion)
  Hydramnios or oligohydramnios
  Multiple pregnancy
  Prematurity
  Premature rupture of membranes

Thus, although presence of one of the above factors does not necessarily mean breech presentation is inevitable, there is sufficient correlation to warrant special attempts to ascertain fetal lie and presentation.

Frank breech presentation is more common in the primigravida and complete or incomplete presentation is more common in the multigravida. There is also difference in the incidence of breech types based on weight (Table 23-1). Overall the incidence of breech presentation by weight demonstrates an inverse relationship (Table 23-2).

DIAGNOSIS

A wise dictum to follow for all patients after 26 weeks' gestation is the assumption that all fetuses are in the breech position until proved otherwise. This may be accomplished by the following:

1. Examine the uterus by the four maneuvers of Leopold (Fig. 4-4). This should yield a 95% rate of diagnosis.
2. Confirm diagnosis by listening to the fetal heartbeat (which should be heard best over the back and usually at or about the level of the umbilicus).
3. Obtain ultrasonographic scan to confirm diagnosis, screen for fetal defects, assess placental placement, and check for multiple gestation or abnormalities in amniotic fluid volume.
4. Use radiography if indicated for critical determinations of breech type.
5. Perform vaginal examination during labor to identify the irregular fetal parts, consisting of the ischial tuberosities, the sacrum, the anus, and possibly the feet. Attempts to determine sex by genital palpation may not be productive.

In all breech presentations position is described by the relationship of the fetal sacrum to the maternal pelvis. Eight positions are possible: sacrum anterior or posterior (SA, SP), right or left sacrum transverse (RST, LST), right or left sacrum anterior (RSA, LSA), right or left sacrum posterior (RSP, LSP).

Table 23-1. Breech type by fetal weight

Breech type	Fetal weight (gm)	
	<2,500	>2,500
Frank	38%	75%
Complete	12%	10%
Incomplete	50%	25%

Table 23-2. Fetal weight and incidence of breech

Fetal weight	Breech incidence
1,000	23%
1,500	12%
2,000	8%
>3,000	3%

DIFFERENTIAL DIAGNOSIS

Differential diagnoses include:
1. Face presentation
2. Fetal anomalies (e.g., vertex anencephaly may be very difficult to exclude by vaginal examination alone)
3. Shoulder presentation
4. Compound presentation

MANAGEMENT

I. External cephalic version

  External cephalic version is a prepartum, external manipulation designed to convert the fetus to a vertex position, thereby averting the breech presentation and its inherent dangers. This maneuver is usually performed prior to the thirty-fourth week of gestation and rarely after the thirty-eighth week. The procedure should be monitored carefully, for if the operator is not experienced more hazard than benefit may result. Primary dangers to the fetus are separation of the placenta and cord entanglement. In recent literature the procedure appears to have a high initial rate of success. It may decrease the incidence of breech presentations at term as well as the number of cesarean deliveries necessary for breech presentations. It can also be accomplished safely and appears to be gaining acceptance in the United States.

  A. Prerequisites
  1. Recent ultrasonographic scan ruling out any contraindications
  2. Reactive nonstress test or negative contraction stress test
  3. Informed consent

  B. Contraindications
  1. Absolute
     a. Multiple pregnancy
     b. Antepartum hemorrhage
     c. Placenta previa
     d. Cesarean section necessary for reasons other than breech presentation
     e. Rupture of membranes
     f. Severe fetal anomalies
  2. Relative
     a. Previous cesarean delivery
     b. Hypertensive states of pregnancy or hypertension
     c. Intrauterine growth retardation

    d. Obesity
    e. Anterior placenta
    f. Rh-negative mother (may be discounted if Rh immune globulin is administered)
  C. Technique
    1. Meet above prerequisites.
    2. Ascertain that contraindications do not exist.
    3. Apply talcum powder to abdomen.
    4. Attempt to gently manipulate the fetus in a "forward somersault."
    5. Monitor FHR every 2 minutes.
    6. Attempt procedure for maximum of 5 minutes per attempt.
    7. Delay repeating procedure for minimum of 3 minutes between attempts (with FHR monitoring).
    8. Monitor FHR after attempt until reactive NST or negative CST is obtained.
  D. Controversies
    There are several points of controversy among authors concerning this procedure, including the following:
    1. Which is the most beneficial maternal position during the procedure
    2. Whether tocolytics can be used safely
    3. Whether analgesics or anesthetics can be used safely
    4. Whether foreward or backward "somersault" is safest and most effective
II. Cesarean section—general measures
  In view of the increased morbidity and mortality in breech presentation and the emphasis on smaller families of maximum quality, a more frequent use of cesarean section is now recommended in breech delivery. However, because of the increased maternal hazard, this procedure must always be performed at the most opportune time by a competent team in a properly equipped hospital. Morbidity associated with the procedure may be less than morbidity with external cephalic version and is definitely less than that associated with breech extraction. Cesarean section should be performed when there is
  A. Any evidence of fetopelvic disproportion
  B. Fetus weighing over 8 lb (3.5 kg) or less than 5.5 lb (2.5 kg)
  C. Gestation of 42 weeks or more
  D. Any prior history of dystocia or injury at previous breech birth
  E. Any abnormality of the first stage of labor
  F. Any need for oxytocin augmentation of labor
  G. Prolonged second stage of labor
  H. Any evidence of fetal distress
  I. Complete or incomplete breech presentation
  J. Intrauterine growth retardation or prematurity
  K. Prolapsed cord
  L. Hyperextension of the fetal head and neck or other abnormalities of attitude
III. Cesarean section—smaller premature infant (under 34 weeks' gestation)
  Breech position is present at labor with approximately 30% of these infants. The relatively large head in comparison to the buttocks increases the chance of entrapment and subsequent trauma and asphyxia. As a result, the chance of death during labor is 16 times more likely than when fetus is in the vertex position (Goldenberg). Many obstetric perinatologists hold that cesarean section is appropriate for most preterm fetuses under the following conditions:
  A. Labor has not progressed to the point of imminent delivery.
  B. Biparietal diameter of the fetal skull is 6.5 cm or more (avoids likelihood of delivering a previable infant).
  C. Capable teams for the procedure and for care of the infant are at hand.
IV. Vaginal delivery
  Although it may be the preferable mode of delivery in certain breech cases, vaginal delivery of the breech presenting fetus must be viewed as a risk procedure and all appropriate precautions must be taken.
  For example, the well-tested guidelines of Collea et al. for vaginal delivery of breech presenting perinates include only:
    Fetuses weighing more than 2,500 gm and less than 3,800 gm
    Frank breech presentation (because cord prolapse is less likely)

Adequate maternal pelvis as shown by x-ray pelvimetry

Their studies indicate the following exclusions from attempted vaginal delivery:

Maternal
Older primigravidas
Obstetric indications for cesarean delivery
Classes B through F diabetes mellitus
Involuntary infertility
Pelvic contracture determined by radiographic pelvimetry
History of difficult or traumatic delivery

Fetal
Congenital anomalies
Nonfrank breech
Estimated weight greater than 3,800 gm or less than 2,500 gm
Floating station
Hyperextension of head and neck or attitude abnormalities

Other criteria may also be applied. For example, assessing the possibility of vaginal delivery may be assisted by the breech scoring index proposed by Zatuchni and Andros (Table 23-3). Configuration and size of pelvis are not directly evaluated in this schema but are indirectly reflected by cervical dilatation, fetal descent, and previous pregnancy. In addition, the scoring index is not useful for patients who are considered for induction because it applies only to patients admitted in labor. If the total score achieved is 3 or less, a cesarean section should be performed. A score of 4 demands careful reevaluation, and a score of 5 or more may justify vaginal delivery. Although this score takes parity into account, other authors have reported the breech presentation in multiparas to be as great a risk as it is in the primipara.

If a vaginal delivery is considered for a breech presentation, there are many critical factors in addition to the "breech index" that determine feasibility. Of paramount importance are the experience and ability of those in attendance.

Other keys to management of labor in breech presentation include the following:

1. Early detection of fetopelvic relations and aberrations, and prediction of whether they will permit vaginal delivery (x-ray pelvimetry and ultrasonographic determination of fetal head size)
   If the biparietal diameter is greater than 9.5 cm vaginal delivery may be ruled out. If it is less than 9.5 cm, further evaluation may be desirable.
2. Determination of the exact position of the extremities (usually accomplished by the same ultrasonographic examination noted above)
   Specifically, extension of the neck and head, fetal size, attitude, position of the legs, and any gross fetal defects need to be detected by radiographs or ultrasonography.
3. Observation for prolapse of cord or for cord complications (a critical step after rupture of membranes)
4. Observation for fetal distress (electronic fetal monitoring)

Table 23-3. Criteria for scoring breech presentations

	Points		
	0	1	2
Parity	Primigravida	Multipara	
Gestational age	39 weeks or more	38 weeks	37 weeks or less
Estimated fetal weight	More than 8 lb (3,630 gm)	7 lb to 7 lb 15 oz (3,176 to 3,629 gm)	Less than 7 lb (3,175 gm)
Previous breech*	None	1	2 or more
Dilatation†	2 cm	3 cm	4 cm or more
Station†	−3 or higher	−2	−1 or lower

From Zatuchni, G.I., and Andros, G.J.: Prognostic index for vaginal delivery in breech presentation at term, Am. J. Obstet. Gynecol. 98:855, 1967.
*Greater than 2,500 gm.
†Determined by vaginal examination on admission.

5. Careful evaluation of labor's progress, in terms of both dilatation and descent of presenting part
6. Immediate delivery by cesarean section if any aberration of labor is observed
7. Use of oxytocin
   The role of oxytocin in breech vaginal delivery remains controversial. The following guidelines are employed by Collea et al., assuming all previous criteria are met:
   a. Premature rupture of membranes with an engaged fetus and no labor
   b. Prolonged latent phase (greater than 10 hr in a primigravida and greater than 6 hr in a multigravida)
   c. Protracted active phase of dilatation (maximum slope less than 1.2 cm/hr in a primigravida and less than 1.5 cm/hr in a multigravida)
8. Minimal use of analgesia
9. Avoidance of early artificial rupture of membranes
10. Vaginal examination at time of rupture of membranes and at onset of labor to rule out cord prolapse
11. Careful monitoring of the mechanisms of labor

Careful attention must be directed to the mechanisms of labor. Characteristically the bitrochanteric diameter engages in the transverse position with the sacrum anterior. The buttocks descends in this or the oblique position until internal rotation occurs at the level of the ischial spines. Then the anterior hip rotates beneath the symphysis pubis and the breech follows the pelvic curve to delivery. If a characteristic pattern is not evident on examination of the presenting part, attempting vaginal delivery needs serious reevaluation.

When the pelvic girdle is delivered the back will again rotate anteriorly to allow the shoulders to engage with the biacromial diameter in the transverse or oblique position. As the shoulders advance into the midpelvis, they rotate into the anteroposterior or oblique position. This course is followed until the anterior shoulder (usually first) emerges from behind the symphysis pubis to be followed by the posterior shoulder.

Meanwhile the head engages in the transverse or oblique position and rotates to occiput anterior at the midpelvis. With descent the occiput engages the symphysis pubis and delivery is accomplished by rotation (flexion) about this point.

Ideal delivery management also includes the following:
1. Minimal anesthesia and delay in giving pudendal block anesthesia until breech is crowning to maintain patient's voluntary expulsive efforts
2. Limited interference during the second stage, delayed as long as possible
3. Loosening and drawing down a short loop of cord when the umbilicus comes into view
4. Prevention of trauma to the head by generous episiotomy
5. Allowing expulsion of fetus to level of umbilicus before manipulating fetus
6. Avoiding hyperextension of fetal neck

The maternal bladder must be emptied and all high-risk preparations must be performed. An experienced obstetrician and an assistant should be scrubbed for vaginal delivery of a breech presenting perinate. Other team members should include an anesthetist or anesthesiologist, an experienced neonatologist, a scrub nurse, a circulating nurse, and a neonatal nurse. The team must keep in mind that the breech presenting perinate has a higher incidence of congenital anomaly. The patient should be cautioned to avoid expulsive efforts until full dilatation of the cervix occurs.

Three methods of vaginal breech delivery of the fetal body include the following:
1. Total breech extraction (in which one and then both of the lower extremities are grasped and used to literally extract the fetus from the uterus) is by far the most hazardous method of vaginal delivery.
2. Spontaneous expulsion (which allows for full delivery of the body without manipulative interference) is the next most hazardous mode of delivery.
3. Assisted breech (in which the fetus is spontaneously expelled to the level of the umbilicus and the remainder extracted) is the least hazardous.

The best mode of delivery for the aftercoming head remains in debate. Some believe that routine use of forceps may protect the head from trauma, but others disagree and recommend manual control of the head.

Opinions on the selection of the proper

anesthetic for breech delivery are as varied as are the approaches to effecting that delivery. One popular method is local infiltration or nerve block for the episiotomy, with general anesthesia for the assisted breech portion of the delivery. However, some physicians urge use of epidural anesthesia. Although most authorities agree that use of as little analgesia and anesthesia as possible is most desirable, they also recognize the need for general anesthesia for total breech extraction.

Maternal and perinatal complications

Maternal morbidity and mortality are related to the increased incidence of premature rupture of membranes seen with breech presentations (a twofold increase) and to trauma because of the increased number of operative deliveries. Morbidity may be associated with cesarean or vaginal delivery. The latter includes lacerations of the maternal perineum, vagina, cervix, and lower uterine segment, an increased number of hemorrhages, and an enhanced infection rate.

Breech delivery may be associated with a perinatal mortality of up to 18% (British Perinatal Study), and thus it is the leading factor in the perinatal death of mature infants. There are numerous factors contributing to the high morbidity and mortality associated with breech delivery, including a twofold increase in fetopelvic disproportion, a twofold increase in dysfunctional labor, and a threefold increase in macrosomia (comparing vertex to breech presentations). There is also an increased incidence of fetal congenital anomalies.

Other factors predisposing the fetus to injury during labor and delivery are as follows:
1. Greater incidence of umbilical cord prolapse (incidence of cord prolapse is 10% with footling, 5% with complete, and 0.5% with frank breech presentations)
2. Pressure on umbilical cord during first stage of labor
3. Increased incidence of placental separation
4. Entrapment of head by cervix
5. Injury of head and neck by rapid descent through birth canal
6. Injury of head and neck by mode of delivery
7. Increased chance of nerve damage because arms are more likely to be swept over head

The most prevalent hazards of breech delivery of the small infant are attributable to the following:
1. Complications of pregnancy (placenta previa etc.)
2. Low birth weight related to complications of pregnancy
3. Injuries associated with low birth weight

In contrast, the large (term or postterm) breech-delivered infant generally is jeopardized by complications of labor, such as the following:
1. Prolapsed cord
2. Uterine dysfunction
3. Hypoxia and trauma during delivery—the consequences of relative fetopelvic disproportion

Perinatal mortality for infants delivered in breech position is 10 to 25 times greater than that for those delivered in vertex position. This difference is largely because of premature birth. However, when statistics are corrected for birth weight, the breech-delivered infant is still at a disadvantage in terms of higher mortality, increased neurologic damage, and subnormal intellectual levels.

Infant morbidity may reach 16%, with nearly half showing signs of permanent injury, primarily the result of asphyxia and intracranial hemorrhage. The breech infant of the multipara may be at equal or greater jeopardy than the infant of the primipara because of the following:
1. Increasing size of subsequent fetuses
2. False sense of security in dealing with a "proved" pelvis

Early identification of breech presentation and related problems is important to outcome. Consultation and more liberal use of cesarean section in borderline cases are necessary to improve outcomes in breech presentations. Repetition of breech presentation occurs in approximately 20% of cases.

Neonatal care

Chapter 9 presents the birth-room attention given to infants who require special care. In addition to birth-room observations outlined in Chapter 8, observe neonate for the following injuries:
1. Fracture of clavicle or humerus; epiphyseal injury
2. Brachial plexus injury (unlikely if Moro reflex is adequate)
3. Fracture dislocation of cervical spine

4. Paralysis of legs (cord injury)
5. Intracranial hemorrhage
6. Occipital osteodiastasis
7. Rupture of liver and spleen

OTHER MALPRESENTATIONS
Transverse lie

When the long axis of the fetus lies at right angles to the long axis of the mother, the presentation is described as a transverse lie. This complication occurs in less than 0.5% of all term gestations. It most frequently is associated with increasing multiparity because of relaxation of the abdominal wall and uterus. Other correlates are bony pelvis contraction, hydramnios, and placenta previa.

The diagnosis is usually readily made by inspection or palpation. Should there be any difficulty in diagnosis by Leopold's maneuvers, confirmation by ultrasonographic or radiographic means should be undertaken. Since this presentation is not amenable to vaginal delivery and there is great hazard of prolapse of the umbilical cord (particularly when fetus is in the back up position) if the patient arrives at the hospital in labor, cesarean section should be performed as soon as feasible. Because of fetal position it is often necessary to perform a low vertical or even classical cesarean delivery. Perinatal mortality is greatly increased with transverse lie, with incidence of about 140:1,000 live births.

Face presentation

When the face of the fetus is the presenting part, it is termed a "face presentation." This condition occurs in only 0.2% of pregnancies. The point for designation of position is the mentum (chin). The diagnosis may be suspected by abdominal examination; however, it is usually confirmed by vaginal examination.

In most cases, x-ray pelvimetry is necessary for adequate pelvic evaluation for vaginal delivery. Indeed, cesarean section will be necessary in nearly all primiparas and many multiparas. If, however, the pelvis is adequate in relation to fetal size, spontaneous delivery or easy low forceps may be anticipated when the mentum is anterior or transverse.

The mentum posterior precludes vaginal delivery, and all fetuses in this position except the very small will require cesarean section. For prevention of maternal morbidity (deep tears in the perineum), wide episiotomy should be performed. Exact clinical correlates have not been developed for this unusual presentation. Perinatal mortality is as high as 70 to 163:1,000 live births if the condition remains unidentified and untreated.

Brow presentation presents roughly the same set of risks as face presentation. However, it occurs less frequently (0.1% of cases).

PROLAPSE OF UMBILICAL CORD

Prolapse of the umbilical cord is a condition in which the funis lies alongside (occult) or lower than the presenting part (overt) in the birth canal. With the overt (or complete) variety, the cord may be contained entirely within the vagina or may protrude through the introitus. The greatest predisposition for cord prolapse occurs when the presenting part does not fill the lower uterine segment and impinges on the cervix. Thus the cord may enter this space and lie alongside or lower than the presenting part.

Overt prolapse occurs in 0.4% to 0.5% of all deliveries. Incidence of occult prolapse of the cord is difficult to ascertain because it is usually asymptomatic unless cord compression occurs. In the Collaborative Perinatal Study carried out by the National Institute of Neurological Diseases and Stroke (NINDS), occult prolapse of the cord was detected in 0.3% to 0.7% of all cases; however, electronic fetal monitoring reveals that approximately one fourth of high-risk patients will have cord compression patterns. Unfortunately, accurate data have not been accumulated concerning the percentage of variable decelerations (cord compression patterns) created by occult prolapse.

Although it occurs infrequently, cord prolapse is an important factor in perinatal wastage because of the great fetal hazard if it does occur. With occult cord prolapse, the normally expected perinatal mortality is doubled, and with overt prolapse it is increased approximately twelvefold.

Diagnosis
CLINICAL CORRELATES

1. Abnormal presentation
   a. Breech
      Footling breech presentation perinates are at greatest risk of cord prolapse; however, all breech presenting fetuses are

at some degree of risk. Overall incidence of this complication with breech presentations is five times greater than with vertex presentations.
   b. Shoulder (transverse lie)
   c. Face
   d. Brow
   e. Transverse
   f. Compound
2. Multiple pregnancy
3. Prematurity (a factor in 45.5% of pregnancies complicated by this condition)
4. Artificial rupture of membranes in presence of a floating presenting part
5. Polyhydramnios and increasing gravidity
   Both conditions correlate with umbilical cord prolapse, although to a lesser degree than the factors noted above.

OCCULT CORD PROLAPSE

Occult cord prolapse is detected most commonly by the presence of variable deceleration in electronic fetal monitoring patterns. Occasionally, sterile vaginal examination may reveal the presence of the umbilical cord along the presenting part.

OVERT PROLAPSE

With complete prolapse the patient may feel the cord slide through the vagina and over the vulva after rupture of the membranes. Usually compression of the cord causes violent fetal activity, obvious to both patient and observer. The cord may be seen or palpated by the patient, an attendant, or a physician during external or internal examination. Auscultation of the fetal heart with a head stethoscope or an electronic fetal monitoring device may reveal fetal distress.

Treatment

1. The patient should be placed immediately in the knee-chest or deep Trendelenburg position.
2. Using aseptic technique, upward pressure should be exerted on the presenting part to relieve cord compression.
3. Repositioning of the cord within the uterus is rarely successful.
4. Careful palpation of the umbilical cord must be performed to ascertain fetal viability. About 17% of pregnant women with this complication have a dead fetus on admission to labor and delivery, and it is possible to err by rushing to deliver the dead fetus.
5. FHR should be monitored continuously until the time of delivery.
6. Delivery should be effected immediately and is most often accomplished by cesarean section with the mother under general anesthesia.
7. Consideration must also be given to other factors that may alter the above management.
   a. If pregnancy is of less than 27 weeks' duration, increasing maternal risk in an effort to save a very immature fetus may be imprudent.
   b. If cervix is nearly or completely dilated and fetal presenting part is well within pelvis, vaginal delivery by use of forceps or vacuum extractor may be accomplished.

Complications

As anticipated, fetal death rates increase with prolapse of the cord. Occult prolapse of the cord in the Collaborative Perinatal Study of the NINDS was not associated with low birth weight infants, whereas overt prolapse of the cord occurred more commonly with low birth weight infants. Perinatal death rates varied between 57 and 185 (per 1,000 births) with occult prolapse of the cord and between 337 and 361 with overt prolapse. There was no consistent increase noted in the risk of neurologic abnormalities at 1 year of age among babies born alive after prolapse of the cord.

VELAMENTOUS INSERTION OF CORD AND VASA PREVIA

In velamentous insertion of the cord its proximal end is attached to the membranes. Fetal vessels then extend across a membranous bridge to the placenta. The abnormality may be the result of growth of the placenta away from the implantation site with concomitant atrophy of villous units in the bare zone about the point of cord insertion. When one or more fetal vessels actually cross the internal os, this variation is called *vasa previa*.
   I. Occurrence
      A. One in 100 singleton placentas
      B. Five to 10 of every 100 twin placentas, with the velamentous insertion

invariably attached to the smaller of the pair
II. Associations
   A. Late abortions
   B. Low birth weight infants
III. Complications
   A. Tear of a bridging vessel
      1. Fetal bleeding ascertained by fetal red blood cells or hemoglobin in vaginal blood
      2. Fetal distress and then fetal death
IV. Therapy imperative to saving offspring
   A. Rapid delivery
   B. Transfusion

BIBLIOGRAPHY

Alexopoulos, K.A.: Importance of breech delivery in pathogenesis of brain damage: end results of long-term follow-up, Clin. Pediatr. **12**:248, 1973.

Allen, J.P., Myers, G.G., and Condon, V.R.: Laceration of the spinal cord related to breech delivery, JAMA **208**:1019, 1969.

Ballos, S., Toaff, R., and Jaffa, A.J.: Deflexion of the fetal head in breech presentation: incidence, management and outcome, Obstet. Gynecol. **52**:653, 1978.

Bean, W.J., Calouje, M.A., Aprill, C.N., et al.: Ultrasound diagnosis of the hyperextended head in breech presentation, JCU **5**:278, 1977.

Benson, W.L., Boyce, D.C., and Vaughn, D.L.: Breech delivery in the primigravida, Obstet. Gynecol. **40**:417, 1972.

Collea, J.V., Chein, C., and Quilligan, E.J.: The randomized management of term frank breech presentation, Am. J. Obstet. Gynecol. **137**:235, 1980.

Collea, J.V., Rabin, S.C., Weghorst, G.R., et al.: The randomized management of term breech presentation: vaginal delivery vs. cesarean section, Am. J. Obstet. Gynecol. **131**:186, 1978.

Faber-Nijholt, R., Huisjes, H.J., Touwen, B.C.L., et al.: Neurological follow up of 281 children born in breech presentation: a controlled study, Br. Med. J. **286**:9, 1983.

Gimorsky, M.L., Petrie, R.H., and Todd, W.D.: Neonatal performance of the selected term vaginal breech delivery, Obstet. Gynecol. **56**:687, 1980.

Gimovsky, M.L., and Petrie, R.H.: Management of the breech presentation, Perinatol. Neonatal. **6**:73, 1982.

Hall, et al.: Breech presentation and perinatal mortality, Am. J. Obstet. Gynecol. **91**:665, 1965.

Hofmeyr, G.J.: Effect of external cephalic version in late pregnancy on breech presentation and caesarean section rate: a controlled trial, Br. J. Obstet. Gynaecol. **90**:392, 1983.

Ingemarsson, I., Westgren, M., and Svenningsen, N.W., et al.: Long-term follow-up of preterm infants in breech presentation delivered by caesarean section, Lancet, **2**:172, 1978.

Karp, L.E., et al.: The premature breech: trial of labor or cesarean section? Obstet. Gynecol. **53**:88, 1979.

Kelsick, F., and Minkoff, H.: Management of the breech second twin, Am. J. Obstet. Gynecol. **144**:783, 1982.

Lyons, E.R., and Papsin, F.R.: Cesarean section in the management of breech presentation, Am. J. Obstet. Gynecol. **130**:558, 1978.

Mann, L.I., and Gallant, J.H.: Modern management of the breech delivery, Am. J. Obstet. Gynecol. **134**:611, 1979.

Niswander, K.R., and Gordon, M.: The women and their pregnancies (The Collaborative Perinatal Study of the National Institute of Neurological Diseases and Storke), Philadelphia, 1972, W.B. Saunders Co.

O'Leary, J.A.: Vaginal delivery of the term breech: a preliminary report, Obstet. Gynecol. **53**:341, 1979.

Ranney, B.: Gentle art of external cephalic version, Am. J. Obstet. Gynecol. **116**:239, 1973.

Rovinsky, J.J., Miller, J.A., and Kaplan, S.: Management of breech presentation at term, Am. J. Obstet. Gynecol. **115**:497, 1973.

Tank, E.S., Davis, R., Holt, J.F., et al.: Mechanisms of trauma during breech delivery, Obstet. Gynecol. **38**:761, 1971.

Zatuchni, G.I., and Andros, G.J.: Prognostic index for vaginal delivery in breech presentation at term, Am. J. Obstet. Gynecol. **98**:854, 1967.

24

Diabetes mellitus

Diabetes mellitus is a general term for a variety of hyperglycemic disorders characterized by hormone-induced metabolic abnormalities; by long-term complications involving large vessels, small vessels, and nerves; and by a lesion of the basement membranes demonstrable by electron microscopy. In 1979, the National Diabetes Data Group (NDDG) divided the primary forms of diabetes (where no associated disease is present) into Type I or insulin-dependent (formerly juvenile-onset) and Type II or insulin-independent (formerly maturity-onset). Secondary forms of diabetes were placed in a third category that included pancreatic disease, hormonal abnormalities, drug-induced diabetes, insulin receptor abnormalities, and genetic syndromes.

Type I diabetes usually begins before the age of 40, often in childhood or adolescence. Onset may be abrupt with polyuria, polydipsia, and weight loss. Body habitus is normal or wasted. Plasma insulin is low or absent. Glucagon levels are high but suppressible with insulin. Patients are ketosis-prone but responsive to insulin.

Type II diabetes usually begins after age 40. The typical patient is obese. Symptoms begin gradually. Plasma insulin levels are normal or high, although they are lower than they should be for the degree of hyperglycemia. Insulin resistance plays a major role in that there is a decrease in the number of insulin receptors, as well as a poorly defined postreceptor defect. Glucagon levels are high and cannot be suppressed with insulin. Patients are not ketosis-prone; however, they are susceptible to nonketotic, hyperosmolar coma.

Diabetes is genetically heterogeneous, and low rates of vertical transmission make it difficult to discern the mechanisms of inheritance. The variable expressivity of Type I diabetes in identical twins suggests the necessity of an interaction between genetic and environmental factors. For example, patients with certain human lymphocyte antigens (HLA) (coded on chromosome 6) may be more susceptible to viral-mediated beta cell injury.

Autoimmunity is also thought to play a role in the etiology of diabetes because islet cell antibodies are frequently present at diagnosis. There are no known HLA relationships with Type II diabetes, yet speculation has focused on chromosome 11, which bears the structural gene for insulin. Extra DNA in the chromosome 11 of Type II diabetics has been found by some but not all laboratories. The presence of this extra DNA suggests the possibility of using this as a marker for Type II disease.

Although diabetes with pregnancy was uncommonly encountered during the preinsulin era, pregnant diabetic patients now account for 1% to 2% of most reported pregnancies. However, most reports emanate from referral centers where complicated cases are concentrated and therefore may not reflect true incidence. The occurrence rate is more likely one in 300 to 400 pregnancies in the United States.

During the preinsulin era, maternal mortality approached 30% and perinatal mortality was 50% to 70%. Fortunately, maternal mortality is now rare and perinatal mortality has fallen to near 5%. To discuss detection and management of diabetes mellitus one must know the classifications of diabetes (see below), the effects of pregnancy on diabetes, and the effects of diabetes on pregnancy.

CLASSIFICATION

Despite the clarity and simplicity of the NDDG classification described above, most obstetricians prefer to use the Priscilla White classification introduced in 1948. This is because it has been widely tested by years of experience and because it has considerable prognostic value (Table 24-1). A modified version of the White classification follows:

Class A Fasting glucose normal with two abnormal values on 3-hr glucose tolerance test

Class B Onset of clinical diabetes after age 20 (duration less than 10 years) or fasting glucose exceeding normal level

Class C Onset of clinical diabetes between the ages of 10 and 19 with duration of 10 to 19 years; no x-ray evidence of vascular disease

Class D Onset of clinical diabetes before the age of 10, or duration of 20 or more years; x-ray evidence of vascular disease in the legs (pelvic arteriosclerosis excluded); retinal changes on funduscopy

Class E Onset of clinical diabetes before the age of 10, or duration of 20 or more years; x-ray evidence of vascular disease in the legs (pelvic arteriosclerosis by x-ray examination); retinal changes on funduscopy

Class F Renal disease

Class R Proliferative retinopathy

Class H Coronary artery disease

Class T Renal transplant

EFFECTS OF PREGNANCY ON DIABETES MELLITUS

Factors of pregnancy interfering with diabetic control and thus enhancing chances of ketoacidosis include the following:

1. Nausea and vomiting of early pregnancy
2. Alterations in carbohydrate tolerance
3. Lowered renal threshold for glucose
4. Increased energy requirement, particularly during labor
5. Anesthesia and possibly cesarean section

The only untoward long-term effect known is worsening of diabetic retinitis during pregnancy resulting in compromise of vision.

Because of increases in the contrainsulin factors (human placental lactogen, estrogen, progesterone, cortisol, and perhaps others) more insulin is usually required during pregnancy. Complicated physiologic interactions make insulin requirements vary so that close observation is necessary. After delivery, about two thirds of the prepregnancy insulin dose is given; however, changes in hormonal status, lactation, diet, and possibly infection may affect insulin needs.

EFFECTS OF DIABETES MELLITUS ON PREGNANCY

Diabetes mellitus exerts many adverse effects on pregnancy. Included are the following:

1. Abortion and infertility—a threefold increase in the abortion rate of insulin-dependent diabetics with a higher incidence of infertility
2. Congenital anomalies—a threefold increase in congenital anomalies among infants born to insulin-dependent diabetics (a 5% to 10% incidence)
3. Increased complication of pregnancy
   a. Hypertensive states of pregnancy—some form develops in approximately 10% to 20% of pregnant diabetics
   b. Polyhydramnios—tenfold increase over nondiabetics
   c. Intrauterine growth retardation—more likely to occur in more severe cases and long-term diabetic
   d. Premature labor and delivery—more likely to occur in the pregnant diabetic with vascular disease
4. Fetal death in utero—most often occurs late in pregnancy and is likely attributable to relative uteroplacental insufficiency
5. Excessive-sized infants (macrosomia)—may be related to imprecise diabetic control, but not all studies confirm this impression; as a consequence of excessive size of the perinate the diabetic mother and baby are at greater risk of the following:
   a. Dystocia
   b. Lacerations
   c. Birth injuries
   d. Cesarean sections
6. Increased neonatal morbidity and mortality because of increased incidence of the following:

Table 24-1. Trends of course of pregnancy by class

Class	A	B	C	D	E	F (Nephropathy)	R (Retinopathy)
Spontaneous abortion rate	N	N	N	+	+++	++++	++++
Hydramnios degree	+	++++	+++	++	++	±	±
Excessive maternal weight gain	+	++++	+++	++	++	0	0
Toxemia (i.e., preeclampsia)	+	++++	+++	++	++	?	Superimposed?
Large placenta	++++	++++	+++	++	+	0	0
Heavy birth weight infant	++++	++++	+++	++	+	0	0
Intrauterine fetal loss	+	++	+	+++	++++	++++	++++
Intrapartum fetal loss	++++	++++	++	+	+	+	+
Neonatal fetal loss	+	++	++	+++	++++	++++	++++
Congenital anomalies	+	+	+	+	+	+	+
Diabetes mellitus intensification	+	++++	+++	+	+	±	+

Modified from White, P.: Med. Clin. North Am. 49:1015, 1965.

    a. Respiratory distress syndrome (25% to 30%)
    b. Hyperbilirubinemia (5% to 40%)
    c. Hypoglycemia (10% to 25%)
    d. Hypocalcemia (25%)
    e. Polycythemia
    f. Renal vein thrombosis
    g. Cardiomyopathy

Table 24-1 details the most common pregnancy complications according to the classification of diabetes. This information is helpful in counseling patients concerning the relative risks of complications they may encounter.

DETECTION OF DIABETES

Since pregnancy enhances propensity for development of diabetes mellitus, it is a propitious time for screening and detection. However, the usual symptoms may not be appreciated in pregnancy, for most pregnant women experience some excessive thirst, hunger, and polyuria and possibly exhibit occasional glycosuria after heavy glucose meals. Although it may not be possible to screen all pregnant women, screening should be used for at least the following criteria:

1. History
   a. Familial diabetes
   b. Previous large baby (weighing 4,000 gm or more)
   c. Habitual abortion
   d. Previous infant with multiple congenital anomalies
   e. Unexplained stillbirths and neonatal deaths
2. Physical examination
   a. Uterus disproportionate for dates (usually larger than expected)
   b. Polyhydramnios
   c. Massive obesity (20% or more heavier than expected for height)
   d. Excessive weight gain with pregnancy
   e. Hypertensive states of pregnancy
   f. Refractory or recurrent candidal vaginitis
   g. Retinopathy
   h. Neurologic disorders
   i. Impairment of renal function
   j. Unexplained vascular disturbances
3. Laboratory
   a. Glycosuria
      Differential diagnoses of sugar in urine during course of pregnancy include lactosuria, low renal threshold for glucose, and diabetes mellitus
   b. Detection by ultrasonography of disproportionate growth for gestation
   c. Refractory or recurrent urinary infections

Screening method

The screening procedure is a blood (or plasma) glucose determination:
1. Fasting—greater than 100 mg/100 ml is suggestive.
2. Two-hour postprandial—positive if

greater than 140 mg/100 ml; 110 to 140 mg/100 ml is suggestive and merits investigation.
3. Study at less than 20 weeks and repeat at 28 to 32 weeks if first test is negative.

This glucose screening must be used in conjunction with the glucose tolerance test if the diagnosis is to be established. Table 24-2 details useful oral glucose tolerance testing limits. However, if the patient's fasting blood glucose determination exceeds 200 mg/100 ml, a glucose tolerance test will be unnecessary and may even be harmful (threat of diabetic coma).

Prerequisites for accurate testing include:
1. 300 gm of carbohydrate in diet for 3 days preceding test
2. Overnight fast prior to test
3. After fasting sample is obtained, administration of 100 gm liquid glucose solution

It is widely accepted that the patient has diabetes mellitus if two or more of the values obtained from this standard 3-hour glucose tolerance test are abnormal. Some authors advocate an intravenous test to obviate the effect of pregnancy on diabetes (slowing absorption of glucose) and because vomiting may occur with an oral test. A fasting plasma glucose determination is made and samples are taken at 20, 30, 40, and 50 minutes after IV administration of 25 gm glucose. The rate of disappearance (k) in %/min is obtained by plotting the values against time on semilogarithmic tables and dividing the time required for the glucose level to fall 50% (T 1/2) into 69.3. Values (k) less than 1.2%/min are known to be more than 2 standard deviations from the mean normal level of 2.1%/min and are considered abnormal.

MANAGEMENT

Care of the pregnant patient must be a team effort with emphasis on patient education, frequent evaluation, attention to detail, individualization of therapy, and continuity of care. Issues in management that arise include control of diabetes, treatment of complications, maternal evaluation, fetal/placental evaluation, and timing for delivery. Goals of management are to:
1. Decrease fetal morbidity and mortality
2. Protect and enhance maternal well-being
3. Maintain fasting blood sugars at 110 mg/100 ml
4. Keep all random blood sugars at 150 mg/100 ml
5. Avoid hypoglycemia
6. Avoid hyperglycemia and ketoacidosis
7. Utilize outpatient management for majority of pregnancy

Control of diabetes
DIET

Although rigid control is necessary for beneficial outcome, extreme dietary restriction, ketosis, and excessive weight gain (over 26 lb) should all be avoided during the course of pregnancy. Even in the obese diabetic, weight loss or severe caloric restriction should be discarded in favor of a controlled weight gain of 20 to 30 lb.

The usual diabetic diet is as follows:

Calories	30 to 35 kcal/kg/day
Carbohydrate	40% to 45% of calories (minimum of 200 gm)
Protein	2 gm/kg/day (100 to 120 gm)
Fat	Remainder of calories (45 to 60 gm)

Slowly digested and absorbed complex carbohydrates (potatoes, bread, beans, and noodle products) are recommended because the blood glucose rises to lower levels, but for a more sustained interval. Concentrated sweets (table sugar, ice cream, pastries, and candies) should be avoided because they are absorbed rapidly and result in greater increments of blood glu-

Table 24-2. Upper limits of normal blood glucose values for detection of diabetes in pregnancy

	Whole blood glucose	Plasma glucose
Screening tests		
Fasting	90 mg/100 ml	105 mg/100 ml
50 gm oral glucose, 1 hr	130 mg/100 ml	150 mg/100 ml
100 gm oral glucose, 2 hr	120 mg/100 ml	140 mg/100 ml
Oral glucose tolerance test		
Fasting	90 mg/100 ml	105 mg/100 ml
1 hr	165 mg/100 ml	190 mg/100 ml
2 hr	145 mg/100 ml	165 mg/100 ml
3 hr	125 mg/100 ml	145 mg/100 ml

cose. Regularity of intake (both time and content) is imperative for reduction of both insulin reactions and hypoglycemia. Total calories should be divided as follows: breakfast, 2/7; lunch, 2/7; dinner, 2/7; and bedtime snack 1/7.

INSULIN GUIDELINES

1. Oral agents should be avoided because of possible teratogenic effects.
2. Insulin requirements may fall one third below prepregnancy needs during first half of pregnancy.
3. Requirements during second half of pregnancy may rise to as much as double prepregnancy needs, and the need for an increase of one U/wk may occur in late pregnancy.
4. Splitting the insulin dose into morning and evening segments given approximately 12 hours apart, the first before breakfast, in 2:1 and 1:1 distributions of intermediate: short-acting insulin permits control superior to that gained with a single dose regimen.
5. Approximating the normal excursion of plasma glucose is ideal (e.g., fasting—less than 90 mg/100 ml, 1 hour postprandial—less than 120 mg/100 ml); however, this goal is unrealistic for many patients. Moreover, some authors have found that moderate control may be as good as tight control. Currently most believe that maintenance of blood glucose levels less than 110 mg/100 ml may reduce perinatal mortality and morbidity, particularly macrosomia with its problem of delivery and increased chance of neonatal hypoglycemia.
6. Home glucose monitoring, after appropriate education, is helpful in adjusting insulin dose to attain this control.
7. Care should be taken to avoid glucose levels below 60 mg/100 ml.
8. Use of insulin in Class A diabetics is controversial. Some believe all Class A diabetics will profit (primarily by having infants of weights closer to normal) if they are empirically started on insulin. Others believe Class A diabetics should have insulin only if their diabetes is not well controlled by diet or if they have previously had a macrosomic infant.
9. When delivery is anticipated cover calorie needs with D5NS at a rate of 100 to 150 ml per hour by infusion. About half of patients require no insulin during labor. If blood sugar exceeds 150 mg/100 ml, decrease level with subcutaneous injections of regular insulin every 4 hours, constant insulin infusion, or addition of 10 to 15 units of regular insulin to each liter of intravenous fluid. Studies with use of the "artificial pancreas" (Biostator), have shown no insulin requirement during the first stage of labor when the glucose infusion rate was constant at 2.55 mg/kg/min.

Treatment of ketoacidosis

Patients with ketoacidosis require intensive team care with monitoring of vital signs, insulin, and intravenous fluids, and serial determinations of blood glucose levels, arterial pH, serum electrolytes, and blood ketones.

Maternal evaluation

Most women with complicated diabetes mellitus in pregnancy require hospitalization. In more severe classifications cardiac and kidney function (including the possibility of urinary infection) should be studied. Special concerns include the following:

1. Because of unfavorable influences on diabetic complications interruption of pregnancy may be considered an option. Certainly sterilization may be warranted in proliferative retinopathy or nephropathy.
2. Emotional distress may cause a change in insulin requirement.
3. Development of toxemia, acidosis, or infection is especially dangerous.
4. Maternal evaluation in the case of a Class A diabetic may be no more complex than including an SMA-12 in the regular prenatal evaluation. However, in Classes B through R evaluation includes SMA-6 and -12, 24-hour urine for creatinine clearance and total protein, urine culture, ECG, chest x-ray examination, serial ultrasonic scans, ophthalmologic examination, and determination of urine threshold for glycosuria.
5. Hospitalization must be used liberally for education, treatment of complications, stabilization, and occasionally for control.
6. The schedule of visits will be predicated by the patient's status, previous reproduc-

tive history, diabetic classification, and other considerations. Thus a plan must be individualized for each patient.
7. The use of hemoglobin A_1C, which initially was promising, has not proved to be of great value in management of diabetes.

Timing of delivery in relation to fetal and placental evaluation
(see Chapter 4)

1. Ultrasonic scan should be used
   a. At less than 20 weeks for detection of fetal anomalies, multiple pregnancy, and placental placement
   b. Serially (every 4 weeks) for fetal growth determinations and detection of hydramnios, fetal edema, and placental enlargement
2. Fetal activity acceleration determination or other biometric testing is recommended to ensure fetal well-being. Testing in classes B through R should be done twice weekly, starting at 32 weeks, or in the case of a prior fetal loss, at least two weeks prior to the time of gestation at which the previous loss occurred. If there is any question about whether values for the less invasive tests are normal, an oxytocin challenge test may be performed. If this, too, is abnormal, perform physiologic maturity testing and consider expeditious delivery.
3. With class A diabetics, studies remain normal, delivery is accomplished when fetus is mature, but not delayed once term has been reached.
4. Complicated class A and classes B through F are most frequently delivered after 37 weeks' gestation, but well before term.
5. Exact timing for delivery is usually determined by physiologic maturity testing of amniotic fluid. However, it should be kept in mind that a more mature L/S ratio is necessary and more PG must be present to afford the same assurance that pulmonary maturity has been reached in infants of the diabetic than in infants of the nondiabetic patient.
6. An elective cesarean section is indicated if:
   a. Vertex if floating
   b. Breech is presenting
   c. Fetal weight is estimated at over 4,000 gm
   d. Complications ensue

Indications for delivery
1. Gestation at or greater than 38 weeks, L/S ratio of 2.5 or more, PG present, and cervix favorable
2. Positive CST
3. Macrosomia (estimated fetal weight of 4,000 gm or more) with lung maturity

Delivery
1. If progress is minimal after 8-hour trial of labor perform cesarean section. (This policy should result in at least a 50% vaginal delivery rate.)
2. Base insulin dose on blood sugar determinations. One-half of patients require no insulin during labor.
3. Infuse D5½NS IV at 125 ml/hr.
4. Coordinate carefully with neonatologists to ensure proper delivery room care of newborn.

Examples of management
Because management for many diabetic patients is complex, examples of typical management are provided.

CLASS A DIABETES
1. Start patient on ADA diet.
2. Obtain double-voided morning urine daily.
3. In addition to usual prenatal laboratory work, obtain an SMA-12.
4. Schedule visits for every 2 weeks until 34 weeks, then weekly.
5. Obtain blood sugar determinations at different times each week.
6. If blood sugars exceed limits noted above or fasting blood sugar is 110 mg/100 ml twice, there is preeclampsia, or mother had previous stillbirth, manage as Class B diabetic.
7. Obtain two ultrasonic scans 4 weeks apart between 16 and 28 weeks.
8. Start NST twice weekly at 38 weeks.
9. Deliver at or near term gestation.
10. Consider using insulin (controversial).
11. If patient spills acetone, increase caloric intake (once hyperglycemia has been ruled out).

CLASSES B THROUGH R DIABETES
1. Consider hospitalization or extensive outpatient evaluation as soon as diagnosis is made.

II. Accurately determine gestational age as early in pregnancy as possible.
III. Obtain baseline laboratory work (in addition to usual prenatal studies) as noted above.
IV. Start patient on ADA diet with the following instructions:
   A. Include 30 to 35 kcal/kg of actual body weight.
   B. Do not exceed 2,600 calories or go below 1,800 calories daily.
   C. Distribute total daily calories between breakfast 2/7, lunch 2/7, dinner 2/7, and a bedtime snack 1/7.
   D. Diet of
      1. 45% to 50% carbohydrate
      2. 30% to 35% fat
      3. 20% to 25% protein
V. Use NPH and regular insulin.
VI. If patient uses more than 40 U/day, split dose as follows:
   A. Give two thirds of dose in morning (before breakfast) and one third of dose approximately 12 hours later.
   B. Give NPH: Regular mix of 2:1 in morning dose and 1:1 in evening dose.
VII. Teach patient to use one of several home glucose testing methods (from finger stick) and to test glucose levels at home once a day on the following schedule: 7 AM, 11 AM, 4 PM, and 9 PM. Have her record these and bring the glucose record at each clinic visit. Have her call if levels are 150 mg/100 ml or higher or 60 mg/100 ml or lower.
VIII. See patient at least every 2 weeks until 30 weeks, then weekly with periodic fasting blood sugar and 2-hour postprandial blood sugar determinations, and Hemoglobin A_1C based on severity of patient's condition.
IX. Perform antepartum fetal surveillance as noted above:
   A. Ultrasonic scans
      1. As early in pregnancy as practical
      2. Every 4 to 6 weeks to follow fetal growth
   B. NST twice weekly started at 32 weeks If NST is not reactive do CST. If CST is positive, consider delivery. If negative, repeat NST the next day.
   C. Amniocentesis at 38 weeks (or earlier in complicated cases) for L/S ratio, PG, and creatinine
X. Deliver according to protocol noted above.
XI. Provide continuity between birth room and neonatal care.

BIBLIOGRAPHY

Burrow, G.N., and Ferris, T.F: Medical complications of pregnancy Philadelphia, 1982, W.B. Saunders Co.

Cousins, L., Rigg, L., Hollingsworth, D., et al.: The 24-hour excursion and diurnal rhythm of glucose, insulin, and c-peptide in normal pregnancy, Am. J. Obstet. Gynecol. **136**:413, 1980.

Coustan, D.R., Berkowitz, R.L., and Hobbins, J.C.: Tight metabolic control of overt diabetes in pregnancy, Am. J. Med. **68**:845, 1980.

Gabbe, S.G.: Application of scientific rationale in the management of the pregnancy diabetic patient, Semin. Perinatol. **2**:361, 1978.

Gabbe, S.G., Mestman, J.H., Freeman, R.K., et al.: Management and outcome of diabetes mellitus, classes B to R, Am. J. Obstet. Gynecol. **129**:723, 1977.

Golde, S.H., Good-Anderson, B., Montero, M. et al.: Insulin requirements during labor: reappraisal, Am. J. Obstet. Gynecol. **144**:556, 1982.

Jovanovic, L., and Peterson, C.M.: Insulin and glucose requirements during the first stage of labor in insulin dependent diabetic women, Am. J. Med. **75**:607, 1983.

Jovanovic, L., Druzin, M., and Peterson, C.M.: Effect of euglycemia on the outcome of pregnancy in insulin dependent diabetic women as compared with normal control subjects, Am. J. Med. **71**:921, 1981.

Kreisberg, R.A.: Diabetic ketoacidosis: new concepts and trends in pathogenesis and treatment, Am. Intern. Med. **88**:681, 1978.

Kulovich, M.V., and Gluck, L.: The lung profile. II. Complicated pregnancy, Am. J. Obstet. Gynecol. **135**:64, 1979.

Leveno, K.J., Hauth, J.C., Gilstrup, L.C., et al.: appraisal of "rigid" blood glucose control during pregnancy in the overtly diabetic woman, Am. J. Obstet. Gynecol. **135**:853, 1979.

Merkatz, I.R., and Adam, P.A.J.: Diabetes in pregnancy, Semin. Perinatol. **2**:287, 1978.

Miller, E., Hare, J.W., Cloherty, J.P., et al.: Elevated maternal hemoglobin A_{1c} in early pregnancy and major congenital anomalies in infants of diabetic mothers, N. Engl. J. Med. **304**:1331, 1981.

Rigg, L., Cousins, L., Hollingsworth, D., et al.: Effects of exogenous insulin on excursions and diurnal rhythm of plasma glucose in pregnant diabetic patients with and without residual B-cell function, Am. J. Obstet. Gynecol. **136**:537, 1980.

Spellacy, W.N., Buhi, W.C., Cohn, J.E., et al.: Usefulness of rapid blood glucose measurements in obstetrics: Dextrostix/reflectance meter system, Obstet. Gynecol. **41**:299, 1973.

25

Infections of the perinate

Neonatal morbidity and mortality from acquired infection exceed morbidity and mortality from all other causes after the first few days of life. The inability of macroglobulin IgM* to be transmitted across the placenta, its lag in reaching optimum levels after birth, and less efficient phagocytosis, undernutrition, and frequent immaturity render the small infant particularly susceptible to invasion by microorganisms. Special precautions for preventing infection, as well as prompt recognition when it occurs, are necessary for optimal management of the infant of low birth weight. Any change in behavior suggesting infection is an indication for treatment with antibiotics after diagnostic procedures have been undertaken. The important task of identifying noninfected infants and avoiding or discontinuing antibiotic therapy when it is not warranted is often overlooked.

PERIOD OF EXPOSURE

I. Infections acquired in utero
   A. Placentally transferred organisms, usually viruses (e.g., rubella), pass directly across the placenta to the fetus.
   B. In ascending infection, microorganisms pass through the cervix, with entry into the amnion encouraged by long labor and premature and prolonged rupture of membranes (Chapter 18). The route of fetal infection is through the respiratory or gastrointestinal tract.

II. Infections acquired during delivery
   A. Generalized infections in which the pathways again are principally the upper airway and gastrointestinal tract
      1. Flora of the maternal genital tract such as group B streptococci
      2. Pathogenic organisms occasionally harbored in the intestinal tract of the mother (e.g., *Listeria monocytogenes, Salmonella* and *Shigella* organisms, *Escherichia coli,* and enteroviruses)
      3. Herpesvirus from maternal genital tract lesions
   B. Local infections
      1. Conjunctiva
         a. Gonococcus infection (profuse purulent discharge by 2 to 4 days of age)
         b. Inclusion conjunctivitis (serosanguineous to yellow-whitish discharge at approximately 1 week)
      2. Oral cavity
         a. Thrush caused by the yeast *Candida albicans*
III. Infections acquired during resuscitation, usually caused by bacteria (e.g., staphylococci and *Diplococcus pneumoniae*) because of contamination from placement of indwelling catheters or endotracheal tubes
IV. Infections from within the nursery by organisms frequently inhabiting the area (e.g., coagulase-negative staphylococci or *Klebsiella-Enterobacter* organisms)
   These infections may be transferred by hands of personnel or spread from contaminated equipment or incubators. The

---

*Although the newborn have a paucity of IgM and bacterial antibodies to gram-negative organisms, they have a surprising resistance to invasion by these organisms.

umbilicus is a receptive site for cutaneous infection leading to sepsis.

BACTERIAL SEPTICEMIA AND OTHER SEVERE INFECTIONS

Sepsis in the neonate can be only suspected prior to the report of a positive blood culture. Treatment delayed for this information may be too late. The newborn's defenses are easily overwhelmed, particularly in the preterm infant because of decreased opsonins in the plasma, reduced level of maternal IgG transferred through the placenta, and lessened efficiency of white blood cell function. There is increasing incidence of bacterial infections in infants at risk because of the general use of invasive techniques in their care and treatment.

Clinical signs suggestive of sepsis or other major infections

1. Change in behavior (i.e., inactivity or irritability)
2. Temperature irregularity
3. Sudden onset of inappropriate apnea
   a. Larger preterm and term infants who show unexpected apnea on the first day of life
   b. Smaller infants who have done well but develop apnea after the first week of life
4. Abdominal distention with decreased tolerance to feedings
5. Evidence of shock (i.e., tachycardia, hypotension, pallor, metabolic acidosis)
6. Intensification of jaundice
7. Increase in rate of respiration with effort in breathing after 24 hours of age, suggesting pneumonia
8. Diarrhea, distention, and shock, suggesting epidemic diarrhea of the newborn
9. Irritability (later seizures), with full fontanel or cranial suture spread, suggesting meningitis

Laboratory aids in determining severe infection

1. Blood smear
   In healthy infants a dramatic rise in total white blood count occurs in first 15 hours of life. With early infection there is a reversal of the normal rise in the neutrophil count. Counts per cubic millimeter that suggest infection are as follows:
   a. First 24 hr: WBC less than 9,000
      Neutrophils less than 4,500
      Absolute bands greater than 1,400
      Ratio of immature to total neutrophils greater than .15
      Platelets less than 100,000
   b. After 4 days: WBC greater than 20,000 or less than 5,000
      Neutrophils greater than 4,500 or less than 1,400
      Bands greater than 500
      Ratio of immature to total neutrophils greater than .12
      Platelets less than 100,000
2. Gastric aspirate
   A single predominant species on smear in addition to an increase in white blood cells may indicate infection.
3. Urine (specimen obtained by suprapubic tap)
   Infection suggested by
   a. Over two white blood cells per low-power field
   b. One or more bacteria per oil-immersion field
4. Spinal fluid examination
   Meningitis suggested by
   a. More than 10 white blood cells/mm^3 (in severe cases, may rise to over 500 white blood cells/mm^3)
   b. Glucose less than 20 mg/100 ml and less than half that of blood glucose level
   c. Evidence of organisms on Gram's stain
5. Chest x-ray film for evidence of infiltrate for consideration of pneumonia
6. Sudden glucosuria and hyperglycemia

Diagnosis

Diagnosis depends on specific organisms growing in cultures of blood, spinal fluid, urine, or stool. Dominant organism grown from umbilicus, nasopharynx, or gastric contents may or may not indicate a specific cause of infection.

Management of bacterial infection

1. Treatment for suspected infection
   a. Begin administering gentamicin and penicillin or ampicillin promptly—a few hours' delay can be fatal.
   b. For infections acquired in a nursery with

a high percentage of resistant organisms, treatment with agents such as cefotaxime should be considered.
   c. Reduce or eliminate oral feedings and give parenteral infusion of fluids, calories, and electrolytes (Chapter 15).
   d. Support infant for shock or respiratory failure if needed.
2. Interpretation of cultures
   a. If cultures are negative, discontinue antibiotics unless signs of possible infection persist.
   b. If blood culture is positive, continue treatment for 10 to 14 days with proper antibiotic agent; treat urinary tract infection or meningitis for a minimum of 2 weeks.
3. Antibiotic drug dosage (Table 25-1)
   Use the higher dosage in meningitis. In preterm infants (and to a lesser extent in those more mature and older) detoxifying enzymes are deficient, and renal function is relatively inefficient. When good urinary excretion is absent even very small doses of some drugs may cause serious reactions. Knowledge of the metabolic fate and prin-

Table 25-1. Antibiotic therapy

Drug	Dose	Indication	Comments
Amphotericin	Test dose 0.1 mg/kg on day 1; increase by 0.1 mg/kg increments to 0.5-1.0 mg/kg/day. Infuse slowly IV over several hours (maximum IV concentration 0.1 mg/ml)	Systemic yeast and fungus infections	Nephrotoxic
Ampicillin	50-100 mg/kg/12 hr for infants <7 days; every 8 hr for infants >7 days; every 6 hr for infants >28 days (IV, IM)	Most gram-positive and gram-negative organisms, *Salmonella, Haemophilus influenzae, Streptococcus faecalis, E. coli,* etc.	
Cefotaxime	50 mg/kg/12 hr for infants <7 days; every 8 hr for infants >7 days (IV)	Most gram-positive and gram-negative organisms	
Gentamicin	*Infants >34 weeks' gestation:* 2.5 mg/kg/12 hr for infants <7 days; every 8 hr for infants >7 days *Infants 28-34 weeks' gestation:* 2.5 mg/kg/18 hr for infants <14 days; 2.5 mg/kg/8 hr for infants >14 days *Infants <28 weeks' gestation:* 2.5 mg/kg/24 hr for infants <14 days; 2.5 mg/kg/12 hr for infants 14-28 days; 2.5 mg/kg/8 hr for infants >28 days (IM or slow IV infusion)	*E. coli, Klebsiella, Enterobacter, Pseudomonas, Proteus*	Nephrotoxic, ototoxic; pharmacokinetic studies recommended when therapy is prolonged
Methicillin	25-50 mg/kg/12 hr for infants <7 days; 25-50 mg/kg every 6 to 8 hr for older infants (IV)	Penicillinase-resistant staphylococci	Nephrotoxic, elevates SGOT, suppresses bone marrow
Nystatin	200,000 units, divided into 4 doses daily (by mouth only)	Oral candidal infection	
Penicillin G	25,000-50,000 U/kg/12 hr for infants <7 days; 25,000-50,000 U/kg every 6 to 8 hr for older infants	Hemolytic streptococci, pneumococci, and some strains of staphylococci	
Vancomycin	15 mg/kg/12 hr for infants <7 days; 15 mg/kg/8 hr for older infants (slow IV infusion over 30-60 min)	Coagulase-negative staphylococci	Nephrotoxic; pharmacokinetic studies recommended

cipal route of excretion is important for estimation of an effective and safe dosage.

MINOR INFECTIONS

1. Pustules, abscesses, and local infections
   a. Open any collection of pus. Make a culture, smear, and Gram's stain of the fluid.
   b. Clean site with alcohol, and expose it to air.
   c. For lesions caused by coagulase-positive staphylococci, sponge area daily with pHisoHex and follow with thorough washing with water.
   d. Segregate infant and observe strict handwashing care.
   e. Isolate babies with multiple infections.
2. Eye discharges
   Eye discharges occur in many healthy premature infants during their nursery course. Prompt and vigorous treatment of pathologic causes is important because the eye may be destroyed or septicemia may occur.
   a. Make a smear and culture of the discharge.
   b. Cleanse the eye and instill broad-spectrum antibiotics every 2 hours (e.g., Neosporin ophthalmic solution, 1 drop in each eye every 2 to 3 hours).
   c. Treat gonorrheal ophthalmia by parenteral penicillin unless organism is penicillin-resistant.
   d. Administer erythromycin locally for inclusion conjunctivitis (intracellular inclusions identified from conjunctival scrapings).
3. Thrush and other candidal infections
   a. Instill nystatin (Mycostatin) in the infant's mouth after feedings for oral mucous membrane involvement.
   b. Apply 1% aqueous gentian violet twice daily when skin surfaces are involved. Gentian violet may also be applied to the buccal cavity.

INFECTIONS WITH GROUP B BETA-HEMOLYTIC STREPTOCOCCI

Group B streptococcal infections are now the leading cause of early neonatal septicemia, surpassing the previously dominant *Escherichia coli*. The organism can be cultured from the vagina of up to 25% of pregnant women and, if present at time of delivery, will be transmitted directly to 40% to 50% of their offspring. The attack rate is low, with an incidence of the disease observed in about 2:1,000 live births. However, mortality ranges between 40% and 75% for these neonates. The attack rate and variations in mortality may depend on the presence or absence of specific type antibody in the mother for transmission to the infant for his protection. Infections of neonates with group B streptococci take two characteristic forms:

I. Early-onset infection from maternal contact is usually attributable to subtype I and appears within 3 days of age and most often within 12 to 24 hours of birth. If initial clinical manifestations are not recognized, survival is unlikely, with a rapid downhill course.
   A. Initial manifestations
      1. Respiratory distress with grunting respiration and cyanosis resembling hyaline membrane disease (present in 90% of cases)
      2. Unexpected early apnea with shock
   B. Associated factors and findings
      1. Premature delivery
      2. Prolonged rupture of membranes with gram-positive cocci on gastric smear
      3. Leukopenia and depressed absolute neutrophil count
      4. X-ray film of chest often showing infiltrates or a picture similar to that seen with hyaline membrane disease
II. Late onset septicemia or meningitis usually occurs at several weeks of age and is most often attributable to subtype III, probably acquired from infant's caretakers. Signs are irritability or lethargy, apnea, failure to nurse, and fever.

Diagnosis

1. Presumptive on basis of gram-positive cocci on bacterial smear of infant's gastric contents, particularly with prolonged membrane rupture
2. Growth of organisms from cultures of blood or cerebrospinal fluid

3. Positive latex agglutination assay (Wellcogen Strep B)

Management

The rapid and overwhelming course of infections due to group B streptococci requires a high degree of suspicion of its early manifestations, prompt diagnostic procedures, and simultaneous introduction of antibiotics (e.g., ampicillin, kanamycin, or gentamicin). In addition, treatment is begun with any two of the associated factors listed above even though the infant appears to be well.

1. Give full critical care support, including maintenance of ventilation and blood pressure.
2. Treat infection with specific antibiotics after appropriate bacterial studies have been done.
3. In cases of suspected or proven infection accompanied by severe neutropenia the use of granulocyte transfusions or exchange transfusions of fresh whole blood may increase survival of infected infants.

VIRAL AND OTHER CONGENITAL INFECTIONS

Recognition and diagnosis of viral infection

1. Factors suggesting viral infection
    a. Small-for-dates infants
    b. Microcephalus and occasionally hydrocephalus
    c. Early jaundice with increased "direct" component of bilirubin
    d. Petechiae, purpura, or vesicular rash
    e. Hepatosplenomegaly, often firm in character
    f. Chorioretinitis, keratitis, conjunctivitis, cataracts, retinopathies, and microphthalmia
    g. Congenital anomalies
    h. Anemia with evidence of hemolysis, thrombocytopenia, disseminated intravascular coagulation (DIC)
2. Diagnosis of viral infection
    a. Obtain history of illness in gravida.
    b. Perform hematocrit, platelet, and reticulocyte counts and fractionation of bilirubin.
    c. Take direct cultures of throat, urine, stool, cerebrospinal fluid, and vesicular fluid (herpesvirus).
    d. Obtain urine specimen for cytology in suspected cases of cytomegalovirus infection.
    e. Perform IgM determination—over 25 mg/100 ml suggests active viral disease.
    f. Test for neutralizing hemagglutinin inhibition and complement-fixing antibodies—repeat test after one month.
    g. Take x-ray films of long bones (rarefactions) and skull (intracranial calcifications).
    h. Perform electrocardiogram for evidence of myocarditis (coxsackie B enterovirus).
    i. Examine retinas for evidence of chorioretinitis or cataracts.

Rubella (German or three-day measles)

Approximately 30% to 50% of fetuses of women who contract rubella during the first 3 months of pregnancy will be adversely affected by the virus. Adequate study of early abortuses might prove involvement to be greater. Whether infants born to women who contract rubella during early pregnancy are obviously defective or not, certainly perinatal mortality is increased, and a high proportion of infants are of low birth weight. In the past, when about 10% of urban and 25% of rural women were not immune to this disease, a substantial number of defective or undersized infants could be expected to be born following rubella epidemics. No correlation apparently exists between severity of maternal rubella and teratogenicity. Fetal damage can occur without obvious illness in the mother. The 1965 rubella epidemic involved many thousands of nonimmune pregnant women and resulted in damage to an extremely large proportion of their offspring during early fetal development.

The rubella virus readily invades the placenta and the fetus during gestation. Viremia during embryogenesis, and perhaps later in pregnancy, may produce signs and symptoms of persistent infection at birth. Appropriate cultures at this time for detection of the rubella virus can prove fetal invasion with or without clinical evidence of disease. Excretion of the virus may persist through the first year despite measurable antibody titer. This continued excretion creates a danger to nonimmunized nursing personnel and babies (Fig. 25-1).

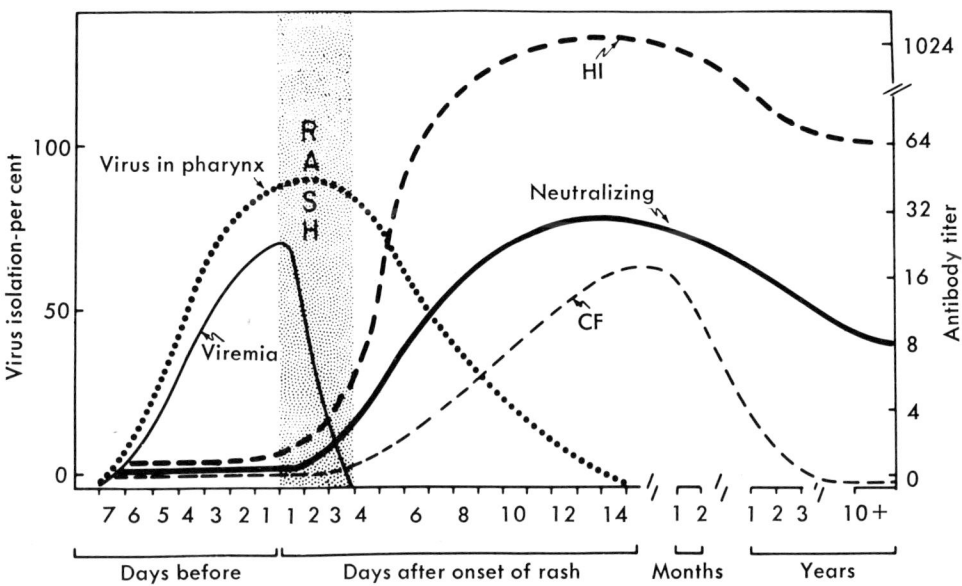

Fig. 25-1. Schematic illustration of the pattern of virus excretion and antibody response during rubella. *HI,* Hemagglutinin-inhibition antibody. *CF,* Complement-fixing antibody. (Modified from Cooper, L.Z., and Krugman, S.: Arch. Ophthalmol. 77:434, 1967.)

I. Diagnosis (after exposure 2 to 3 weeks previously)
   A. In the child or adult, rubella causes no specific lesion but (in order of possible occurrence) it can cause
      1. Low-grade fever and slight malaise that coincide with eruption
      2. Lymphadenopathy (postcervical, postauricular)
      3. Fleeting, fine, maculopapular rash (face to trunk to extremities)
      4. Leukopenia
      5. Occasionally arthropathy or encephalitis, or both
   B. In the neonate *rubella syndrome* is a congenital infection.
      1. Teratogenic effects
         a. Intrauterine growth retardation
         b. Congenital heart disease, hypoplasia of myocardium
         c. Sensorineural deafness (occasional anomalies of the cochlear duct, organ of Corti)
         d. Cataract or glaucoma, or both
         e. Neonatal purpura ("blueberry muffin baby")
         f. Dermatoglyphic abnormalities (unusual fingerprints, palmar creases, skin folds)
      2. Systemic involvement with or without malformation
         a. Adenitis, hepatitis, hepatosplenomegaly, jaundice
         b. Anemia, thrombocytopenia with petechial hemorrhages
         c. Areas of rarefaction in metaphyses of bones and irregularities of the epiphyseal lines of long bones shown by x-ray examination
         d. Encephalitis, meningitis
         e. Myocarditis (ECG changes)
         f. Eye lesions (iridocyclitis, retinopathy)
         g. Pneumonia (interstitial type)
      3. Later effects
         a. Reduced growth, failure to thrive
         b. Multiple physical and behavioral handicaps

When the pregnant woman contracts rubella—confirmed by a rise in hemagglutinin-inhibition (HI) antibody over a

2-week period—during the first trimester, incidence of malformation in the infant is about 35%, 25% when in the second month, and 10% when in the third month. After the fourth month, abnormalities, except for hearing defects, are uncommon. (Congenital rubella has not been implicated as a cause of skeletal defects such as cleft palate, meningomyelocele, or phocomelia.)
II. Laboratory tests
   A. A rapid rubella virus HI test and an IgM fluorescent antibody test are diagnostic.
   B. Culture of the rubella virus from nasopharyngeal washings is possible but difficult.
   C. Leukopenia that is present early may be followed by an increase of plasma cells.
   D. Delayed hypersensitivity reaction with impaired cellular immunity is noted.
III. Treatment for neonate with congenital rubella
   A. Strict isolation for as long as pharyngeal virus shedding or virus excretion in the urine persists
   B. Ophthalmologic consultation to avoid blindness from glaucoma or cataracts
   C. Use of immunized nursery attendants
   D. Multidisciplinary care, since early recognition and treatment of handicaps will improve child's chances of maximal development
IV. Prevention
   A. Live attenuated rubella vaccine is highly effective and usually results in lasting immunity except for later gross exposure in an occasional individual. The vaccine should be given to all children before puberty. A pregnant woman in the immediate family may be a contraindication to use the vaccine because of theoretical teratogenicity of the attenuated virus.
   B. Susceptible females (no HI antibody present) may be purposefully exposed or vaccinated provided they are not pregnant and will not conceive for at least 2 months after inoculation.
   C. Immune serum globulin (gamma globulin) will not prevent rubella. Although it may suppress outward evidence of the disease, the pregnant woman may develop a subclinical rubella with its many congenital complications.
   D. First-trimester therapeutic abortion, when permissible, should be seriously considered in bona fide cases.

Herpes simplex virus infection

Herpesvirus infection in the neonate commonly is acquired by contact with the mother's infected birth canal (usually herpesvirus type 2). Though occasional case reports of intrauterine malformations and congenital infection of the infant have been published, transplacental passage of the virus appears to be infrequent.

The risk of acquisition of the virus by the neonate in a genitally infected mother may be as high as 50%. Approximately 90% of herpesvirus infection in infants is caused by herpesvirus type 2, most likely because of the greater chance of contact, since this virus has a predilection for the genital area.

Incubation period for herpesvirus is apparently between 4 and 21 days.
I. Signs
   Typically in an infection acquired at birth, the infant will be asymptomatic for several days. Then the following may be observed:
   A. Lethargy
   B. Febrile episodes
   C. Mottled skin
   D. Hepatosplenomegaly
   E. Poor feeding
   F. Seizures
   G. Disseminated intravascular coagulation (DIC)
   H. Vesicular lesions on skin and scalp
   In addition to these symptoms, a congenitally infected neonate may demonstrate the following at birth:
   I. Growth retardation
   J. Microcephaly
   K. Intracranial calcifications

L. Microphthalmia
   M. Chorioretinitis
   N. Inclusion bodies in urine
II. Laboratory results commonly observed in herpesvirus infections include the following:
   A. Elevated IgM
   B. Abnormal cerebrospinal fluid values
   C. Abnormal liver function studies
   D. Abnormal coagulation panel compatible with DIC (Chapter 31)
III. Diagnostic aids
   The disease is often difficult to diagnose on basis of clinical symptoms alone unless characteristic skin lesions are visible (small vesicles usually grouped and surrounded by erythema).
   A. Identification of characteristic multinucleated giant cells and intranuclear inclusions visible on a smear obtained from scrapings of vesicles, fixed with alcohol, and stained with Papanicolaou's stain
   B. Isolation of virus from vesicle fluid, throat washing, urine, blood, or cerebrospinal fluid
   Specimen on a swab placed in Leibowitz-Emory transport medium can be shipped to a virus laboratory at room temperature. Other specimens for virus culture must be frozen or stored in dry ice during transport. Typical cytopathic changes are visible on tissue culture within 2 to 9 days.
   C. Diagnosis by serologic assay, that is, inhibition, passive hemagglutination assay, detection of IgM antibodies, or enzyme-linked immunosorbent assay (ELISA)
IV. Management
   Antiviral agents now available include vidarabine (Ara-A) and acyclovir. Their use has shown a low incidence of toxicity and a decrease in mortality and morbidity in infections with herpesvirus.
   Dosage for vidarabine is 15 mg/kg/day administered IV over a 12-hour period for 5 to 10 days. Acyclovir is infused IV over 60 minutes in doses of 5 to 15 mg/kg at 8-hour intervals for 5 to 10 days.
   A. Infants suspected to be infected with herpesvirus or delivered vaginally of a mother with active herpes progenitalis or by cesarean section to a mother with active lesions and rupture of membranes lasting more than 4 hours:
      1. Segregate infant from nursery for duration of hospitalization or a maximum of 21 days (maximum length of incubation period).
      2. Allow mother-infant contact only in infant's own room and under strict isolation procedures (gown and gloves).
      3. Require personnel caring for infant to wear gown and gloves.
   B. Infants delivered by cesarean section of a mother with active herpesvirus whose membranes were not ruptured or ruptured less than 4 hours before birth:
      1. Infant may be kept in nursery after thorough washing.
      2. Mother-infant contact is allowed in mother's room with gown and glove technique.
      3. Mother is not allowed to have contact with other infants.
V. Prognosis
   Mortality for newborns with the disease, whether herpesvirus type 1 or 2, is 50% to 70%. Infants with localized involvement have a better prognosis. Outcome for surviving infants is frequently complicated by abnormal neurologic development.
VI. Prevention
   A. Identify mothers with genital lesions from herpesvirus before delivery by taking cultures in suspect cases.
   B. Deliver infants of mothers with positive cultures from genital lesions by cesarean section to avoid inoculation. (Cesarean section within 4 hours after rupture of membranes probably is warranted.)
   C. Prohibit contact with any neonate by personnel with active herpetic lesions.

Cytomegalovirus infection

The cytomegalovirus (CMV), by far the most common among those known to cause congenital infections, is reported to occur in 1% to 2% of all pregnancies in the United States. In contrast to other infectious agents, such as rubella, this virus can infect the fetus despite maternal immunity, although maternal immunity seems to lessen severity of infection in the fetus. Primary maternal infection with CMV carries a 50% risk of vertical transmission to the offspring with a greater chance of symptoms at birth and long-term handicap of the child.

1. Signs (at or within 24 hours of birth)
   a. Jaundice
   b. Hemolytic anemia
   c. Thrombocytopenia with generalized petechiae
   d. Hepatosplenomegaly
   e. Central nervous system disease (including cerebral calcification)
   f. Chorioretinitis
   g. Retarded growth
2. Diagnostic aids
   a. Immunofluorescence (IgM)
   b. Specific intracellular inclusion bodies
      An "owl-eye" halo appearance in the shed epithelial cells of a urine concentrate stained with hematoxylin-eosin may be seen. The saliva may also contain these cells. Pleocytosis is not uncommon in spinal fluid, in which similar inclusion bodies may also be found.
   c. Rising antibody titers
   d. Virus isolation from urine, throat, or cerebrospinal fluid
3. Treatment
   No effective prophylactic or therapeutic measures have been discovered.
   a. Give symptomatic, supportive treatment.
   b. Ensure parental support.
   c. Isolate infant while in nursery and avoid his or her contact with pregnant women until virus excretion ceases.
4. Prognosis
   Mortality from cytomegalovirus infection is relatively low (less than 10%), especially in those infants who are asymptomatic at birth. Although earlier reports suggest a high incidence of handicaps in survivors, more recent studies have shown a more favorable prognosis. Sensorineural hearing loss was observed in approximately 10% to 15% of children with congenital CMV infections, but there was a paucity of other developmental handicaps. The differences in outcomes of the various studies may be explained by differences in populations studied (i.e., differences in degree of infection in infants, in socioeconomic backgrounds of mothers, etc.). More information is needed to better delineate risk to the perinate.
5. Prevention
   Development of a cytomegalovirus vaccine now under investigation offers hope for prevention of the potentially devastating effects of a primary CMV infection in pregnant women.

Syphilis

Pregnancy complicated by untreated early syphilis is a major cause of midtrimester abortion, fetal death in utero, or premature labor and delivery the world over. Whether the neonate will show stigmas of congenital syphilis depends on when the mother contracts the disease. If infection occurred less than 1 to 2 years prior to the conception, the fetus probably will be seriously affected. When onset of the disease coincides with conception or is very early in pregnancy, a deformed, congenitally afflicted, and premature infant probably will eventuate. Whether a woman who contracts syphilis during the second half of a pregnancy will deliver a diseased offspring or one that is unaffected has not been determined.

A serologic test for syphilis such as the Rapid Plasma Reagin (RPR) at the first obstetric visit is essential for identification of the syphilitic mother. The symptoms of syphilis may be unnoticed during pregnancy; even the secondary nonpruritic rash may be insignificant. Tertiary syphilis rarely complicates pregnancy.

The severity of untreated early syphilis is diminished by pregnancy in many women. Gestation will not modify relapses after insufficient treatment, however, nor will it alter late syphilis.

I. Signs
   Congenital syphilis in the neonate can present a major diagnostic problem. Clinical findings are frequently absent. A

primary stage is absent, since *Treponema pallidum* is introduced directly into the fetal circulation.
  A. Early stage (under 2 years of age)
    1. Vesicular bullous cutaneous lesions
    2. Mucous membrane lesions (affected nose and pharynx produce "snuffles")
    3. Osteochondritis
    4. Hepatosplenomegaly
    5. Hemolytic anemia
    6. Abnormal cerebrospinal fluid findings (up to 50% of infants)
  B. Late congenital syphilis (over 2 years of age)
    In the majority of cases disease is latent except for a reactive serologic test for syphilis. The following signs may be present:
    1. Interstitial keratitis
    2. Hutchinson's tooth
    3. Eighth-nerve deafness
    4. Neurosyphilis
    5. Bone involvement with sclerotic gummatous lesions, as in saber shin, destruction of nasal septum, or rhagades
II. Diagnostic aids
  A. Identify *Treponema pallidum* in serum from lesions by dark-field examination.
  B. Perform IgM specific fluorescent treponemal antibody-absorption test (FTA-ABS test). This is diagnostic, since IgM does not cross the placenta. The test will be positive, usually before clinical symptoms occur; therefore it is very useful.
  C. Since VDRL and regular FTA-ABS tests are usually for IgG antibodies, they are not diagnostic unless repeated titers demonstrate a rise.
III. Treatment of infant
  A. Infant with negative RPR
    1. When mother is adequately treated and there is no suspicion of reinfection, no treatment is indicated.
    2. When mother with early disease is not adequately treated, treat the asymptomatic infant with 50,000 U/kg of benzathine penicillin and follow with monthly RPR titers for 3 months.
  B. Infant with positive RPR
    1. When mother is adequately treated and infant is asymptomatic but RPR titer is higher than that of mother, treat infant as described below.
    2. When mother is not treated or is inadequately treated and infant is asymptomatic and has an RPR titer equal to or less than that of mother, treat with 50,000 U/kg of benzathine penicillin and follow with monthly RPR titers for 3 months.

  If infant is symptomatic or asymptomatic with RPR titer higher than that of his mother, perform lumbar puncture and obtain x-ray films of long bones. If cerebrospinal fluid is abnormal or infant has signs of congenital syphilis, treat with penicillin G 100,000 U/kg in 2 or 3 divided doses IV or IM for 10 days.
  If baby is asymptomatic and cerebrospinal fluid is normal, treat with one dose benzathine penicillin 50,000 U/kg IM and follow with monthly titers until RPR is negative.
IV. Prognosis
  Although treatment may cure the infection, outcome for fetus depends on damage inflicted by *Treponema* prior to treatment, which may result in abortion, stillbirth, neonatal death, or a live but defective infant. Treatment of mother within first trimester should prevent fetal infection, and a full dose of penicillin to the infected mother after the first 3 weeks of the infection should cure fetal infection. However, treatment of congenital syphilis in its late stage will not reverse defects such as deafness, keratitis, and bone disease.

Toxoplasmosis

Placental transfer of the parasite *Toxoplasma gondii* to the fetus in the nonimmune gravida is increasingly common.

Although 20% to 30% of women have positive titers during pregnancy, the infection is likely to have antedated pregnancy, with the parasite in the encysted form and not dangerous to the fetus. As many as 2 to 7 per 1,000 women acquire the active disease in pregnancy, 30% to 40% of whom have infected infants. Transmission of infection is reported to increase with gestation. Identification of positive titers during pregnancy in women with previous negative titers suggests a proliferative disease dangerous to the fetus.

I. Signs
   A. Early
      1. Hepatosplenomegaly with jaundice
      2. Chorioretinitis and microphthalmia
      3. Lethargy or convulsion, or both
   B. Later
      1. Hydrocephalus or microcephalus
      2. Mental retardation
      3. Cerebral calcification
II. Diagnosis
   A. IgM fluorescent antibody test may be positive.
   B. A Sabin-Feldman dye test remains elevated for many months, in contrast to the passively transferred antibody from the mother.
III. Therapy of congenital toxoplasmosis
   Therapy is difficult because parasite may never be completely eliminated. Drugs recommended at present are effective against proliferative form of toxoplasma, but they may not eradicate encysted form.
   A. Infants with symptoms at birth should be treated with pyrimethamine (1 mg/kg every 2 to 3 days orally or IV) and sulfadiazine (50 to 100 mg/kg/day orally in 2 daily doses). Treatment should be continued for 3 weeks. Pyrimethamine is a folic acid antagonist; monitoring of white blood cell and platelet counts is advised. Treatment courses may have to be repeated 3 to 4 times during the first years of life.
   Administration of steroids may alleviate some of the inflammatory processes of the disease (e.g., chorioretinitis).
   B. Healthy-appearing newborns in whom definite serologic diagnosis has not yet been confirmed, but whose mothers definitely acquired an infection during pregnancy, should receive one course of treatment until results are obtained from laboratory test.
IV. Treatment of acute maternal infections
   Active disease in the mother has been treated with pyrimethamine and sulfonamides with a significant reduction in the incidence of congenitally infected infants. Treatment with these drugs during the first trimester should be avoided because of possible teratogenic effects.
V. Prevention
   Routine screening of women for evidence of active disease is now done in several states. Through such a program, along with treatment of the newly infected mother, death or damage to their infants may be avoided.

Coxsackievirus disease

The coxsackievirus, type A or B (each of which includes many serotypes) causes an acute, influenza-like enteric or respiratory illness in adults. It also affects the fetus by (1) transplacental passage of the submicroscopic agent or (2) exposure of the neonate to diseased individuals. Occasionally the mother and attendants will have no clinical evidence of a viral disorder. Coxsackievirus may cause fetal malformations and is very serious for the premature infant. Several days after birth the newborn infant with the disease will have a cough, loose stools, fever, and tachycardia. Meningoencephalitis or myocarditis may develop. Neonatal death is often attributable to circulatory collapse or respiratory failure. Routine laboratory studies reveal no typical abnormalities. The virus may be isolated from throat washings or stools. Only symptomatic therapy is available. Prognosis depends on extent of the disease.

Tuberculosis

Congenital tuberculosis is rare. Neonates born of mothers with tuberculosis have no specific affinity for the disease. It is essential to segregate the mother with pulmonary tuberculosis from her infant, however, to avoid neonatal acid-fast infection.

Patients undergoing treatment for tuberculosis should strictly avoid conception until the disorder has been inactive for 2 to 5 years, depending on severity. All obstetric patients should have chest x-ray examinations as soon as gestation is confirmed. Women who have arrested pulmonary tuberculosis should have chest films taken every 3 months during pregnancy and 6 months after delivery.

Isoniazid and para-aminosalicylic acid probably are not teratogenic in the doses usually given for chemotherapy of tuberculosis.

Listeriosis

Modern surveys have shown that up to 4% of pregnant women harbor *Listeria monocytogenes* in the cervix or vagina. Invasion of the placenta occasionally occurs, with influenza-like symptoms in the mother and the possibility of early delivery. A dirty brown amniotic fluid has been noted in instances of listeriosis.

Infants infected either through direct invasion or from birth contamination may be seriously jeopardized. Mortality and morbidity are high, particularly from central nervous system complications.

1. Clinical findings
   a. Fetal involvement with scattered foci of necrosis (granulomatosis infantiseptica) indicate disease.
   b. Delayed infection of the newborn infant—vomiting, lethargy, and cardiorespiratory symptoms—often indicates listeriosis.
2. Diagnosis
   a. Positive fluorescent antibody test is diagnostic.
   b. Culture nasopharynx, stomach contents, and meconium (sometimes liquid) for gram-positive pleomorphic bacteria—*do not confuse with diphtheroids*.
   c. Perform spinal tap to identify listeriosis.
3. Treatment
   a. Treat vigorously with penicillin or ampicillin while awaiting results of specific drug-sensitivity tests.
   b. Maintain observation for sequelae of disease after dismissal from hospital.

BIBLIOGRAPHY

Ablow, R.C., Driscoll, S.G., Effmann, E.L., et al.: A comparison of early-onset group B streptococcal neonatal infection to the respiratory-distress syndrome in the newborn, N. Engl. J. Med. **294**:65, 1976.

Baker, C.J., and Barrett, F.F.: Transmission of group B streptococci from mother to neonate, J. Pediatr. **83**:919, 1973.

Baker, C.J., and Kasper, D.L.: Correlation of maternal antibody deficiency with susceptibility to neonatal group B streptococcal infection, N. Engl. J. Med. **294**:753, 1976.

Baker, C.J. and Rench, M.A.: Commercial latex agglutination for detection of Group B streptococcal antigen in body fluids, J. Pediatr. **102**:393, 1983.

Barett-Connor, E.: Current status of the treatment of syphilis, West. J. Med. **122**:7, 1975.

Bryson, Y.J.: The use of acyclovir in children, Pediatr. Infect. Dis. **3**:345, 1984.

Chien, L., Whitley, R., Nahmias, A., et al.: Antiviral chemotherapy and neonatal herpes simplex virus infection: a pilot study-experience with adenine arabinoside (ara-A), Pediatrics **55**:678, 1975.

Chin, K.C., and Fitzhardinge, P.M.: Sequelae of early-onset Group B hemolytic streptococcal neonatal meningitis, J. Pediatr. **106**:819, 1985.

Christensen, R.D., Bradley, P.P., and Rothstein, G.: The leucocyte left shift in clinical and experimental neonatal sepsis, J. Pediatr. **98**:101, 1981.

Christensen, R.D., Rothstein, G., Anstall, H.B., et al.: Granulocyte transfusions in neonates with bacterial infection, neutropenia, and depletion of mature marrow neutrophils, Pediatrics **70**:1, 1982.

Desmonts, G., and Couvreur, J.: Congenital toxoplasmosis: a prospective study of 378 pregnancies, N. Engl. J. Med. **290**:1110, 1974.

Edwards, M.S., Rench, M.A., Haffar, A.A., et al.: Long-term sequelae of Group B streptococcal meningitis in infants, J. Pediatr. **106**:717, 1985.

Eichenwald, H.F., and McCracken, Jr., G.H.: Antimicrobial therapy in infants and children, J. Pediatr. **93**:337, 1978.

Feigin, R.D.: The perinatal group B streptococcal problem: more questions than answers, N. Engl. J. Med. **294**:106, 1976.

Florman, A.L., Gershon, A.A., Blackett, P.R., et al.: Intrauterine infection with herpes simplex virus, JAMA **225**:129, 1973.

Franciosi, R.A., Knostman, J.D., and Zimmerman, R.A.: Group B streptococcal infections, J. Pediatr. **82**:707, 1973.

Frenkel, J.K.: Congenital toxoplasmosis: prevention or palliation, Am. J. Obstet. Gynecol. **141**:359, 1981.

Handsfield, H.H.: Prevention of congenital syphilis, JAMA **252**:1750, 1984.

Hanshaw, J.B.: Herpes virus hominis infections in the fetus and newborn, Am. J. Dis. Child. **126**:546, 1973.

Hanshaw, J.B., and Dudgeon, J.H.: Viral disease of the fetus and newborn, Philadelphia, 1978, W.B. Saunders Co.

Harner, R.E., Smith, J.L., and Israel, C.W.: The FTA-HBS test in late syphilis, JAMA **203**:545, 1968.

Herrmann, K.L., Halstead, S.B., Brandling-Bennett, A.D., et al.: Rubella immunization: persistence of antibody four years after a large-scale field trial, JAMA **235**:2201, 1976.

Idsoe, O., Guthe, T., and Willcox, R.R.: Penicillin in the treatment of syphilis: the experience of three decades, Bull. WHO **47**(suppl.), 1972.

Katz, S.L.: The possible relationship of viruses, other than rubella and cytomegalovirus, to the etiology of birth defects, Birth Defects **4**:57, 1968.

Kimball, A.C., Kean, B.H., and Fuchs, F.: Congenital toxoplasmosis: a positive study of 4048 obstetric patients, Am. J. Obstet. Gynecol. **111**:211, 1971.

Kumar, M.L., Nankervis, G.A., Jacobs, I.B., et al.: Congenital and postnatally acquired cytomegalovirus infections: long-term follow-up, J. Pediatr. **104**:674, 1984.

Leff, R.D., Andersen, R.D., and Roberts, R.J.: Simplified gentamicin dosing in neonates: a time- and cost-efficient approach, Pediatr. Infect. Dis. **3**:208, 1984.

Manroe, B.L., Weinberg, A.G., Rosenfeld, C.R., et al.: The neonatal blood count in health and disease. I. Reference values for neutrophilic cells, J. Pediatr. **95**:89, 1979.

Mascola, L., Pelosi, R., Blount, J.H., et al.: Congenital syphilis, JAMA **252**:1719, 1984.

McCracken, G.H.: Pharmacological basis for antimicrobial therapy in newborn infants, Am. J. Dis. Child. **128**:407, 1974.

McCracken, G.H., and Kaplan, J.M.: Penicillin treatment for congenital syphilis: a critical reappraisal, JAMA **228**:855, 1974.

McCracken, G.H., Threlkeld, N.E., and Thomas, M.L.: Pharmacokinetics of cefotaxime in newborn infants, Antimicrobial Agents Chemother. **21**:683, 1982.

Modlin, J.F., Brandling-Bennett, A.D., Witte, J.J., et al.: A review of five years' experience with rubella vaccine in the United States, Pediatrics **55**:20, 1975.

Monif, G.R.G., Egan, E.A., Held, B., et al.: Correlation of maternal cytomegalovirus infection during varying stages of gestation with neonatal involvement, J. Pediatr. **80**:17, 1972.

Nahmias, A.J.: The TORCH complex, Hosp. Pract. **9**:65, 1974.

Overall, J.C., Jr.: Neonatal bacterial meningitis, J. Pediatr. **76**:499, 1970.

Overall, J.C., Jr., and Glasgow, L.A.: Virus infections of the fetus and newborn infant, J. Pediatr. **77**:315, 1970.

Overall, J.C., Jr., Whitley, R.J., Yeager, A.S., et al.: Prophylactic or anticipatory antiviral therapy for newborns exposed to herpes simplex infection, Pediatr. Infect. Dis. **3**:193, 1984.

Plotkin, S.A.: Prevention of cytomegalovirus disease, Pediatr. Infect. Dis. **3**:1, 1984.

Plotkin, S.A., and Starr, S.E., editors: Symposium on perinatal infections, Clinics in Perinatology, Philadelphia, 1981, W.B. Saunders Co.

Rawls, W.E., Desmyter, J., and Melnick, J. L.: Serologic diagnosis and fetal involvement in maternal rubella, JAMA **203**:627, 1968.

Remington, J.S., and Klein, J.O., editors: Infectious diseases of the fetus and newborn infant, Philadelphia, 1976, W.B. Saunders Co.

Rowan, D.F., McCraw, M.F., and Edward, R.D.: Virus infections during pregnancy (ECHO, Coxsackie), Obstet. Gynecol. **32**:356, 1968.

Saigal, S., Lunyk, O., Larke, R.P.B., et al.: The outcome in children with congenital cytomegalovirus infection, Am. J. Dis. Child. **136**:896, 1982.

Schaad, U.B., McCracken, G.H., and Nelson, J.D.: Clinical pharmacology and efficacy of vancomycin in pediatric patients, J. Pediatr. **96**:119, 1980.

Skinner, W.E.: Routine rubella antibody titer determinations in pregnancy, Obstet. Gynecol. **33**:301, 1969.

Srinivasan, G., Ramamurthy, R.S., Bharathi, A., et al.: Congenital syphilis: a diagnostic and therapeutic dilemma, Pediatr. Infect. Dis. **2**:436, 1983.

Stagno, S., Pass, R.F., Dworsky, M.E., et al.: Congenital cytomegalovirus infection the relative importance of primary and recurrent maternal infection, N. Engl. J. Med. **306**:954, 1982.

Stagno, S., Reynolds, D.W., Lakeman, A., et al.: Congenital CMV infection: consecutive occurrence due to viruses with similar antigenic compositions, Pediatrics **52**:788, 1973.

Van Dyke, R.B., and Spector, S.A.: Transmission of herpes simplex virus type 1 to a newborn infant during endotracheal suctioning for meconium aspiration, Pediatr. Infect. Dis. **3**:153, 1984.

Section III SPECIFIC PROBLEMS OF THE NEONATE

26

The very low birth weight baby

We have included this chapter to emphasize a leading challenge in perinatal health care and the need to focus on preventive medicine as well as comprehensive support when birth is inevitable.

GENERAL CONSIDERATIONS
Mortality

Although very low birth weight (VLBW) infants (those weighing less than 1,500 gm) represent less than 1% of live births, they now contribute almost 60% of all neonatal deaths (Table 34-1) and represent a major factor in infant mortality in the United States. Progress has been made in perinatal care, and infants weighing less than 1,000 and even 800 gm at birth now have a significant chance of intact survival. In a 1983 study by Hoskins et al., of 106 infants weighing less than 1,000 gm at birth, 72 (68%) survived. Of survivors, 9 (13%) had neurologic handicaps and 2 (3%) were blind at follow-up. Other 1983 VLBW infant studies show that of surviving infants weighing less than 800 gm at birth at three different institutions between 67% and 81% were normal. Despite improved outcome for VLBW infants the overall goal must be to effect better pregnancy education and identification of those at risk and to increase access to prenatal and perinatal care and so reduce the incidence of births of VLBW infants.

Morbidity

Although VLBW infants admitted to tertiary centers now have a survival rate of approximately 70%, the number of survivors with serious handicaps (10% to 20%) may have risen because of the increased number of survivors weighing under 1,000 gm. Mechanical ventilation and improved methods of nutritional support have improved the chance of living for infants already compromised by asphyxia, shock, or hypothermia. Irreversible damage cannot be predicted in advance so that full support must be initiated as the infant's right. However, a time limit for continued critical care should be considered for the infant who shows no improvement or serious deterioration (see Chapters 30 and 35).

Economic costs

Approximately half the beds in tertiary centers are now used by infants who weighed under 1,500 gm at birth. The extended days of critical care necessary for these infants requires approximately 5,000 beds daily in the United States. At a cost of approximately $2,000 per day, the yearly expense of critical care alone for these smaller infants could reach 1 billion dollars a year.

Social cost

We found in a study of 100 small infants that approximately one fourth of VLBW infants were born to teenagers and another fourth to older single or separated women. For the most part these infants were unplanned, often rejected, and likely to become dependent on government support.

APPROACHES TO PREVENTION
(see also Chapter 37)

Reduction in percentage of VLBW infants born can be accomplished through better education and pregnancy control starting with the teenager. Sweden's low neonatal mortality is primarily because of the very low percentage of infants born weighing under 1,500 gm. In

Japan the percentage of births to young mothers (less than 20 years of age) is 1.1, while it is 14.8 in the United States; Japan's infant mortality is only 6.2, while the U.S. rate is 11.2 (Demographic Yearbook, 1983, United Nations).

Other efforts to use include the following:
1. Expand skills in detection of threatened early labor and promptly inhibit labor when feasible. Lauersen et al. have shown that beta-mimetic agents can delay labor in 90% of selected women and extend pregnancy an average of 44 days. This delay in delivery could lower mortality of 29-week fetuses from approximately 30% to less than 5%.
2. Transfer to a regional center those women with threatened labor at 32 weeks or less.
3. Avoid undue pessimism regarding neonatal outcome. Although the very immature fetus is at increased risk for death and injury, fetal size and maturity have been underestimated in the majority of instances, which has allowed a too casual approach to initial care of VLBW infants at birth.

SPECIFIC PROBLEMS OF THE SMALL NEONATE
Hypoxia and hyperoxia

Use of continuous monitoring of oxygen tension has revealed that tissue levels in the preterm infant fluctuate greatly with recurrent and prolonged periods of both hypoxia and hyperoxia often unrecognized by clinical observation. Reduction in respiratory exchange, short of apnea, is frequently and easily induced by the many treatments and procedures incidental to standard care. Periods of hypoxemia may last for many minutes after handling of the infant, resulting in fatigue and inactivity, as well as relaxation of the ductus arteriosus, increasing left-to-right shunting of blood. The effects of these stressful episodes of hypoxemia may necessitate further diagnostic studies. Continuous sensitive care by neonatal nurses is required.

A most serious accompaniment of hypoxia is its effect on the fine vascular structure of the small infant's cerebral vessels. This injury along with vascular engorgement associated with hypercapnia, hyperosmolality, and overcorrection of hypotension places the infant at risk for periventricular hemorrhage (PVH) (p. 289). Papile has observed from CT scans of the head that nearly 50% of all infants under 1,500 gm exhibit evidence of cerebral hemorrhage. A majority of these die and nearly half of the survivors develop hydrocephalus. Intensive care supported by mechanical ventilation has increased survival and delayed death so that hyaline membrane disease has been superseded by intraventricular hemorrhage as the main cause of death.

Hyperoxia is equally hazardous. In a recent study permanent damage to the retina (see the discussion on retrolental fibroplasia on p. 262) was observed in as many as 15% of smaller surviving infants with one fourth of those being blind. For support of metabolic processes, the preterm infant may require a Pa_{O_2} of 50 to 70 mm Hg. Maintaining this level often requires supplemental oxygen; thus the chance of hyperoxia is increased during periods of improved ventilation. Every effort must be made to prevent extended periods of hyperoxia (greater than 90 mm Hg), but spasm of retinal arteries and capillary obliteration may occur at lower levels of oxygenation.

A high oxygen concentration usually given in conjunction with intermittent positive pressure ventilation, causes direct damage to the pulmonary tissues. Because many immature infants in tertiary centers require this support, approximately 20% show x-ray evidence of fibrosis of the lungs known as bronchopulmonary dysplasia (BPD).

Hypoglycemia and hyperglycemia
(see Chapter 32)

The possibility of development of hypoglycemia because of the delayed feeding of small premature infants is high (Fig. 12-1). On the other hand, these infants are usually unable to metabolize more than 0.35 gm/hr or 8 gm/day during the first days of life. Thus a solution of D10W at 100 ml/kg/day can overload a VLBW infant's glucostatic mechanism with dangers of hyperosmolality and osmotic diuresis. Careful periodic monitoring of serum glucose levels (Dextrostix) is a necessary screen.

Starvation and dehydration

Delays in supplying fluid and calories to premature infants born in the fifties have been blamed for much of the later handicapping found in these infants. Hypoglycemia, hypernatremia, acidosis, and hyperbilirubinemia as a result of this practice were not always recognized even as recently as 15 years ago. Delays in achieving positive nitrogen balance, another likely cause of impaired development in these infants, may have been on the basis of suspended brain cell division at a critical period of growth. Parenteral nutrition or transpyloric feeding is usually necessary for supporting nutrition in the stressed infant.

BIBLIOGRAPHY

Bennett, F.C., Robinson, N.M., and Sells, C.J.: Growth and development of infants weighing less than 800 grams at birth, Pediatrics **71**:319, 1983.

Drew, J.H.: Immediate intubation at birth of the very low-birth-weight infant, Am. J. Dis. Child. **136**:207, 1982.

Dweck, H.S., and Cassady, G.: Glucose intolerance of very low birthweights, 1,100 grams or less, Pediatrics **53**:189, 1974.

Fuchs, V.R., and Perreault, L.: Expenditures for reproduction-related health care, JAMA **255**:76, 1986.

Hirata, T., Epcar, J.T., Walsh, A., et al.: Survival and outcome of infants 501 to 750 gm: six year experience, J. Pediatr. **102**:741, 1983.

Hoskins, E.M., Elliot, E., Shennan, A.T., et al.: Outcome of very low–birth weight infants born at a perinatal center, Am. J. Obstet. Gynecol. **145**:135, 1983.

Jung, A.L., and Streeter, N.S.: Total population estimate of newborn special-care bed needs, Pediatrics **75**:993, 1985.

Koops, B.: Retinopathy of the premature: magnitude of the problem today, Clin. Res. **26**:108A, 1978.

Lauersen, N.H., Merkatz, I.R., Tejani, N., et al.: Inhibition of premature labor: a multicenter comparison of ritodrine and ethanol, Am. J. Obstet. Gynecol. **127**:837, 1977.

Lee, K.S., Paneth N., Gartner, L.M., et al.: The very low-birth-weight rate: principal predictor of neonatal mortality in industrialized populations, J. Pediatr. **97**:759, 1980.

Lubchenco, L.O.: The high risk infant. In Schaffer, A.J., editor: Major problems in clinical pediatrics, Philadelphia, 1976, W.B. Saunders Co.

Pape, K.E., Buncic, R.J., Ashby, S., et al.: The status at two years of low-birth-weight infants born in 1974 with birth weights of less than 1,001 gm, J. Pediatr. **92**:253, 1978.

Papile, L.A., Burstein, J., Burstein, R., et al.: Incidence and evolution of subependymal and intraventricular hemorrhage: a study on infants with birth weights less than 1,500 gm, J. Pediatr. **92**:529, 1978.

Pomerance, J.J., Ukrainski, C.T., Ukra, T., et al.: Cost of living for infants 1,000 grams or less at birth, Pediatrics **61**:908, 1978.

Walker, D.J.B., Vohr, B.R., and Oh, W.: Economic analysis of regionalized neonatal care for very low-birth-weight infants in the state of Rhode Island, Pediatrics **76**:69, 1985.

27

Identification and management of respiratory problems

Between 5% and 10% of newborn infants have some respiratory difficulty after birth, the incidence of which is inversely related to their maturity. The fact that pulmonary problems are the leading cause for neonatal deaths lends importance to the need for prompt diagnosis and treatment of any respiratory difficulty. The skilled care necessary for such infants often requires their referral to a regional center.

Signs indicating respiratory distress are not always caused by pulmonary disorders, however. Disease of the central nervous system, congenital anomalies of the heart or gastrointestinal tract, and manifestations of shock must be considered in the differential diagnosis.

RECOGNITION OF RESPIRATORY DISTRESS

The following signs are commonly observed in infants with disease of the respiratory system, as well as in certain nonpulmonary problems.

Tachypnea

A respiratory rate of over 60 respirations/min indicates tachypnea. Respiratory rates should be evaluated only when the infant is sleeping or resting. Tachypnea is the most common sign of abnormal ventilation and is found in many respiratory disorders. It is a common sign of heart failure and early shock as well.

Intercostal retractions

Retractions of subcostal and intercostal tissues, as well as the sternum, demonstrate the infant's difficulty in stabilizing his thorax to improve lung inflation. This instability of the thoracic wall leads to increased excursion of the diaphragm, evident as abdominal protrusion during inspiration, the "seesaw" pattern of respiration. Retractions indicate inadequate filling of the lung with air, as in hyaline membrane disease (HMD), but also may result from obstructions of the upper airways.

Grunting

Almost pathognomonic of HMD, grunting is manifested by the infant trying to exhale against a closed and then partially closed glottis. As the infant grunts, he emits a groaning or whining sound during expiration. Grunting is an infant's attempt to maintain maximum alveolar expansion and better gas exchange.

Flaring of the nares

Flaring of the nares is an inspiratory widening of the nostrils. It is observed frequently in infants with significant respiratory distress.

Cyanosis

Cyanosis should be evaluated under bright daylight or daylight fluorescent light while the infant is quiet. Central cyanosis is defined as a bluish discoloration of the mucous membranes and tongue, as well as the skin, and signifies arterial unsaturation. Cyanosis of pulmonary origin, such as hypoventilation, diffusion difficulties, and ventilation/perfusion unevenness, will be relieved by increasing the inspiratory oxygen concentration. Failure of cyanosis to disappear while the infant is breathing pure oxygen indicates significant right-to-left shunts. Although more common in congenital heart disease, such shunting may accompany severe HMD, as well as persistence of the fetal circulation (primary pulmonary hypertension).

Respiratory depression or apnea

Respiratory depression manifested by shallow and irregular respiration interposed with prolonged apneic episodes and cyanosis is the most serious sign of impending catastrophe in the newborn. Its etiology may be pulmonary or nonpulmonary.

Blood gas changes

Hypoxemia (P_{AO_2} less than 50 mm Hg) and hypercarbia (P_{CO_2} over 45 mm Hg) are common in respiratory distress. Nonpulmonary conditions such as congenital heart disease will manifest hypoxemia but often with somewhat low P_{CO_2} (under 35 mm Hg). Acidosis (pH less than 7.3 or a base deficit of more than -5) is often observed with reduced gas exchange. Hypercarbia, in most acute respiratory problems, will lower the pH, resulting in "respiratory acidosis." Factors leading to impaired oxygen transport to tissues will cause metabolic acidosis, primarily through accumulation of lactic acid. Some of these factors are hypoxemia, insufficient cardiac output, vasoconstriction, hypotension, anemia, and abnormal hemoglobin.

GENERAL MANAGEMENT OF RESPIRATORY DISTRESS

Promptness in offering care for stabilization of the infant with respiratory distress is a critical factor in determining the outcome. Respiratory failure may occur acutely, requiring early diagnosis and precise management. The correction of inadequate oxygenation and hypercarbia is the first goal of treatment.

Initial care

1. Place infant under radiant heat or in Isolette and maintain skin temperature between 36° and 36.5° C (97° and 98° F).
2. Attach cardiorespiratory monitor.
3. Administer sufficient oxygen with a hood to relieve cyanosis until blood gas results are obtained; then maintain P_{AO_2} between 50 and 70 mm Hg (or 45 and 50 mm Hg when warmed heel capillary blood is used). Humidify O_2 if 30% or more is given.
4. Ease infant's respiratory efforts by elevating his shoulders slightly with a folded towel.
5. Ensure patent airway and use suction whenever secretions accumulate. Suction secretions from the nose with a bulb syringe and from the oropharynx with Fr 8 or 10 suction catheter. For intubated infants give airway care as outlined in discussion of mechanical ventilation (p. 260).
6. Ventilate infant's lungs with bag and mask if cyanosis persists, despite oxygen given by hood, or if repeated apnea occurs. Consider instituting transpulmonary distending pressure or endotracheal intubation and mechanical ventilation.
7. Insert umbilical artery catheter (Chapter 10) if infant appears to be critically ill or requires significant amounts of oxygen (over 40%).
8. Obtain x-ray films of chest and abdomen to ascertain diagnosis as well as to verify correct catheter position.
9. Monitor blood pressure with Doppler method or by a transducer from arterial catheter. If infant appears to be in shock, manage appropriately (Chapter 29).
10. Administer parenteral fluids by peripheral vein or umbilical vessel catheter (Chapter 15).
11. Determine the following data on admission:
    a. Weight, length, head circumference
    b. Hematocrit, hemoglobin level
    c. Blood type and cross matching for fresh packed cells
    d. Serum sodium, potassium, chloride, calcium, and bilirubin if infant appears jaundiced
    e. Blood gas measurements
12. Correct anemia if hematocrit is less than 45%; transfuse infant with fresh packed cells (10 ml/kg will raise hematocrit about 5%).
13. Correct acidosis when necessary.
14. If major infection is suspected, obtain necessary cultures and administer antibiotics.

Continued care

1. Monitor heart rate or heart and respiratory rates continuously until infant's condition has stabilized sufficiently and apneic episodes no longer occur.

2. Use flow sheet kept at infant's bedside for all blood gas results, laboratory data, concentration of oxygen, constant positive airway pressure (CPAP), ventilator settings, and so forth (See Appendix F).
3. Monitor blood gases frequently, correct any acidosis promptly, and maintain Pa_{O_2} and Pco_2 in their normal ranges.
4. Observe infant's hematocrit serially and avoid anemia. During acute phase of illness, maintain hematocrit above 45%; in chronic cases, above 35%.
5. Carefully monitor fluid intake and output, weigh infant at least daily, monitor serum electrolytes daily, and watch infant's nutritional state. In acute respiratory distress, infants tend to retain fluids and may require only 60 to 80 ml/kg to maintain hydration. During acute phase of disease it is best not to feed infant orally. Consider parenteral nutrition instead (Chapter 17).
6. Removal of central catheters
   a. Remove arterial catheter as soon as infant can be maintained under 30% O_2 and his condition has sufficiently stabilized so that frequent arterial sampling for blood gases is no longer needed.
   b. Remove central venous catheter whenever pressure monitoring can be discontinued or this avenue is no longer needed for emergency support. Never leave catheter in place solely for purpose of administering fluids.

Oxygen therapy

Increased inspiratory oxygen concentrations are usually needed in management of respiratory disorders, after significant asphyxiation, during shock, and so forth. Although this therapy may be lifesaving, it is potentially dangerous and therefore requires skill in its administration.

Clinical assessment of hypoxia in a neonate is extremely inaccurate. Cyanosis may not necessarily mean there is hypoxemia, as is the case in polycythemia. Conversely, an infant who appears to be noncyanotic may be hypoxic, as in the case of anemia.

ADMINISTRATION OF OXYGEN

1. Monitor and record at least hourly the concentration of inspired oxygen. The use of air-oxygen blenders requires certainty of their accuracy.
2. For the use of an oxygen concentration over 30%:
   a. Humidify and warm oxygen.
   b. Use hood* placed over infant's head.
   c. Monitor hood temperature to prevent hypothermia or hyperthermia of infant.
   d. Use gas flow of at least 2 L/min to prevent accumulation of carbon dioxide.

MONITORING OF BLOOD OXYGEN LEVEL IN THE INFANT

Serial assessment of oxygenation, particularly in the preterm infant, is absolutely necessary to avoid extremes in the partial pressure of systemic arterial blood (Pa_{O_2}). Although a range of Pa_{O_2} of 50 to 80 mm Hg is desirable, this range is difficult to maintain. With levels below 45 mm Hg oxygenation of tissues may not be adequate, but, on the other hand, with tensions over 90 mm Hg there are dangers of retrolental fibroplasia and, with high concentrations of inspired oxygen, toxic effects on the lung. Intermittent blood gas sampling is the mainstay in controlling oxygen therapy (see next section). However, necessary delays in identification of excessive peaks and valleys in oxygen tensions occur, and they are not always recognizable from clinical observation. Development of the transcutaneous continuous oxygen monitor for measurement of oxygen tensions directly through the skin (TcP_{O_2}) is an important aid in the care of smaller infants who are susceptible to numerous factors that interfere with oxygenation.

Advantages and disadvantages of the transcutaneous oxygen monitor (TcP_{O_2}) follow:
1. Advantages
   a. Prevention of extended periods of hypoxia (e.g., undetected apnea)
   b. Aids in education of care givers concerning infant's sensitivity to overhandling (e.g., vigorous suctioning of respiratory tract)
   c. Better control of assisted ventilation and of weaning infant from it
   d. Early identification of any problem causing acute deterioration of the infant (e.g., air leaks)

---

*A hood equipped with a lid allows suctioning without excessive falloff in ambient oxygen (oxygen is heavier than air).

e. Avoidance of overcorrection of abnormal tensions detected from blood samples because of the necessary delays in processing and reporting of serial specimens
2. Disadvantages
   a. Possibility in infants in shock of impaired peripheral perfusion resulting in reduced TcP_{O_2} compared to Pa_{O_2}
   b. Need for meticulous care, calibration, and application of electrode
   c. Skin burns from electrode

Continuous monitoring of oxygen saturation by a transcutaneous technique is another aid in oxygen therapy and is helpful in the prevention of hypoxemia in the infant.

Sampling for blood gases

Blood gas and pH determinations are usually obtained from the aorta through an umbilical artery catheter, from an arterialized "heel stick" after thorough warming of a foot, or from puncture of a radial or temporal artery.

AORTIC SAMPLES

1. Technique of sampling
   a. With a clean syringe, aspirate contents of catheter (approximately 1 ml).
   b. With a tuberculin syringe—its dead space filled with heparin—slowly aspirate 0.3 ml of blood, preventing air bubbles from entering the syringe.
   c. Cap syringe, rotate it in the hands to enhance mixing, and place it entirely in ice water. Send it to the laboratory at once for processing.
   d. Inject previously aspirated catheter contents into patient to prevent unnecessary blood loss.
   e. Flush catheter with 1 ml 5% dextrose solution containing 1 unit of heparin per milliliter of solution.
   f. Keep record of amounts of blood withdrawn for sampling and amounts of fluid used for flushing.
2. Advantages
   a. Accurate arterial values are obtained.
   b. Sampling can be done frequently without disturbance to the infant.
3. Disadvantages
   a. Complications from an aortic catheter are common enough to avoid this approach except in infants with moderate to severe respiratory distress.
   b. Right-to-left shunting through the ductus arteriosus leads to lower oxygen tension in postductal vessels. Sampling from preductal sources occasionally (right temporal or radial artery) will offer a check on Pa_{O_2} values in the retinal vessels.

HEEL-STICK SAMPLES

1. Technique of sampling
   a. Warm infant's foot by immersing it in warm water (40° C) for 5 minutes or wrapping it in a warm moist towel.
   b. Rub heel with 70% alcohol on a cotton pledget and dry.
   c. Puncture heel with a Bard-Parker No. 11 or Redi-Lance blade, sufficiently deep to obtain free flow of blood.
   d. Discard first drop and rapidly collect blood free of air bubbles in proper capillary tubes.
   e. Insert metal sliver into capillary tube.
   f. Seal ends of tube tightly.
   g. Mix blood by sliding magnet over capillary tube, which will move metal sliver through blood.
   h. Place capillary tube in ice water and take to laboratory for processing.
2. Advantages
   a. Samples can be obtained repeatedly for prolonged periods.
   b. Safety from complications associated with arterial catheters.
3. Disadvantages
   a. P_{CO_2} is up to 10 mm Hg higher in sick infants.
   b. P_{O_2} values above 45 mm Hg may be significantly lower than arterial values. In fact, levels above 60 mm Hg may reflect dangerously high arterial levels—a factor to be considered in avoiding retrolental fibroplasia.
   c. Crying of infant will distort blood gas results.
   d. Infant may be exhausted by this procedure, especially if it is repeated frequently.

PERIPHERAL ARTERIAL SAMPLES

1. Technique of sampling
   a. Identify vessel with use of a transilluminator or by palpation of pulse.
   b. Prepare skin over vessel.
   c. With heparin solution, fill dead space of a

tight-fitting tuberculin syringe, using a firmly attached 25 gauge needle.
  d. Insert needle with bevel up into vessel against direction of blood flow.
  e. Withdraw blood slowly with gentle suction on syringe. (A bubble-free sample of 0.3 ml is necessary.)
  f. Hold cotton pledget firmly over vessel for 5 minutes to prevent formation of a hematoma that might make further sampling difficult if not impossible.
  g. Seal syringe and place it in ice water for determination of blood gas levels.
2. Advantages
  a. Ability to obtain accurate arterial values
  b. Avoidance of use of central catheter
3. Disadvantages
  a. Repeated frequent sampling is difficult and often impossible.
  b. Crying of infant will distort blood gas results.

FREQUENCY OF SAMPLING

1. Whenever using oxygen, blood gas samples should be obtained at least every 4 to 6 hours.
2. More frequent determinations are necessary during acute stage of respiratory diseases and less frequent determinations in stabilized chronic conditions.

Treatment of acidosis

Treatment of acidosis is important to the infant's prognosis. When pH is normalized, pulmonary and peripheral vascular resistance is lowered, leading to increased blood flow through the lungs and tissues, improvement in myocardial contractility, and maintenance of cell metabolism.

RESPIRATORY ACIDOSIS

Respiratory acidosis (P_{CO_2} over 45 mm Hg; normal, 35 to 40 mm Hg) is caused by impaired elimination of CO_2 because of underventilation in relation to perfusion of the lung. This type of acidosis should be treated only by improvement of ventilation and not by administration of sodium bicarbonate, which would lead to an increase in P_{CO_2} and further worsen acidosis.

METABOLIC ACIDOSIS

Metabolic acidosis is usually caused by impairment of oxygen transport to tissues and subsequent accumulation of lactic acid. Other factors, such as renal immaturity or failure, also may lead to development of this type of acidosis.

Sodium bicarbonate is the buffer of choice to correct the acidotic state. Tromethamine (THAM) is not often recommended because of its potential effects of raising serum osmolarity and depressing the respiratory center.

1. Calculation of dose of sodium bicarbonate ($NaHCO_3$) for correction of acidosis
  a. Calculate base deficit (mEq/L) from nomogram using pH and P_{CO_2} (see Fig. 27-1).
  b. Multiply base deficit (mEq/L) × infant's weight (kg) × 0.4 to obtain mEq of $NaHCO_3$ needed for correction of acidosis.
2. Administration of $NaHCO_3$
  a. Dilute $NaHCO_3$ with equal amounts of sterile water to lower osmolarity.
  b. Infuse solution parenterally; to prevent tissue damage, never infuse faster than 1 mEq/min. Avoid administration through improperly placed catheter.
  c. Do not exceed dose of 8 mEq/kg/24 hr because of possible hypernatremia and subsequent intracranial hemorrhage.
3. In cases of severe asphyxiation, do not wait for a blood gas result, but give $NaHCO_3$ parenterally 2 to 4 mEq/kg of infant's weight.

METHODS OF VENTILATORY ASSISTANCE

Treatment of failing respirations with continuous transpulmonary distending pressure or assisted intermittent ventilation, or both, has become widely practiced in neonatal intensive care centers. Success of these techniques depends on the availability of a skilled neonatal team and laboratory support throughout a 24-hour day.

Continuous transpulmonary distending pressure

Therapy using continuous transpulmonary distending pressure (CDP) is helpful in conditions where lung compliance is decreased and alveolar collapse leads to poor oxygenation. Through maintenance of CDP, alveolar stability is improved and results in a diminished alveolar oxygen difference and rise in $P_{A_{O_2}}$ (Fig. 27-2). This concept was used first by Gregory and associates, who applied a continuous positive airway pressure (CPAP) in spontaneously breathing infants with hyaline membrane disease (HMD). Since then this method has become widely accepted. The Pa_{O_2} and minute ventilation are not affected significantly unless alveoli are overdistended by an inappropriately high pressure, which leads to a decrease in pulmonary blood flow and cardiac output, reduced minute ventilation, and deterioration of the patient's condition. Therefore care must be taken by observation of results of serial blood gas and arterial or central venous pressure measurements to guard against possible overdistention of alveoli.

Conditions with hypercarbia are ill-suited for this therapy because they require an improvement in ventilation. Continuous transpulmonary distending pressure can be helpful in infants with HMD requiring 50% to 60% or

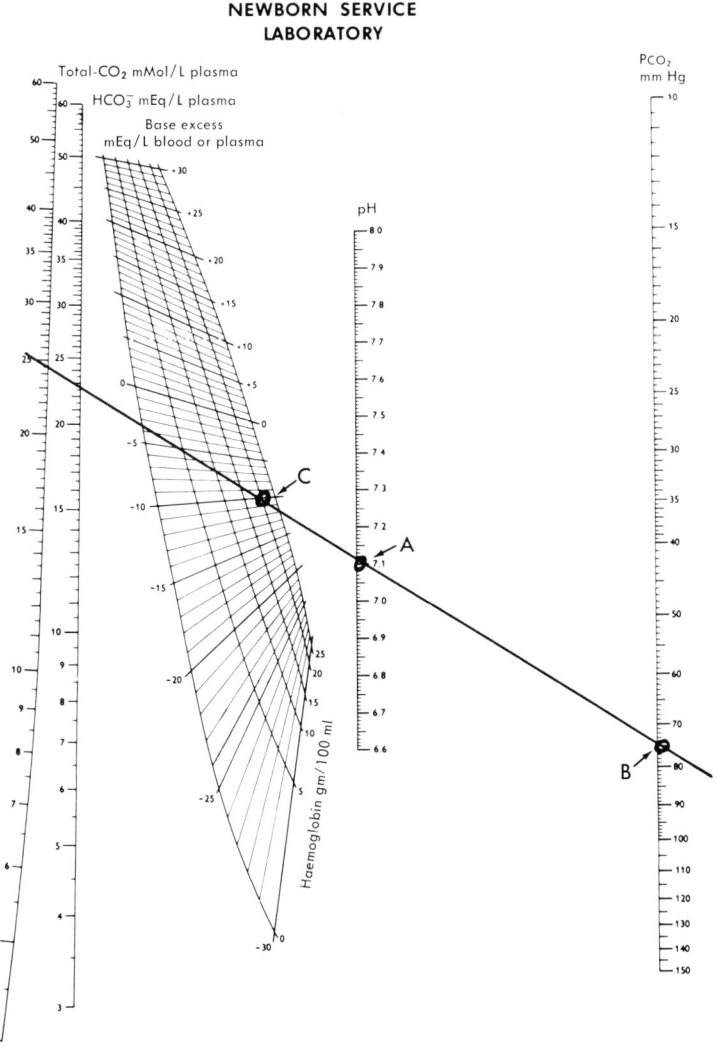

Fig. 27-1. Acid-base nomogram (adapted from Siggaard-Andersen; copyright Radiometer), with an example of plotted data from a sick infant. Base excess can be computed when hemoglobin and any two of the following parameters are known: blood pH, P_{CO_2}, plasma bicarbonate, or total carbon dioxide content of plasma. The values (pH at point **A** and P_{CO_2} at point **B** in this example) are plotted on their scales, and a straight line is drawn through these points across all columns. The base excess is read on the grid line representing the amount of the patient's hemoglobin (**C**). (From Korones, S.B.: High-risk newborn infants: the basis for intensive nursing care, ed. 3, St. Louis, 1981, The C.V. Mosby Co.)

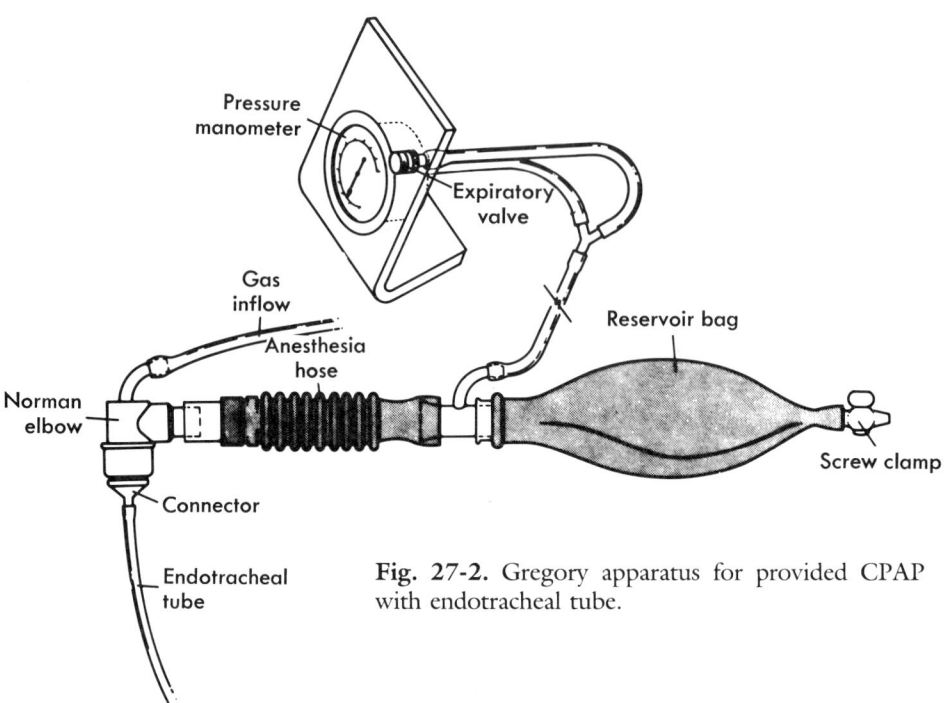

Fig. 27-2. Gregory apparatus for provided CPAP with endotracheal tube.

more of O_2 to maintain P_{AO_2} of 50 mm Hg or to ease severe retractions when lesser amounts of oxygen are needed. This method may also be used for infants with frequent apnea resistant to easy stimulation.

TYPES OF DISTENDING PRESSURE

1. Continuous negative pressure (CNP)
   Alveolar collapse is diminished by application of a constant negative pressure around the infant's body up to the neck by means of a small negative-pressure chamber. This method has proved successful even though access to the infant is limited; however, intubation is not needed. Venous return to the heart is not diminished. Pressures of -5 to -8 cm H_2O are sufficient with milder disease; in more severe cases, pressures of -10 to -12 cm H_2O may be required.
2. Continuous positive airway pressure (CPAP)
   Alveolar collapse is diminished by application of a constant positive pressure to the infant's airway.

MODES OF CONTINUOUS POSITIVE AIRWAY PRESSURE (CPAP)

1. Head chamber
   a. Advantage: intubation not needed
   b. Disadvantages: suctioning infant's airway is difficult; neck seals frequently leak; gastric distention must be avoided by placement of orogastric tube
2. Mask CPAP
   a. Advantages: no need to intubate; easy to apply
   b. Disadvantages: infants sometimes "fight" mask; very small premature infants may tolerate mask poorly; risk of intracranial hemorrhage may be increased; gastric distention must be prevented by placement of orogastric tube; leaks occur at pressures of 8 to 10 cm H_2O
3. Nasal prongs (Argyle)
   a. Advantages: prongs are easy to apply; there is no need to intubate infant.
   b. Disadvantages: stabilization is difficult at times; use is limited to low pressure needs because transmission of higher pressures is prevented by flow resistance within nosepiece; gastric distention must be avoided by placement of orogastric tube.
4. Nasopharyngeal tube (Portex endotracheal tube advanced through one nostril into nasopharynx only)
   a. Advantages: tube is applied easily; pressure transmission is better than with nasal prongs; there is less irritation to infant; intubation can be avoided.
   b. Disadvantages: nasal erosion can occur;

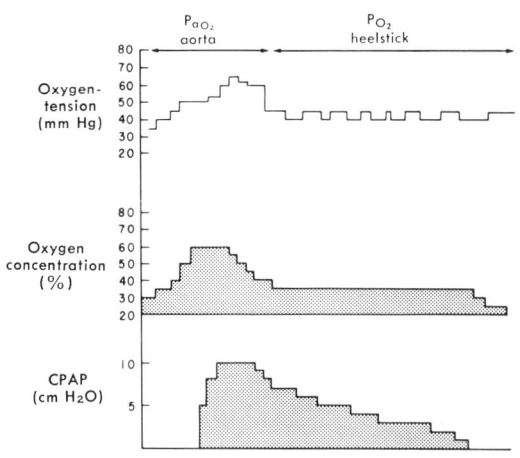

Fig. 27-3. Increasing amounts of ambient oxygen were required to raise arterial oxygen tension to acceptable values (50 mm Hg). CPAP was introduced to avoid administration of high concentrations of oxygen to this preterm infant, thereby maintaining the oxygen tension at a lower $F_{I_{O_2}}$. As the infant recovered, first the oxygen concentration and then the CPAP were reduced gradually, with oxygen tension being maintained within an acceptable range.

gastric distention must be avoided by placement of orogastric tube.
5. CPAP by intubation (Fig. 27-2)
   a. Advantage: pressure can be applied more consistently without variance or leakage problems.
   b. Disadvantage: intubation requires the skill and constant presence of an experienced team to avoid complications from this method (extubation, tube obstruction, faulty tube placement).

In summary, any method leaves something to be desired, and the choice must be made according to personal belief and circumstances where this therapy is used. Continuous transpulmonary distending pressure without intubation, such as the use of nasal prongs, has the advantage of greater safety to the patient and should be the preferred mode whenever possible.

METHOD (Fig. 27-3)

1. Start with the same amount or 10% more oxygen than that used before CPAP was initiated.
2. Warm and humidify air-oxygen mixture if more than 40% oxygen is given or infant is intubated.
3. Maintain gas flow from nebulizer through CPAP equipment between 4 and 6 L/min.
4. Set pop-off valve at 20 cm H_2O for safety.
5. Apply initial pressure of about 4 to 5 cm H_2O (1 mm Hg = 1.3 cm H_2O). If there is no significant improvement of Pa_{O_2} after 15 minutes, increase pressure by 2 cm H_2O increments until desired result is obtained. (Maximal pressure should not exceed 10 to 12 cm H_2O in larger infants; 6 to 8 cm H_2O in infants weighing less than 1.5 kg.)
6. Inflate infant's lungs several times every 30 minutes to prevent CO_2 accumulation and to prevent the development of atelectasis.
7. As infant's condition improves, Pa_{O_2} may rise significantly. Maintain normal oxygen tensions by decreasing O_2 concentration gradually in 5% to 10% increments until less than 40% is administered (blood gas determinations may be needed as often as every 30 minutes).
8. At this point lower CPAP gradually by increments of 1 to 2 cm.
9. After pressure of 2 cm is reached, place infant's head under a hood, giving the same amount or 10% more oxygen than before; observe carefully, and monitor blood gases.
10. While using CPAP, carefully monitor infant for signs of pulmonary overdistention by watching for an increase in P_{CO_2} and central venous pressure, or a decrease in pH, Pa_{O_2}, and arterial pressure. In such a case gradually lower end-expiratory pressure. Administration of volume expanders may aid in correction of hypotension.
11. Always be on the alert for sudden development of pneumothorax (discussed later in this chapter), signaled by clinical deterioration of patient.

Mechanical ventilation

Prolonged use of ventilators for neonates should be reserved for intensive care centers, where continuous team care can be given. Criteria for ventilation vary somewhat among centers. Hypoxemia (PA_{O_2} less than 50 mm Hg) when more than 60% O_2 is used and there is failure to improve with the use of transpulmonary distending pressure, particularly with P_{CO_2} over 65 mm Hg, generally indicates the need for mechanical ventilation. When P_{CO_2} is elevated but less than 65 mm Hg, the decision to ventilate will rest on other factors such as the rate of rise of P_{CO_2}, pH, O_2 requirement, and the frequency of apnea or bradycardia.

TYPES OF VENTILATION USED

1. Intermittent negative pressure ventilation (INPV)
   Although offering the advantage of avoiding intubation, this mode confines infant to a sealed chamber, limiting access to him and subjecting him to cooling. This method is usually not satisfactory for small preterm infants.
2. Intermittent positive pressure ventilation (IPPV)
   IPPV can be accomplished with several types of ventilators.
   a. Volume-controlled ventilators will deliver a predetermined fixed volume at set rates independent of ranges in pulmonary compliance and resistance.
   b. Pressure-controlled ventilators—with this type, predetermined pressures will terminate the inspiratory phase regardless of volume delivered, a situation that can lead to significant under-ventilation if pulmonary compliance decreases.
   c. Time-cycled ventilators allow independent adjustments in duration of inspiratory and expiratory phase. This type of ventilator also allows spontaneous inspiration by the infant, making possible "intermittent mandatory ventilation" and gradual weaning.
   d. Ventilation with bag and mask—this is best limited to short-term needs. It offers the advantage of not requiring nursing staff care for an intubated infant, but demands in nursing time and difficulty in controlling quality of ventilation are disadvantages.

GENERAL GUIDELINES IN MECHANICAL VENTILATION

Since each ventilator model functions differently, precise instructions for their use go beyond the limits of this book and must be learned in an intensive care nursery.

The following are general guidelines only, to be followed whenever mechanical ventilation is given by intermittent positive pressure (IPPV).

Endotracheal tubes

Technique of intubation, as well as that of tube fixation, has been discussed in detail in Chapter 10.
1. Tubes should be of uniform diameter and made of radiopaque nontoxic material.
2. Intubation can be performed by nasotracheal or orotracheal mode, although we prefer the latter, since it eliminates trauma to nasal passage.
3. A snug fit should be avoided to minimize trauma to trachea.

Airway care

1. Always use humidified gases warmed to body temperature.
2. Give chest physiotherapy followed by suctioning at regular intervals (i.e., every 1 to 4 hours) depending on amount of secretions, as follows:
   a. Give chest physiotherapy to all parts of lung by vibration (using hands or electric toothbrush) and percussion with cupped hands.
   b. Increase inspired oxygen concentration by 10% prior to suctioning to minimize hypoxia.
   c. Instill 0.25 ml of sterile saline into endotracheal tube to facilitate removal of secretions; ventilate infant's lung for a few breaths.
   d. Perform suctioning with sterile precautions; use end-hole catheter (Fr 5 or 6 catheter for 2.5 to 3 mm tube; Fr 8 catheter for larger tubes). This procedure is exhausting to infant; therefore do not prolong therapy unnecessarily.
   e. Suction secretions from each mainstem bronchus by turning infant's head first to one side while suctioning and then to the other. Be sure to ventilate infant's lung for a few breaths between suctionings to minimize hypoxia.

3. Change infant's position every few hours. Never leave infant flat on his back because this leads to underventilation of parts of his lung.

Starting mechanical ventilation

Since each infant's need vary considerably, suggestions made are general in nature. Choice of settings for the following are to be considered.

RESPIRATORY RATE

For most infants with respiratory failure, rates chosen should be in the range of 25 to 35 inflations per minute. Rates considerably faster than these may enhance development of interstitial air, especially when peak- and end-inspiratory pressure are relatively high. Infants who suffer from minimal hypercarbia without severe acidosis or hypoxemia may require lower initial rates to lessen the chance of overventilation and respiratory alkalosis.

PEAK INSPIRATORY PRESSURE (PIP)

The cause of respiratory failure will determine to a great extent what pressure range may be required to ensure adequate inflation of the lung. Conditions resulting in low compliance of the lung, such as HMD, usually require inflationary pressures above the normal range. In small preterm infants weighing less than 1,500 gm we start at 20 cm H_2O and in larger infants, at 25 cm H_2O. Higher pressures may be needed, depending on the level of P_{CO_2}. Infants with relatively normal lung compliance, such as in cases of apnea of prematurity and sepsis without pneumonia, should require inspiratory pressures in the range of only 8 to 15 cm H_2O.

Initial assessment of adequacy of chosen pressure should rely on observation of chest wall movement and evidence of breath sounds by auscultation.

TIME OF INSPIRATION AND EXPIRATION (I:E RATIO)

Generally an I:E ratio of 1:2 is used. Mounting evidence indicates that, as inspiratory time is prolonged, especially when using a "square" form of ventilation in contrast to the more conventional "wave" form, oxygenation is improved. Yet, overdistention of alveoli can be caused by prolonging the I:E ratio. Therefore start with a ratio of less than one, but consider an increase to 1:1 in an infant with HMD if oxygenation is insufficient while you are using high concentrations of oxygen.

POSITIVE END-EXPIRATORY PRESSURE (PEEP)

The use of distending pressure is helpful in infants with HMD and when cardiac failure complicates this disease. Again caution is necessary to avoid alveolar overdistention. If CPAP was used for the infant before, we would usually maintain a similar end-expiratory pressure while using the ventilator. Pressures used are in the range of 2 to 6 cm H_2O in most instances.

Assessment of adequacy of ventilation

In addition to close observation for over-all improvement in chest wall movement, breath sounds, and color of the infant, serial blood gas determination and blood pressure recordings are vital for assessing adequacy of ventilation. Use of transcutaneous monitoring of $TcPO_2$ and $TcCO_2$ has improved the ability to more closely assess the ongoing ventilatory needs of infants with respiratory distress.

1. Initial analysis should be obtained 10 to 15 minutes after ventilation of the infant has been started.
2. Frequency of analyses usually ranges from 15 minutes to 4 hours. Blood gas analyses should not be obtained immediately before or after chest physiotherapy, suctioning, or change in ventilator setting to allow accurate assessment.
3. P_{CO_2} should be maintained between 36 and 42 mm Hg and $P_{A_{O_2}}$ between 50 and 70 mm Hg.
4. Increases in ventilator rates and pressures lead to decrease of P_{CO_2} and increase in $P_{A_{O_2}}$, whereas lower settings have opposite effects.
5. An exception applies to overdistention of alveoli, for which a small decrease in PIP, I:E ratio, or PEEP should lead to improvement of blood gas values.
6. Any change in ventilation should be made in small increments, always followed by blood gas assessment.
7. All settings with changes and blood gas results are to be recorded on flow sheets (see Appendix F).

Weaning from ventilator

1. As the infant's condition improves, settings for all parameters gradually are decreased.
2. Oxygen concentration is lowered in 5% to

10% increments, and when it is reduced to 35% to 40%, end-expiratory pressure is gradually lowered, 1 to 2 cm H_2O at a time.
3. PIP is lowered gradually to values approximating the normal range (10 to 15 cm H_2O for infants weighing less than 1,500 gm, and 15 to 20 cm H_2O for larger infants).
4. Respiratory rate is then decreased slowly, with P_{CO_2} and Pa_{O_2} maintained in normal ranges.
5. Once infants are breathing spontaneously, extubation can be considered.

Extubation

Extubation should be undertaken only when the infant tolerates spontaneous breathing well for several hours.

PROCEDURE

1. Suction airways and ventilate infant's lungs for several minutes.
2. Cut sutures; loosen tape around endotracheal tube.
3. Withdraw tube while holding maximum inflation of chest, using anesthesia bag.
4. Place infant in an environment with 10% more oxygen than was used before extubation.
5. Ensure proper humidification of inspired gases.
6. Continue chest physiotherapy and intermittent suctioning of the nasopharynx.

Do not feed infant by nipple or gavage until at least 8 to 12 hours after extubation to allow vocal cord approximation (until infant is able to cry). Feeding may then be considered if infant's condition is stable.

COMPLICATIONS ARISING FROM OXYGEN THERAPY AND MECHANICAL VENTILATION
Retinopathy of prematurity

Also called retrolental fibroplasia (RLF), retinopathy of prematurity was first reported in 1942. It may cause myopia and permanent partial or total loss of vision. Its occurrence apparently is related to the following:
1. Immaturity of infant's retina
2. Oxygen tension in arterial blood
3. Duration of oxygen therapy
4. Deficiency of endogenous antioxidants
5. Carbon dioxide levels in blood

The very immature infant with frequent apneic episodes is most susceptible to this disease, especially when given an excessively high oxygen concentration. An oxygen tension higher than is necessary for physiologic requirements that is sustained for several hours may cause irreversible vasoconstriction of the retinal arteries. Neovascularization of part or all of the retina follows; in severe cases vascularization of the vitreous occurs also. Retinal hemorrhage, partial or total retinal detachment, and cicatrix formation within the vitreous lead to the disastrous permanent disability.

Fortunately most changes detected are mild and do not lead to blindness.

The precise level of oxygen tension and time required to cause this disease are not known but certainly relate to the maturity of the infant. However, the disease has been reported (although rarely) in preterm infants who never received additional oxygen. Nevertheless, close monitoring of Pa_{O_2} in all premature infants receiving supplemental oxygen is of utmost importance. Arterial oxygen tensions should range between 50 and 70 mm Hg, and arterialized heel-stick tensions are more safely kept between 45 and 50 mm Hg.

Whether continuous monitoring of oxygen tensions with transcutaneous oxygen electrodes will help limit this complication has yet to be demonstrated. Administration of vitamin E to infants at risk of developing RLF has been shown to minimize severity of the disease, but exact dosages and safety of such treatment have not yet been determined.

All preterm infants who received oxygen should have an ophthalmologic examination using indirect ophthalmoscopy before discharge from the hospital and again several months later. Photocoagulation and cryotherapy have been used with varying success for infants with severe retinopathy in attempts to diminish retinal detachment.

Bronchopulmonary dysplasia

Bronchopulmonary dysplasia (BPD) was described by Northway and colleagues in infants with severe HMD treated with positive-pressure ventilators and high inspiratory oxygen concentrations. The disease resembles Wilson-Mikity syndrome (pulmonary dysmaturity) in many ways. Findings include the following:
1. Difficulty in weaning an infant with

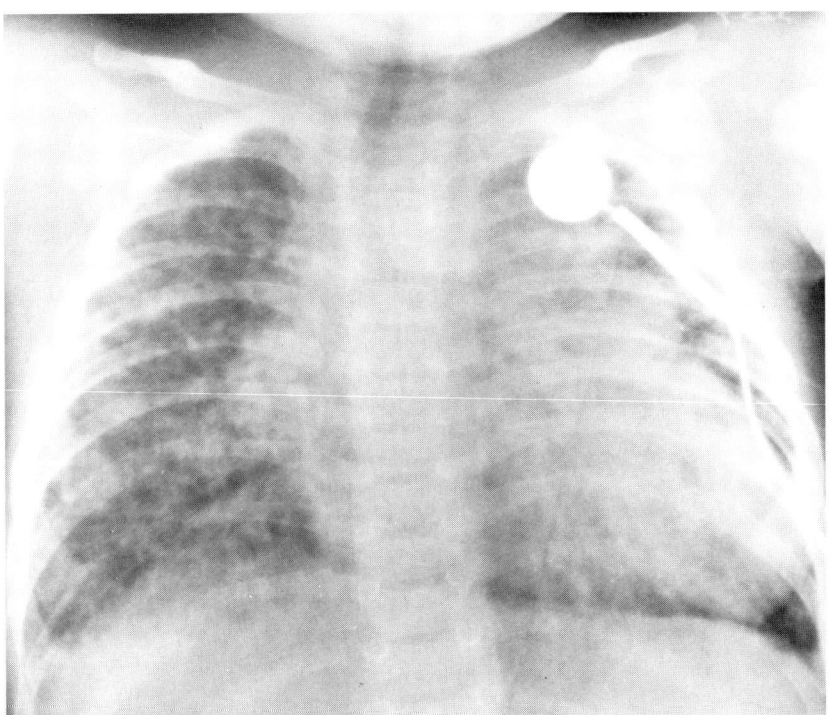

Fig. 27-4. Bronchopulmonary dysplasia after exposure to high concentrations of oxygen in conjunction with positive-pressure ventilation.

HMD from a positive-pressure respirator (frequently the first indication)
2. X-ray changes (Fig. 27-4)
    a. First findings of typical HMD may change to opacification of lung fields with obliteration of heart border during first week of life.
    b. Between 10 and 20 days of age increasing coarse cystic changes are visible bilaterally.
    c. These findings are persistent for weeks, gradually changing to emphysematous areas bilaterally with depression of diaphragms.
3. Increased or persistent tachypnea and labored respirations
4. Oxygen dependency for weeks

BPD has a mortality of 30% to 50%. Development of cor pulmonale and heart failure can complicate recovery. An important factor in development of this disease seems to be administration of oxygen in high concentrations (over 60%) and mechanical ventilation with positive pressure. Ventilation modes resulting in alveolar overdistention and with accumulation of interstitial air are especially related to increased occurrence of BPD. The high frequency of BPD in infants treated with positive-pressure respirators, in contrast to its virtual absence when negative-pressure respirators are used, may point to a more complicated etiology.

The use of minimal oxygen concentrations compatible with satisfactory oxygen tensions and mechanical ventilation with modes that limit destructive alveolar overdistention will lessen occurrence of BPD. This attention to management is especially important because specific treatment is not yet available. However, furosemide (Lasix) and, in cases with symptoms of bronchospasm, bronchodilators are helpful in management of BPD and are drugs commonly used for this disease.

Pneumothorax

Pneumothorax is seen in 10% to 40% of infants whose lungs are ventilated. However, it is also observed as a spontaneous event, occurring after resuscitation with positive pressure, or after

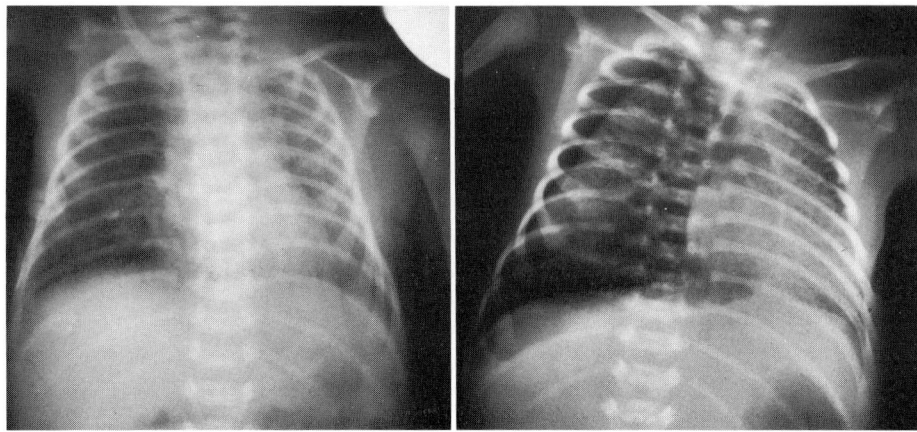

Fig. 27-5. Emphysema of right lung (left radiograph), which has developed into serious tension pneumothorax shown in right film.

aspiration by the infant of tenacious materials, such as meconium and mucus. Overdistention of alveoli, causing their rupture, and accumulation of interstitial air probably are initiating events. Pneumothorax is associated with an increased risk of intraventricular hemorrhage in preterm infants.

Spontaneously occurring pneumothorax may be undetected but can be associated with considerable respiratory distress. Pneumothorax under tension (Fig. 27-5) usually leads to rapid deterioration of the infant's condition.
Signs encountered include the following:
1. Increasing respiratory difficulty
2. Hypoxemia, hypercarbia, acidosis
3. Elevation of central venous pressure
4. Fall in arterial pressure
5. Decrease of breath sounds to auscultation over involved side
6. Increase in transillumination over involved side

Transillumination is helpful in prompt detection of a major air leak and will allow immediate intervention and so diminish the chance of severe deterioration of the infant's condition.

MANAGEMENT OF PNEUMOTHORAX

In cases when symptoms are minimal and oxygen requirements are low, observation only is required. Nevertheless, these infants should be placed in environments where early intervention can be undertaken. A chest tube should be placed when pneumothorax is associated with significant respiratory distress, with air under tension (mediastinal shift, diaphragmatic depression), or when there are even small collections in infants treated with a ventilator.

NEEDLE ASPIRATION OF PNEUMOTHORAX

Placement of a chest tube can be time consuming and inconvenient (e.g., during transport), yet prompt relief may be urgent for infant survival. For this we use an intravenous catheter to reduce the chance of laceration of the lung.

The procedure is as follows:
1. Prepare skin with povidone-iodine (Betadine) followed by alcohol.
2. Connect 22-gauge intravenous catheter to 3-way stopcock attached to a 20 ml syringe.
3. With stopcock turned off, insert needle in second intercostal space in midclavicular line or fourth space in anterior axillary line.
4. Open stopcock toward syringe and aspirate any air present.
5. Turn stopcock off and withdraw intravenous catheter once chest tube is placed. During transport, attachment of intravenous catheter or chest tube to a Heimlich flutter valve will prevent reaccumulation of air.

CHEST TUBE PLACEMENT FOR PNEUMOTHORAX

Although use of small catheters is helpful for immediate relief, larger tubes are required for prolonged placement to prevent their obstruction and subsequent reaccumulation of intrapleural air.

Optimal air evacuation is achieved with the tube placed anteriorly from either an incision at the fourth to fifth intercostal space in the midaxillary line or at the second intercostal space in the midclavicular line. The latter position is chosen in the very small infant to ensure positioning of all holes of the chest tube within the pleural cavity.

1. Prepare skin as usual.
2. Obtain a chest tube, preferably one such as the Dekanatel* trocar catheter. The trocar will be helpful in guiding the catheter to the desired position. Use Fr 10 catheters for infants of less than 1,500 gm birth weight, Fr 12 for larger infants, or whenever a large air leak is suspected, since a wider diameter will enhance evacuation of air.
3. Make a small incision in skin, just long enough to allow a snug fit around chest tube. Place mattress suture across incision. Leave ends untied.
4. Dissect intercostal muscles with a curved hemostat, sliding it over the rib to avoid intercostal vessels.
5. Insert trocar catheter (with trocar lubricated and both trocar and tube bent to aid anterior placement) through incision until it has penetrated the pleura.
6. Carefully remove trocar, holding tube in place. For infants who are breathing spontaneously, be sure to occlude catheter promptly when removing trocar to prevent sucking of air during inspiration. Connect catheter to underwater seal or suction, and open chest tube. For infants whose lungs are ventilated with positive pressure the above precautions are less critical.
7. Secure chest tube with a suture placed through skin and blue ridge supplied for this purpose with the Dekanatel trocar catheter. Previously placed mattress suture should be tied once and left. It will be used to occlude incision with a double knot once chest tube is removed.
8. Coat insertion site with antibiotic ointment, and cover it with a small dressing.
9. Connect chest tube to underwater seal or suction using negative pressure of 10 to 15 cm.
10. Obtain chest film.
11. Milk tube frequently to prevent obstruction.

REMOVAL OF CHEST TUBE

Removal of chest tubes can usually be accomplished 48 to 96 hours following placement or when air bubbles are no longer observed to come from chest tube and a chest x-ray film shows full expansion of lung. Observation of no further reaccumulation of air while tube is connected to underwater seal is another assurance of removal readiness.

Pneumomediastinum

Infants with pneumomediastinum usually are managed by observation only unless survival of the infant is in question. Needle aspiration of air from the mediastinum can be performed by insertion of the needle parallel to the sternum under the xiphoid bone until air is aspirated. Larger catheters can be placed in the same location.

Pneumoperitoneum

Pneumoperitoneum, a rare complication, is seen occasionally after resuscitation with bag and mask and during prolonged ventilation. Abdominal distention and worsening of the infant's respiratory status suggest this complication. Air enters the peritoneal cavity, usually by dissection down the aortic sheath from a pneumomediastinum or through a perforation of the stomach (especially after bag resuscitation). An x-ray examination of upright abdomen will show air under the diaphragm. Immediate relief can be obtained by aspiration of air with a needle. Careful evaluation with contrast studies is necessary to rule out a perforated gastrointestinal tract. Surgical exploration may be needed on occasion.

Pneumopericardium

Fortunately a rare occurrence with mechanical ventilation, pneumopericardium can be fatal unless detected early and treated immediately. The infant usually deteriorates very quickly with

---

*Howmedica, Inc., 110 Jericho Turnpike, Floral Park, N.Y. 11001.

decreasing arterial pressure, narrowing of pressure difference, and rapid heart rate. Tamponade eventually will lead to a cardiac output too low for survival.

Transillumination of the anterior chest wall may aid in establishing the diagnosis. Although a chest x-ray film is diagnostic, prompt intervention before a film can be taken usually is required to save the infant's life.

Insertion of a Fr 22 intravenous catheter underneath the xiphoid parallel to the sternum and aspiration of air from the pericardial sac will promptly result in improvement of the infant's condition. Connection to continuous prolonged suction may be needed.

CAUSES OF RESPIRATORY DISTRESS IN THE NEONATE
Hyaline membrane disease (respiratory distress syndrome)

The onset of respiratory distress in a preterm infant during the first few hours of life, followed by the familiar expiratory grunt first noted after 3 to 6 hours of age, is generally indicative of hyaline membrane disease (HMD). The name refers to the pink-staining fibrinoid deposits that line the alveolar ducts, which are observed at autopsy examination. The precise mechanism of formation is obscure, but the disease, with its interference with alveolar ventilation, is responsible for as many as 12,000 infant deaths each year in the United States. From 20% to 30% of those with the established disease die. Affected males have nearly double the mortality of female infants.

  I. Associated factors
   A. Insufficient surfactant production associated with prematurity
   B. Asphyxiation during labor and delivery, further diminishing surfactant levels
   C. Presence of acidosis, hypoxemia, hypovolemia, and hypothermia
  II. Pathophysiology
   Diminished surfactant production in lung parenchyma is insufficient to maintain alveolar stability, causing progressive alveolar collapse. Resulting hypoxemia, acidosis, and shock lead to vasoconstriction of the pulmonary arteries and pulmonary hypoperfusion. The following events apparently occur:
   A. Reduction in lung compliance (lung stiffness) and a consequent increase in the work of breathing—these changes reduce alveolar ventilation and further decrease gaseous exchange.
   B. Right-to-left shunts—these may occur outside the lungs at ductus arteriosus or foramen ovale sites: additionally, intrapulmonary shunts result in bypass of the alveoli.
   C. Effusion of plasma through the capillary walls, with fibrin deposits in the alveoli and alveolar ducts (hyaline membranes)—this leads to airway obstruction and further compounds the problem.
   Many other factors have been implicated, including elevated circulating catecholamines, bradykinin deficiency, and disseminated intravascular coagulation.
  III. Gross and microscopic pathology
   A. Gross changes observed in infants dying of this disease include:
    1. Resorption atelectasis with distended terminal bronchioles
    2. Lung sections resembling liver in color and consistency
   B. Microscopic findings
    1. Pink-staining fibrinoid deposits adjacent to the aerated portions of the terminal bronchioles and alveolar ducts (hyaline membranes)
    2. Pulmonary vascular engorgement, often with frank hemorrhage
  IV. Clinical features
   A. Moderately severe cases
    1. Gradual increase in respiratory rate (over 60 respirations/min)
    2. Intercostal retraction
    3. Expiratory moan or grunt, sternal and costal retraction, flaring of nares
    4. Fine rales heard at end of inspiration, with reduced air exchange
    5. Foam appearing in the mouth and on the lips (pulmonary edema)
    6. Cyanosis when infant is in room air

7. Baby inactive, assuming a frog-like position
  B. Severe cases
    1. Hypotonia, hypotension, peripheral edema
    2. Cyanosis requiring higher concentrations of oxygen to clear
    3. Apneic periods
  Recovery is indicated by a gradual improvement in respiratory symptoms and blood gas values. Complications include patent ductus arteriosus, cerebral and pulmonary hemorrhages, and air leaks.
V. Laboratory observations
  Changes in blood gas and pH determinations are not specific for hyaline membrane disease and are frequently abnormal, but they serve as an important guide to the seriousness and progress of the disease
  A. Falling pH (under 7.25)
  B. Rising P_{CO_2} (over 45 mm Hg)
  C. Falling PA_{O_2} (under 50 mm Hg)
VI. Chest x-ray examination (Fig. 27-6)
  A. A reticulogranular pattern of the lung can be expected, or opacification of both lung fields in severe cases.
  B. The radiolucent bronchial airway (air bronchogram) extends beyond the heart border because of the air-filled bronchial tree outlined by opacified perihilar areas.
VII. Management
  A. Offer initial and continued care as outlined in this chapter.
  B. Maintain PA_{O_2} between 50 and 70 mm Hg (45 to 50 mm Hg arterialized capillary blood).
  C. Correct acidosis.
  D. Use CPAP if infant is hypoxic in 60% or more oxygen or exhibits deep retractions in 45% oxygen.
  E. Initiate ventilation if CPAP trial is not successful, the infant becomes apneic, or P_{CO_2} rises.
  F. Expect recovery to take anywhere from 1 to several weeks, depending on severity of disease and complications.
  G. Delay oral feeding. Consider parenteral nutrition. We prefer the delay of gastric feedings until the following have occurred:
    1. Infant's respiratory rate is less than 60 respirations/min
    2. Infant has been extubated for

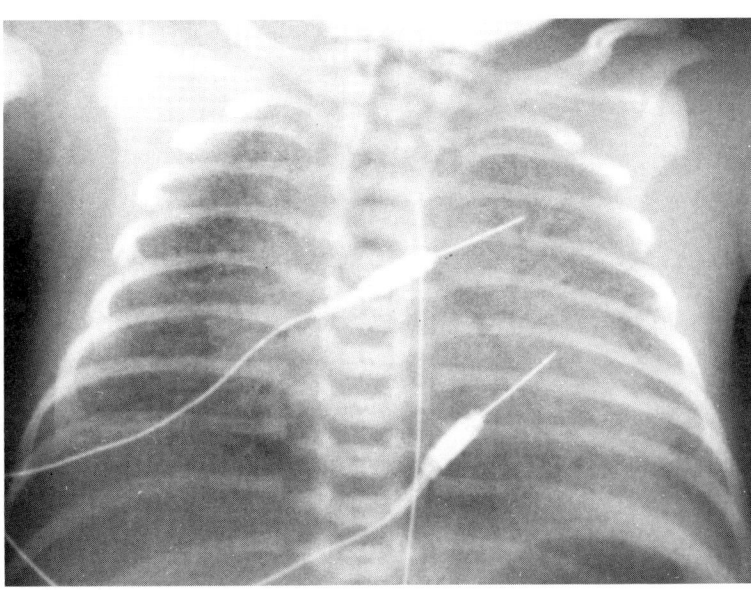

Fig. 27-6. Reticulogranular pattern of lung fields in hyaline membrane disease (idiopathic respiratory distress syndrome).

12 to 24 hours (exceptions are long-term respirator cases)
3. Infant shows functioning gastrointestinal tract (no distention, normal bowel sounds)

VIII. Sequelae

Survival in severe cases is usually followed by later normality, but there is a possibility of later neurologic complication.

IX. Prevention

A. Delay delivery when possible until term or until L/S ratio or rapid surfactant test (RST) indicates maturity unless risks to premature infant are less hazardous than complications of pregnancy.

B. Give dexamethasone to mother before premature delivery of an infant to aid maturation of fetal lungs when L/S ratio or RST indicates prematurity (see Chapter 4).

C. Give optimum care at delivery with prompt resuscitation, amelioration of metabolic acidosis, and avoidance of hypovolemia and chilling.

Apnea of prematurity

Apnea is primarily an extension of periodic breathing in the immature infant with his decreased sensitivity to carbon dioxide and oxygen. When apnea persists beyond 10 seconds, bradycardia is likely, and if respirations do not resume in another 20 seconds, cyanosis will develop, accompanied by asphyxia. (See also the discussion on monitoring for apnea, Chapter 14.)

Approximately 30% of infants less than 32 week's gestation (1,750 gm) at birth and nearly all infants of less than 30 weeks' gestation have apneic periods. Other causative factors include the following:

1. Temperature variations—above or below thermoneutral level (skin temperature 36°C or 97°F)
2. Airway obstruction, such as by mucus or milk
3. Vasovagal response to feedings
4. Hypoglycemia, hypocalcemia
5. Sepsis or meningitis
6. Intracerebral hemorrhage
7. Hyaline membrane disease

MANAGEMENT

1. Monitor respiration and heart rate. Heart rate monitoring alone may be sufficient, since bradycardia follows apnea in most cases. Some infants, however, may have a fixed heart rate during apnea, so that monitoring of respiration also becomes necessary.
2. Prevent dehydration and temperature irregularities that might increase frequency of apnea.
3. Position infant on abdomen or side to minimize apnea. Avoid neck flexion and keep infant's head in line with his trunk.
4. Treat apnea in its early stages by gentle stimulation; the use of oscillating waterbeds has been helpful in many cases.
5. Suction secretions from nasopharynx if cyanosis persists, and resuscitate infant with bag and mask if there is no response to stimulation, using the same air-oxygen mixture administered to the infant before resuscitation. Avoid hyperoxemia by careful monitoring of infant's Pa_{O_2}.
6. Consider intubation or the use of nasal prongs with a continuous transpulmonary distending pressure (1 to 4 cm H_2O), which acts as a "lung stabilizer" for infants with frequent apnea. This procedure is particularly useful when the infant does not tolerate repeated bag and mask ventilation.
7. In cases of refractory apnea not relieved by the above measures, consider administration of aminophylline parenterally or theophylline orally in doses starting with a 5 mg/kg loading dose followed by 2 mg/kg doses given at 6- to 8- hour intervals. Serum levels between 10 and 14 µg/ml are usually therapeutic.
8. Consider overnight monitoring with complete cardiorespirogram of infant with history of repeated apnea prior to discharge. Some infants may eventually have to be sent home with a monitor to avoid unnecessary prolongation of hospitalization. This should be considered only if all other medical problems are resolved and the infant's respiratory pattern fails to mature as expected.
9. Mechanical ventilation should be instituted in severe cases refractory to above treatment. Because of the compliant lungs in typical apnea of prematurity, pressures must be kept low.

Meconium aspiration syndrome

Fetal aspiration, in which meconium-contaminated amniotic fluid and other particulate matter enter the lungs, is probably the result of hypoxia in utero, accompanied by increased fetal respiratory activity. These events may occur either gradually, as in placental insufficiency with chronic fetal distress, or abruptly from any sudden interruption of maternal-fetal oxygen transport, as occurs with cord prolapse or placental separation.

Meconium staining of amniotic fluid is observed at birth in 9% to 16% of all deliveries. In about half of these meconium is found in the trachea, and up to 20% of infants with meconium-stained fluid delivered develop significant disease. Thick meconium, when aspirated by the infant, will partially or totally obstruct minor and major airways.

Results of this aspiration are development of pulmonary atelectasis or emphysema, depending on the degree of obstructions. Pneumothorax may occur and cause further distress to the infant.

CLINICAL FINDINGS

1. Increase in inspiratory effort and tachypnea
2. Medium to gross rales resulting from aspirated debris in the bronchi
3. Hypoxemia, hypercarbia, and acidosis
4. Chest x-ray film showing evidence of diffuse, coarse infiltration with generally overexpanded lung fields from trapped air and occasionally presence of pneumomediastinum or pneumothorax (Fig. 27-7).

PREVENTION OR AMELIORATION OF SEVERE ASPIRATION

Early knowledge of meconium passage during pregnancy and labor will alert the physician and midwife to possible fetal distress and subse-

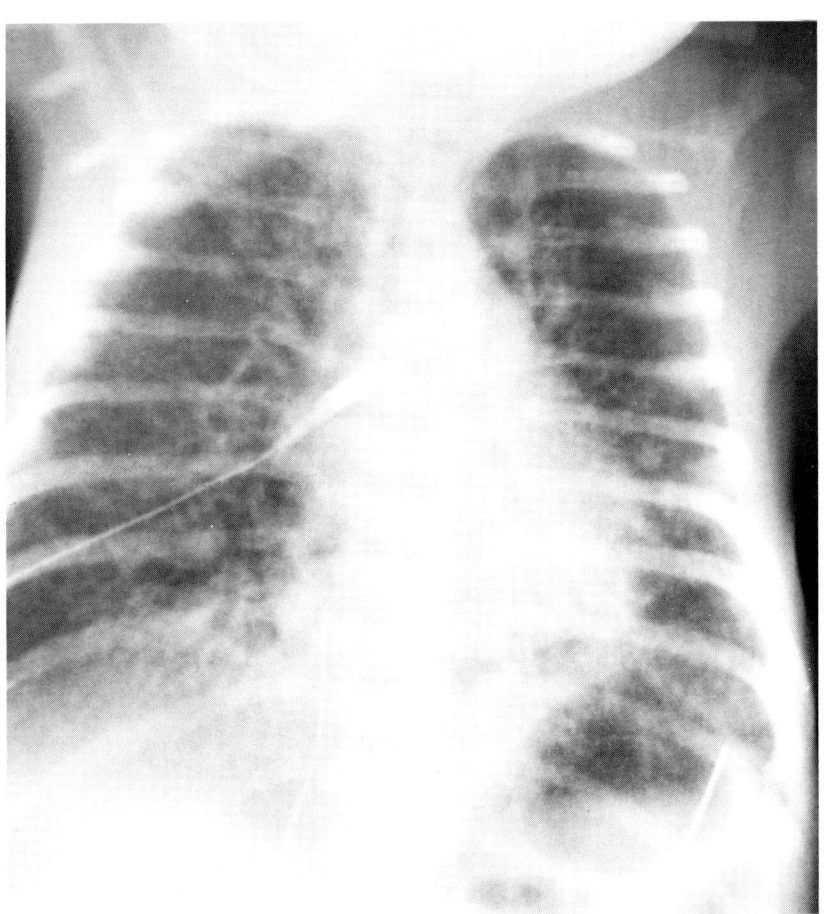

Fig. 27-7. Meconium aspiration syndrome associated with severe respiratory distress.

quent fetal aspiration of amniotic fluid. Prompt attention at delivery will prevent aspiration or deeper inhalation of meconium with the first breaths and thus significantly reduce the incidence of severe aspiration.

1. As soon as the head is delivered, suction fluid from oropharynx and nose with large catheter (Fr 10) and remove as much meconium as possible.
2. As soon as the infant is delivered, unless he is crying vigorously and has good color, view trachea with laryngoscope and thoroughly remove any meconium present by suction with large catheter. In infants with copious amounts of sticky meconium, perform lavage of the trachea with 1 to 2 ml of saline solution, followed by suction.
3. While performing the above procedures, maintain warmth under radiant heating, monitor vital signs, and supply oxygen close to face. Avoid use of positive pressure until airway is cleared.

MANAGEMENT OF SYMPTOMATIC INFANTS

1. Offer full intensive care.
2. View and suction trachea as above unless certain of thorough suctioning.
3. Carefully observe pulmonary and acid-base status and treat accordingly. Be prepared for development of air leaks.
4. Administer antibiotics if bacterial invasion is suspected or pneumonia is present on x-ray examination.
5. Consider ventilatory support with any clinical deterioration.

Persistent pulmonary hypertension

Also called persistence of fetal circulation, persistent pulmonary hypertension (PPH) is the result of the continuation or reestablishment of pulmonary vasoconstriction that is present in the fetal state. The result is a large right-to-left shunting of blood mimicking cyanotic congenital heart disease. The disorder is usually seen in term or postterm infants with a history of fetal distress, meconium aspiration, or depression at birth. It does, however, also occur in preterm infants suffering from hyaline membrane disease. Infants suspected of having PPH may be very difficult to treat and should be referred promptly to a tertiary neonatal center.

CLINICAL MANIFESTATIONS

1. Tachypnea, often with retractions beginning at birth
2. Cyanosis or borderline Pa_{O_2} often unrelieved by even high concentrations of oxygen
3. Worsening of condition with agitation, crying, or stress
4. Chest x-ray film showing signs of meconium aspiration, mild cardiomegaly, HMD, or no significant abnormalities at all
5. Evidence of right-to-left shunt by simultaneous sampling of preductal and postductal arterial blood (i.e., right radial artery and umbilical artery) showing higher Pa_{O_2} in the preductal sample (This can also be accomplished with the simultaneous use of two TcO_2 monitors placed close to the right shoulder and on the abdomen.)
6. PCO_2 that is usually normal but pH that may be low because of metabolic acidosis from tissue hypoxemia

CARDIOLOGIC EVALUATION

The most important diagnosis to exclude in neonates with possible PPH is cyanotic congenital heart disease. The diagnosis of PPH cannot always be made by the above-mentioned difference in Pa_{O_2}, especially in the infant whose ductus arteriosus is closed.

Echocardiography is the best noninvasive technique for diagnosing PPH. This technique can demonstrate the prolongation of systolic time intervals found in infants suffering from PPH.

Cardiac catheterization to measure pulmonary arterial pressure is a highly invasive procedure and should be considered only in cases when the diagnosis remains unclear and the infant is not responding to therapy.

INITIAL MANAGEMENT

1. Offer full intensive care.
2. Attempt to achieve optimal oxygenation by:
   a. Placing infant in environment with high concentrations of oxygen
   b. Ventilating infant's lungs mechanically
   c. Offering more specific therapy to achieve pulmonary vasodilation (see below)
   d. Maintaining optimal cardiac output
      This usually requires placement of catheters in both the inferior vena cava and the umbilical artery and close following of

respective pressures. Administration of colloid and/or vasopressor drugs may be needed.
  e. Keeping infant well sedated to minimize agitation
  f. Considering use of muscle relaxants in cases when high ventilator settings are needed

SPECIFIC THERAPY

PPH has been shown to improve dramatically when infants are hyperventilated. The resulting hypocarbia (PCO_2 range 25-30 mm Hg) will cause pulmonary arterial vasodilation and increase in systemic PA_{O_2}. This therapy is recommended for those infants not responding adequately to conventional management. For some infants who do not respond to hyperventilation or those with severe primary lung disease other than PPH, medication with tolazoline should be attempted. This potent vasodilator, although not specific for the pulmonary vasculature, has been helpful in many instances. Systemic hypotension is a frequent complication that requires vigorous treatment. Tolazoline is administered with a loading dose of 1 to 2 mg/kg IV over several minutes followed by a continuous infusion of 1 to 2 mg/kg/hr IV. Use of the drug should be discontinued if increased oxygenation is not achieved or systemic pressures cannot be maintained at more than 50 mm Hg in a term infant.

Transient tachypnea of newborn

Transient tachypnea occurs primarily in mature infants with no specific antenatal events, although maternal sedation and delivery by cesarean section may be associated factors. Its incidence has been reported to account for up to 30% of all cases of respiratory distress. The pathogenesis appears to be the delayed absorption of fetal lung fluid trapped in the interstitial spaces and engorged periarterial lymphatics (insufficient fall in pulmonary vascular pressure). Outcome is invariably favorable after a course of several hours to several days.

Differentiation of transient tachypnea from hyaline membrane disease or aspiration syndromes is usually easy because of its mild, self-limited course and different appearance on chest x-ray films.

CLINICAL FEATURES

1. Elevated respiratory rates (up to 120 respirations/min) in the absence of significant retractions or rales
2. Occasionally cyanosis in room air, always relieved with additional oxygen
3. Chest x-ray film demonstrating normal findings or prominent hilar markings with peripheral streaking, suggestive of fluid engorgement and slight hyperaeration of lungs

MANAGEMENT

1. Close observation with monitoring of vital signs
2. Administration of oxygen to prevent central cyanosis
3. Support with parenteral fluid during symptomatic stages

Pulmonary hemorrhage

Pulmonary hemorrhage is a nonspecific disorder with many possible causes. It may be found in as many as 10% of autopsies performed on premature infants, infants who were small for dates, or stillborn infants. Asphyxia appears to be a common denominator. Pulmonary hemorrhage rarely occurs as a primary disease but more frequently is observed in severely ill infants as a complication of hyaline membrane disease, patent ductus arteriosus, or sepsis with disseminated intravascular coagulation.

CLINICAL SIGNS

1. Bloody froth in the mouth or nose after sudden cyanotic episode
2. Chest retraction, tachypnea, and cyanosis

TREATMENT

1. General supportive care is indicated.
2. Any clotting defect should be identified and transfusion of fresh whole blood or plasma considered.

Pulmonary dysmaturity

First described by Wilson and Mikity in 1960, pulmonary dysmaturity occurs in small premature infants, usually after the first week of life. Etiology is obscure and not necessarily related to oxygen therapy. The disease resembles bronchopulmonary dysplasia (Fig. 27-4), in which infants have been subjected to high O_2 concentrations while using a positive-pressure venti-

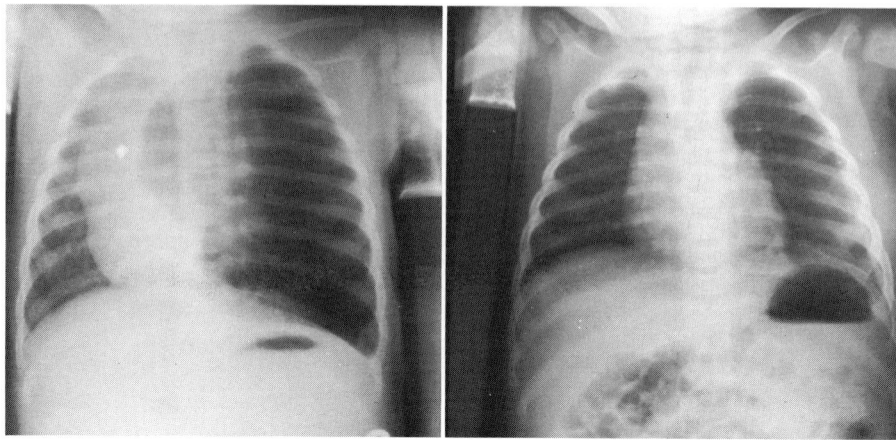

Fig. 27-8. Lobar emphysema with depressed diaphragm and displaced mediastinum (left film). After lobectomy, the lung has returned to its normal position (right film).

lator for severe RDS. Mortality is approximately 30%.

CLINICAL FEATURES

1. Tachypnea, mild retractions, occasionally apnea
2. Elevated Pco_2 in severe cases and hypoxemia in room air
3. Reduced functional residual capacity and vital capacity
4. Bilateral diffuse coarse cystic changes and hyperaeration of lung fields, revealed by chest x-ray films
5. Symptoms that increase in severity over several weeks and gradually improve after several months
6. Hyperaeration of lung base during recovery phase, demonstrated by x-ray films (Cystic changes disappear gradually, and x-ray films will appear normal between 6 months and 2 years of age.)
7. Cor pulmonale, a complicating factor in some severe cases

MANAGEMENT

1. Administration of oxygen if necessary to prevent hypoxemia
2. General supportive measures

Respiratory distress and congenital anomalies of the respiratory tree

Congenital anomalies of the respiratory tree are infrequent, but this possibility should be considered when respiratory difficulty has its onset in the birth room. Respiratory effort accompanied by cyanosis, sometimes with wheezing, choking, or gasping, and excessive mucus requires definitive investigation of the airway and its structures. Lesions may be intrinsic or may encroach on the respiratory passage or lung parenchyma from without. A lateral x-ray film of the airway as well as an anteroposterior x-ray film of the chest is mandatory as an emergency procedure. Fluoroscopy of the esophagus with barium swallow and angiography may be warranted. The following is a partial list of such defects*:

1. Choanal atresia (Chapter 33)
2. Tracheal or laryngeal stenosis, or webs
3. Mediastinal masses
4. Congenital lung cysts and lobar emphysema (Fig. 27-8)
5. Agenesis and hypoplasia of lungs
6. Esophageal atresia, with or without tracheoesophageal fistula (Chapter 33)
7. Diaphragmatic hernia (Chapter 33)
8. Malformation of the great vessels, including vascular ring
9. Phrenic nerve and vocal cord paralyses

---

*More definitive approaches can be found in these valuable books: Scarpelli E.M., Auld, P.A.M., and Goldman, H.S.: Pulmonary disease of the fetus, newborn, and child, Philadelphia, 1978, Lea & Febiger; Caffey, J.: Pediatric x-ray diagnosis, ed. 7, Chicago, 1978, Year Book Medical Publishers, Inc.

BIBLIOGRAPHY

Adamson, T.M., Hawker, J.M., Reynolds, E.O.R., et al.: Hypoxemia during recovery from severe hyaline membrane disease, Pediatrics **44**:168, 1969.

Allen, R.W., Young, A.L., and Lester, P.D.: Effectiveness of chest tube evacuation of pneumothorax in neonates, J. Pediatr. **99**:629, 1981.

Auld, P.A.M.: Oxygen therapy for premature infants, J. Pediatr. **78**:705, 1971.

Avery, M.E., and Fletcher, B.D.: The lung and its disorders, ed. 3, Philadelphia, 1974, W.B. Saunders Co.

Brumley, G.W.: The critically ill child: the respiratory distress syndrome of the newborn, Pediatrics **47**:758, 1971.

Bucciarelli, R.L., Egan, E.A., Gressner, I.H., et al.: Persistence of fetal cardiopulmonary circulation: one manifestation of transient tachypnea of the newborn, Pediatrics **58**:192, 1976.

Cassady, G.: Transcutaneous monitoring in the newborn infant, J. Pediatr. **103**:837, 1983.

Chernick, V., and Reed, M.H.: Pneumothorax and chylothorax in the neonatal period, J. Pediatr. **76**:624, 1970.

Chernick, V., and Vidyasagar, D.: Continuous negative chest wall pressure in hyaline membrane disease: one year experience, Pediatrics **49**:753, 1974.

Daily, W.J.R., Klaus, M., and Meyer, H.B.P.: Apnea in premature infants. I. Monitoring, incidence, heart rate changes, and an effect of environmental temperature, Pediatrics **43**:510, 1969.

DeLeon, A.S., Elliott, J.H., and Jones, D.B.: The resurgence of retrolental fibroplasia, Pediatr. Clin. North Am. **17**:309, 1970.

Duc, G.: Assessment of hypoxia in the newborn, Pediatrics **48**:469, 1971.

Farrell, P.M., and Wood, R.E.: Epidemiology of hyaline membrane disease in the United States: analysis of National Mortality Statistics, Pediatrics **48**:167, 1976.

Finnegan, L.P., McBrine, C.S., Steg, N.L., et al.: Respiratory distress in the newborn, Am. J. Dis. Child. **119**:212, 1970.

Fitzhardinge, P.M., Pape, K., Arstikaitis, M., et al.: Mechanical ventilation of infants of less than 1,501 gm birth weight: health, growth and neurologic sequelae, J. Pediatr. **88**:531, 1976.

Fox, W.W., and Duara, S.: Persistent pulmonary hypertension in the neonate: diagnosis and management, J. Pediatr. **103**:505, 1983.

Gregory, G.A., Gooding, C.A., Phibbs, R.H., et al.: Meconium aspiration in infants: a prospective study, J. Pediatr. **85**:848, 1974.

Gregory, G.A., Kitterman, J.A., Phibbs, R.H., et al.: Treatment of the idiopathic respiratory distress syndrome with continuous positive airway pressure, N. Engl. J. Med. **284**:1333, 1971.

Haworth, S.G., and Reid, L.: Persistent fetal circulation: newly recognized structural features, J. Pediatr. **88**:614, 1976.

Hill, A., Perlman, J.M., and Volpe, J.J.: Relationship of pneumothorax to occurrence of intraventricular hemorrhage in the premature newborn, Pediatrics **69**:144, 1982.

Hittner, H.M., Godio, L.B., Rudolph, H.J., et al.: Retrolental fibroplasia: efficacy of vitamin E in a double blind clinical study of preterm infants, N. Engl. J. Med. **305**:1365, 1981.

Hittner, H.M., Godio, L.B., Speer, M.E., et al.: Retrolental fibroplasia: further clinical evidence and ultrastructural support for efficacy of vitamin E in the preterm infant, Pediatrics **71**:423, 1983.

Hobel, C.J., Oh, W., Hyvarinen, M.A., et al.: Early versus late treatment of neonatal acidosis in low-birth weight infants: relation to respiratory distress syndrome, J. Pediatr. **81**:1178, 1972.

Huch, R., Huch, A., Albani, M., et al.: Transcutaneous P_{O_2} monitoring in routine management of infants and children with cardiorespiratory problems, Pediatrics **57**:681, 1976.

Hunt, C.E.: Capillary blood sampling in the infant: usefulness and limitations of two methods of sampling compared with arterial blood, Pediatrics **51**:501, 1973.

Johnson, J.D., Malachowski, N.C., Grobstein, R., et al.: Prognosis of children surviving with the aid of mechanical ventilation in the newborn period, J. Pediatr. **84**:272, 1974.

Kamper, J.: Long-term prognosis of infants with severe idiopathic respiratory distress syndrome. I. Neurologic and mental outcome, Acta Paediatr. Scand. **67**:61, 1978.

Kamper, J.: Long-term prognosis of infants with severe idiopathic respiratory distress syndrome. II. Cardiopulmonary outcome, Acta Paediatr. Scand. **67**:71, 1978.

Kao, L.C., Warburton, D., Sargent, C.W., et al.: Furosemide acutely decreases airways resistance in chronic bronchopulmonary dysplasia, J. Pediatr. **103**:624, 1983.

Kattwinkel, J., Fleming, D., Cha, C.C., et al.: A device for administration of continuous positive airway pressure by the nasal route, Pediatrics **52**:131, 1973.

Kattwinkel, J., Nearman, H.S., Fanaroff, A.A., et al.: Apnea of prematurity, J. Pediatr. **86**:588, 1975.

Kinsey, V.E., Herold, H.J., Kalina, R.E., et al.: $P_{A_{O_2}}$ levels and retrolental fibroplasia: a report of the cooperative study, Pediatrics **60**:655, 1977.

Koops, B.L., Abman, S.H., and Accurso, F.J.: Outpatient management and follow-up of bronchopulmonary dysplasia, Clin. Perinatol. **11**:101, 1984.

Krauss, A.N., Klain, D.B., and Auld, P.A.M.: Chronic pulmonary insufficiency of prematurity, Pediatrics **55**:55, 1975.

Krauss, A.N., Levin, A.R., Grossman, H., et al.: Physiologic studies on infants with Wilson-Mikity syndrome, J. Pediatr. **77**:27, 1970.

Northway, W., Rosan, R.C., and Porter, D.: Pulmonary disease following respirator therapy, N. Engl. J. Med. **276**:357, 1967.

Peabody, J., and Philip, A.: Disorganized breathing: an important form of apnea and cause of hypoxia, Pediatr. Res. **11**:540, 1009, 1977.

Peabody, J., Gregory, G., et al.: Failure of conventional monitoring to detect hypoxia, Clin. Res. **25**:1902, 1977.

Porat, R.: Care of the infant with retinopathy of prematurity, Clin. Perinatol. **11**:123, 1984.

Reynolds, E.O.R., Robertson, N.R.C., and Wigglesworth, J.S.: Hyaline membrane disease, respiratory distress, and surfactant deficiency, Pediatrics **42**:758, 1968.

Rigatto, H., and Brady, J.P.: Periodic breathing and apnea in preterm infants, I. Evidence for hypoventilation possibly due to central respiratory depression, Pediatrics 50: 202, 1972.

Rigatto, H., and Brady, J.P.: Periodic breathing and apnea in preterm infants. II. Hypoxia as a primary event, Pediatrics 50:219, 1972.

Rigatto, H., Brady, J.P., and de la Torre Verduzco, R.: Chemoreceptor reflexes in preterm infants. I. The effect of gestational and postnatal age on the ventilatory response to inhalation of 100% and 15% oxygen, Pediatrics 55:604, 1975.

Rigatto, H., Brady, J.P., and de la Torre Verduzco, R.: Chemoreceptor reflexes in preterm infants. II. The effect of gestational and postnatal age on the ventilatory response to inhaled carbon dioxide, Pediatrics 55:614, 1975.

Rothberg, A.D., Marks, K.H., and Maisels, M.J.: Understanding the Pleurevac, Pediatrics 67:482, 1981.

Schapiro, R.L., and Evans, E.T.: Surgical disorders causing neonatal respiratory distress, Am. J. Roentgenol. 114: 305, 1972.

Schreiner, R.L., and Kisling, J.A.: Practical neonatal respiratory care, New York, 1982, Raven Press.

Shannon, D.C., Gotay, F., Stein, I.M., et al.: Prevention of apnea, bradycardia in low-birthweight infants, Pediatrics 55:589, 1975.

Simmons, M.A., Adcock, E.W., III, Bard, H., et al.: Hypernatremia and intracranial hemorrhage in neonates, N. Engl. J. Med. 291:6, 1974.

Smith, P.C., and Daily, W.J.R.: Mechanical ventilation of newborn infants, IV. Technique of controlled intermittent positive-pressure ventilation, Anesthesiology 34: 127, 1971.

Stahlman, M.E., Hedvall, G., Dolanski, E., et al.: A six-year follow-up of clinical HMD, Pediatr. Clin. North Am. 20:433, 1973.

Stern, L.: The use and misuse of oxygen in the newborn infant, Pediatr. Clin. North Am. 20:447, 1973.

Thibeault, D.W., Grossman, H., Hagstrom, J.W.C., et al.: Radiological findings in the lungs of premature infants, J. Pediatr. 74:1, 1969.

Vohr, B.R., Bell, E.F., and Oh, W.: Infants with bronchopulmonary dysplasia, Am. J. Dis. Child. 136:443, 1982.

28

Neonatal hyperbilirubinemia and prevention of kernicterus

Jaundice in the newborn, a common sign of potential trouble, is primarily caused by unconjugated bilirubin, a breakdown product of hemoglobin (Hgb), after its release from hemolysed red blood cells. The rate of hemolysis and the red cell mass available (increased by placental transfusion) affect the amount of bilirubin formed. Normally 1 ml of blood per kilogram of the perinate's body weight (1% of circulating blood) is hemolysed daily, yielding 0.15 gm of Hgb. This amount of Hgb produces 5 mg of bilirubin, to which is added another milligram or so from other heme pigments. This amount of bilirubin can normally be conjugated in the liver with glucuronide by glucuronyl transferase and be excreted into the bile as the water-soluble direct reacting form of bilirubin. However, with overproduction of bilirubin or reduction in glucuronide conjugation, bilirubin levels will increase and jaundice will be noted when serum levels of approximately 6 mg/100 ml are reached. If untreated, 10% to 20% of preterm infants will have peak bilirubin levels above 12 mg/100 ml and be at risk for kernicterus. The very immature and stressed infant is often at risk at even lower levels.

Kernicterus is the result of free unconjugated bilirubin entering brain tissue and causing neurotoxic damage. Between 2% and 16% of all autopsied preterm infants show this type of injury. Bilirubin encephalopathy and neurologic deficits in survivors can be reduced by (1) avoiding stressful events in the perinatal period that enhance bilirubin neurotoxicity, (2) supporting the binding of bilirubin to albumin molecules to reduce amounts of free, easily diffusable bilirubin, and (3) limiting the rise in bilirubin levels. Although skin color is a poor measure of bilirubin amounts, twice-daily inspection for jaundice under white light will identify a possible problem.

CONDITIONS ASSOCIATED WITH INCREASED BILIRUBIN LEVELS
Factors leading to overproduction of unconjugated bilirubin

1. Physiologic factors
   a. Red blood cell destruction (1% to 1.4%/24 hr, depending on percentage of fetal hemoglobin)
   b. Amount of additional blood received from placenta
2. Hemolytic disease of the newborn or erythroblastosis fetalis (p. 276), which is the result of maternal isoimmunization to a fetal blood group antigen
3. Enclosed hemorrhage (e.g., cephalhematoma, ecchymosis from bruising [breech delivery], pulmonary bleeding, ingestion of placental or maternal blood with melena)
4. Resorption of bilirubin* from meconium

---

*Beta-glucuronidase found in the intestinal wall can hydrolyse the bilirubin glucuronide in meconium, allowing free bilirubin produced to be absorbed into the bloodstream. Although most bilirubin is cleared by the placenta during fetal life, up to 200 mg (0.5 to 1 mg/gm of meconium) has accumulated in the term infant.

when its elimination is delayed because of intestinal obstruction, delayed onset of feeding, and intestinal hypomotility in the small premature infant
5. Increased production of nonhemoglobin heme secondary to low caloric intake
6. Congenital red blood cell abnormality with hemolysis (spherocytosis)
7. Congenital enzyme deficiency (e.g., glucose-6-phosphate dehydrogenase deficiency, hexokinase deficiency)
8. Drug-induced hemolytic anemia mediated through an enzyme deficiency, such as when large amounts of a vitamin K analog are given to mother or infant
9. Infection-induced hemolysis (more likely to intensify jaundice after 3 days of age)

Factors delaying or interfering with bilirubin conjugation into water-soluble direct reacting form

1. Immaturity of, or defects in, glucuronyl transferase enzyme system
2. Metabolic factors such as asphyxia, hypoglycemia, hypothermia, or decreased thyroid activity
3. Increased lipase activity or presence of maternal steroid Pregnanediol, both present in human milk
4. Hepatic cell damage caused by infection or drugs

Factors leading to impaired excretion of bilirubin

Factors that affect bilirubin excretion lead to accumulation of conjugated bilirubin (serum level over 2 mg/100 ml), as well as unconjugated bilirubin. Water-soluble conjugated or direct reacting bilirubin is not encephalotoxic and does not enter brain tissue. Many physicians subtract direct reacting bilirubin from total bilirubin in judging the need for exchange transfusion.
  1. Hepatitis caused by viral, bacterial, protozoal, or toxic agents
  2. Biliary duct obstruction (congenital or caused by inspissation), malformation of bile canaliculi
  3. Hypoxia
  4. Inborn errors of metabolism causing liver disease (i.e., galactosemia)
  5. Cholestasis related to parenteral nutrition

WHEN TO INVESTIGATE CLINICAL JAUNDICE

1. Jaundice appearing in first 24 hours
2. Serum bilirubin greater than 10 mg/100 ml by 36 hours of age
3. Bilirubin levels rising at a rate greater than 3 mg/12 hr
   (All the above situations suggest a hemolytic process and the possibility that an exchange transfusion may be required.)
4. Preterm infants with bilirubin levels over 6 mg/100 ml and term infants with levels over 15 mg/100 ml—levels usually not found until after 48 hours, having multiple causes
5. Bilirubin levels failing to subside after 6 days or jaundice persisting after 10 days
6. Sudden accentuation of jaundice after 3 to 4 days

DIAGNOSTIC APPROACH TO EXCESSIVE JAUNDICE AND HYPERBILIRUBINEMIA

1. Complete family and pregnancy history (including breast feeding) and physical examination
2. Capillary blood for direct and indirect reacting bilirubin levels plus hematocrit
3. Peripheral smear for variations in red cell morphology and a reticulocyte count (greater than 7% suggests excessive fetal red cell losses)
4. Coombs' test and cross match of infant's cells with maternal serum to detect abnormal antibodies when infant and mother are of same type; blood typing of mother and baby
5. Observation and appropriate cultures for suspected infection
6. Special tests for enzyme deficiencies and galactosemia when indicated

ERYTHROBLASTOSIS FETALIS

Sensitization of the mother (isoimmunization) occurs after incompatible blood administration or after one or more pregnancies in which fetal erythrocytes have escaped into the maternal circulation. The mother produces antibodies that cross the placental barrier to cause agglutination and hemolysis of fetal red blood cells.

Because of the widespread administration of RhoGAM (Appendix H) to women who are Rh negative, serious cases of isoimmunization, once a significant cause of perinatal death, are now rare. In addition, screening of maternal blood serum in early pregnancy for antibodies (Appendix H) and identification, if present, of the specific blood group antigen will alert the physician to offer appropriate management. Serial amniocentesis (Appendix H) will indicate severity and possible need for early delivery or fetal transfusion, or both.

Management of infant at delivery

Severe erythroblastosis will often require early exchange at lower levels of bilirubin in anticipation of its rapid rise.
1. Clamp cord promptly.
2. Collect tube of cord blood (allow clotting) for typing, Coombs' test, and blood serum bilirubin level determination.
3. Obtain tube of oxalated cord blood for hemoglobin count and smear for identification of immature red cell forms (nucleated red blood cells and spherocytes).
4. Place infant under radiant heat; observe for color, edema, and hepatosplenomegaly; support infant in general with full intensive care as indicated in Chapter 14.
5. See p. 279 for type of blood to be used.

ABO incompatibility

More common than isoimmunization from the Rhesus group, but much less severe, is ABO incompatibility. This occurs when type A or B fetal red blood cells cause a type O mother to develop specific antibodies. The newborn may show a weakly positive direct Coombs' test. Cord bilirubin is usually less than 4 mg/100 ml and any hyperbilirubinemia can usually be treated with phototherapy as outlined on p. 278. Exchange transfusions are required in occasional cases only. Ongoing hemolysis may cause anemia and justifies serial hematocrit studies until stable.

KERNICTERUS

The clinical manifestations of kernicterus (bilirubin encephalopathy) appear during the first week of life. Generalized hypotonia and depression of reflexes may be followed by hypertonia and seizures. These signs are likely to be followed by death or serious neurologic sequelae in survivors. Evidence exists that hyperbilirubinemia without the clinical picture of kernicterus may retard development, and in susceptible immature preterm infants, serum bilirubin levels as low as 9 to 12 mg/100 ml may be associated with brain cell staining from bilirubin entry. These infants may have either been stressed so that their susceptibility to the disease is increased or have low albumin concentrations or limited binding sites on the albumin molecule for bilirubin binding. Measurement of unbound or free bilirubin has proved difficult for clinical assessment.

Factors interfering with albumin binding

1. Reduced albumin levels (albumin less than 3 gm/100 ml)
2. Presence of drugs (e.g., sulfonamides and salicylates) that take up binding sites on the albumin molecule
3. Free fatty acids, possibly increased by hypoglycemia, hypothermia, and use of parenteral fat, that may displace bilirubin from binding sites
4. Acidosis

Factors that stress the infant

The following are factors that may increase susceptibility (particularly for the immature infant) to the neurotoxic effect of bilirubin by (1) enhancing its passage across the blood-brain barrier and (2) reducing cellular integrity:
1. Perinatal asphyxia (pH under 7.20)
2. Unstable physiologic condition of newborn indicated by Apgar score of 3 or less at 5 minutes
3. Hypothermia (temperature less than 35° C)
4. Deterioration of infant's condition as indicated by clinical signs

Although the precise effects of these insults are indeterminate, the increased risk may be sufficient to justify treatment at lower levels of bilirubin.

Prevention of kernicterus

Although expert perinatal care for the infant at risk will decrease susceptibility to kernicterus, the main goal is that of limiting peak bilirubin levels. Recent information (Pearlman, et al.) indicates that kernicterus, as shown by autopsy examination, is virtually absent when bilirubin levels have been controlled. Nevertheless, staining of the basal ganglia has been found in VLBW infants whose serum bilirubin levels were no different than levels in similar yet unaffected infants. The clinical courses of these infants did not differ from those of larger infants indicating that the VLBW infants would be at increased risk for kernicterus.

The two modes of therapy that are in general use to control bilirubin levels are phototherapy and exchange transfusions. Therapy with phenobarbital has also been found useful in lowering bilirubin levels. However, the slowness of action (approximately 2 to 3 days) limits the usefulness of this drug for most cases of neonatal hyperbilirubinemia.

PHOTOTHERAPY

Phototherapy applied to unclothed infants is accepted by most physicians as standard treatment for nonhemolytic hyperbilirubinemia when the unclothed skin is exposed to wavelengths of 400 to 500 nm. Unconjugated bilirubin is decomposed into colorless compounds excreted in the bile. Either daylight or blue fluorescent lights are effective. We add blue-light tubes emitting relatively more light in the effective wavelengths to the panel when significant jaundice is present and place them at 60 cm from the infant. Phototherapy will reduce peak bilirubin levels by 25% to 50%. The intensity of light in the therapeutic range should be measured daily to assure an adequate dose of phototherapy (Bilimeter, Olympic Surgical Co., Seattle). *Starting phototherapy for hyperbilirubinemia obligates the physician to begin considering possible causes.*

When to start phototherapy (Fig. 28-1)

1. Very small infants at the first sign of jaundice
2. Any preterm infant with jaundice by 24 hours of age (including laboratory workup)
3. Stressed preterm infants when bilirubin level reaches 6 to 7 mg/100 ml (zone D)
4. Healthy preterm infants (zone C)
5. Term infants whose bilirubin level exceeds 15 mg/100 ml (zone B)

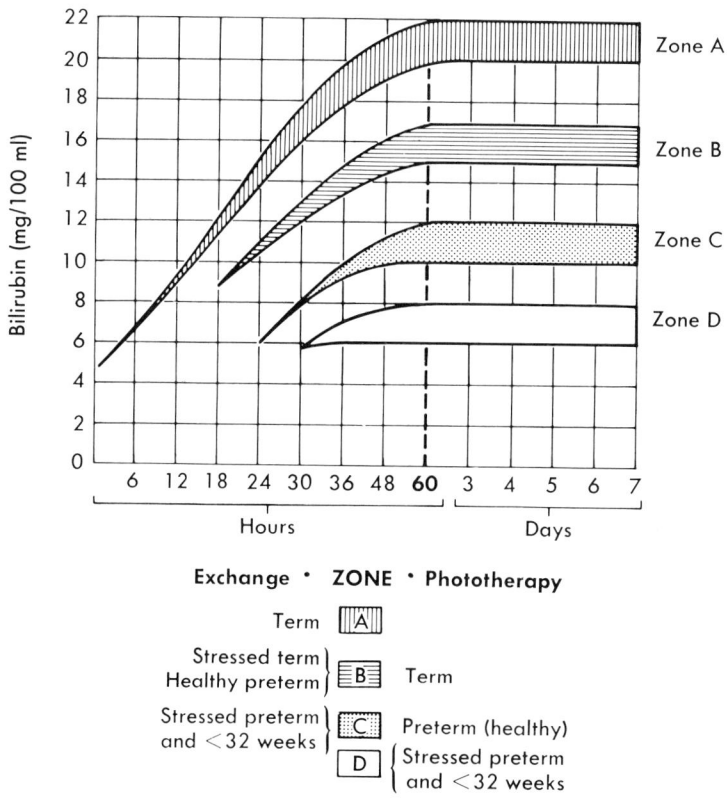

Fig. 28-1. Guide for treatment of hyperbilirubinemia by phototherapy and exchange transfusion depending on serum bilirubin levels and risk of infant for kernicterus. It is assumed that the direct reacting fraction of bilirubin is less than 2 mg/100 ml.

We are unwilling to initiate therapy for healthy mature infants with nonhemolytic bilirubinemia under this level and will discharge them with a level of 13 to 15 mg/100 ml after 48 hours of age if daily bilirubin determinations can be made. Measurements may be discontinued when bilirubin falls under 13 mg/100 ml. However, the physician should be informed if jaundice persists beyond 1 week. Overuse of phototherapy delays discharge, increases parental anxiety (and separation), and raises medical costs.

Observation of infants receiving phototherapy

1. Determine bilirubin level every 12 hours (degree of bilirubinemia cannot be estimated from skin color) and 12 hours after discontinuance of phototherapy (rebound effect).
2. Monitor infant's temperature and body weight more frequently.
3. Perform hematocrit reading during and after phototherapy to detect possible anemia.

Hazards of phototherapy

1. Suppression of jaundice may limit an important sign of sepsis, hemolytic disease, or hepatitis.
2. Higher levels of bilirubin than are suggested by skin color may be present.
3. Although the bilirubin rise in mild erythroblastosis may be controlled, hemolysis continues and may be followed by unrecognized anemia.
4. Damage to retinas may occur without eye protection.
5. An increase in the infant's body temperature may require adjustments in incubator control.
6. Dehydration from increased evaporation through skin may occur.
7. Thermistors in incubators equipped with servo control should be screened from direct radiation.

EXCHANGE TRANSFUSION

Exchange transfusion is used for (1) treatment of hemolytic disease (except in mild cases) and (2) excessive bilirubinemia not controlled by phototherapy in preterm infants. Because exchanges are now seldom required in the community hospital, the procedure is best performed in a secondary or tertiary hospital.

When to exchange blood for excessive bilirubinemia (Fig. 28-1)

1. Exchange transfusions are performed for stressed preterm infants when confirmed bilirubin values rise into zone C or above.
2. Exchange transfusions are performed for severely stressed term infants and healthy preterm infants when serum bilirubin values plot in zone B or above.
3. Exchange transfusions are performed for most term infants in zone A, most of whom will have erythroblastosis fetalis. The guidelines in Fig. 28-1 allow individual consideration for each case, which requires experience and knowledge of the total picture. It is assumed that total bilirubin includes no more than 1 to 2 mg/100 ml of the direct reacting fraction and that laboratory error is no more than 5%. Waiting for zones to be reached before an exchange is accomplished requires that matched blood be available in advance. A difficult matching of blood may delay the procedure and enhance the risk of kernicterus.

Type of blood to be used

1. Packed cells or partially sedimented cells are used for the anemic and often anoxic infant in the birth room. These infants have usually suffered severe hemolytic disease. Fresh O-negative blood previously cross-matched with the mother's serum is required.
2. Fresh whole blood is used for the standard exchange. Preferred blood contains no antibody to the infant's red blood cells (i.e., Rh-negative blood for infants with erythroblastosis attributable to Rh factor, or blood containing little or no anti-A or anti-B for infants with an ABO incompatibility ["low" titer type of blood], or red cells of the infant's type resuspended in fresh A-B plasma).
3. Albumin-primed exchange
   When the bilirubin level is excessive (usually 15 to 20 mg/100 ml:
   a. Give 1 gm/kg of body weight of salt-poor albumin (25%) 60 minutes before the exchange.
   b. Follow the exchange with the same therapy—1 gm binds 16 mg of bilirubin.
   WARNING: An increase in venous pressure may be contraindication because

protein has an oncotic effect and expands blood volume.

Technique of exchange transfusion

1. Remove properly identified donor unit from refrigerator at least an hour before using to allow warming to room temperature. Heating blood to body temperature too rapidly may damage red cells. Short coils placed in water bath at 36° C or the Hamilton Bloodwarmer are used most frequently for warming during exchange.
2. Restrain infant under thermistor-controlled overhead warmer. Attach heart rate monitor.
3. Have a team skilled in resuscitative techniques at bedside, as well as a circulating nurse.
4. Take 60 to 90 minutes for total exchange time, using 5 to 10 ml aliquots. A leisurely approach:
   a. Allows closer observation of infant
   b. Permits greater diffusion of bilirubin into vascular space
   c. Enhances metabolization of citrate in anticoagulated blood, thus reducing acid load
5. Place a radiopaque catheter into an umbilical vessel (Chapter 10), ensuring proper position (thoracic inferior vena cava, thoracic aorta, or aortic bifurcation) by obtaining x-ray films.
6. Attach 3-way stopcock and syringe to proximal end of catheter (disposable exchange transfusion sets contain all necessary attachments).
7. Monitor pressures (central venous or arterial), keeping venous pressures between 5 and 10 cm H_2O. Keep arterial pressures in normal range (Chapter 29).
8. At beginning of exchange, obtain blood from catheter for hematocrit and bilirubin determinations.
9. Keep accurate record during exchange transfusion, noting each successive amount of blood removed and replaced, vital signs of infant, and drugs given.
10. Monitor infant's cardiac rate and electrocardiogram continuously.
11. Observe respirations and skin color, as well as color of withdrawn blood.
12. Maintain infant's blood temperature and oxygen requirements.
13. Inject slowly 0.5 ml calcium gluconate (10%) diluted with saline solution after each 100 ml of blood is exchanged.
    a. Calcium lessens general irritability and irregularity of the heart.
    b. Too rapid an injection slows the heart.
14. Exchange at least 170 ml of blood/kg of body weight.
15. Consider hypoglycemia in erythroblastosis and screen with Dextrostix test if baby's condition is less than excellent.
16. Obtain blood for determination of hematocrit and bilirubin levels at end of procedure. Consider preparing a new unit of blood for possible repeat exchange.

Complications of exchange transfusions

1. Heart failure from hypervolemia or hypovolemia
2. Bradycardia or cardiac arrest from low pH of donor blood (acidosis), hyperkalemia (old blood), rapid injection of calcium, or faulty catheter position
3. Hypocalcemia from citrate binding
4. Hypothermia and increased blood viscosity from cold blood or external chilling
5. Air emboli entering heart from air leaks in system or suction through catheter when negative venous pressure develops on sudden inspiratory effort
6. Thrombotic emboli entering pulmonary vein
7. Sepsis from infected cord stump or contaminated equipment
8. Intensification of hypoglycemia
   Be prepared to give 5 ml of 10% glucose, followed by a glucose infusion.
9. Thrombocyte depletion after repeated exchange transfusions

Although occurrence of the above complications may be as infrequent as 1%, occurrence varies with the experience of the team performing the procedure. Therefore exchange transfusion should be undertaken by persons thoroughly familiar with this technique.

BIBLIOGRAPHY

Behman, R.E., Brown, A.K., Currie, M.R., et al.: Preliminary report of the committee on phototherapy in the newborn infant, J. Pediatr. **84**:135, 1974.

Cremer, R.J., Perryman, P.W., and Richards, D.H.: Influence of light on the hyperbilirubinemia of infants, Lancet **1:**1094, 1958.

Giunta, F., and Rath, J.: Effect of environmental illumination in prevention of hyperbilirubinemia of prematurity, Pediatrics **44:**162, 1969.

Harper, R.G., Sia, C.G., and Kierney, C.M.P.: Kernicterus 1980, Clin. Perinatol. **7:**75, 1980.

Lucey, J., Ferreiro, M., and Hewitt, J.: Prevention of hyperbilirubinemia of prematurity by phototherapy, Pediatrics **41:**1047, 1968.

Maurer, H.M., Shumway, C.N., Draper, D.A., et al.: Controlled trial comparing agar, intermittent phototherapy, and continuous phototherapy for reducing neonatal hyperbilirubinemia, J. Pediatr. **82:**73, 1973.

Odell, G.B.: Neonatal hyperbilirubinemia. In Oliver, T.K., editor: Monographs in neonatology, New York, 1980, Grune & Stratton, Inc.

Pearlman, M.A., Gartner, L.M., Lee K., et al.: Absence of kernicterus in low-birthweight infants born 1971 through 1976: comparison with findings in 1966 and 1967, Pediatrics **62:**460, 1978.

Pierson, W.E., Barrett, C.T., and Oliver, T.K., Jr.: The effect of buffered and non-buffered ACD blood on electrolyte and acid-base homeostasis during exchange transfusion, Pediatrics **41:**802, 1968.

Silberberg, D.H., Johnson, L., and Ritter, L.: Factors influencing toxicity of bilirubin in cerebellum tissue culture, J. Pediatr. **77:**386, 1970.

Sisson, T.R.C., Kendall, N., Glauser, S.C., et al.: Phototherapy of jaundice in newborn infants. I. ABO blood group incompatibility, J. Pediatr. **79:**904, 1971.

29

Cardiovascular problems

This chapter presents only the most serious and common cardiovascular problems that require prompt attention. Cardiovascular adjustments at birth are discussed in Chapter 8. Suspicion of significant cardiovascular disease justifies referral to a tertiary center for further evaluation, which may include echocardiography, cardiac catheterization, and possibly surgery. At least two per 1,000 liveborn infants have severe congenital heart disease (CHD). Approximately half of these infants survive.

Signs of serious cardiovascular disease include the following:
1. Central cyanosis
2. Congestive failure
3. Shock
4. Change in quality of pulses or precordial activity
5. Irregular cardiac rhythm
6. Cardiac murmurs with other evidence of abnormality
7. Abnormal ECG
8. Chest x-ray film revealing abnormal cardiac silhouette and increase or decrease in pulmonary vascularity

CYANOSIS

Most causes of cyanosis of the newborn are associated with respiratory distress or failure, which are discussed in Chapter 27. Unexpected cyanosis or the gradual appearance of a dusky hue is likely to be associated with cardiovascular problems and requires investigation and support.

Skin color must be observed under white light or daylight when the infant is quiet and in a thermoneutral environment. Central cyanosis must be differentiated from peripheral cyanosis, which usually persists from birth and may last for several days. It is usually confined to the extremities, does not involve the mucous membranes, and is intensified by a continued cool environment.

Central cyanosis is pathologic and defined as cyanosis of skin, tongue, and mucous membranes in the presence of 3 gm or more of reduced hemoglobin in arterial blood. Infants with severe anemia are unlikely to show cyanosis even with low oxygen saturation, whereas infants with polycythemia may be cyanotic with adequate levels of oxygen saturation.

Fetal hemoglobin has an increased affinity for oxygen, and the premature infant may not show cyanosis at arterial oxygen tensions of less than 40 mm Hg even though this level falls within the hypoxic range.

Some normal infants may not be relieved of central cyanosis until 10 to 20 minutes after birth.

Causes of central cyanosis

1. Pulmonary diseases (Chapter 27)
2. Congenital heart disease
   Breathing may be rapid, but it is not distressed unless there is heart failure.
   a. Right-to-left shunt and diminished or increased pulmonary blood flow without heart failure (e.g., tetralogy of Fallot, pulmonary atresia, tricuspid atresia, or transposition of great vessels)
   Breathing is deep and slightly increased in frequency.

b. Congenital heart disease with heart failure (e.g., large patent ductus arteriosus or myocarditis)
3. Polycythemia
   The heart may be enlarged. See p. 294 for treatment.
4. Shock and sepsis
   Hypovolemia and septic shock lead to intense vasoconstriction and can be associated with central as well as peripheral cyanosis.
5. Central nervous system
   Breathing is likely to be slow and shallow, with reduced ventilation and lowered P_{AO_2}.
   a. Intracranial hemorrhage or abnormality
   b. Meningitis or meningoencephalitis
   c. Perinatal asphyxia and shock
   d. Narcosis from maternal medication
6. Miscellaneous causes (e.g., hypoglycemia, methemoglobinemia)

Diagnostic observations and procedures

1. Observe baby for breathing pattern.
2. Auscultate heart, determine liver size, and check peripheral pulses and blood pressure of all extremities.
3. Obtain x-ray film of chest and electrocardiogram.
4. Obtain hematocrit, blood glucose, and serum calcium levels.
5. Perform analysis of blood gases, including arterial oxygen tension.
6. Repeat blood gas determinations after placing infant in 100% oxygen for several minutes. Failure of oxygen tension to rise over 50 mm Hg (may reach 400 mm Hg in normal term infants) indicates presence of large right-to-left shunt of the circulation. Blood may be bypassing the lungs (intracardiac shunt) or the alveoli (intrapulmonary shunt) compatible with congenital heart disease, hyaline membrane disease, or persistence of fetal circulation.
7. Consider spinal tap and study for sepsis.

CARDIAC FAILURE

Heart failure may simulate disorders of other organs or systems, and other disease entities may appear with some of the clinical signs of heart failure. The closer the time of birth to the time at which heart failure becomes apparent, the more critical its nature. Clinical deterioration or failure to improve within 12 hours of treatment usually is an indication for cardiac catheterization and angiocardiography.

Associations

1. Structural heart disease (most common cause) attributed to errors of embryogenesis in the first 2 months of gestation (e.g., transposition of the great vessels, hypoplastic left heart)
2. Myocarditis attributed to invasion of heart by viral organisms (e.g., Coxsackie B viruses, infection with bacterial sepsis, or damage from bacterial toxins)
3. Respiratory disease with increased vascular resistance (e.g., hyaline membrane disease or pneumonia)
4. Polycythemia or circulatory overload in overtransfusion or twin-to-twin transfusion
5. Anemia, as with hydrops fetalis
6. Arrhythmias caused either by congenital heart block (less than 80 beats/min) or by paroxysmal atrial tachycardia (180 to 300 beats/min)
7. Miscellaneous conditions, including hypoglycemia, cerebral or hepatic arteriovenous fistula, glycogen storage disease, hypertension, and endocardial fibroelastosis

Clinical features

1. Common signs are tachypnea (60 to 100 respirations/min at rest), tachycardia (150 to 180 beats/min at rest), fatigue or difficulty with feeding, enlarging liver (3 to 5 cm below the costal margin), and pulmonary rales or rhonchi.
2. Less common signs are systemic edema, elevated venous pressure, inappropriate sweating, a gallop rhythm, and pulsus alternans.
3. Chest x-ray examination often discloses enlargement of heart (cardiothoracic index of over 75%), changes in cardiac contour, or diminished or engorged pulmonary vasculature.
4. Electrocardiogram may indicate hypertrophy of one or more chambers, abnormalities of the mean QRS axis, and rhythm disturbances.

Noncardiac diseases simulating heart failure

1. Cardiomegaly of hypoglycemia in the newborn

2. Central cyanosis with heart murmurs in respiratory disease (e.g., idiopathic respiratory distress)
3. Liver enlargement from specific conditions (e.g., fetal viral invasion, galactosemia, or neuroblastoma)
4. Tachypnea from metabolic acidosis or minor pulmonary disorders (e.g., transient tachypnea of the newborn)
5. Peripheral edema observed in oliguria caused by renal failure, hypoalbuminemic states, and lymphedema
6. Factitious cardiomegaly from an apparent wide mediastinal shadow caused by a chest deformity or an x-ray film taken during expiration

Management

1. Offer intensive care, with skin temperature maintained at 36° C (97° ± 1° F), oxygen concentration between 30% and 35%, ECG monitoring, and an inclined plane position (head raised at an angle of 10 to 20 degrees).
2. Digitalize patient (for dosage, see Appendix G). Observe for
   a. Bradycardia (discontinue digitalis when heart rate is under 100 beats/min)
   b. Signs of heart block, multiple ectopic beats
   c. Hypokalemia
3. Maintain fluid and nutritional support. Volume of fluid given should be limited during the acute phase (i.e., 80 to 120 ml/kg/day).
4. Consider use of diuretics (e.g., furosemide [Lasix]) 1 mg/kg of body weight, IM or IV.
5. Obtain consultation for consideration of early cardiac catheterization, angiocardiography, and possible surgery.

SHOCK

Shock is defined as a state of inadequate circulating blood volume resulting in decreased perfusion and oxygenation of tissues. Prompt identification and treatment are urgent.

Varieties of shock

1. Hypovolemic shock
   a. Severe blood loss secondary to rupture of umbilical cord, abruptio placentae, twin-to-twin transfusion, or disconnected arterial line
   b. Loss of plasma into extravascular spaces
   c. Loss of body water by persistent vomiting or diarrhea or by evaporative skin losses
2. Cardiogenic shock caused by
   a. Myocardial failure from severe hypoxemia
   b. Cardiac arrythmias
   c. Mechanical restriction of cardiac function from tamponade, tension pneumothorax, or excessive levels of transpulmonary distending pressure
3. Septic shock in which overwhelming infections impair peripheral arterial resistance caused by released toxins
4. Miscellaneous types of shock, including adrenal insufficiency and severe hypoglycemia

Signs of shock

1. Tachycardia
2. Tachypnea
3. Pallor (especially after blood loss)
4. Poor filling of blanched skin, indicating poor tissue perfusion
5. Hypotension (see Fig. 29-1 for range of normal blood pressure)
6. Decreasing urinary output
7. Hypothermia
8. Apnea
9. Metabolic acidosis
10. Hypoglycemia
11. Evidence of coagulation defects

Management of shock

Shock is not a static state; attention to the infant therefore has to be continuous.

1. Place infant in an Isolette or radiant warmer, keeping skin temperature at 36° C (97° F).
2. Monitor infant's heart rate, as well as arterial and, if possible, venous pressure; measure urinary output.
3. Correct metabolic acidosis by administering sodium bicarbonate; continue to monitor blood gases as a measure of effectiveness of therapy.
4. Offer oxygen and assisted ventilation if needed to prevent hypoxemia.
5. Maintain optimal cardiac output and perfusion.
   a. Consider administration of volume expanders (blood, fresh frozen plasma, or Plasmanate 10 to 20 ml/kg) if capillary filling is poor or infant is hypotensive

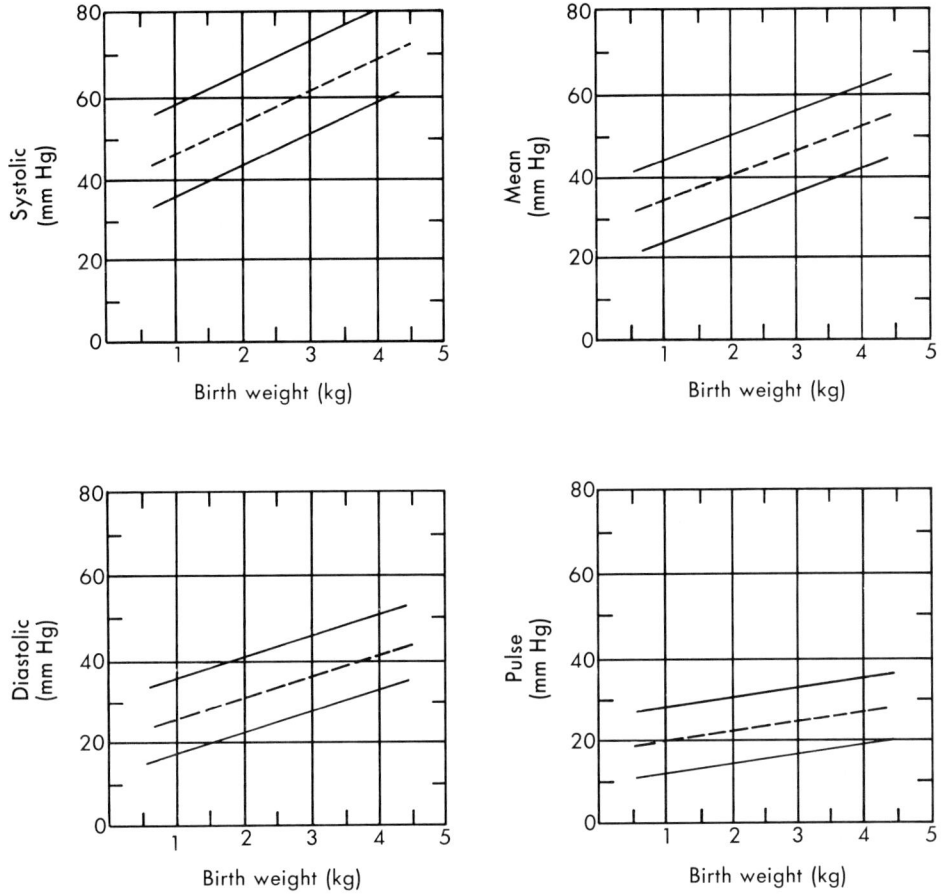

Fig. 29-1. Linear regressions *(broken lines)* and 95% confidence limits *(solid lines)* of systolic *(top left)*, diastolic *(bottom left)*, mean *(top right)*, and pulse pressure *(bottom right)* on birth weight in 61 healthy newborn infants during the first 12 hours after birth. (From Versmold, H.T., Kitterman, J.A., Phipps, R.H., et al.: Pediatrics **67**:607, 1981.)

(Fig. 29-1). Larger doses may be required if hypovolemia is severe, indicated by tachycardia, hypotension, or low central venous pressure (less than 4 cm H_2O).

b. If perfusion or systemic pressures remain inadequate, administer adrenergic drugs such as dopamine and/or dobutamine (infusion into vein or artery at 5 to 10 μg/kg/min). Dopamine not only directly improves cardiac output but also selectively improves renal perfusion and helps reestablish or maintain urine output, which is frequently reduced in shock. However, in doses over 10 μg/kg/min, dopamine may show increasing α-adrenergic effects, leading to vasoconstriction and decreased tissue perfusion and urine output, as well as metabolic acidosis. Dobutamine can be used in addition to dopamine when higher doses are required, since it does not have the α-adrenergic effect of dopamine.

c. If infant becomes bradycardiac, use atropine 0.01 mg/kg IV or eprinephrine (1:10,000 dilution) 0.5 to 1.0 ml IV. For continuing inadequacy of heart rate, infuse isoproterenol 0.2 to 0.5 μg/kg/min IV.

6. Carefully measure urine output. If less than 1 to 2 ml/kg/hr, assess adequacy of cardiac output at stated above.

7. Administer antibiotics if infection is suspected.

8. Promptly correct any other problems that might lead to shock (i.e., pneumothorax, pneumopericardium, overexpansion of lung from inappropriately high ventilator settings, hypoglycemia, etc.).

PAROXYSMAL SUPRAVENTRICULAR TACHYCARDIA (PST or PAT)

Paroxysmal supraventricular or atrial tachycardia (PST or PAT) is the most frequently occurring type of tachyarrhythmia. In absence of major structural defects, the prognosis is good. Development of PST may begin in fetal life or in the first few days after birth.

Clinical manifestation

1. PST may be suspected during fetal life when FHR is over 200 beats/min, not otherwise explained. Fetal PST may be lethal or give rise to hydrops. Consider early delivery if L/S ratio is favorable, or give digoxin to gravida for possible conversion of fetal tachycardia to sinus rhythm.
2. Listlessness and pallor, which may culminate in tachypnea and other signs of heart failure, may indicate PST during newborn period.

ECG tracing demonstrates a ventricular rate of over 180 beats/min, a fixed R-R interval, and an abnormal P wave.

Management

If infant is tachycardic, obtain ECG for diagnosis. If skin color and systemic pressure are normal, no intervention may be needed, and the symptoms may subside spontaneously. If tachycardia persist or infant shows signs of impeded cardiac output, the following should be considered:

1. Noninvasive maneuvers eliciting a vagal reflex bradycardia (i.e., deep catheter suctioning through nasal passages or icepack placed on infant's face)
2. Digitalization of infant
   Give one-half total digitalizing dose parenterally (Appendix G). Conversion usually occurs in 2 hours.
3. Use of cardioversion with DC counter shock
   Because this is a dangerous procedure, it should be performed in a neonatal center unless infant is moribund and unlikely to survive the transport. Five to 20 watt-seconds are used under ECG monitoring. Repeat procedure if not successful.

PATENT DUCTUS ARTERIOSUS (PDA)

In the preterm infant, particularly in the very immature, delay in closure of the ductus is to be expected. For most of these infants no clinical signs are evident except for a systolic murmur in the upper left sternal border transmitted to the back. This murmur disappears as "term" is reached. Increase in the flow through the ductus, (especially from left to right, as seen in hyaline membrane disease) may overburden both the heart and the lung and result in deterioration of the infant or difficulty in weaning him from the ventilator.

Incidence of PDA increases with the immaturity of the infant. A majority of very low birth weight infants recovering from hyaline membrane disease develop serious signs of the disease. Excessive fluid administration apparently aggravates the condition.

The presence of symptoms of PDA significantly increase the risk of intraventricular hemorrhage in the preterm infant and also have been linked to necrotizing enterocolitis. PDA, therefore, has some rather serious implications for infants and should be treated promptly.

Clinical manifestations

1. Deterioration of infant's condition while infant is using ventilator or inability to wean infant from it
2. Tachypnea and feeding limitations in a previously well infant

Signs to note

1. Enhancement of systolic murmur and heart activity
2. "Bounding" peripheral pulses that may be observed in the groin
3. Cardiomegaly and increased pulmonary vascular markings from left-to-right shunting of blood
4. Congestive failure

Diagnosis

Methods used to verify presence of symptomatic PDA include the following:

1. Doppler evaluation showing evidence of significant reverse flow during diastole in major arteries (i.e., brachial artery)
2. Echocardiography demonstrating an enlarged left atrium or large left atrial/aortic diameter ratio

3. Contrast echocardiography showing left to right flow through the ductus

Cardiac catheterization is rarely used because of the risks associated with this invasive procedure.

Management

1. Initial stabilization includes the following:
   a. Sufficient oxygenation given by mechanical ventilation, if necessary
   b. Digitalization
   c. Administration of furosemide 1 mg/kg every 12 hours IM or IV
   d. Restriction of fluid to 90 to 120 ml/kg/day parenterally
2. Closure of ductus performed by administration of indomethacin or surgical ligation

Use of indomethacin, a prostaglandin synthetase inhibitor, has become the favored approach, since it is usually successful. Because of its nephrotoxicity it should not be given to infants with significant renal impairment. Surgical ligation is performed for those infants who do not respond to the drug or who are not able to receive it.

Ductus dilatation

In duct-dependent congenital heart disease in infants with pulmonary atresia, tricuspid atresia, and related conditions, an open ductus arteriosus often is the only source of pulmonary blood flow. Prostaglandin E, which can produce a powerful dilatation of the ductus arteriosus, should be infused parenterally for temporary dilatation of the ductus to promote stabilization in preparation for successful shunt surgery.

BIBLIOGRAPHY

Bucciarelli, R.L., Egan, E.A., Gressner, I.H., et al.: Persistence of fetal cardiopulmonary circulation: one manifestation of transient tachypnea of the newborn, Pediatrics **58**:192, 1976.

Cotton, R.B., Stahlman, M.T., Bender, H.W., et al.: Randomized trial of early closure of symptomatic patent ductus arteriosus in small preterm infants, J. Pediatr. **93**:647, 1978.

Freed, M.D., Heyman, M.A., Lewis, A.B., et al.: Prostaglandin E$_1$ in infants with ductus arteriosus-dependent congenital heart disease, Circulation **64**:899, 1981.

Friedman, W.F., Hirschklau, M.J., Printz, M.P., et al.: Pharmacologic closure of patent ductus arteriosus in the preterm infant, N. Engl. J. Med. **295**:526, 1976.

Garson, A., Gillette, P.C., and McNamara, D.G.: Supraventricular tachycardia in children: clinical features, response to treatment, and long-term follow-up in 217 patients, J. Pediatr. **98**:875, 1981.

Gersony, W.M., Peckham, G.J., Ellison, R.C., et al.: Effects of indomethacin in premature infants with patent ductus arteriosus: results of a national collaborative study, J. Pediatr. **102**:895, 1983.

Haworth, S.G., and Reid, L.: Persistent fetal circulation: newly recognized structural features, J. Pediatr. **88**:614, 1976.

Heymann, M.A., and Rudolph, A.M.: The ductus arteriosus: Proceedings of the Seventy-fifth Ross Conference of Pediatric Research, Columbus, Ohio, 1978, Ross Laboratories.

Johnson, G.L., Breart, G.L., Gewitz, M.H., et al.: Echocardiographic characteristics of premature infants with patent ductus arteriosus, Pediatrics **72**:864, 1983.

Kitterman, J.A., Edmunds, L.G., Gregory, G.A., et al.: Patent ductus arteriosus in premature infants, N. Engl. J. Med. **287**:473, 1972.

Lees, M.H.: Heart failure in the newborn infant, J. Pediatr. **75**:139, 1969.

Lees, M.H.: Cyanosis of the newborn infant, J. Pediatr. **77**:484, 1970.

Lewis, A.B., Freed, M.D., Heyman, M.A., et al.: Side effects of therapy with prostaglandin E$_1$ in infants with critical congenital heart disease, Circulation **64**:893, 1981.

McCarthy, J.S., Zies, L.G., and Gelband, H.: Age-dependent closure of the patent ductus arteriosus by indomethacin, Pediatrics **62**:706, 1978.

Merritt, T.A., Disessa, T.G., Feldman, B.H., et al.: Closure of the patent ductus arteriosus with ligation and indomethacin: a consecutive experience, J. Pediatr. **93**:639, 1978.

Nadas, A.S., and Tyler, D.C.: Pediatric cardiology, ed. 3, Philadelphia, 1972, W.B. Saunders Co.

Neal, W.A., Bessinger, F.B., et al.: Patent ductus arteriosus complicating respiratory distress syndrome, J. Pediatr. **86**:127, 1975.

Roberts, N.K., and Gelband, H.: Cardiac arrhythmias in the neonate, infant and child, New York, 1977, Appleton-Century-Crofts.

Serwer, G.A., Armstrong, B.E., and Andersson, P.H.W.: Noninvasive detection of retrograde descending aortic flow in infants using continuous wave doppler ultrasonography, J. Pediatr. **97**:394, 1980.

Versmold, H.T., Kitterman, J.A., Phibbs, R.H., et al.: Aortic blood pressure during the first 12 hours of life in infants with birth weight 610 to 4220 grams, Pediatrics **67**:607, 1981.

30

Serious neurologic disorders

In the prematurely born infant, neurologic development appears to continue unabated as it would have in the intrauterine environment, unless adversely affected by critical events.

Sensory stimulation from incubator motors, bright lights, circulating air, and flow from cool humidified air-oxygen mixtures may cause hyperactivity of the infant during the first days of life. Whether such stimulation induces harm is not known, but such an abnormal environment is in distinct contrast to the relative sensory isolation and protection found in the warm, dark confines of an intrauterine fluid compartment.

More serious are the insults of hypoxia, metabolic aberrations, and infections. The newborn, particularly when immature, is easily injured by such events. Intracranial birth injury and kernicterus (p. 277), however, are now infrequent because of preventive measures. Meningitis (p. 237) occurs in one in every 250 preterm infants born.

CENTRAL NERVOUS SYSTEM (CNS) DISORDERS
Seizures

Seizures are common in all neonatal intensive care units and of the most serious consequence during the neonatal period. Death follows in perhaps 30% of preterm infants who have seizures, and approximately 30% of survivors (depending on etiology) have permanent neurologic residua. The preterm infant is most susceptible to seizures or subtle seizure activity, which must be recognized, since this activity further potentiates brain injury from hypoventilation and asphyxia.

RECOGNITION
1. Subtle signs (more likely to be seen in the preterm infant because of less well organized central nervous system)
   a. Tonic horizontal deviation of eyes
   b. Repetitive blinking and fluttering of eyelids
   c. Disorganized orobuccolingual movements
   d. "Rowing" movements of upper limbs, pedaling of lower limbs, or posturing of a limb
   e. Apnea and cyanosis
2. Increased tone of body, usually generalized with limbs held in extension and resisting flexion
3. Clonic movements characterized by jerking of one or another limb, which may migrate to another body part in an unordered fashion

Jitteriness or tremulousness are not seizures but are rhythmic movements that cease with gentle passive flexion. Jittery infants have been stressed in a less serious way than those with seizures.

ETIOLOGIC FACTORS
1. Perinatal asphyxia
   Anoxia during labor and the first minutes of life is the most common central nervous system insult resulting in permanent cellular damage in infants who exhibit seizures from it. Seizures are typically manifested within the first 12 to 24 hours of life.
2. Intracranial hemorrhage
   Seizures from gross hemorrhage, attributable to birth injury from tears of membranes

and blood vessels, are now infrequent. Periventricular hemorrhage, common in the small preterm infant (see following section), usually occurs within 1 to 3 days after a hypoxic event, with seizures usually following within 4 hours of a major hemorrhage. Subarachnoid bleeding has a better prognosis.
3. Metabolic derangements (see Chapter 32) Precise blood levels of either glucose or calcium low enough to initiate seizures and the time frame for low levels of blood glucose to produce neuronal damage are not known. Asphyxia tends to potentiate the effect of metabolic insults. Nevertheless, serum calcium under 7 mg/100 ml and blood glucose under 30 mg/100 ml require treatment.
4. Cerebral infections (e.g., bacterial meningitis, transplacental viral invasion with meningoencephalitis, cytomegalovirus disease, rubella, herpes simplex)
5. Developmental malformations (e.g., cerebral agenesis, porencephalia)
6. Miscellaneous factors
   a. Other electrolyte disorders that may cause seizures: hypernatremia (sodium over 148 mEq/L), hyponatremia (sodium under 125 mEq/L), and hypomagnesemia (magnesium under 1 mEq/L)
   b. Inborn errors of metabolism (e.g., galactosemia, maple syrup urine disease, pyridoxine deficiency)
   c. Hyperviscosity of blood
   d. Narcotic withdrawal after maternal addiction
   e. Kernicterus (bilirubin encephalopathy)

DIAGNOSIS AND MANAGEMENT

1. Obtain blood for glucose, calcium, and sodium level determinations (in addition, urea nitrogen, phosphorus, magnesium, potassium, and plasma amino acid level measurements may be necessary).
2. If Dextrostix test on first drop of blood is under 40 mg/100 ml, infuse by push 5 ml/kg D10W followed by a continued infusion rate of 3 to 4 ml/kg/hr (Chapter 32). One must avoid sudden increases in serum osmolarity by excessive glucose administration.
3. If hypoglycemia is not present and seizures persist, give phenobarbital 10 mg/kg IV slowly. Repeat once in 15 to 30 minutes if needed. Phenytoin 10 mg/kg IV may be needed if phenobarbital does not arrest seizure activity. Daily maintenance dose of phenobarbital to maintain serum levels between 15 to 25 µg/ml is 5 mg/kg.
4. Obtain cerebrospinal fluid for cell numbers, protein, glucose, and blood. If fluid is bloody and fails to clear, intraventricular hemorrhage is most likely. If white cell numbers are over 10 cells/mm^3 with a predominance of polymorphonuclear neutrophil leukocytes and the glucose level is less than half that of the blood, bacterial meningitis is likely and a smear and culture should be obtained.
5. If serum calcium is under 7 mg/100 ml, give 1 to 2 ml/kg of 10% calcium gluconate diluted half with water by slow push IV (see also p. 300).
6. For magnesium level under 1.5 mEq/L, give 0.1 to 0.2 mg/kg of 50% magnesium sulfate IM.

Further investigation may include an electroencephalogram, ultrasonographic examination of the head, and a computerized-tomographic (CT) brain scan.

PERIVENTRICULAR AND INTRAVENTRICULAR HEMORRHAGE

Intracerebral hemorrhage is probably the most frequently encountered cause of serious neurologic disturbance in the immature infant. In recent years periventricular hemorrhage (PVH) extending into the ventricles (IVH) has superseded the importance of other brain hemorrhages (subdural, subarachnoid, and intracerebellar). PVH, according to Papile, is found by computerized-tomographic scan observation in nearly 45% of all infants weighing under 1,500 gm.

Intracerebral hemorrhage is a leading cause of death in low birth weight infants. More tragically, nearly 60% of infants surviving periventricular and intraventricular hemorrhages have significant handicaps. Larger hemorrhages are more likely to cause neurologic deficits.

Ventilator support has been considered a factor in etiology, but hypoventilation with apnea and respiratory failure from hyaline membrane disease that demanded the use of mechanical support are more likely factors. Asphyxial episodes increase susceptibility to hemorrhage, with hypoxia as a likely factor in weakening vascular endothelial integrity and elevating PCO_2 to cause venous congestion from an increase of cerebral blood flow. Excessive support of blood volume for hypotension with volume expanders may play a role. In any event, increased intracranial pressure with engorgement of cerebral vessels and rupture of capillaries leads to leakage of blood into the subependymal germinal layer. Later breakthrough of the hemorrhage into the ventricular system is presumed to occur.

Clinical signs

In catastrophic cases infants show inactivity, apnea, general flaccidity, and seizures. Hypotension, bradycardia, and failure of homeostatic control of temperature, glucose, and water are followed by severe metabolic acidosis and anemia.

In less serious states in which recovery is likely, one sees less dramatic changes as those listed above but observes alterations in behavior and activity, particularly aberrations in eye and limb movements.

In serious cases, a sudden drop in hematrocrit level and a full anterior fontanel may be observed. Spinal fluid obtained by lumbar puncture is commonly bloody and does not clear. Up to 50% of intracerebral hemorrhages, however, fail to cause any specific symptoms and may therefore be missed.

In those infants suffering from larger intraventricular hemorrhage progressive hydrocephalus may develop, which will cause further brain damage. The first clinical sign of this complication is an enlarging head (an increase in head circumference of 1.3 cm or more per week).

Diagnosis

Ultrasonographic examination of the head carried out through the anterior fontanel is the method of choice for diagnosis of PVH and IVH. Advantages of this method are that it is noninvasive and can be performed at the bedside. A computerized-tomographic brain scan is another approach allowing accurate diagnosis, but it is not a bedside procedure and has the disadvantage of exposing the infant to radiation.

Management

1. Prompt correction of coagulation defects, if present, with fresh frozen plasma and treatment of shock are indicated in infants who show acute deterioration. In cases of massive hemorrhage death is likely and extended respiratory support is often futile.
2. Infants should be followed with intermittent ultrasonographic examinations of the head. Repeated lumbar puncture for drainage of cerebrospinal fluid may be indicated for those infants whose examinations show significant increases in ventricular size. A shunt is performed if hydrocephalus remains progressive.

HYDROCEPHALUS AND MICROCEPHALUS

Head measurements should be recorded at birth and charted longitudinally on a growth graph (Fig. 30-1). Thus a baseline is established for determination of the rate of growth. Any measurement above or below 2 standard deviations (S.D.) of the mean for the infant's gestational age suggests an abnormality. Infants who have suffered fetal undernutrition may have a head circumference well below the 3rd percentile and yet develop normally, particularly if growth of the head accelerates into the normal channels of growth during the first year. Relative macrocephaly in comparison with other measurements is common in the low birth weight infant because of the tendency for preferential brain growth. Seldom is such a head measurement above the mean for the gestational age.

Hydrocephalus

Evidence of an abnormally large head or rapid increase in head circumference suggests obstruction of cerebrospinal fluid flow. Frequent causes are intracerebral hemorrhage, congenital or acquired infections, or anomalies of the brain. Observe the infant for the following:

1. Fullness or bulging fontanel
2. Early spreading of the cranial sutures,*

---

*Infants severely undernourished during fetal life may show spreading of sutures on the basis of "catch-up" growth in brain-cell size with optimum postnatal nutrition. A widened sagittal suture at birth is seen in severely undergrown and dysmature infants who have suffered from insufficient calcium deposition.

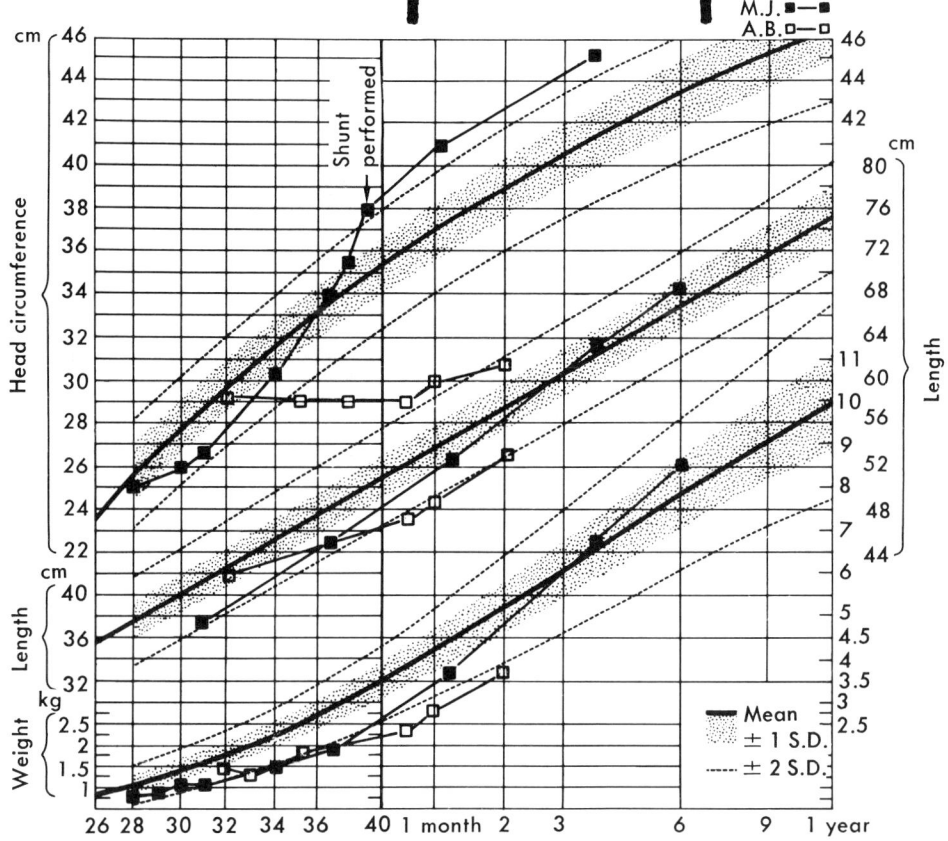

Fig. 30-1. Infant M.J., ■, shows a rapid increase in head circumference from 33 to 38 cm during a period of 3 weeks, a result of obstructive hydrocephalus secondary to intracranial hemorrhage. Infant A.B., □, represents growth retardation attributable to herpes-virus encephalitis. Head circumference has slowed proportionately more than growth in length, presumably from brain cell damage. (From Babson, S.G., and Benda, G.I.: J. Pediatr. **89:**814, 1976.)

which normally override in the premature infant after birth and stay thus for the first 3 to 4 weeks of life

3. Excessive head growth (more than 1.2 cm/wk during a 3-week period)
4. Asymmetric or extensive transillumination

Microcephalus or failure of normal head growth

Microcephalus at birth (head size less than 2 S.D.) suggests the possibility of cerebral dysgenesis, fetal meningoencephalitis, or general craniostenosis. Inadequate head growth suggests, in addition to the above, perinatal asphyxia with brain-cell damage, acquired infection (e.g., herpesvirus), nutritional failure, or the many causes of failure to thrive, including metabolic defects.

Failure of adequate growth is suggested by the following:

1. Continued overlapping of the sutures in the preterm infant after 3 weeks of age
2. Longitudinal increase in head circumference under 0.7 cm/wk (preterm)
3. Head size disproportionately small for length

See Fig. 30-1 for excessive and diminished growth in head size.

BIBLIOGRAPHY

Babson, S.G., and Henderson, N.B.: Fetal undergrowth: relation of head growth to later intellectual performance, Pediatrics **53:**890, 1974.

Hambleton, G., and Wigglesworth, J.S.: Origin of intraventricular hemorrhage in the preterm infant, Arch. Dis. Child **51**:651, 1975.

Holden, K.R., Mellits, E.D., and Freeman, J.M.: Neonatal seizures. I. Correlation of prenatal and perinatal events with outcomes, Pediatrics **70**:165, 1982.

Kenny, J.D., García-Prats, J.A., Hilliard, A.J., et al.: Hypercarbia at birth: a possible role in the pathogenesis of intraventricular hemorrhage, Pediatrics **62**:465, 1978.

McInerney, T.K., and Schubert, W.K.: Prognosis of neonatal seizures, Am. J. Dis. Child. **117**:261, 1969.

Mellits, E.D., Holden, K.R., and Freeman, J.M.: Neonatal seizures. II. A multi-variable analysis of factors associated with outcome, Pediatrics **70**:177, 1982.

Papile, L.A., Munsick-Bruno, U., and Schaefer, A.: Relationship of cerebral intraventricular hemorrhage and early childhood neurologic handicaps, J. Pediatr. **103**:273, 1983.

Papile, L.A., Burstein, J., Burstein, R., et al.: Incidence and evolution of subependymal and intraventricular hemorrhage: a study of infants with birth weights less than 1,500 gm, J. Pediatr. **92**:529, 1978.

Rose, A.L., and Lombroso, C.T.: Neonatal seizure states: a study of clinical, pathological, and electroencephalographic features in 137 full-term babies with a long-term follow-up, Pediatrics **45**:404, 1970.

Towbin, A.: Central nervous system damage in the human fetus and newborn infant, Am. J. Dis. Child. **119**:529, 1970.

Volpe, J.J.: Neonatal periventricular hemorrhage: past, present and future, J. Pediatr. **92**:693, 1978.

Volpe, J.J.: Neurology of the newborn, Philadelphia, 1981, W.B. Saunders Co.

31

Hematologic problems

ANEMIA

Pallor, although a common sign of asphyxia or illness, usually is caused by anemia (often secondary to blood loss) occurring before, during, or after delivery.

A hematocrit reading obtained several hours after birth is a valuable baseline measurement in cases of potential blood loss. This initial value is usually higher than the cord level, depending on the volume of placental transfusion with a necessary readjustment of plasma volume, as well as the degree of sludging of cells if capillary blood is used (stasis usually from chilling). Any fall in hematocrit value during the first few hours of life is an indication of recent blood loss.

Early anemia
CAUSES

1. Blood loss before or during birth is usually attributable to
   a. Fetomaternal transfusion (confirmed by the Kleihauer fetal hemoglobin test, using a blood smear)
   b. Occult bleeding from tearing of aberrant fetal vessels leading from the cord to the placenta (velamentous insertion of cord)
   c. Placental tearing or membrane laceration (placenta previa, vasa previa, respectively)
   d. Placenta transection at cesarean section
   e. Twin-to-twin transfusion (parabiotic twins)
   f. Rupture of spleen or tear of capsule of liver
2. Blood loss after birth can occur from
   a. Holding of infant above level of placenta with cord unclamped
   b. Birth trauma with loss of blood into infant's own body spaces (e.g., intracranial hemorrhage, mutiple cephalohematoma, and subcapsular hemorrhage of the liver)
   c. Slipped tie from cord stump
   d. Coagulation defects from insufficient clot-forming factors such as thromboplastin and prothrombin, which are synthesized in the liver and dependent on vitamin K for production
   e. Thrombocytopenia from maternal platelet antigen sensitization or severe infection
   f. Coagulation defects produced by maternal ingestion of drugs such as coumarin
3. Anemia attributable to hemolytic diseases
   a. Erythroblastosis fetalis
   b. Spherocytosis and congenital nonspherocytic hemolytic anemia
   c. Drug-induced disorders such as may be caused by vitamin K analogs given in excess to the mother or the infant
   d. Glucose-6-phosphate dehydrogenase deficiency and other red blood cell enzyme defects

TREATMENT

1. Transfuse infant's blood with whole blood or packed cells (10 to 20 ml/kg) at the following indications:
   a. Immediately after birth if the neonate is pale, hypotonic, and in shock
   b. During the first 24 hours if the infant's hematocrit value is below 35% to 40% (12 to 13 gm/100 ml of hemoglobin; higher levels for distressed infants)

Infants with respiratory distress syndrome should have blood transfused at levels of less than 45% (hemoglobin under 14 gm/100 ml)
  c. Toward end of first week if hematocrit value is below 30% to 35% (10 to 12 gm/100 ml of hemoglobin)
2. Perform serial hematocrits
  a. Every 60 minutes for suspected blood loss, since a measurable progressive fall (from plasma dilution) indicates blood loss and possible necessity of transfusion
  b. Every other day after exchange transfusion until infant's condition is stabilized

Delayed anemia
CAUSES

I. Physiologic anemia of prematurity (after age of 4 weeks)
   A. The premature baby begins life with a hemoglobin level somewhat lower than that of the term infant. The postnatal fall is exaggerated by the following:
      1. Greater body growth
      2. Somewhat shorter red blood cell life span
      3. Delay in onset of erythropoiesis
   B. The more immature premature infant will show a hematocrit value fall to as low as 20% to 25% (6 to 8 gm/100 ml of hemoglobin) by 6 to 7 weeks of age. At this time a rapid increase in reticulocytes checks this fall, raising the total hemoglobin mass and finally the hemoglobin level itself.
II. Blood loss
   A. Iatrogenic loss from blood sampling
   B. Chronic loss (e.g., bowel disease)
III. Infection
IV. Insufficient exogenous iron, usually after 2 months of age
V. Vitamin E deficiency

TREATMENT AND PREVENTION

A hematocrit is obtained every day or two for infants with acute illness and once a week for those at medium risk.
  1. Record volume of blood removed, particularly in the small preterm infant.
  2. Administer 2 mg/kg elemental iron orally daily by 2 months of age to prevent iron-deficiency anemia.
  3. Give 20 to 30 mg of elemental iron orally daily for treatment of iron-deficiency anemia.
  4. Give 25 IU of Aquasol E daily to preterm infants weighing under 1,500 gm at birth.

NEONATAL HYPERVISCOSITY

Neonatal hyperviscosity is observed during the first few days of life and occurs when red cell volume is excessively high in relation to plasma volume, causing reduced blood flow and hypoxemia to body tissues. Hyperviscosity is observed in approximately 5% of all neonates but is infrequent in the preterm infant. Newborns with this disorder are subject to complications such as renal vein thrombosis and necrotizing enterocolitis. Increased risk for abnormal neurologic findings has been found by some authors on follow-up studies of such infants.

Controversy does exist about the disease itself and criteria for its diagnosis and treatment. Nevertheless, it is current opinion that all infants be screened for hyperviscosity at 4 to 8 hours of age.

Ramamurthy demonstrated a linear relationship between blood viscosity and umbilical venous hematocrit (Hct_{uv}). In his study, 94% of neonates had normal viscosity with Hct_{uv} of less than 63%. Hct_{uv} is obtained only when an initial capillary hematocrit reading (Hct_c) is higher than 70% and a subsequent peripheral venous hematocrit reading (Hct_v) is higher than 65% (by experience Hct_c is higher than Hct_v, and Hct_v is higher than Hct_{uv}).
  1. Associations
     a. Hypervolemia from excessive placental transfusion, maternofetal transfusion, or twin-to-twin transfusion
     b. Increased erythropoiesis resulting in a high amount of hemoglobin and found in small-for-dates infants, those with dysmaturity, infants of diabetic mothers, and those who have had chronic fetal distress
  2. Symptoms
     a. Grunting respirations (hypervolemia)
     b. Tachypnea
     c. Lethargy
     d. Poor feeding
     e. Cardiac decompensation
     f. Hyperbilirubinemia
     g. Cyanosis
     h. Seizures
     i. Abdominal distention

j. Bloody stools
k. Oliguria, hematuria

MANAGEMENT

An exchange transfusion is the procedure of choice for infants with blood hyperviscosity. Reduction of the infant's hematocrit to approximately 55% is the goal. The following formula can be used for estimation of blood volume to be replaced by plasma.

Estimated exchange volume =
$$\frac{\text{Blood volume}^* \times (\text{Observed Hct} - \text{Desired Hct})}{\text{Observed Hct}}$$

1. Prepare umbilical area with iodine.
2. Place umbilical catheter into either inferior vena cava or lower abdominal aorta, or (when previous two options are not possible) into umbilical vein just until blood return is observed.
3. Withdraw blood in 5 ml aliquots and replace it with equal amounts of Plasmanate or fresh plasma to desired exchange volume.
4. Before removing catheter, repeat hematocrit to ensure that red cell volume was lowered the desired amount.

BLEEDING OR SKIN HEMORRHAGE

When a newborn shows evidence of bleeding, one must determine whether he is sick or well or has received vitamin K prophylaxis and whether there is a family history of bleeding problems, maternal infection, or drugs taken that could be associated with bleeding. If the infant is sick, the condition suggests liver disease or disseminated intravascular coagulation; if well, immune-mediated disease, vitamin K deficiency, or isolated clotting deficiencies are suggested. Because most serious bleeding problems are associated with thrombocytopenia, an immediate screen of platelet numbers should be made. Multiply the number of platelets seen on each oil-immersion field by 15,000 (10 to 15 per field are normal).

Thrombocytopenia

The clinical expression of thrombocytopenia in the neonate is dramatic and extensive. Unlike the occasional petechiae visible on the scalp and face of an otherwise normal infant after vaginal delivery, petechial hemorrhages of thrombocytopenia are visible over the entire body. Platelet counts are usually below 50,000 cells/mm^3 and are often less than 10,000 cells/mm^3.

1. Associations
   a. Overwhelming infections (e.g., cytomegalovirus infection, rubella, toxoplasmosis, herpesvirus infection, and bacterial sepsis)
   b. Severe erythroblastosis fetalis
   c. Platelet depletion after repeated exchange transfusions
   d. Maternal drugs inducing thrombocytopenia in the fetus (e.g., thiazides)
   e. Autoimmune thrombocytopenia
   f. Congenital leukemia
   g. Disseminated intravascular coagulation
2. Management
   Besides specific treatment, such as antibiotics in sepsis, platelet transfusions may be given to reduce the bleeding tendency. Transfusions are advisable if the platelet count is under 10,000 cells/mm^3. Complete exchange transfusion with freshly drawn whole blood is another alternative in such cases.

Disseminated intravascular coagulation

Disseminated intravascular coagulation (DIC) is an uncommon but serious disorder in the newborn in which the equilibrium between microclot formation and destruction in the vascular system is disturbed. Thrombocytes are rapidly removed from the circulation, leading to a bleeding diathesis. DIC is not a clinical entity but is secondary to multiple insults to the neonate resulting in tissue injury.

1. Associations
   a. Overwhelming infections, viral and bacterial
   b. Respiratory distress syndrome
   c. Shock associated with other disorders
2. Clinical signs
   a. Increased bleeding tendency (e.g., from heel-sticks)
   b. Bleeding from umbilicus, trachea, or gastrointestinal tract
3. Diagnostic aids
   Consumption of clotting factors in DIC leads to abnormalities in the coagulation system. The disorder should be strongly

---

*Infants blood volume = 80 ml × weight (kg)

suspected if the following associations are found:
a. Decreased numbers of platelets
b. Evidence of red blood cell damage on smear (e.g., schistocytes)
c. Prolonged partial thromboplastin time
d. Prolonged prothrombin time (greater than 30 seconds)
e. Fibrinogen deficiency (less than 1 gm/100 ml)
f. Positive fibrin split products
4. Management
a. Therapy should be directed against primary cause (sepsis, shock).
b. Administration of fresh frozen plasma (10 ml/kg) at 12- to 24-hour intervals will aid in restoration of clotting function.
c. Platelet transfusions are indicated when infant's thrombocyte count is under 10,000 cells/mm^3.

Vitamin K deficiency

The ability of a neonate to synthesize and use vitamin K is dependent on gestational as well as chronologic age. Lack of vitamin K or impaired liver function leads to impaired synthesis of coagulation factors II, VII, IX, and X and to increased bleeding tendency in a neonate evident in a prolonged prothrombin time. Prothrombin time normally is prolonged during the first 3 to 4 days in term infants and the first 10 to 14 days in preterm infants.

1. Causes
   a. Antibiotic treatment eliminating normal gastrointestinal flora
   b. Diarrhea and malabsorption
   c. Deficient intake of vitamin K when infant is fed with certain commercial milks
   d. Lack of vitamin K supplementation during prolonged parenteral fluid therapy.
   e. Maternal use of drugs causing vitamin K deficiency in the infant (i.e., coumadin derivatives and certain anticonvulsants)
2. Management
   Administer vitamin K_1 (not vitamin K analogs, which may cause hyperbilirubinemia) 0.5 to 1 mg, after birth to every neonate; also administer when vitamin K deficiency is suspected.

BIBLIOGRAPHY

Black, V.D., Lubchenco, L.O., Luckey, D.W., et al.: Developmental and neurologic sequelae of neonatal hyperviscosity syndrome, Pediatrics **69**:426, 1982.

Brans, Y.W., Shannon, D.L., and Ramamurthy, R.S.: Neonatal polycythemia. II. Plasma, blood, and red cell volume estimates in relation to hematocrit levels and quality of intrauterine growth, Pediatrics **68**:175, 1981.

Glader, B.E., and Buchanan, G.R.: The bleeding neonatate, Pediatrics **58**:548, 1976.

Goldberg, K., Wirth, F.H., Hathaway, W.E., et al.: Neonatal hyperviscosity. II. Effect of partial plasma exchange transfusion, Pediatrics **69**:419, 1982.

Goldman, H.I., and Amadio, P.: Vitamin K deficiency after the newborn period, Pediatrics **44**:745, 1969.

Hathaway, W.E., Mull, M.M., and Pechet, G.S.: Disseminated intravascular coagulation in the newborn, Pediatrics **43**:233, 1969.

Meutzer, W.C.: Polycythemia and the hyperviscosity syndrome in newborn infants, Clin. Haematol. **7**:63, 1978.

Oski, F.A., and Naiman, J.L.: Hematologic problems in the newborn, Philadelphia, 1982, W.B. Saunders Co.

Ramamurthy, R.S., and Brans, Y.W.: Neonatal polycythemia. I. Criteria for diagnosis and treatment, Pediatrics **68**:168, 1981.

Stiehm, E.R., and Clatanoff, D.V.: Split products of fibrin in the serum of newborns, Pediatrics **43**:770, 1969.

Wirth, F.H., Goldberg, K.E., and Lubchenco, L.O.: Neonatal hyperviscosity. I. Incidence, Pediatrics **63**:833, 1979.

Yao, A.C., and Lind, G.: Placental transfusion, Am. J. Dis. Child. **127**:128, 1974.

32

Metabolic problems

The premature infant is less able to maintain physiologic homeostasis than is the full-term infant. Particularly, the immature infant has difficulty in maintaining glucose and sodium homeostasis during the first week of life. Another handicap is in hydrogen ion control. The lungs and kidney have limited reserves in their capacities for this function. Respiratory and metabolic acidosis may often occur.

The kidneys are anatomically deficient in their complement of glomeruli and tubular components until after 35 weeks of gestational age. In addition to a limitation in the excretion of acid, the premature infant is handicapped in the abilities to concentrate and dilute electrolytes, clear urea, and excrete phosphate when faced with heavy feeding loads or stressed by fluid restrictions.

Many enzyme systems of the immature infant are developed only in proportion to gestational age, for example, the conjugation of bilirubin, the regulation of blood glucose, and the metabolization of tyrosine. Nevertheless, these enzymatic and organ systems, faced with the challenge of early extrauterine life, may mature in advance of the biologic time clock.

HYPOGLYCEMIA OF THE NEWBORN

Hypoglycemia (during the newborn period) is present when the blood glucose level falls below 30 mg/100 ml. This disorder prevails among preterm infants, especially those suffering from intrauterine growth retardation. Symptomatic hypoglycemia occurring at lower blood glucose levels is a preventable syndrome and may have damaged as many as 5,000 infants born in past years in the United States. Persistent hypoglycemia is rare.

I. Incidence
Fig. 12-1, p. 109, shows the percentage of infants by weight and gestational age who could develop hypoglycemia if not fed or given glucose infusions soon after birth.
II. Pathogenesis
  A. Decreased rate of entry of glucose into blood, usually from insufficient glycogen and fat stores (e.g., in infants who are premature, dysmature, or small for gestational age)
  B. Increased rate of removal of blood glucose, which occurs in the following conditions:
    1. Asphyxial conditions
    2. Hypothermia
    3. Hyaline membrane disease (breathing effort and hypoxia)
    4. Hypermetabolism (the undergrown infant with increased cell numbers per unit of weight)
    5. Temporary hyperinsulinism in infants of diabetic mothers or infants with erythroblastosis fetalis
  C. Interruption of glucose infusions
    1. During exchange transfusions
    2. During blood transfusions
    3. Infiltration or discontinuance of infusion (rebound hypoglycemia)
III. Signs
  A. Irritability, tremors, eye-rolling, seizures, and coma
  B. Apnea and cyanosis
  C. Listlessness and poor feeding
IV. Diagnosis
A checked quantitative blood glucose

level below 30 mg/100 ml indicates hypoglycemia. Specimens drawn must be placed in ice unless processed immediately because the level falls rapidly at room temperature.

V. Management
   A. Give 5 to 10 ml/kg of a 10% glucose solution IV by push.
   B. Continue infusion of 10% to 15% glucose solution at 4 ml/kg/hr.
   C. Add 2 to 3 ml of 10% calcium gluconate and 2 to 3 mEq of sodium chloride per 100 ml of infused fluid.
   D. Feed infant when he is asymptomatic.
   E. Reduce parenteral glucose gradually after blood glucose levels have remained over 50 mg/100 ml and feedings have been established (never reduce infusion abruptly, or a hypoglycemia reaction may result).
   F. Give hydrocortisone, 5 mg/kg of body weight, or adrenocorticotropic hormone (ACTH) (4 units every 12 hours) if blood glucose fails to rise above 30 mg/100 ml after 6 hours or if symptoms of hypoglycemia persist.
   G. Monitor therapy with longitudinal blood glucose determinations.

Prevention

Nurses should be trained in identification of risk groups, and thus seizures from hypoglycemia should not occur in a nursery. The following groups are particularly susceptible:
1. Undergrown or undernourished infants (below the 10th percentile of the Lubchenco grid [Fig. 12-1])
2. Premature infants, particularly those weighing under 2,000 gm at birth or suffering from hyaline membrane disease
3. Infants subjected to fetal distress and asphyxia during labor and delivery
4. Infants born after prolonged gestation, especially those showing signs of dysmaturity (peeling of skin with loss of subcutaneous fatty tissue)
5. Infants who are large for gestational age, particularly infants of diabetic mothers

Serial screening of all infants at risk by peroxidase reagent strips (Dextrostix) should be done in the first hours of life and every 4 to 6 hours thereafter until glucose level is well stabilized at over 50 mg/100 ml. Infants with a low Dextrostix reading and a corroborative laboratory determination of under 30 to 40 mg/100 ml require an intravenous glucose infusion or an increase in the amount given if infusion has already been started. Offer early feeding (at 2 hours of age) to infants at risk for hypoglycemia and continue feeding at 3-hour intervals, if tolerated (see Chapters 12, 15, and 16.)

Hypoglycemia of infants with erythroblastosis fetalis

Erythroblastosis fetalis, for reasons not known, is accompanied by hyperplasia of the islands of Langerhans in the pancreas, and hypoglycemia is observed on occasion. Hyperinsulinemia similar to that seen in infants of diabetic mothers apparently is the cause of hypoglycemia that typically occurs on the first day of life or after an exchange transfusion with citrated blood. The incidence of hypoglycemia is higher in infants with more severe disease.

1. Treatment
   Confirmed hypoglycemia should be managed as previously suggested.
2. Prevention
   a. Monitor blood glucose by Dextrostix, as suggested for infants of diabetic mothers.
   b. Feed infants early and frequently to ensure good caloric and carbohydrate intake.
   c. Ensure constant glucose infusion during and especially several hours after an exchange transfusion with citrated blood to prevent rebound hypoglycemia.

Infants of mothers with diabetes and gestational diabetes

The failing competence of the placenta often observed after 36 weeks of gestation imposes fetal deprivation on some infants, as well as the risk of fetal death (Chapter 24).

I. Complications
   Increased morbidity and neonatal mortality are based on the following complications:
   A. Hyaline membrane disease, the most important complication, may have its genesis in the increased exposure to

intrauterine asphyxia, the method of delivery (cesarean section in preterm infants), and a disordered metabolic state. Tachypnea, not always caused by hyaline membrane disease, is recognized in as many as 50% of infants of diabetic and prediabetic mothers. Delayed maturation of the fetal lung (in class A, B, and C diabetic mothers) is another factor explaining the occurrence of hyaline membrane disease in infants delivered close to term.

B. Hypoglycemia caused by temporary hyperinsulinism (a response of the normal fetal pancreas to the higher maternal glucose level; infants of mothers whose glucose levels during the last 2 months of pregnancy were maintained in the normal range have less hyperinsulinism) should be suspected in the following:
1. Infants of mothers with overt diabetes
2. Infants of mothers with gestational diabetes
3. Infants who are oversized for gestation or have the appearance of an infant of a diabetic mother IDM (i.e., soft skin, abundance of subcutaneous fatty tissue, and round "tomato" face, as well as being large for gestational age)

In the past, when conditions of mothers with diabetes were less well controlled and their infants were not as well cared for, more than 50% of infants of diabetic mothers had hypoglycemia. Moreover, up to 10% of infants of diabetic mothers had symptoms of hypoglycemia, tremors, apnea and cyanosis, and seizures. Usually blood glucose levels return to normal by 8 hours of age, but persistent hypoglycemia may have continued when fetal malnutrition was present.

C. Lethal congenital anomalies occur in 2% to 3% of all infants of diabetic mothers.
D. Hypocalcemia and hypomagnesemia, with a range of symptoms indistinguishable from hypoglycemia, may occur.
E. Hyperbilirubinemia, hyperkalemia, and hyperphosphatemia may be seen.

II. Treatment
A. Have competent assistance at delivery.
B. Resuscitate infant promptly, with maintenance of warmth, support of blood volume, and correction of metabolic acidosis.
C. Offer full incubator care, regardless of infant's weight.
D. Feed 10% glucose three times every 2 hours, then formula if tolerated.
E. Screen hourly with Dextrostix for 8 hours and then every 4 hours until 24 hours of age.
F. Administer parenteral glucose when there is a confirmed serum glucose level below 30 mg/100 ml.
G. Offer continuous parenteral infusion of 10% to 15% dextrose (80 ml/kg/24 hr) to any infant whose mother has established diabetes and who suffered from asphyxia during labor and delivery or shows signs of respiratory distress. Continue infusion until infant has sufficient oral intake; then gradually taper rate of infusion.

HYPERGLYCEMIA

Hyperglycemia indicates a serum glucose level over 125 mg/100 ml. This frequent disorder is usually transient. Because glucose easily enters the brain, generalized swelling and possible damage may occur. Hyperglycemia when accompanied by significant glycosuria will cause osmotic diuresis and possible dehydration.

1. Factors associated with hyperglycemia
   a. Prematurity
      The immature infant frequently demonstrates intolerance to rapid infusion of dextrose solutions during the first few days of life. Because of increased insensible water loss, these infants often require large amounts of parenteral fluid to avoid excessive weight loss. Infusions of over 0.4 gm/kg/hr (i.e., 100 ml of 10% glucose/kg/24 hr) might not be metabolized by the immature infant during this early period.
   b. Severe stress (e.g., septic shock, severe respiratory distress syndrome with shock, or intracerebral hemorrhage)

Transient hyperglycemia frequently accompanies these diseases and normally improves as the primary condition is controlled.
   c. Rapid infusion of dextrose solution
      As infants are treated for dehydration or shock, and fluids are administered rapidly, hyperglycemia may result, especially when 10% dextrose is used.
2. Treatment
   If hyperglycemia is observed, reduce glucose load by decreasing rate of glucose infusion or concentration of glucose solution administered.
3. Prevention
   a. Check urine glucose every 4 to 8 hours with Clinistix or Clinitest.
   b. Perform Dextrostix if Clinitest result is 1+ or more.
   c. Reduce glucose load if blood glucose values exceed 125 mg/100 ml.
   d. Limit glucose infusion rate to 0.3 to 0.4 gm/kg/hr in the small preterm infant during the first days of life.

HYPONATREMIA

Hyponatremia indicates a serum sodium level under 125 mEq/L. It may damage the central nervous system and be the cause of seizures.
1. Factors associated with hyponatremia
   a. Asphyxiation or severe respiratory distress syndrome causing inappropriate secretion of antidiuretic hormone (ADH), with loss of sodium in the urine
   b. Water intoxication
   c. Certain oliguric states
   d. Diarrhea
   e. Adrenal insufficiency
   f. Treatment of mother with low-salt diets and diuretics
2. Symptoms
   a. Lethargy
   b. Apneic episodes
   c. Shock
3. Treatment
   a. Over a 12- to 24-hour period, administer a quantity of sodium in mEq equal to 60% × kilograms of body weight × mEq of the serum sodium deficit below 135 mEq/L.
   b. Recheck serum sodium level.
   c. Limit fluid intake if inappropriate secretion of ADH is suspected.

HYPERNATREMIA

Hypernatremia indicates a serum sodium level over 148 mEq/L and is dangerous because it causes a shift of water away from the brain (since sodium does not cross readily into the central nervous system). This leads to pressure differences within the system, causing dilatation and possible rupture of capillaries in the brain. Occasionally this condition leads to acute tubular necrosis of the kidney.
1. Etiology
   a. Excessive sodium administration, especially of sodium bicarbonate during resuscitation and treatment of acidosis
   b. Insufficient fluid administration
   c. Dehydration caused by increased insensible water loss of the small preterm infant or by hyperthermia or diarrhea
2. Symptoms
   a. Lethargy
   b. Extreme irritability on stimulation
   c. Seizures
3. Treatment
   a. Reduce serum sodium values slowly (24 to 48 hours).
   b. Replace any fluid deficit (over 10% loss of body weight) (in addition to maintaining usual fluid requirements) with 5% glucose solution containing NaCl 4 mEq/kg during the first 24 hours. Plain glucose solution encourages brain edema and cerebrovascular complications.
   c. Gradually adjust fluid intake to approximately 125 to 170 ml/kg/24 hr, and electrolytes (sodium, potassium, and chloride) to 2 to 3 mEq/kg/24 hr on the basis of serial electrolyte determinations.

HYPOCALCEMIA

Approximately 30% of preterm infants weighing less than 2,000 gm at birth will have serum calcium levels of less than 7 mg/100 ml before 48 hours of age if untreated.
1. Factors predisposing infants to hypocalcemia include the following:
   a. Relative hypoparathyroidism caused by suppressed function of the fetal para-

thyroid from transferred maternal parathyroid hormone

This function improves gradually after birth.
   b. Decreased renal capacity for phosphorus excretion

   This handicap is accentuated with increased phosphorus loads, such as in infants who are fed cow's milk. Phosphorus retention depresses serum calcium levels, leading to the classical neonatal tetany seen at 6 or 7 days of life.
   c. Preterm delivery, rendering the infant deficient in calcium
2. Factors further adding to the risk of hypocalcemia
   a. Stress such as asphyxia, which tends to cause increased corticosteroid and thyrocalcitonin release, which may result in lowered serum calcium
   b. Treatment of acidosis with bicarbonate, which tends to decrease the ionized portion of serum calcium
   c. Exchange transfusions with citrated blood, temporarily causing binding of serum calcium with citrate
   d. Low calcium intakes, especially seen in prolonged parenteral infusion when insufficient calcium is given
3. Signs commonly observed
   a. Twitching of extremities
   b. Jitteriness, especially during handling of infant
   c. High-pitched cry
   d. Seizures
   e. Prolonged Q-T segment on electrocardiogram
4. Diagnosis
   a. Serum calcium level under 7 mg/100 ml (3.5 mEq/L)
   b. Corresponding rise in serum phosphorus to over 8 mg/100 ml
5. Treatment
   a. Symptomatic infants or infants not receiving oral feedings should receive 2 ml/kg of 10% calcium gluconate, slowly IV, diluted equally with 5% glucose. (Continued requirements may range between 4 to 7 ml/kg/24 hr for several days.)
   b. Nonsymptomatic infants receiving oral feedings should be offered calcium gluconate or calcium lactate, 1 to 3 gm daily in divided doses. Therapy may have to be continued from several days to 2 or 3 weeks and gradually discontinued.
6. Prevention

   Addition of 3 ml of 10% calcium gluconate to each 100 ml of dextrose infusion from the first day of life while serum levels are monitored will minimize hypocalcemia.

HYPOMAGNESEMIA

1. Blood serum levels are under 1 mEq/L to produce signs.
2. Incidence is infrequent.
3. Associations are newborns undergoing exchange transfusion (citrate-binding), infants of diabetic mothers, and those who are small for dates.
4. Signs are irritable behavior extending into tetany and indistinguishable from signs of hypocalcemia.
5. Suspect hypomagnesemia when serum calcium levels are low but phosphorus levels are normal.
6. Treat with 0.2 ml/kg of a 50% solution of magnesium sulfate IM.

HYPERMAGNESEMIA

1. Blood serum levels are over 5 mEq/L.
2. Incidence is infrequent.
3. Disorder is found in infants whose mothers were treated with magnesium sulfate for toxemia.
4. Signs are profound central nervous system depression with a decrease in sensitivity of motor end plates and apnea.

BIBLIOGRAPHY

Altstatt, L.B.: Transplacental hyponatremia in the newborn infant, J. Pediatr. **66**:985, 1965.

Barrett, C.T., and Oliver, T.K., Jr.: Hypoglycemia and hyperinsulinism in infants with erythroblastosis fetalis, N. Engl. J. Med. **278**:1260, 1968.

Battaglia, F.C., Prystowsky, H., Smisson, C., et al.: Fetal blood studies. XIII. The effect of the administration of fluids intravenously to mothers upon the concentrations of water and electrolytes in plasma of the human fetuses, Pediatrics **25**:2, 1960.

Brown, D.R., and Salsburey, D.J.: Short-term biochemical effects of parenteral calcium treatment of early-onset neonatal hypocalcemia, J. Pediatr. **100**:777, 1982.

Clarke, P.C.N., and Carre, I.J.: Hypocalcemic hypomagnesemic convulsions, J. Pediatr. **70**:806, 1967.

Cornblath, M., Joassin, G., Weisskopf, B., et al.: Hypoglycemia in the newborn, Pediatr. Clin. North Am. **13**:905, 1966.

Dweck, H.S., and Cassady, G.: Glucose intolerance in infants of very low risk weight, Pediatrics **53**:189, 1974.

Feldman, W., Drummond, K.N., and Klein, M.: Hyponatremia following asphyxia neonatorum, Acta Paediatr. Scand. **59**:52, 1970.

Finberg, L.: Hypernatremic dehydration in infants, N. Engl. J. Med. **289**:196, 1974.

Griffiths, A.D.: Association of hypoglycaemia with symptoms in the newborn, Arch. Dis. Child. **43**:688, 1969.

Lipsitz, P.J., and English, I.C.: Hypermagnesemia in the newborn infant, Pediatrics **40**:856, 1967.

Lubchenco, L.D., and Bard, H.: Incidence of hypoglycemia in newborn infants classified by birth weight and gestational age, Pediatrics **47**:831, 1971.

Pildes, R.S., Cornblath, M., Warren, I., et al.: A prospective controlled study of neonatal hypoglycemia, Pediatrics **54**:5, 1974.

Raivio, K.O., and Osterlind, K.: Hypoglycemia and hyperinsulinemia associated with erythroblastosis fetalis, Pediatrics **43**:217, 1969.

Salle, B., David, L. Glorieux, F., et al.: Hypocalcemia in infants of diabetic mothers, Acta Paediatr. Scand. **71**:573, 1982.

Simmons, M.A., Adcock, E.W., Bard, H., et al.: Hyponatremia and intracranial hemorrhage in neonates, N. Engl. J. Med. **291**:6, 1974.

Tsang, R.C., Chen, I., Hayes, W., et al.: Neonatal hypocalcemia in infants with birth asphyxia, J. Pediatr. **84**:428, 1974.

Tsang, R.C.: Neonatal magnesium disturbances: a review, Am. J. Dis. Child. **124**:282, 1972.

33

Major congenital anomalies and developmental defects

Of all infants born, 0.5% to 1% have a congenital anomaly severe enough to end in death or require surgery to avoid death. Another 1% require definitive attention to avoid morbidity and handicapping. Careful observations in the birth room or nursery will identify most of these conditions. Our approach to the serious signs of congenital abnormalities is to alert physicians and nurses to key signs of these serious disorders and to present an early management plan or emergency support requirements. We will group the discussion among infants (1) having respiratory distress at birth, (2) developing increasing cyanosis disproportionate to the degree of respiratory distress, (3) showing early signs of intestinal obstruction, (4) having midline defects, or (5) demonstrating significant congenital anomalies including endocrine and metabolic disorders. Although the percentage of congenital defects rises with the degree of immaturity, the majority of defects occur in the term infant of over 38 weeks in gestational age. Major congenital defects are now the leading cause of death in term births where perinatal care is of good quality. With the fall in other causes of neonatal mortality, they now account for over 25% of all deaths.

ANOMALIES ASSOCIATED WITH RESPIRATORY DISTRESS AT BIRTH

When there is difficulty establishing respiration at birth, particularly in the mature infant, and meconium aspiration has been ruled out, one must consider intrinsic obstruction of the respiratory tree or encroachment upon it. The establishment of an airway by intubation must be followed by an anteroposterior (and lateral) x-ray examination of the neck and chest. Any wheezing, choking, or gasping efforts by the infant in an attempt to breathe freely suggest possibility of the following: choanal atresia; laryngeal, tracheal, or bronchial webs or stenosis; external masses in neck (lymphangioma, hygroma, thyroid enlargement); mediastinal masses; phrenic or vocal cord paralyses; malformation of great vessels with vascular ring; congenital pulmonary disease, including pneumonia; pleural collections of fluid (chyle, hydrops); lung cysts; esophageal atresia with or without tracheoesophageal fistula; and diaphragmatic hernia. The first and last two items mentioned are discussed here because they are more likely to be encountered than the other anomalies.

Choanal atresia

Bilateral obstruction of the choanae is rare but should be suspected when cyanosis at birth is dramatically abolished with crying. With ending of the cry, chest retractions recur with absence of nasal flaring. Diagnosis is confirmed by failure to pass an Fr 8 catheter into the nasopharynx. In routine checks for nasal patency, intermittent compression of each nostril and observing or listening for air movement will identify obstruction.

Immediate relief is offered by placement of an oral airway. Gavage feedings will be required until surgical repair of the obstruction, which is usually performed during the neonatal period for bilateral atresia.

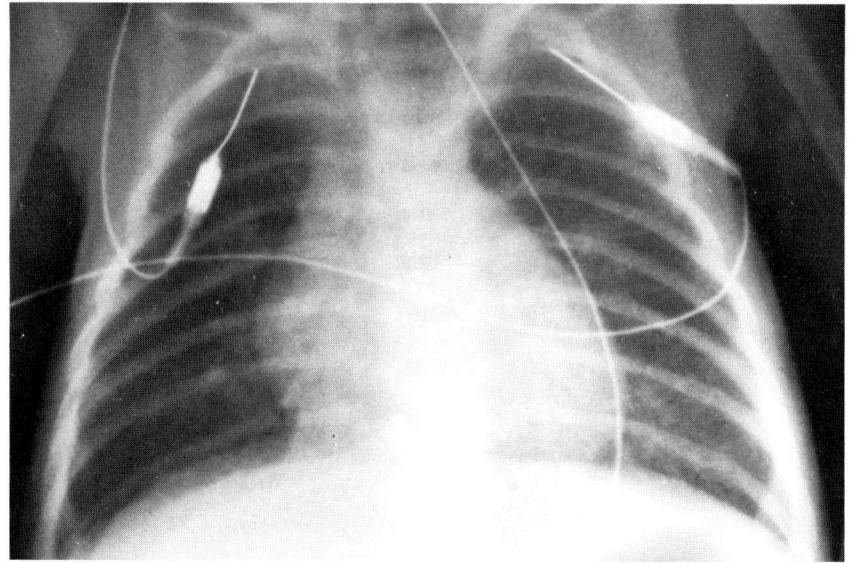

Fig. 33-1. Esophageal atresia with tracheoesophageal fistula. Note dilated and air-filled upper atretic segment of esophagus clearly outlined by its increased radiolucency.

Esophageal atresia with tracheoesophageal fistula

Esophageal atresia with tracheoesophageal fistula (TEF)* occurs in one to two of 3,000 infants born as an isolated defect and should be diagnosed promptly.

CLINICAL MANIFESTATIONS

1. Evidence of polyhydramnios in the mother
2. Respiratory distress from birth with retraction of rib cage, choking, and cyanotic episodes
3. Excessive flow of saliva from mouth
4. Hoarse cry
5. Evidence of dilated upper esophagus on x-ray film of chest

DIAGNOSTIC APPROACH

1. Inability to advance radiopaque Fr 10 catheter passed into esophagus to its full length into the stomach (tube length equal to that of distance from bridge of nose to xiphoid of sternum) will quickly alert physician to presence of an obstruction.
2. With catheter in place, perform x-ray examination of chest and neck, which will reveal tip of catheter located in upper part of esophagus; Fig. 33-1 demonstrates air-filled pouch without catheter.

Missed diagnoses have occurred when too small a catheter is passed, only to curl up in the pouch giving the operator the false sense of having reached the stomach. To confirm stomach placement, one should feel the catheter through the abdominal wall, listen for gurgle on blowing a puff of air through the catheter, or test stomach contents for acidity with Nitrazine paper. Occasionally stomach contents are alkaline from dilution of swallowed amniotic fluid.

After determination of obstruction, the following procedures are instituted:

1. Tertiary center is contacted for transfer of infant.
2. Double-lumen catheter is placed in pouch for continuous or frequent intermittent suctioning.
3. Infant is kept in raised position to avoid gastric reflux of acid materials into lung.
4. Positive pressure ventilation is avoided, if possible, because connection of lower end of esophagus with trachea allows overdistention and possible rupture of stomach. Distention may be so great that emergency gastrostomy is necessary.

---

*Other defects are not uncommon with TEF. Particularly one looks for Vater's association: vertebral defects, imperforate anus, and radial bone and renal dysplasia.

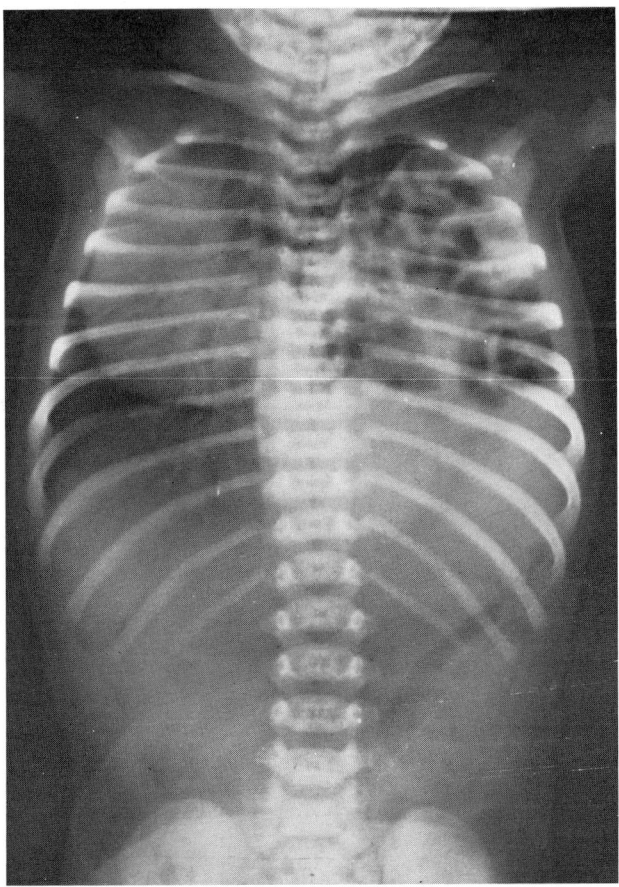

Fig. 33-2. Diaphragmatic hernia in which early recognition and prompt surgery resulted in survival.

Although rare, esophageal atresia is sometimes seen with no fistula present.

Feeding an infant with esophageal atresia leads to disaster, just as does an insufficient emptying of pooled secretions from the pouch. Babies with respiratory distress syndrome or the small preterm infant who has the malformation may have to be managed temporarily with esophageal suction and gastrostomy to gain time and have a more vigorous infant before operation. Mortality should be less than 5% in infants in the absence of other congenital anomalies.

Diaphragmatic hernia

Diaphragmatic hernia (DH) occurs in one of every 2,200 newborns and is the failure of pleuroperitoneal folds to fuse completely, resulting in abdominal viscera moving into the thorax. This problem alone is serious enough and is further aggravated by the increasing compression of lung tissue from accumulation of gastrointestinal air (intensified by mask ventilation). An added hazard is the long-standing occupation of viscera in the chest cavity, which prevents lung growth and results in pulmonary hypoplasia that is more severe on the side of the hernia. The impaired capacity of the lung and resistance to ventilation raises the chance of lung rupture. Complicating chances for recovery of infants with DH is the frequent coexistence of persistent pulmonary hypertension (see p. 270).

CLINICAL MANIFESTATIONS

1. Significant respiratory distress and cyanosis
2. Decreased breath sounds over involved part of thorax (usually left side); often bowel sounds will be audible instead
3. Shift of cardiac impulse to the right
4. Scaphoid abdomen

5. X-ray film of chest revealing loops of bowel in thorax with mediastinal shift away from involved side (Fig. 33-2); at birth with no air yet in bowel, an x-ray film may give appearance of dense opacification of involved side of chest.

SUPPORTIVE CARE

1. Ventilation by endotracheal tube with minimum pressures (less than 30 cm H_2O) if color cannot be maintained by oxygen alone or PCO_2 rises above 60 mm Hg
2. Maintenance of continuous gastric suction
3. Provision of glucose infusion and external warmth
4. Transfer of infant directly to an operating room for surgical relief of hernia in critical cases

Postoperative care demands tertiary hospital support because of continuing respiratory problems and often extended parenteral alimentation requirements. Mortality is high because of delay in recognition, failure to maintain respiratory support, presence of pulmonary hypertension and hypoplasia, or too aggressive replacement of viscera in a limited abdominal space.

CYANOSIS AND CONGENITAL HEART DISEASE

Central cyanosis, present in any nondistressed infant or deemed more severe than would be expected to accompany any respiratory distress the infant might have, should be considered congenital heart disease (CHD) until proved otherwise. Oxygen administration usually fails to relieve cyanosis. Because of the increasing proportion of infants whose cardiac defects can be corrected or improved by skilled team care, the aggressive approach to diagnosis in suspected congenital heart disease is often taken and results in the transfer of thousands of infants each year to regional neonatal centers. Approximately 2.2 per 1,000 live born infants have severe congenital heart disease, of whom approximately one half now survive. On p. 282 a discussion of cyanosis and it differential diagnosis is presented.

INTESTINAL OBSTRUCTION

Although specific anomalies of the gut are infrequent and in the range of one for every 3,000 to 20,000 births, collectively they are frequent enough to justify a definitive search in the birth room (Chapter 8), particularly in infants with reduced birth weights.

I. Signs of intestinal obstruction
  A. Hydramnios
     Amniotic fluid may accumulate because of an imbalance in its circulation caused by mechanical interruption in high intestinal or esophageal obstruction in the fetus. This prevents fluid swallowed by the fetus from being absorbed through the gut into the maternal circulation.
  B. Excessive gastric aspirate
     Fluid (clear or green stained) obtained from the stomach in excess of 15 to 20 ml indicates possible intestinal obstruction.
  C. Bile-stained vomitus
     Because this sign does not occur in the normal infant, its presence indicates intestinal obstruction until proved otherwise. Differential diagnoses include swallowed amniotic fluid contaminated with meconium and a relaxed pyloric sphincter in the very prematurely born infant.
  D. Abdominal distention
     This early postnatal sign is the result of accumulation and delay in the passage of swallowed air. In high intestinal obstruction the abdomen may be scaphoid. Paralytic ileus may distend the abdomen similarly and can be the result of infection, asphyxia, or shock.
  E. Obstipation
     This later sign is more significant if the infant's abdomen is distended or the meconium is abnormal in color and consistency.
II. Diagnostic procedures
  A. Specific physical examination includes the following:
    1. Carefully palpate abdomen for masses (volvulus), doughy intestinal loops (meconium ileus), and scaphoid abdomen (diaphragmatic hernia).
    2. Digitally explore the anus to detect imperforate anus, meconium plug syndrome, or the "white meconium" of intestinal atresia.
    3. Pass a soft Fr 10 radiopaque cath-

eter into the stomach. Failure of the catheter to pass into the stomach indicates esophageal obstruction, and the catheter will demonstrate the level of obstruction on x-ray examination. Note amount and color of stomach contents.
B. Radiograph of abdomen
Gas patterns (contrast material may not be indicated) on an x-ray examination of the upright abdomen may indicate the level of an intestinal obstruction as follows:
1. Air extending as far as the pyloric end of the stomach indicates a pyloric web.
2. Air extending to the second portion of the duodenum ("double-bubble") suggests duodenal atresia, annular pancreas, or incomplete intestinal rotation.
3. Air extending to midgut indicates jejunal or ileal obstruction.
4. Minute bubbles of air intermixed in meconium in intestinal loops (ground-glass appearance) suggest meconium ileus.
5. Distention of colon by gas supported by a dilated bowel in the flank area indicates the possibility of aganglionic megacolon, meconium plug syndrome, or imperforate anus.
6. Free air in the abdomen (pneumoperitoneum) signifies gastrointestinal perforation or (rarely) pulmonary air leaks.
C. A barium enema may indicate one of the following:
1. Microcolon (small intestinal obstruction)
2. Malrotation of the intestine (ectopic position of cecum)
3. Hirschsprung's disease
This is identified by a narrowed zone leading into a dilated colon. Barium must be diluted and injected minimally, or this clue will be obscured by an overriding dilated opaque bowel pattern. Later film will show delayed evacuation of barium and occasionally ragged ulcers of enterocolitis.

III. Initial treatment of specific surgical diseases
All infants who are suspect for gastrointestinal emergencies should have full supportive care, gastric suction, prompt x-ray examination, and, when a surgical condition is likely, full team care, including a pediatric surgeon.

Duodenal atresia

Duodenal atresia occurs about once in every 5,000 deliveries. The incidence is increased in infants with Down's syndrome (8%). The obstruction sometimes is the result of external constriction of the duodenum from an annular pancreas.

CLINICAL MANIFESTATIONS

1. History of polyhydramnios in the mother
2. Bile-stained vomiting
3. Mild or no distention of upper abdomen
4. Evidence of "double bubble" on x-ray examination of abdomen indicating the dilated stomach and proximal part of the duodenum with absence of air in remainder of intestine

INITIAL MEASURES

1. Decompress stomach by inserting orogastric tube for drainage.
2. Correct any dehydration, hypoglycemia, or electrolyte imbalance with parenteral fluids.

Correction can usually be accomplished with surgical resection of the atretic segment and reanastomosis.

Malrotation with volvulus

Lack of proper fixation of the mesentery of the small bowel is the usual cause for twisting loops of intestine, which are usually found in the proximal small bowel. This complication can occur without specific reason or after previous surgery as a result of band formation.

MANIFESTATIONS

1. Bile-stained vomiting occurs.
2. Abdomen may be severely distended or not distended at all; initially, there is evidence of tenderness over the intestinal mass.
3. Infant frequently appears to be critically ill and may be in shock.
4. X-ray examination of the abdomen may reveal striking absence of air in the gut. Sometimes a fluid-filled distended loop of

intestine may be seen. A barium enema usually shows the cecum in the upper right or central abdomen.

INITIAL MEASURES

An infant with volvulus presents an emergency and usually requires prompt surgery to prevent necrosis of large parts of the intestine caused by strangulation of its circulation.

1. Insert orogastric tube for decompression.
2. Vigorously support infant's circulatory status and treat shock if present.
3. Continue administration of parenteral fluids.

Jejunal and ileal atresia

Jejunal and ileal atresia are believed to arise after an ischemic insult to part of the small intestine during fetal life.

MANIFESTATIONS

1. Significant abdominal distention
2. Bilious vomiting
3. X-ray evidence of distended loops of bowel with air-fluid levels
   Barium enema will show a microcolon in cases of distal ileal atresia.

Resection of the atretic segment will usually allow full recovery. Management of shock and proper stabilization may be necessary prior to surgery for severely ill infants.

Meconium ileus and meconium peritonitis

Cystic fibrosis frequently causes impaction of viscous meconium in the small intestine leading to its obstruction and sometimes rupture in utero. Meconium then will enter the peritoneal cavity and calcify after delivery. Bacterial colonization of the ileum may also cause peritonitis.

MANIFESTATIONS

Symptoms are similar to those seen in ileal atresia in addition to the following:

1. Abdomen feels pasty and is usually distended from loops of bowel impacted with the sticky meconium.
2. Rectal examination will reveal limited amounts of whitish meconium.
3. X-ray examination demonstrates tiny soap-like bubbles in meconium-filled intestinal loops and characteristic absence of air-fluid levels. In cases of meconium peritonitis, calcification may be seen in the abdomen.

A barium enema will show a microcolon.

THERAPY

Therapy includes elimination of the meconium by surgery. Nutritional support and long-range planning will have to be made if cystic fibrosis is proved to be the underlying cause.

Hirschsprung's disease (megacolon)

Early abdominal distention and an empty rectum at birth suggest a neurogenic failure of intestinal propulsion because of a lack of ganglion cells in an intestinal segment. The atonic area is most often found as a narrowed rectosigmoid segment. Sometimes it is felt as a narrowing on digital examination and can be identified with a barium enema (if sparingly used). Occasionally diarrhea rather than lack of stool will be the presenting sign.

Diagnosis is confirmed by a rectal biopsy that shows a reduction in ganglionic cells.

Treatment, as with all cases of intestinal obstruction, should be performed in a neonatal center. The early appearance of a newborn who is, except for his distention, apparently normal should not delay diagnosis and surgery. Colostomy avoids the complications of enterocolitis and shock.

Imperforate anus

Failure of differentiation of the urogenital sinus and cloaca during embryologic development results in imperforate anus. It is encountered once in about 20,000 births.

MANIFESTATIONS

Signs will vary depending on the presence or absence of a fistula.

1. There is failure to pass meconium within 24 hours of age. (If a large perineal or vaginal fistula is present, meconium may pass through it without difficulty.)
2. Abdominal distention, usually present, may not develop if decompression can occur through a large fistula.
3. Normal anus is absent. Fistulas may be observed on the perineum or vagina. In male infants a fistula may enter the bladder or urethra and lead to meconium-stained urine.

4. X-ray examination will help to determine the type of lesion present.

THERAPY

Creation of a colostomy for initial decompression is the usual procedure unless the disruption of a thin rectal membrane allows an easy correction or a perineal fistula is sufficiently large for evacuation of stool. Total correction to achieve a functional anus with continence is attempted at a later stage.

Meconium plug syndrome

Delay in passage of meconium more commonly is the result of overdry meconium, capped often with a mucus plug, which is not expelled by peristaltic action. Infants frequently are small for dates.

MANIFESTATIONS

1. Delay of meconium passage
2. Abdominal distention
3. Absence of any other signs indicating severe illness

Diagnosis usually is made by rectal examination, which will often result in passage of the sticky "plug" followed by normal-appearing meconium. On occasion a barium enema may be indicated when rectal examination does not provide relief. The enema itself, while demonstrating the patency of the colon, will be therapeutic, causing expulsion of the firm meconium. Recovery is uneventful.

ABDOMINAL WALL DEFECTS
Omphalocele

Occurring once in about 6,000 births, omphalocele results from failure of intestinal contents to return to the abdominal cavity during embryologic development.

MANIFESTATIONS

The infant is born with a protrusion of part of the intestines and viscera through a widened umbilical ring. The mass is covered by a layer of peritoneum and amnion, which sometimes ruptures at delivery.

INITIAL THERAPY

1. Cover mass with sterile gauze soaked in saline solution warmed to body temperature.
2. Cover gauze with plastic sheeting.
3. Monitor temperature of infant frequently to keep it in the normal range.
4. Place nasogastric tube for decompression.

Repair of the lesion may be simple if the defect is small. Often, however, prolonged therapy is required, including mechanical ventilation and parenteral nutrition. Recovery may be complicated by sepsis and adhesions, as well as the presence of other major congenital defects, such as congenital heart disease or intestinal atresia.

Gastroschisis

Gastroschisis is seen less frequently than omphalocele and differs from the above in that embryologic development is complete with the exception of an abdominal wall defect just lateral to the umbilicus.

MANIFESTATIONS

1. Intestines and viscera protrude through the abdominal wall.
2. The lesion is not covered by a membrane.
3. The umbilical cord originates just lateral to the wall defect.

INITIAL TREATMENT

The same measures advised under omphalocele apply to this lesion. In small extrusions surgical repair can be easy. Larger defects are a formidable problem requiring prolonged intensive care. Fluid losses can be extensive, and prompt replacement of water and electrolytes is often necessary.

Exstrophy of bladder and cloaca

Exstrophy of the bladder or the cloaca is rare and requires protective care similar to that needed in other midline defects. The frequency of occurrence of other anomalies presents the need for thorough multidisciplinary consultation and family counseling.

Myelomeningocele

Failure of closure of the spinal canal with associated abnormalities of the spinal cord and nerve roots occurs once in every 2,000 to 4,000 births in the United States, and in up to 1% of births in Ireland and Wales. When paralysis is present with lack of sphincter control, thorough counseling of parents is mandatory for decision making. This must include discussion of the complications of hydrocephalus, mental retardation, and the possibility of wheelchair existence. The countless operations necessary and the crippling nature of the disease is a coping problem often beyond the strengths of the family. One should take time for the parents to adjust to the problem so they can make a thoughtful decision.

Appearance of increased levels of alpha-fetoprotein in the amniotic fluid around 16 weeks allows early diagnosis of cranial (anencephaly) or other spinal column defects and offers a new approach in prenatal diagnosis of subsequent pregnancies, which present a much higher risk of producing infants with similar defects. These include encephalocele, hydranencephaly, and anencephaly.

MULTIPLE CONGENITAL DEFECTS

A child with multiple congenital anomalies may represent a recognizable pattern of malformation. If so, a diagnosis can possibly be made. We recommend, as aids in the attempts to diagnose the condition of such a child, use of D.W. Smith's *Recognizable Patterns of Human Malformations* (Philadelphia, 1982, W.B. Saunders Co.), as well as D. Bergsma's *Birth Defects Compendium* (New York, 1979, A.R. Liss, Inc.). Infants with multiple congenital anomalies for whom diagnosis has not been made must have emergency karyotyping. Karyotyping is important for two reasons. The first is that if the child does have a chromosomal problem, a diagnosis can be made. Most parents are relieved when they learn of a diagnosis, even if it has a poor prognosis. The other point is that more congenital anomalies produced by a partial trisomy or deletion defect of a chromosome can now be found. In this situation the child's problem may be the result of a balanced translocation of chromosomes in the parents. It is important to counsel parents that subsequent children or those of their relatives can be produced with chromosome defects.

An infant found with three or more minor anomalies has a 90% chance of having a major defect. Whenever one major defect is found, others should be suspected. Stillborn infants and neonates who die should be evaluated for congenital anomalies, particularly those who are disproportionate or have an odd appearance. There are a number of chondrodystrophies, such as achondrogenesis, thanatophoric dwarfism, or osteogenesis imperfecta, that are incompatible with life and lead to death shortly after birth. These children all have short arms and legs or fractures. Our recommendation for evaluation of these children includes photographs (preferably color slides or pictures), total body x-ray examination, karyotyping, a careful physical examination, and a detailed autopsy.

When three or more systems are malformed, the chances of chromosomal defect is high. The family deserves and needs compassionate attention and complete genetic counseling when all information is at hand.

Down's syndrome

This well-known disease occurs once in 650 births. Fifty percent of children with this condition are produced by women over 35 years of age. Because it is a chromosomal abnormality, prenatal diagnosis can detect the condition prior to the twentieth week of pregnancy. We recommend that all women who are pregnant at 35 or over undergo amniocentesis at approximately 16 weeks after the first day of the last menstrual period.

When such a condition is recognized in the birth room (or later), we recommend that the parents together be told promptly of the possibility of Down's syndrome, pending karyotyping. Although genetic counseling will be necessary, the physician who knows the family best should be the one to first inform them of the medical suspicion.

In Down's syndrome, the following signs occur more frequently than others: pallor, skin marmoration, flat facial profile, flattened nasal bridge, round head shape, excessive neck skin, oblique palpebral fissures, blunt inner palpebral angles, Brushfield's spots around the periphery of the iris, intermittently protruding tongue, which is more pointed than thickened, hyperflexibility of joints, simian crease, and small size for gestational age, including size of the head. X-ray studies show dysplasia of the pelvis and middle phalanx of the little finger. Most of these clinical and radiologic findings occur in over 70% of infants with Down's syndrome.

METABOLIC, ENDOCRINE, AND MISCELLANEOUS DEFECTS

Infants who fail to thrive (in the presence of good care and nutrition), have prolonged jaundice, persistent vomiting, unexplained depression or irritability of the central nervous system (to the point of seizures), or acetonuria must be considered to have a metabolic disease. These include disorders of amino acid synthesis, frequently with aminoaciduria (phenylketonuria, tyrosinemia), defects in urea cycle with hyperammonemia (argininosuccinicaciduria), disorders of organic acids resulting in metabolic acidosis (propionicacidemia, congenital lactic acidosis), defects in the metabolism of sugars (galactosemia, fructosemia), and disorders of lipid and glucose metabolism. The reader is referred to the excellent discussions in Behrman's *Neonatal Perinatal Medicine* (St. Louis, 1983, The C.V. Mosby Co.), Avery's *Neonatology* (Philadelphia, 1981, J.B. Lippincott Co.) and Bergsma's *Birth Defects Compendium* (New York, 1979, A.R. Liss, Inc.) for further information in these areas.

One can identify some errors of metabolism (for example, phenylketonuria, maple syrup disease, and galactosemia) by finding reducing substances in the urine (a positive Clinitest and a positive Phenistix) and by analyses of dried blood samples collected on filter paper (Guthrie). Unexplained bizarre behavior of the neonate requires a thorough investigation with the inclusion of metabolic studies on urine and blood sent to a regional metabolic laboratory. Early diagnosis may be the only chance of intact survival.

Hypothyroidism

Congenital hypothyroidism (one per 3,000 to 5,000 births) can be detected by blood screen for T_4 blood levels. Clinical recognition may be difficult, but consideration of this treatable disease is important before permanent neurologic damage occurs. The subtle changes suggesting hypothyroidism are hypothermia, prolonged jaundice, poor feeding, umbilical hernia, a large anterior fontanel, and sluggish behavior. Coarsening of facies with puffed eyelids, generalized edema, enlarged tongue, protruding abdomen, and constipation may not occur until later.

Ambiguous genitalia

This condition is an emergency medical problem because one must identify in such infants the possibility of congenital adrenal hyperplasia (and potential salt losses) and also assign the appropriate sex for rearing. An infant with a small or vestigal phallus that appears insufficient for performing the male role requires prompt consultation. Such an infant is best reared as a female, even though proved to be male by karyotype. Problems of intersexuality require effective teamwork among pediatrician, urologist, endocrinologist, and geneticist for appropriate gender assignment, reconstruction, and hormonal treatment. If the opportunities are missed, tragedy and psychologic handicapping can result.

Abdominal masses

Besides midline defects, other obvious or palpable enlargements are to be considered. These include cystic kidneys, hydronephrosis, hydrometrocolpos, bladder enlargements, liver cysts and tumors, ovarian cysts, and retroperitoneal tumors. The involvement of the urogenital system is so frequent that urologic study is urgent so that correctable defects are not neglected.

Cleft palate or lip

These defects (one per 600 births) should not be missed in the birth room and their presence should be promptly conveyed to both parents, preferably by the physician closest to the family. Although cleft palate may interfere with feeding efficiency and require special feeding methods, good results with surgical correction justify encouragement from the physician. Presence of other defects can cloud the future, however. Early consultation with a plastic surgeon and speech therapist establish a necessary support program. The use of the team concept as supplied by crippled children's services is the ultimate in team care. Seldom is the lip closed before 2 weeks or the palate before 12 months of age.

Dislocated or subluxated hips

Every infant must have his hips abducted with the legs held in the flexed position to make sure the head of the femur is firmly held in the acetabulum. If the femoral head is posteriorly displaced or can be made to slip in or out of the socket, a special splint is necessary to hold the hips in abduction and in appropriate location. In subluxation of the hips, with the upper leg held firmly between thumb and forefingers, one feels a "click" as the unstable head slides across the posterior ridge of the acetabulum. X-ray films may not be helpful when there is insufficient ossification in the newborn period and initial treatment depends on clinical experience.

Fetal alcohol syndrome
See Chapter 2.

SUMMARY

At the birth of a definitely or possibly defective child a plan of action is required. Diagnosis is often difficult and full use of specialized centers, including a genetic and metabolic laboratory, and consultative advice are often necessary. The physical examination should emphasize tonus, vigor, responsiveness, and careful body measurements for possible disproportion and undergrowth for gestational age. Appropriate x-ray films and EEG tracings are often helpful. History should include a pedigree, mother's health, results of other pregnancy experience, complete knowledge of pregnancy course and status at birth, maternal alcoholism, aberrant drug habits, and unusual therapeutic requirements (for example, anticonvulsant drugs and antimetabolites), which may affect development.

Defective fetuses require similar history and examination in detail by clinicians as well as by the pathologist. Dysmorphic infants or fetuses require blood for karyotyping, and if blood cannot be obtained from the fetus, skin biopsy for fibroblast karyotyping will do.

Particular clinical findings suggesting birth defects or fetal disease are small or low-set ears (Potter's, Down's, or Goldenhar's syndromes), large tongue (cretinism, Beckwith-Wiedemann syndrome), abnormal scalp hair or hypotonia (central nervous system malformations), skin rash and enlarged liver and spleen (fetal infection, storage disease), and lymphedema (Turner's syndrome). The eyes should be evaluated for cataracts (galactosemia), for clouding of the cornea (congenital glaucoma, fetal infection), and for microphthalmia, defects that are often overlooked.

The birth of an infant with a congenital malformation presents complex challenges to the physician who will care for the affected child and his family. Drotar and colleagues demonstrated five stages of parental reactions (anger, denial, sadness, adaptation, and reorganization) in dealing with a congenitally malformed child. Early crisis counseling from the first days of life is crucial in the development of parental attachment and adjustment. As soon as the infant is born, the newborn should be shown to the parents. Physical contact minimizes the estrangement that can develop and helps to emphasize the normal aspects of the infant. The continued interest of physician in the infant's progress and arrangements for necessary studies and consultations is essential. The parents are in need of help, and his humaneness and sympathetic concern are vital ingredients to successful parent-infant interaction.

BIBLIOGRAPHY

Adams, M.M., Erickson, J.D., Layde, P.M., et al.: Down's syndrome, JAMA **246**:758, 1981.

Avery, G.B.: Neonatology, Philadelphia, 1981, J.B. Lippincott Co.

Behrman, R.E.: Neonatal perinatal medicine, ed. 2, St. Louis, 1983, The C.V. Mosby Co.

Bergsma, D.: Birth defects compendium, New York, 1979, A.R. Liss Inc.

Burton, B.K., and Nadler, H.L.: Clinical diagnosis of inborn errors of metabolism in the neonatal period, Pediatrics **61**:398, 1978.

Council on Scientific Affairs: Maternal serum α-fetoprotein monitoring, JAMA **247**:1478, 1982.

Drotar, D., Baskiwicz, A., Irvin, N., et al.: The adaptation of parents to the birth of an infant with a congenital malformation: a hypothetical model, Pediatrics **56**:710, 1975.

Gross, R.H., Cox, A., Tatyrek, R., et al.: Early management and decision-making for the treatment of myelomeningocele, Pediatrics **72**:450, 1983.

Kalter, H., and Warkany, J.: Congenital malformations: etiologic factors and their role in prevention, N. Engl. J. Med. **308**:424, 1983.

Klein, M.D., Kosloske, A.M., and Hertzler, J.H.: Congenital defects of the abdominal wall, JAMA **245**:1643, 1981.

Macfarlane, M.T., Lattimer, J.K., and Hensle, T.W.: Improved life expectancy for children with exstrophy of the bladder, JAMA **242**:442, 1979.

Smith, D.W.: Recognizable patterns of human malformation, ed. 3, Philadelphia, 1982, W.B. Saunders Co.

34

Perinatal mortality

The perinatal period in its broadest definition extends from 20 weeks of completed gestation through 27 days of postnatal life.

Neonatal and fetal mortality per 1,000 live births are similar in the United States (Fig. 34-1), and the figures together represent perinatal mortality. A steady decline in both fetal and neonatal death rates has occurred during the past 30 years. The rate of reduction has doubled in the decade of the seventies, mostly because of increasing sophistication of perinatal care rather than any significant drop in numbers of low birth weight infants born, which suggests that our ability to give critical care around the period of birth has surpassed efforts toward prevention of prematurity. Despite reductions in perinatal mortality, the overall rate in the United States is still 25% above perinatal mortality in the states with the lowest rates.

FETAL MORTALITY

Identification of the pregnancy at high risk and better surveillance of the fetus are keeping pace with advances in neonatal care. The 30% of deaths that are primarily preventable now are those that occur in association with maternal disease, such as diabetes and toxemia, and those resulting from disproportion or malposition. These preventable fetal deaths usually involve infants weighing over 2,500 gm born at term, and, thus they contribute thousands to the perinatal toll. Approximately 40% of fetal deaths, however, are the result of defects of the placenta or cord—factors often undiscovered until delivery unless detected by awareness of interrupted fetal growth. The 15% to 20% of deaths resulting from fetal defects are, in the main, not salvageable.

NEONATAL MORTALITY

States and countries with the lowest mortalities have less than 6 neonatal deaths per 1,000 live births. Mortality is inversely proportional to birth weight as shown for the state of Oregon in Table 34-1. Also shown is the percentage of infants born and the mortality per 1,000 live births for each birth weight group. Note that 5.1% of all infants (the low birth weight groups) contribute to 70% of all neonatal mortality. Mortality figures for 1983 are 67% below those reported 19 years ago in the first edition of this book. Progress is being made—neonatal mortality was 5.5 in 1983. Note that over 55% of neonatal mortality now occurs in infants who weigh under 1,500 gm.

Associations of neonatal deaths

Improved care during the perinatal period and avoidance of complications of pregnancy and labor have markedly reduced death and morbidity. Asphyxia, a leading causative factor in respiratory distress syndrome and cerebral palsy, and birth injury, often the result of unresolved fetal malposition, have been strikingly diminished. As neonatal mortality approaches 5 per 1,000 live-born infants, approximately 2 per 1,000 will die from lethal congenital anomalies. This rate appears to have stabilized and is the result of severe defects incompatible with life (e.g., anencephaly, trisomies, hypoplastic left heart). The other main contribution to neonatal mortality is extreme immaturity, principally be-

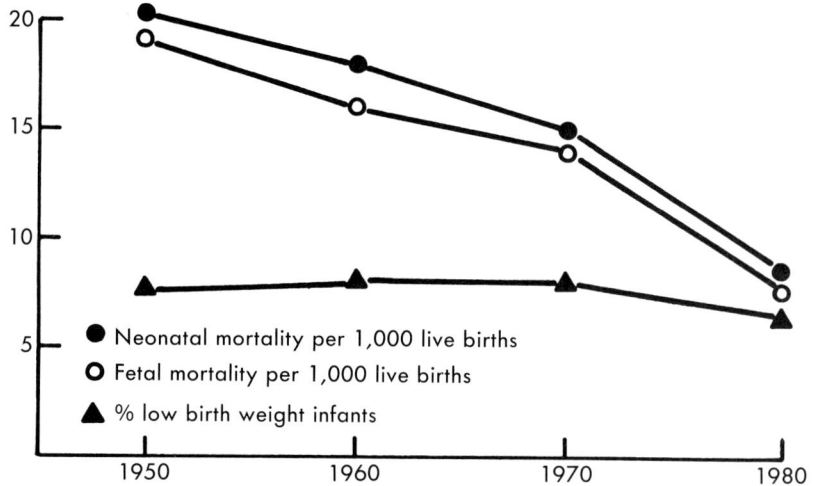

Fig. 34-1. Downward reduction in fetal and neonatal mortality in relation to percentage of low birth weight infants in the United States.

Table 34-1. Neonatal death rates per 1,000 live births by birth weight group in Oregon during 1983 (41,047 total total live births)

Birth weight groups (gm)	Death rate in each weight group	Percentage of total births	Death rates for total births
Low birth weight			
less than 500	970.6	0.08	0.8
500-999	493.4	0.37	1.8
1,000-1,499	136.6	0.45	0.6
1,500-1,999	42.0	0.99	0.4
2,000-2,499	9.8	3.23	0.3
TOTAL	77.7	5.10	3.9
Birth weight over 2,500 gm			
2,500-2,999	3.5	12.50	0.5
3,000-3,499	1.5	34.90	0.5
3,500-3,999	0.7	33.10	0.2
4,000-4,499	1.3	11.70	0.15
4,500-and up	1.8	2.70	0.05
TOTAL	1.5	94.90	1.4
GRAND TOTAL		100.00	5.4†

*Data from Vital Statistics Center of Oregon State Health Division.
†Includes five deaths with no weight.

cause of infants weighing under 1,000 gm at birth. This group represents less than half of one percent of all births but contributes about 2.5 deaths per 1,000 live-born infants. These two sources of death now account for over 75% of all neonatal mortality in population areas with exemplary perinatal care. Any further significant reductions in neonatal mortality must depend on preventive measures.

LOW BIRTH WEIGHT INFANTS AND MORTALITY

The incidence of small infants (under 2,500 gm) is a practical measure of maternal health and affects comparisons of neonatal mortality and morbidity of any population. Nevertheless, the traditional separation of newborns into "term" and "premature" on the basis of weight above and below 2,500 gm has little biologic significance. In some parts of the world, where living conditions are substandard, there are more mature infants (over 37 weeks' gestation) than preterm infants weighing between 2,000 and 2,500 gm.

In more fortunate groups for whom fetal growth is optimal, a greater number of prematurely born infants may weigh over than under 2,500 gm. Finally, neonatal mortality does not become minimal until after 3,000 gm in birth weight has reached (Table 34-1). The World Health Organization has been instrumental in introducing the term "low birth weight" for infants weighing less than 2,500 gm in place of the term "premature." This appellation recognizes the small, mature infants with their special problems and requirements but lessens the emphasis on the prematurely born, per se. Incorrect conclusions can be drawn from so-called "premature" baby studies, depending on the number included who are undergrown.

As several studies have shown, the main difference in neonatal mortality rates between

Table 34-2. Comparison of neonatal mortality with percentages of very low birth weight infants born in various populations

Population groups	Percentage of infants weighing under 1,500 gm	Neonatal mortality*
Sweden (1982)	0.6	4.2
United States (1982)	1.2	7.7
White (U.S.) (1982)	0.9	6.8
Black (U.S.) (1982)	2.5	13.1
Mothers 25-29 yr (1983-1984)	0.7	4.6
Mothers under 20 yr (1983-1984)	1.2	7.3

*Rate per 1,000 live births.

population groups is the percentage of very low birth weight (VLBW) infants born. Because infants weighing under 1,500 gm now account for most neonatal mortality, it is worthwhile to compare neonatal mortality with the incidence of VLBW infants born. Table 34-2 demonstrates the significant association of VLBW infants born with neonatal mortality rates, comparing rates in the United States and Sweden, rates among black and white populations of the United States, and rates for women of low and higher maternal age from the state of Oregon. Because nearly 50% of infants weighing under 1,500 gm die (circa 1980), each 0.5% increase in birth numbers of this immature group increases the neonatal mortality by 2.5 per 1,000 live births. See also Table 1-5.

The fact that reduction in the low birth weight rate (Fig. 34-1) in the United States has not kept pace with the steady improvement in perinatal mortality suggests that better maternity and nursery care has superseded improvements in social, educational, and economic conditions—factors related to the incidence of low birth weight infants in any area.

SUMMARY

The low birth weight infant contributes the major share to perinatal mortality and morbidity. The higher rates of jeopardy for each lower birth weight group are apparent. Often overlooked is the fact that, in terms of numbers, about 30% of all perinatal deaths occur after 37 weeks of gestation has been achieved and, in terms of weight, after 2,500 gm has been reached.

Much emphasis has been placed in recent years on the more rapid decrease in infant mortality in certain other advanced countries of the world over decreases in the rate in the United States. The most recent ranking places the United States in seventeenth place (1983). This poor showing is discomfiting because more money is spent on health per person in the United States than in any of these countries. Medical deficiencies are only partly responsible, however. Although in many areas of medical sophistication the United States is second to none, it is estimated that 25 million Americans receive inadequate or little, if any, health care.

Reduction of immaturity by the advancement of fetal age—when this is possible—must be the initial aim in management. Neonatal mortality for infants born at 28 weeks could be lowered 80% by increasing gestational age to 32 weeks, assuming fetuses have been developing normally. Moreover, extension of gestation and increase in maturity would also sharply reduce the likelihood of physical or mental handicap in survivors. This goal is difficult to achieve because the cause of early birth is often unknown and cannot usually be anticipated and so prevented. On the other hand, certain complications of pregnancy still require early delivery if fetal death is to be avoided.

The second goal of management is reduction of overall perinatal mortality and improvement in the quality of survivors by optimal use of physician and nursing skills, particularly in the recognition and management of acute and chronic fetal stress. The expansion of regional perinatal centers to provide intensive care of the fetus and newborn at risk has markedly reduced perinatal mortality.

Although there has been reduction in the risk of injury and later handicapping of newborns, salvage of greater numbers of very immature infants, particularly those weighing under 1,000 gm, has added to the numbers of newborns who are at the highest risk. Certainly, mere survival of these infants is not good enough.

The final and obviously the most important goal is reduction of the number of low birth weight infants born—both preterm and undersized. Social and educational advancement, encouragement of welcome and wellborn infants, and prevention of unintended pregnancies are necessary correlates to reaching this goal. Continued research in human reproduction and behavior is urged. Embryologists, pathologists, sociologists, psychologists, cultural anthropologists, and many others must join in the quest.

BIBLIOGRAPHY

Behrman, R.E., Babson, S.G., and Lessel, R.: Fetal and neonatal mortality in white middle-class infants, Am. J. Dis. Child. **121**:486, 1971.

Erickson, T.D., and Bjerkedal, T.: Fetal and infant mortality in Norway and the United States, JAMA **247**:987, 1982.

Geijerstam, G.: Low birth weight and perinatal mortality, Public Health Rep. **84**:939, 1969.

Gruenwald, P.: Perinatal death of full-sized and full-term infants, Am. J. Obstet. Gynecol. **107**:1022, 1970.

Guyer, B., Wallach, L.A., and Rosen, S.L.: Birthweight-standardized neonatal mortality rates and the prevention of low birth weight: how does Massachusetts compare with Sweden? N. Eng. J. Med. **306**:1230, 1982.

Lee, K., Paneth, N., Gartner, L.M., et al.: The very low-birth-weight rate: principal predictors of neonatal mortality in industrialized populations, J. Pediatr. **97**:759, 1980.

Lee, K., Paneth, N., Gartner, L.M., et al.: Neonatal mortality: an analysis of the recent improvement in the United States, Am. J. Public Health **70**:15, 1980.

Lilien, A.A.: Term intrapartum fetal death, Am. J. Obstet. Gynecol. **107**:595, 1970.

Lubchenco, L.O.: The high risk infant, Philadelphia, 1976, W.B. Saunders Co.

Lubchenco, L.O., Searles, D.T., and Brazie, J.V.: Neonatal mortality rates: relationship to birth weight and gestational age, J. Pediatr. **81**:814, 1972.

Public health aspects of low birth weight, WHO Techn. Rep. Ser. No. 217, 1961.

Thompson, J.: Perinatal mortality in retrospect and prospect, Scott. Med. J. **14**:89, 1969.

Usher, R.: Clinical implications of perinatal mortality statistics, Clin. Obstet. Gynecol. **14**:885, 1971.

Wallace, H.M.: Factors associated with perinatal mortality and morbidity, Clin. Obstet. Gynecol. **13**:13, 1970.

Wegman, M.E.: Annual summary of vital statistics—1984, Pediatrics **76**:861, 1985.

Section IV PERINATAL OUTCOME

35

Growth and development of the low birth weight infant: neurologic deficits

NEONATAL GROWTH AND DEVELOPMENT
Growth
Growth of the preterm infant after birth dramatically slows from the fetal rate.
1. Weight
   a. Birth weight loss averages 10% to 15% for all weight groups. The low weight is reached at 4 to 6 days of age.
   b. Birth weight is regained in 1 to 3 weeks, depending on maturity and nutritional intake.
   c. Infants suffering fetal undernutrition lose less weight and regain their birth weight more rapidly, especially if they are fed early.
   d. By 40 weeks of postmenstrual age,* body weight is as much as 1,000 gm below that expected had the infant been delivered at term. This discrepancy may be reduced by attention to nutritional intake during the first ten weeks of life.
2. Length
   a. Growth in length slows during the first week of extrauterine life.
   b. Growth in body length is resumed at the fetal rate about the third week of life if adequate nutrition is available (more than 1 cm/wk).
   c. By 40 weeks of postmenstrual age the very premature infant can be as much as 3 to 5 cm shorter than expected length had he been born at term.
3. Head circumference
   a. A lesser lag occurs in the rate of head growth. During the first few days of life an infant's head may decrease between 0.5 and 1.0 cm in circumference, with an accompanying overlapping of the sagittal suture.
   b. The later weekly growth increase is often as much as 0.9 to 1.1 cm. Increase in head size at a rate above 1.2 cm/wk suggests hydrocephalus (Fig. 35-1). Frequently the rate of head growth of the preterm or small-for-dates infant will surpass that projected for the fetus. This temporarily more rapid increase in size, as well as a slight separation of the sutures, may be confused with hydrocephalus. However, the rate of head growth is seldom over 1.2 cm/wk. An increase in transillumination may be noted along with pitting pedal edema in the very immature infant. Salt excess or low protein intake may be responsible for this pseudohydrocephalus, but head growth by 2 months of corrected age will resume at an appropriate rate.
4. Cellular growth
   Much interest has focused on growth as a function of cell size and numbers. Cell division is more active during intrauterine life and then gradually slows after birth, depending on the organ system. Each system has its own biologic time clock for

---
*Postmenstrual age refers to the combined gestational period (fetal) and postnatal age. As in the measurement of gestational age, the time is reckoned from the first day of the last menstrual period. Conception occurs approximately 2 weeks later, a date seldom known.

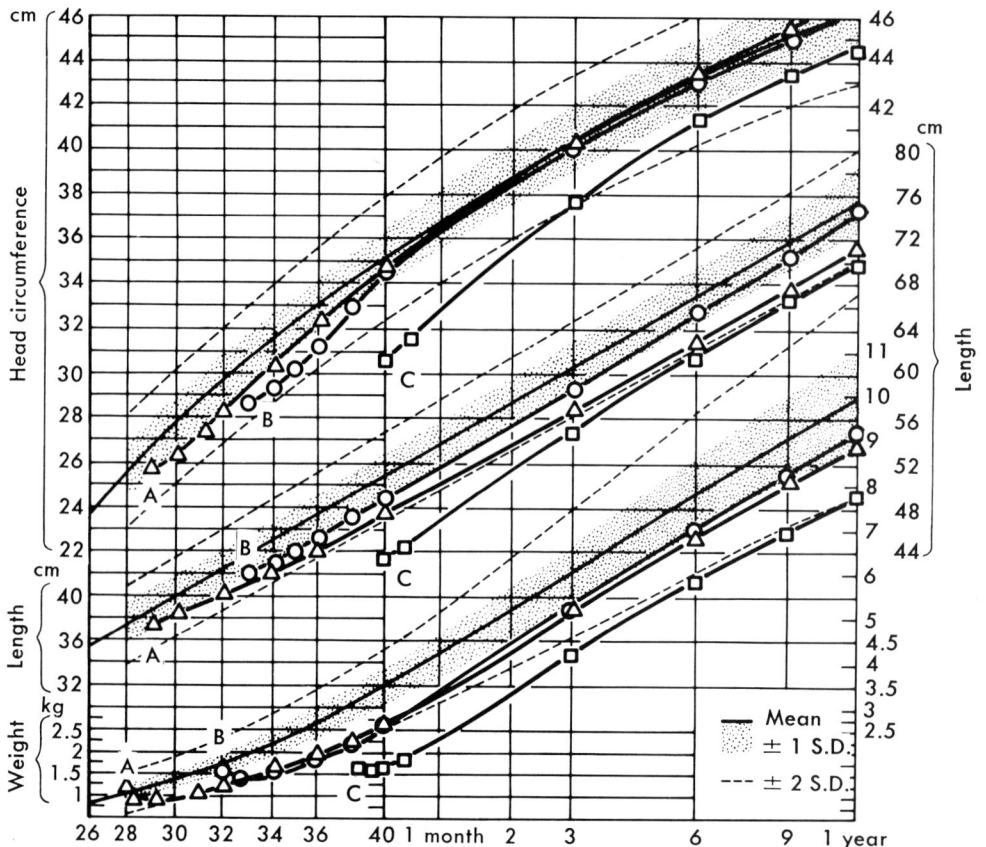

Fig. 35-1. Mean growth curves of three groups of low birth weight infants plotted in three parameters. At birth very premature, *A,* and moderately premature, *B,* infants are both appropriate in size for gestation; full-term infants are severely undergrown, *C*. (Redrawn from Babson, S.G.: J. Pediatr. 77:11, 1970.)

growth. Severe limitation in nutrition may reduce cell numbers as well as cell size. Cellular division and growth in the brain is critical before and after birth, and although knowledge of long-term effects of undergrowth in the human fetus and neonate is limited, sufficient nutrition must be provided whenever possible to support maximum cerebral development.

Development

Neuromuscular development of the preterm infant appears to keep pace with that of his fetal counterpart in utero, if neither severe limitation in nutrition nor cerebral injury has occurred. The following longitudinal observations help to establish the infant's postmenstrual age and, in retrospect, substantiate gestational age at birth.

1. Nipple sucking may be adequate for taking all feedings by 33 to 34 weeks.
2. The infant, in response to elicitation of the Moro reflex, will exhibit an extension of arms, followed by some flexion response, during the thirty-fifth week.
3. Tonus of neck muscles may be sufficiently developed so that the following can be observed:
   a. At 36 weeks the wakeful infant can hold the head firmly when infant is pulled forward by arms from supine position.
   b. At 37 weeks the infant can raise the head from the mattress momentarily when in the prone position.
4. After 38 weeks the infant will fix his eyes on the observer's face and follow its movements; in addition the infant will have a vigorous cry and regular respiration and will maintain body temperature.
5. After 40 weeks the infant will turn the

head in following an object. This response establishes the likelihood of vision and eye movement coordination.
6. Infants at term will blink in response to a loud noise and the older preterm infant will startle at a metallic tap on an incubator wall.

At the time of discharge from the hospital the prospect of favorable later development will be supported by appropriate neuromuscular and neurosensor responses, a vigorous demand for feedings, a satisfactory neurologic examination, and normal-appearing retinas.

POSTNATAL GROWTH AND DEVELOPMENT
Longitudinal growth

Despite a generally more optimistic prognosis, the growth lag suffered by preterm infants at birth may never be made up entirely. Nearly all longitudinal studies indicate a continued difference in height and weight compared with standard populations. Nevertheless, caution must be used in such evaluations because prematurity data include children who may show reduced growth as a result of (1) central nervous system injuries or deficiencies, (2) suboptimal nutrition, and (3) low birth weight from intrauterine growth retardation.

After exclusion of the seriously handicapped, we must conclude that prematurely born children do not differ importantly from other children in later growth.

Fig. 35-1 demonstrates growth through the first year of life in three groups of low birth weight infants in weight, length, and head circumference, corrected for gestational age. Infants in group A were small and premature, those in group B were moderately premature and also appropriate in size, and those in group C were all under 2,000 gm at birth and born at term.

Curves for length and weight in these low birth weight infants parallel but remain below curves of growth considered normal for the fetus and infant; those in the undersized group of infants were reduced the most.

Head circumference in the groups of preterm infants, after an initial lag, increases at an accelerated rate, so that their growth curves may approach or temporarily surpass the expected mean curve for fetal growth. Thereafter, head circumference follows the expected pattern observed in normal infants.

In the infant having suffered fetal undergrowth all measurements at birth are proportionately reduced (Fig. 35-1), with head size usually the least restricted, apparently because of preferential brain growth. One may expect some catch-up in growth in well-fed infants. However, by the age of 6 months most of the readjustment from undergrowth (as well as from overgrowth, see Fig. 11-3) has occurred, and from this time on most infants will follow the established channels of growth.

Neuromuscular, sensory, and social responses

In approximately 80% of survivors even the very immature infants will develop normally. One should expect the following responses by 6 months of corrected age (postnatal age − weeks of prematurity). For example, an infant born at 27 weeks of gestational age (13 weeks early) must have reached 9 months of postnatal age to have a corrected age of 6 months.
1. Grasps objects well that are held in different locations
2. Transfers objects from hand to hand
3. Sits with support and rolls over
4. Laughs responsively and babbles
5. Differentiates people and prefers his mother
6. Turns readily at sounds

At 12 months of corrected age the infant:
1. Pulls self to a standing position and takes a few steps with support
2. Says a few meaningful words
3. Has a well-developed pincer grasp in obtaining and eating small bits of food
4. Releases objects on request
5. Adjusts posture when being dressed

NEUROLOGIC AND INTELLECTUAL DEFICITS

The factors that influence mortality of the fetus and neonate also increase the likelihood of problems in the survivor. In general, the lower the birth weight, the greater the incidence of later handicaps. One third to one half of infants weighing under 1,500 gm were once reported to have moderate to severe problems. Although it is likely that fetal asphyxia, trauma, and delay in resuscitation are primarily responsible for

most later handicaps, it is now clear that other factors must be considered, including the following:
1. Developmental defects with greater incidence of anomalies
2. Postnatal insults that may result from the following:
   a. Delay in instituting nutritional requirements
   b. Biochemical aberrations (e.g., hypoglycemia, hyperbilirubinemia, acidosis)
   c. Later asphyxia from complications of care (e.g., problems of mechanical ventilation, monitoring failure)
3. Low social environment with the following:
   a. Cultural impoverishment
   b. Substandard feeding habits
   c. Increased likelihood of genetic inadequacy
   d. Poor physical and intellectual nurturing and stimulation

Nevertheless, asphyxia is the usual common denominator and carries a substantial but often unpredictable burden for the infant, depending on its severity, duration, and the resistance of the infant (maturity and nutritional state). Prolonged hypoxia can produce definite cerebral lesions (periventricular leukomalacia). However, severe asphyxia per se, before or after birth, may leave the brain unscathed.

In the monkey, less than 10 minutes of complete postnatal anoxia apparently does little in the way of physical damage to the brain or later behavior. A longer period of anoxia increases the chance of damage, with the certainty of permanent change after 15 minutes of apnea. In human studies, effects from apnea observed after birth are difficult to interpret, since an unknown period of asphyxia is likely to have been present prior to birth.

The complications and problems of infants who were small for dates or oversized at birth are discussed in Chapter 12. The smaller preterm infants, particularly those who weigh under 2,000 gm at birth, will be discussed in this chapter. In addition to these groups, other newborns at risk have a considerably increased chance of impairment in later development. They also require careful longitudinal observations. This miscellaneous group includes infants with (1) fetal asphyxia, prolonged resuscitation, or low Apgar scores at 5 minutes; (2) suspected or diagnosed intracranial hemorrhage; (3) severe respiratory distress or sepsis; (4) neonatal seizures, hypotonia, and inattention to sound or visual stimuli; (5) suspected or diagnosed congenital malformations, hereditary disease, or fetal infection; and (6) families with serious social or mental health problems.

Intellectual development

The reduced intellectual ability of children who are born prematurely is well known. The more immature an infant is at birth, the greater the likelihood of a deficit. The relationship of prematurity to complications of pregnancy that contribute to asphyxial damage, the greater susceptibility to trauma of the early born, and delays in feeding and metabolic support may be the factors primarily responsible. The increased frequency of women with a lower socioeconomic background to bear preterm infants and the cultural impoverishment that may be present also play a role in these intellectual deficits. Inadequate school performance may be noted even when intelligence is in the normal range. Nevertheless, there appears to be a definite improvement in later intellectual functions of preterm infants who have been supported by full intensive care methods throughout the perinatal period.

Neurologic deficits

In the past, nearly 40% of patients enrolled in cerebral palsy clinics were infants of low birth weight. Over 75% of children with spastic diplegia were born early. Longitudinal observations of infants who were very premature at birth have demonstrated in the past that approximately 10% to 15% have some degree of cerebral palsy. However, mental retardation and speech deficiency are not the rule in these children.

The incidence of cerebral palsy and other neurologic defects has been reduced in recent years to 5% to 10%, which suggests improvement in the care of preterm infants.

The following observations suggest cerebral palsy:
1. History of difficulty in sucking or swallowing
2. Gradual increase in extensor tone, such as displayed by the following:

a. Extension of head when ventrally suspended
   b. Resistance to dorsiflexion of feet
   c. Difficulty in sitting alone
   d. Adductor spasm on abduction of legs
   e. Toe walking with tightening of heel cords
3. Asymmetry of movements, particularly in hand action and fisting
4. Hyperreflexia with sustained clonus
5. Hypotonia with increased range of motion

Vision and hearing

Strabismus has occurred in the past in 10% to 15% of lower weight groups of children who had been preterm infants. Refractive errors likewise are more common. Retinopathy of prematurity is almost exclusively a disorder of the smaller preterm infant, leading to blindness in 5% to 10% of surviving infants who weighed less than 1,000 gm at birth.

Hearing impairment occurs in about 5% of these infants, either singly or with other defects; however, ototoxic drugs, as well as viral invasion, may play a part in pathogenesis.

Behavior disorders

Incoordination, distractibility, a short attention span, and emotional instability, often referred to as "minimal brain syndrome," are observed occasionally. Lack of confidence, shyness, and overdependence may be recognized. Some of these variations may reflect subtle injury to the central nervous system, whereas others may stem from the parents' overconcern for, or at times rejection of, the infant.

Nevertheless, the great number of preterm infants, regardless of size at birth, are remarkably well adjusted and normal in behavior. Their prematurity may be used as an excuse for common variations of behavior in the general school population.

Health and illness

Preterm infants have greater risk of acquiring infectious disease during the first year of life. The number of their hospital admissions for severe respiratory disease is several times that of mature control infants. Unexplained crib deaths are two to three times more common in preterm than in term infants.

CHILD ABUSE

The low birth weight infant who was prematurely born is three times more likely to be subjected to physical and emotional abuse and neglect than the average infant. Insufficient attention to nutritional requirements and the practice of poor hygiene are not uncommon. The following associations may intensify child abuse:

1. Prolonged separation of mother and infant directly after birth
2. Warnings by family friends and physicians of the possibility of death or defect
3. Unplanned pregnancy and unwanted child
4. Stressful intrafamily relationships

The physician and nurse should be aware of these factors surrounding birth and the possibility that the infant might be subconsciously or overtly rejected. Child neglect can be reduced if the perinatal team emphasizes the following:

1. Stress the positive and optimistic aspects to woman with a pregnancy at risk.
2. Prepare mother for the possibly frightening exposure to intensive care nursery.
3. Have mother and father enter the nursery and touch their infant as soon after birth as possible. This necessary binding with eye-to-face contact may overcome a tenuous maternal tie. In case of neonatal transport, wheel infant into mother's room for similar contact.
4. Explain reasons for each type of equipment (e.g., phototherapy lights, eye protection, monitor attachments).
5. Continue to maintain contact with parents during and after hospital stay.
6. Interview parents of high-risk neonates during hospital stay for possible stressful states. The social worker and public health nurse are necessary members of the professional team in alleviation of problems contributing to the instability of the family unit.

LONGITUDINAL ASSESSMENTS

The frequency of sequelae seen in prematurely born and growth-retarded infants, as well as in those at risk for other reasons, requires careful serial observations for early identification of handicapping defects. Examination should include the following:

1. Growth measurements and plotting in relation to gestational age (Fig. 11-2) This procedure is necessary in identification of any disproportion in growth.
2. Developmental screening such as the Denver Development Screening Test (by W.K. Frankenburg and J.B. Dodds, University of Colorado Medical Center)
3. Neurologic examination, especially for tonus, reflex behavior, vision, eye muscle coordination, hearing, and sound production, including speech development

Motor delay must always be interpreted with caution, particularly in children who were extremely premature. Also, signs of increased tone through 6 months of postnatal age may not be significant. Some delay can be compatible with later normality. The following signs, however, are prejudicial to normal development: (1) history of difficult feeding, (2) irritability, (3) hypertonia with stiffening of body, and (4) hypotonia.

Gross changes in neurologic behavior require multidisciplinary examinations (speech, intelligence, hearing, vision, and so forth) because several areas of handicapping are likely. Complete care includes counseling of parents, arrangements for remedial care, planning for education, and use of appropriate physician and paramedical personnel and public health facilities, together with the crippled children's services.

Children who demonstrate minor deviations from accepted standards of development or who show variations in behavior pattern (short attention span, clumsiness, and so forth) may need much more attention than they often get. In these situations the family should receive continued and interested support from the physician, and the child should have encouragement, particularly in his feeling of self-worth.

BIBLIOGRAPHY

Babson, S.G.: Growth of low birth weight infants, J. Pediatr. **77**:12, 1970.

Babson, S.G., and Henderson, N.B.: Fetal undergrowth: relation of headgrowth to later intellectual performance, Pediatrics **53**:890, 1974.

Churchill, J.A., Masland, R.L., Naylor, A.A., et al.: The etiology of cerebral palsy in preterm infants, Dev. Med. Child Neurol. **16**:143, 1974.

Davies, P.A., and Davis, J.P.: Very low birth weight and subsequent head growth, Lancet **11**:1216, 1970.

Davies, P.A., and Tizard, J.P.M.: Very low birth weight and subsequent neurological defect, Dev. Med. Child Neurol. **17**:3, 1975.

Drillien, C.M.: Later development and follow-up of low birth weight babies, Pediatr. Ann. **1**:44, 1972.

Francis-Williams, J., and Davies, P.A.: Very low birth weight and later intelligence, Dev. Med. Child Neurol. **16**:709, 1974.

Fitzhardinge, P.M.: Early growth and development in low birthweight infants following treatment in an intensive care nursery, Pediatrics **56**:126, 1975.

Fitzhardinge, P.M.: Follow-up studies on low birth weight infants, Clin. Perinatol. **3**:503, 1976.

Grunnet, M.L., Curless, R.G., Bray, P.F., et al.: Brain changes in newborns from an intensive care unit, Dev. Med. Child Neurol. **16**:320, 1974.

Hack, M., Fanarott, A.A., and Merkatz, I.R.: The low-birth-weight infant-evolution of a changing outlook, N. Engl. J. Med. **301**:1162, 1979.

Klein, N., Hack, M., Gallagher, J., et al.: Preschool performance of children with normal intelligence who were very-low-birth-weight infants, Pediatrics **75**:531, 1985.

Lubchenco, L.O., Bard, H., Goldman, A.L., et al.: Newborn intensive care and long-term prognosis, Dev. Med. Child Neurol. **16**:421, 1974.

Lubchenco, L.O., Delivoria-Papadopoulos, M., Butterfield, L.J., et al.: Long-term follow-up studies of prematurely born infants. I. Relationship of handicaps to nursery routines, J. Pediatr. **80**:501, 1972.

Lubchenco, L.O., Delivoria-Papadopoulos, M., and Searls, D.: Long-term follow-up studies of prematurely born infants. II. Influence of birth weight and gestational age on sequelae, J. Pediatr. **80**:509, 1972.

Nickel, R.E., Bennett, F.C., and Lamson, E.N.: School performance of children with birth weight of 1000 g or less, Am. J. Dis. Child. **136**:105, 1982.

Saigal, S., Rosenbaum, P., Stoskopt, J.B., et al.: Outcome in infants 501 to 1000 gm birth weight delivered to residents of the McMaster Health Region, J. Pediatr. **105**:969, 1984.

Stahlman, M.E., Hedvall, G., Dolanski, E., et al.: A six-year follow-up of clinical HMD, Pediatr. Clin. North Am. **20**:433, 1973.

Stewart, A.L., and Reynolds, E.O.: Improved prognosis for infants of very low birth weight, Pediatrics **54**:724, 1974.

Stewart, A.L., Turcan, D.M., Rawlings, G., et al.: Prognosis for infants weighing 1000 g or less at birth, Arch. Dis. Child. **52**:97, 1977.

Wiener, G.: The relationship of birth weight and length of gestation to intellectual development at ages 8 to 12 years, J. Pediatr. **76**:694, 1970.

36

Regionalization and guidelines for perinatal care

The regionalization of perinatal care is now an established fact in many areas of North America. Organization of such care for the fetus and neonate at high risk is advocated by major medical groups, including the American Medical Association. Pregnant women whose fetuses have been identified as being at increased risk of death or damage are referred increasingly to perinatal centers for full perinatal team support. Approximately 5% to 10% of all deliveries will be at high risk, and another 10% to 25% will be at moderate risk. Criteria for identifying those at risk are given in Chapter 2.

Unfortunately, not all of those at risk are identifiable prior to labor or even delivery. Unsuspected complications or premature labor continue to occur in primary hospitals, resulting in the deliveries of jeopardized infants and the need for special care. Although some maternity units are of sufficient size and have the capability to offer 24-hour intensive neonatal coverage, most hospitals do not. Therefore an emergency plan should be formulated for transport of an infant in distress to a perinatal center when the infant's condition does not stabilize or improvement fails to occur. Neonates at high risk are best transferred by a specialized physician-nurse transport team capable of providing full intensive care in transit.

LEVELS OF CARE

Infants in severe respiratory distress and those with major congenital defects require, in most instances, transport to a neonatal center that offers what has come to be called "tertiary care." Infants in moderate distress born in a primary or smaller community hospital often require transfer to an intermediate or secondary hospital capable of giving continuing specialized care. Special care units must not be developed indiscriminately, since staffing requirements are demanding in terms of numbers as well as skills.

The concept of regionalization for obstetric and neonatal care, designed to reduce maternal and infant mortality and morbidity, represents an obstetric and newborn health care system composed of three distinct types of facilities.

The highest-level facility is the *regional perinatal center,* which is fully equipped to handle any type of obstetric or newborn problem. Serving patients having complications beyond the treatment capability of other facilities, the regional center would become the focal point for referral and consultation for those patients requiring specialized care not available at other hospitals.

A second level of care would be provided by the *intermediate or larger community hospital,* which should serve the bulk of obstetric and newborn patients. It should be capable of offering continuing special care, with only a small number of unusual or complicated problems referred from it to the regional center.

The third and final type of facility, the *small community or rural hospital,* providing a sharply limited amount of care, is nonetheless necessary in locations where geographic and population factors limit access to other facilities. Pregnancies should be carefully screened for risk problems for appropriate management and possible delivery at higher level facilities.

SMALL COMMUNITY OR RURAL HOSPITAL (PRIMARY CARE)

The continuing move to consolidate smaller maternity units and develop perinatal centers allows for better care of risk patients, as well as affording the unanticipated infant at risk (up to 40% of problem babies) a better chance for optimal care and intact survival. Most hospitals in smaller communities will of necessity have an insufficient number of deliveries to give more than temporary intensive care. Approximately 75% of infants born are fortunately at the lowest risk—those born at term (40 ± 2 weeks' gestation) and weighing between 3,000 and 4,000 gm at birth. Unless these babies show disability, they may be placed in the regular nursery or discharged after an observation period of 4 to 6 hours near the nurses' station or in a mother-infant recovery area.

Responsibilities of community hospital

Sufficient facilities and skilled personnel must be available for adequate resuscitation and initial intensive care of any unexpectedly sick or distressed infant until he is stabilized or has been placed in the care of a transport team. In addition, special care must be available for the 10% to 20% of infants who are at medium risk (see Chapter 12). These infants include the following:

1. Large- and small-for-dates infants
2. Preterm infants (34 to 37 weeks' gestation)
3. Dysmature or undergrown infants who demonstrate no asphyxia at birth and who can accept early feedings
4. Infants with depressed Apgar scores (4 to 6) whose conditions have improved on admission to the nursery

These infants are at increased risk until good health is demonstrated, and any hospital that has a maternity department should be capable of providing the basic care outlined.

Transfer of infants to regional center

(See Chapter 13.)

Of infants born in the smaller community hospital, 3% to 6% require transfer to a hospital giving continuing specialized care. Approximately one third of these infants need the team support of a tertiary center. These include those who are severely depressed at birth, demonstrate increasing respiratory distress, show significant congenital anomalies, are under 32 weeks' gestation, or weigh less than 1,500 gm. In addition, a small percentage will develop the following problems not evident at birth that often require transfer:

1. Delayed respiratory distress (e.g., aspiration, pneumothorax, pneumonia)
2. Apneic or cyanotic spells (e.g., those with congenital heart disease or sepsis)
3. Disorders of behavior and activity, including vomiting, abdominal distention, and hypotonia
4. Seizures and sepsis
5. Hemorrhage or pallor
6. Jaundice before 24 hours of age or bilirubin over 15 mg/100 ml

Special care requirements and facilities

The nursery area can serve as an admission, recovery, observation, and special-procedure area for infants at increased risk. These babies are preferably placed near the nurses' station. At least 2 feet of space is needed between units.

1. Medical, nursing, and paramedical personnel at all times should have the following skills:
    a. Ability to resuscitate infant by positive-pressure methods and to intubate infant if necessary
    b. Ability to infuse $NaHCO_3$, glucose, blood, Plasmanate, or other blood volume expanders through an umbilical vessel for temporary support
    c. Ability to give known monitored concentration of oxygen by hood sufficient to control central cyanosis and to record these levels
    d. Ability to ensure an appropriate thermal environment for infant from time of birth
    e. Knowledge in using simple monitoring equipment, phototherapy for otherwise well babies, and Dextrostix testing, particularly for distressed or inappropriately grown infants
    f. Ability to identify significant variations from the usual during first 4 to 6 hours of life (transitional care)

In addition, personnel should ensure that there is access by phone to a regional center for consultation regarding problems and a prearranged plan with a trans-

port center for the immediate transfer of sick newborn infants.
2. Utilities
   a. Oxygen, compressed air, and suction availability
   b. Electrical equipment—sufficient 120-volt outlets to a common ground (half on hospital emergency power circuit)
   c. Washbasins—one for each four to six patients, with foot or knee controls
3. Equipment
   a. Incubators or radiant warming systems: at least one radiant warmer in the labor and delivery suite, at least two (preferably four) incubators or warmers for each 100 infants born per month, for transitional care
   b. A warmed nebulized oxygen source and hood (not less than two per 50 infants born per month)
   c. Oxygen analyzer
   d. Heart rate or heart rate and apnea monitors (two per 100 deliveries per month)
   e. Phototherapy units (two per 100 deliveries per month)
   f. A means of blood pressure measurement
   g. An accurate scale, ideally one calibrated in grams
   h. Resuscitation and stabilization equipment and medications (see Chapter 9)

Obstetric requirements are dependent on the capabilities of the medical and nursing staff and on the size of the maternity unit. Because women at high risk often will be referred to the nearest maternity center for delivery, emphasis is placed on the following:

1. Early identification of the pregnancy at high risk to allow primary physician to share in management with staff at the center
2. Established communication arrangement, particularly in evaluation of impending labor and delivery
3. Emergency transport service with capability for management of women in threatened labor
4. Availability of electronic fetal monitor for those cases in which intrapartum distress may develop

LARGER COMMUNITY HOSPITALS FOR CONTINUING SPECIAL CARE (INTERMEDIARY CARE)

Centers for special care should be planned to meet patient, medical, community, and regional needs. Intermediate hospitals should provide a standard of care sufficient for most of the contingencies encountered by an obstetric or newborn service. The care provided should be of high quality and in no way inferior to comparable services available at the regional center. Because of rising costs and falling birth rates, consolidation of maternity services is necessary for maximum efficiency in providing quality service. Ideally a minimum of 2,000 infants should be delivered each year to offer efficient continuing care to both fetus and neonate at high risk. However, a more limited number of deliveries is justified when the hospital, by its geographic character, supplies special services to adjacent rural hospitals. An organized system of communication and transport for interchange of patients at risk is required.

Specific obstetric requirements

I. Obstetric personnel and staffing
   A. A staff physician-in-charge who is knowledgeable in perinatal technology
   B. In-house 24-hour obstetric and anesthesia coverage
   C. A specially trained obstetric registered nurse on each shift, with an adequate number of circulating nurses trained in obstetric nursing
   D. Programs for special and ongoing training and staff meetings to ensure high standards of perinatal care
II. Facilities and services
   A. Sufficient space and equipment to permit the following:
      1. FHR monitoring (more than one unit)
      2. Cesarean section performed within 20 minutes or less of decision to perform procedure (emergency section room)
      3. Emergency transfusion of O-negative blood within 20 minutes or less of decision to transfuse
      4. Closely monitored postdelivery or postoperative recovery room

5. Resuscitation capability in delivery an section room
B. Hospital services available on a 24-hour basis including:
1. Full laboratory support, with blood bank
2. Rapid surfactant test
3. Respiratory therapy and radiologic services
4. Ultrasonography
5. Serial estriol level testing
6. Social service

Specific neonatal requirements

A minimal unit of at least four intensive care infant beds is required to justify the specialized care program outlined. The following basic recommendations are in addition to the emergency and observational care that are suggested for the primary hospital:

I. Pediatric personnel and staffing
  A. A physician-in-charge who has had special training or experience in neonatal care, on call 24 hours a day
  B. A registered nurse trained in neonatal care on each shift
  C. Paramedical personnel trained in respiratory therapy and in engineering and electronic supervision
  D. Nurse-patient ratio of 1:3 (may vary from 1:2 to 1:4)
  E. A committee responsible for planning and maintaining standards of care, policy, and regular review of the special care service, with particular attention paid to infection control
  F. Programs for special and ongoing training of key personnel
  G. Public health nurse and social worker consultation services
II. Utilities
  A. Two outlets each per patient for oxygen; one each for compressed air and suction
  B. Eight to ten 110-volt outlets per patient module, with half of outlets on hospital emergency power circuit
  C. 220-volt outlet per room for portable x-ray unit
  D. Adequate, convenient washbasins
III. Equipment
  A. Four intensive care beds of the Isolette type or four open radiant warmers per 100 deliveries per month; additional modules if infants are admitted from regional hospitals
  B. Ward services
    1. Adequate resuscitation equipment
    2. Hematocrit centrifuge
    3. T-S (total solids) meter
    4. Glucose monitoring (urine and blood)
    5. Transillumination light (and darkroom)
    6. X-ray view box
IV. Laboratory capabilities (24 hours)
  A. pH, P_{CO_2}, and P_{O_2} determinations
  B. Bilirubin measurement, direct and indirect
  C. Microelectrolyte determination
  D. Assessment of coagulation status, microhematologic service, blood typing, minor incompatibility detection
V. Special diagnostic and supportive service
  A. Immediately available x-ray services
  B. Blood bank
  C. Respiratory therapy (therapist on call, responsible for maintenance of equipment)
  D. Electroencephalograph and electrocardiograph recorders with newborn leads
  E. Rapid infant transport without heat loss (Chapter 13)
VI. Medical services
  A. Gavage feeding
  B. Exchange transfusion
  C. Parenteral fluids
  D. Umbilical artery catheterization
  E. Temporary ventilator support

REGIONAL CARE CENTERS (TERTIARY CARE)

Regional care centers provide the ultimate in perinatal care for the very high–risk pregnancy and neonate.

Approximately 5% to 10% of women have sufficiently critical problems in pregnancy to be delivered with a full perinatal team in attendance. These conditions include eclampsia, severe diabetes, hydramnios, severe bleeding, premature rupture of membranes at less than 35 weeks' gestation, premature labor at less than 32 weeks' gestation, and heart disease.

Between 2,000 and 6,000 births in an area are necessary to justify 24-hour in-house coverage by a skilled staff and to make a hospital economically viable. Fifteen-minute cesarean section time, emergency fetal scalp blood gas and pH determination capability, B-scan ultrasonography, and 1-day estriol and rapid surfactant tests are among the requirements of such a center, in addition to those mentioned for the intermediary center.

Approximately 2% to 3% of newborns require the most critical care. This care covers infants requiring extended ventilatory assistance, cardiac catheterization, neonatal surgery, genetic and metabolic evaluation, and prolonged parenteral alimentation.

For a perinatal regional center to be designated as a tertiary facility, it must draw from a pregnancy population sufficient to maintain skills of the team and ancillary personnel in the care of the high-risk perinate. For example, an available pregnancy population of approximately 5,000 to 10,000 is necessary to maintain expertise in (1) preterm delivery of infants of less than 32 weeks' gestational age and (2) extended ventilatory support for infants with severe respiratory distress. Between 10,000 and 15,000 may be necessary to support neonatal surgery, and 15,000 to 20,000 to maintain a team that can diagnose and treat congenital heart disease. To maintain a team for genetic diagnosis or fetal transfusion for severe isoimmunization should require a pregnancy population of 25,000 to 50,000.

Personnel and staffing requirements

1. A neonatologist on stand-by call
2. In-house physicians on 24-hour call capable of providing emergency life-support measures including pediatric resident and anesthesiologist; perhaps also a neonatal nurse specialist
3. Registered nurses on each shift who have had at least 3 months' training in specialized neonatal care
4. Ability to have one-to-one nurse-patient ratio for extremely sick infants
5. Emergency consultative services (perinatal hotline) and a physician-nurse team for organized transport of infants between hospitals, involving ground and air travel—available 24 hours a day and 7 days a week
6. When neonatal care is offered in the subspecialties (e.g., cardiology or surgery), an appropriate team that has been organized in detail and that has access to diagnostic facilities, so that total care for these special problems can be integrated in the center
7. Clearly defined administrative responsibilities

Recommended facilities and services (in addition to the requirements of other specialized nurseries)

1. Incubators or open-air warmers with eight to ten electrical outlets, and two oxygen, compressed air, and suction outlets for each unit
2. An area of 60 to 100 square feet for each intensive care module
3. Cardiorespiratory and central blood pressure monitoring
4. Capacity for delivering continuous positive airway pressure (CPAP) or continuous negative pressure (CNP) and intermittent positive-pressure breathing (IPPB) or intermittent negative-pressure breathing (INPB), with constant support by respiratory therapists
5. Complete 24-hour emergency radiologic services and laboratory support for blood gas and microelectrolyte determinations; the capability to perform blood coagulation studies and serum and urine osmolarity tests
6. Ability to offer prolonged parenteral alimentation and to prepare parenteral nutritional fluids under controlled conditions
7. Educational programs for center personnel as well as for physicians and nurses from referring hospitals
8. Full-time social service and public health nurse support
9. Follow-up studies of former patients to evaluate methods of care and mortality and morbidity

BIBLIOGRAPHY

American Academy of Pediatrics, American College of Obstetricians and Gynecologists: Guidelines for perinatal care, Evanston Ill., Washington, D.C. 1983.

Blackman, L.R., and Brown, A.K.: Recommended standards for hospital nursery services, Augusta, Ga., 1973, Medical College of Georgia.

Brans, Y.W.: Planning a perinatal center: from vision to reality, Clin. Perinatol., **10**:3, 1983.

Dinermon, B.: Obstetric services in the central area of Los

Angeles County, 1973, Comprehensive Health Planning Council of Los Angeles County.

Lucey, J.F.: Why we should regionalize perinatal care, Pediatrics **52:**488, 1973.

Merenstein, G.B.: Regionalization of perinatal care, Milit. Med. **140:**193, 1975.

Merkatz, I.R., and Johnson, K.G.: Regionalization of perinatal care in the United States, Clin. Perinatol. **3:**271, 1976.

Russell, K.P., Gardiner, S.H., and Nichols, E.E.: A conceptual model for regionalization and consolidation of obstetrical and gynecologic services, Am. J. Obstet. Gynecol. **121:**756, 1975.

Ryan, G.M.: Toward improving the outcome of pregnancy, Obstet. Gynecol. **46:**375, 1975.

Sunshine, P., editor: Regionalization of perinatal care, Report of Sixty-sixth Ross Conference, Columbus, Ohio, 1974, Ross Laboratories.

Swyer, P.R.: The regional organization of special care for the neonate, Pediatr. Clin. North Am. **17:**761, 1970.

The National Foundation–March of Dimes, Committee on perinatal health: toward improving the outcome of pregnancy—recommendation of the regional development of maternal and perinatal health services, 1976.

Section V PREVENTION

37

Prevention of high-risk pregnancies

In the United States perinatal mortality accounts for 55,000 deaths each year, or about 1.5% of all pregnancies that reach 20 weeks' gestation. In a 1971 study the Committee on Perinatal Welfare of the Massachusetts Medical Society held that one third of the deaths at the time were preventable. Maternal factors were attributable in 30%, obstetric problems in 46%, and pediatric factors in 40% of deaths. With the developments in perinatal care already established in the 1970s, Schneider maintained (as reported at the Sixty-sixth Ross Conference, 1974) that two thirds of neonatal deaths and half of fetal deaths were preventable, as indicated by his studies in the Wisconsin perinatal program. A similar avoidability probably applies to perinatal morbidity, an important factor in that significant handicaps develop in 7% of the infant survivors of the neonatal period.

The residuals of having been born too soon or too small have been widely publicized and include cerebral palsy, mental retardation, and sensory defects. The enormity of this problem is apparent, and the need to confront the factors relating to prematurity, fetal undergrowth, and defective development is still urgent. Too often, adverse effects of pregnancy and birth have reduced the normal infant to an inferior one, physically and mentally.

Extension in regionalization of perinatal care (Chapter 36) and cooperation between practicing physicians and health experts have developed organized levels of care with the result that neonatal mortality in a number of states has been reduced to less than 6 deaths per 1,000 deliveries.

Reduction in the percentage of live-born neonates who weigh under 1,500 gm has not been achieved. This group accounts for over half the neonatal mortality in the United States; yet it represents only 1% of all live-born infants. The fact that Sweden, on a percentage basis, has less than half the number born in this weight group may indicate the social and educational achievements of the Scandinavian population.

What share of the U.S. tax dollar should be spent on full maternity and nursery care programs, with emphasis on the quality of life, compared to tax money now spent on rehabilitation services, such as mental health and retardation centers and crippled children's programs, services so often necessary as the result of deficiencies in some part of pregnancy experience?

As an aid to sharper development of goals, the United States should examine the working programs of Norway. The objectives of the Family and Child Welfare Services there have been described to be "for the protection and support of families and the rising generation" or, more specifically, "keeping down infant mortality, preventing illness and death in pregnancy and during delivery, ensuring children's healthy development and helping to protect mothers from the many strains of bearing and rearing children."*

Our objective in this book has been to lessen such frequent and unfortunate events by detailed care of the fetus and neonate. These last pages summarize the broad approach necessary to reduce prematurity and high-risk pregnancy.

---

*From Evang, K.: Health services in Norway, Oslo, 1960, Norwegian social policy; Lougholm, M.: Family and child welfare in Norway, Oslo, 1961, Norwegian Joint Committee on International Social Policy. Twenty years later Norway was in the lowest group among the countries of the world in neonatal mortality.

SOCIOECONOMIC IMPROVEMENT

Better education and employment opportunities could improve the lots of under-privileged persons. A rise in the standard of living will improve the general health of a population and will sharply decrease the percentage of low birth weight infants born. Efforts to reduce the dropout rate from high school should fortify achievement of these goals. Ill-timed pregnancy at this period should not cause discontinuation of education.

Position in society, with its many implications, has been the most important factor pertaining to the availability and quality of obstetric-pediatric care in the United States. Knowledge of needs and desires and of how these can best be met is a primary determinant in the receipt of medical service.

SOCIOMEDICAL MEASURES

1. Ensure the emotional and physical health of adolescents. Adolescent medicine, a subspecialty, seeks to improve the fitness of teenagers. Preparation for marriage and family life must be a feature of this "medical" function.
2. Promote desirable attitudes toward life and parenthood. The physician should assume some responsibility for the well-being of girls and boys during and soon after puberty, when long-standing habits and basic convictions develop, and mothers- and fathers-to-be set their life-styles in community living.
3. Guide the young in sexual behavior, pregnancy responsibility, and family planning. Family planning is far more than birth control. It also includes an understanding of reproductive physiology and pathology, infertility, and social aspects of sex; premarital and genetic counseling; breast and genital cancer detection; pregnancy timing and spacing; therapeutic abortion and sterilization; demography; and research in human reproduction. Ideally, these and related educational services should be available in every community.
4. Extend immunization programs in anticipation of pregnancy. Immunization of all individuals against rubella before puberty will virtually eliminate this critically teratogenic disease. Early poliomyelitis and measles immunization must continue.
5. Educate the public regarding general as well as reproductive health effects of use of alcohol, tobacco, narcotics, and other street drugs.

OBSTETRIC MEASURES

The high-risk obstetric patient calls for very special knowledge by physician and nurse, sophisticated laboratory facilities, and trained, available technical assistance, as well as interdisciplinary collaboration. The success of complete maternity care is to be measured not only by the salvage of life and the improvement in standards of health of mothers and babies, but also by diminished fears, difficulties, and discomforts that have to be faced to some extent by every woman who embarks on motherhood. The following measures to prevent prematurity and high-risk pregnancy should be taken:

1. Improve the timing, quality, and quantity of preconceptional care. Preventive medicine anticipates and corrects problems to avoid complications. The patient and her husband should be in the best possible health before starting a family. Problems to be controlled or treated range from diabetes mellitus to genital tract abnormalities. Correction of nutritional deficits includes attention to anemia, obesity, and underweight. These conditions are frequent and too often remain uncorrected even when pregnancy is well advanced.
2. Encourage earlier preconceptual and prenatal care. Advantages for the unborn may be explained through secondary education, reinforced at the time of premarital examinations, fully developed with preconceptual visits, and reinforced when the diagnosis of pregnancy is established.
3. Identify high-risk patients early (before pregnancy, if possible) for planning for pregnancy, evaluation, treatment, and sympathetic counseling. Many of the risk factors have been discussed and include poor previous pregnancy outcome; previous undersized or oversized babies; overnutrition and undernutrition of the gravida; very early or advanced age of gravida; out-of-wedlock pregnancy; infertility and endocrinopathy; and stress or anxiety of woman.
4. Effect therapeutic abortion in women who cannot carry fetuses to viability and those with serious problems that will irremedia-

bly adversely affect their offspring. Other indicators for interruption of pregnancy include health and mental disorders and serious familial metabolic diseases and chromosomal aberrations such as Down's syndrome, which may be discovered by tissue culture obtained by antenatal diagnosis. Obviously each elective abortion represents a tragedy not limited to just the fetus and the mother. It represents a societal failure to pave the way to successful reproduction (see next section, "Prevention of Unwanted Pregnancy").

5. Offer counseling services when familial defects are known or have occurred. Many couples will voluntarily limit conception when crippling hereditary disease is likely.
6. Strictly forbid use of substances known to harm the fetus, (e.g., tobacco, alcohol, heroin, etc.). Cigarette smoking increases fetal and neonatal jeopardy and results in undersized neonates. Alcohol is associated with fetal alcohol syndrome. The deleterious effects of addicting substances are well known.
7. Deliver better obstetric care through expanded medical resources of referral, diagnosis, consultation, and treatment. The team approach is required to avoid fetal casualty and control occurrence of serious residuals and sequelae of many serious conditions that occur in pregnancy. Such disorders include urinary tract infection, cardiopathies, toxemia, and many other conditions that may require hospital admission and readmission for study, therapy, and rest.
8. Expand regional centers for specialized and complete maternity and nursery services, particularly for the perinate in jeopardy. Establishment of such centers should be of the highest priority. The following benefits would accrue: (1) training of specialized personnel, who are in short supply in this field; (2) demonstration and participation in specialized perinatal care for the physician and nurse in the regional care area; and (3) cooperation between regional centers and local hospitals for the transfer of pregnant women (and sometimes their infants) who are at high risk (twinning, toxemia, etc.).
9. Implement care to include migratory, underprivileged persons. There are many patients who do not "belong" but who need medical attention or special care. Seasonal farm workers and alienated youth are examples.
10. Diagnose twinning by the twenty-sixth week of gestation to institute special care.
11. Supervise adequacy of diet. Controlling the quantity and quality of nutrients is important to fetal health. Avoid undernutrition during the third trimester, even in obese women. Seek special dietary support (e.g., the WIC Program) for the young gravida and those women considered to be undernourished.
12. Obtain homemaker assistance; bed rest is important for cardiac, multiple pregnancy, and chronic abortion patients. Many threatening disorders of pregnancy are associated with uterine hyperirritability. Bed rest may be both prophylactic and therapeutic during pregnancy.
13. Eliminate abortogenic infections (i.e., syphilis, listeriosis, mycoplasma infections, brucellosis, toxoplasmosis, cytomegalovirus, rubella, and malaria). Treat and cure bacteriuria, vaginitis, and cervicitis.
14. Institute expectant, informed management of second- and third-trimester uterine bleeding problems. Far more mischief results from radical than from conservative treatment of antepartum bleeding. Maternal hemorrhage or premature birth is a high price to pay for an impulsive direct diagnosis of placenta previa, for example.
15. Avoid ill-timed, early induction of labor or cesarean section. The duration of pregnancy is often uncertain. If dates alone are used to time the termination, an immature neonate may be delivered. With the tests now available to determine fetal maturity and size, elective termination of pregnancy resulting in a preterm infant should not occur.
16. Administer Rh_o (D) immune globulin to all Rh-negative unsensitized mothers, antenatally at 26 to 28 weeks and as indicated after each delivery or abortion.
17. Advise on future pregnancy. Short pregnancy spacing (under one year) is inimical to the health of the mother and the following child. Rates for prematurity, perinatal mortality, and even infant death after leav-

ing the hospital of birth, are significantly increased when the interpregnancy period is less than six months.

PREVENTION OF UNWANTED PREGNANCY—TO BE WELCOME AND WELLBORN

Although improvement in general health and more sophisticated obstetric care carry a high priority, prevention of unwanted pregnancy is most important. Unwelcome pregnancies contribute significantly to the current increase in population problems and proportionately more to perinatal death and morbidity than do planned and expected pregnancies.

In 1965 the National Fertility Study indicated that 17% of births among the nonpoor were the result of unwanted pregnancies compared with 42% of births among the poor, or nearly one fourth of all births in the United States. We believe these figures are a very conservative estimate of the situation in 1986. Approximately 90% of teenage pregnancies are admitted mistakes. Reversing these figures could significantly improve the outcomes of conception, the safety of the intrauterine environment, and the quality of life.

I. Sequelae of unwanted pregnancy
   A. An increase in congenital anomalies, prematurity, and undersized newborns results from unwanted pregnancies. Eighty-five percent of all small babies of white mothers admitted to the neonatal Intensive Care Center of the University of Oregon Health Science Center were unplanned and unwanted. Rejection appeared to persist in 36% of these cases, even with professional counseling.
   B. The battered child, whether the victim of psychologic or physical trauma, is more likely to be the result of an unplanned and unwanted pregnancy. The part parental rejection may play in underachievement and delinquency may be considerable.
II. Associations of unplanned pregnancy
   Unplanned pregnancy stems from the failure to use a contraceptive method effectively. Of the 12,000 abortions performed in the state of Oregon in 1983, only 30% of the women reported the use of a contraceptive method. Factors that relate to these failures are numerous but include the following:
   A. Lack of knowledge
   B. Unconcern for the consequences of sexual intercourse
   C. Religious beliefs
   D. Difficulty in obtaining, or unavailability of, contraceptives
   E. Early dating and emotional immaturity
   F. Poor relationships with parents
   G. Personality conflicts
   H. Efforts to hold the male's affection
   I. Drug abuse, principally alcohol
   J. Personal irresponsibility
III. What can be done
   Some positive methods to be considered for reducing the number of unplanned pregnancies are as follows:
   A. Education of children and adolescents by specially trained teachers on family life, human responsibility, sexual behavior, drug abuse, and venereal disease to supplement and support information gained in the home
   B. Education (school, news media) of parents in family living, for themselves as well as their children; these presentations should include information about the following:
      1. Each parent's responsibility as an individual and as a member of society
      2. The advantage of planning a family at an optimum time, considering parental age, number of children, and spacing
   C. Wider availability and dissemination of knowledge of contraceptives and birth control techniques; training of more public health nurses and paramedical personnel in these details; establishment of Planned Parenthood type of clinics in each community
   D. Establishment of clinics that offer free testing for early pregnancy, particularly for the teenager; the early identification of pregnancy will encourage the following:
      1. Appropriate early prenatal care

2. Guidance in dealing with an unwanted or ill-advised pregnancy
E. Liberally applied and available abortion; this often-questioned procedure has gained popular support and may be necessary even after better techniques in birth control are developed and people are willing to accept and use them
F. Financial advantages aimed at reducing the incidence of unwanted pregnancy but benefiting the wanted child
G. More easily available sterilization

Sophistication about sexual behavior, wider use of contraception and abortion, and the high standard of living in the Scandinavian countries may account for their reduced numbers of infants who weigh under 1,500 gm.

The advancement of science, and medicine in particular, has been a major factor in the control of disease and pestilence, which has upset the balance of nature in population control of man. Medical personnel must be more forceful in helping to solve the tragedy of overpopulation.

The overcrowding of cities and the increasing public and private costs of rearing and educating children have emphasized the urgency of reproductive restraint and the responsibilities of parenthood. It is the first time in human history that we are able to depend on the quality of care, nutrition, and education to control population growth rather than rely on pestilence and famine for the restraint of unlimited reproduction.

Families should be created purposefully and intentionally, not accidentally or regretfully. Our world is too small and too complex for any but wanted children who will be loved.

As said in Shakespeare's *Julius Caesar* (Act III, Scene 1):

> How many ages hence
> Shall this our lofty scene be acted o'er,
> In states unborn and accents yet unknown!

BIBLIOGRAPHY

Abernethy, V., and Abernethy, G.L.: Identification of adolescent girls at high risk for unwanted pregnancy, Am. J. Orthopsychiatry **44**:442, 1974.

Benson, R.C.: Direction, innovation, exploration: an obstetric triptych, Am. J. Obstet. Gynecol. **110**:151, 1971.

Gold, E.M., and Ballard, W.M.: The role of family planning in prevention of pregnancy wastage, Clin. Obstet. Gynecol. **13**:145, 1970.

Hunscher, H.A., and Tompkins, W.T.: The influence of maternal nutrition on the immediate and long-term outcome of pregnancy, Clin. Obstet. Gynecol. **13**:130, 1970.

Larsson, G.: Prevention of fetal alcohol effects, Acta Obstet. Gynecol. Scand. **62**:171, 1983.

Page, E.W.: Pathogenesis and prophylaxis of low birth weights, Clin. Obstet. Gynecol. **13**:79, 1970.

Vaux, K.: Who shall live? Philadelphia, 1970, Fortress Press.

Wallace, H.M.: Factors associated with perinatal mortality and morbidity, Clin. Obstet. Gynecol. **13**:13, 1970.

Wallace, H.M., Goldstein, H., and Erickson, A.: Comparison of infant mortality in the United States and Sweden, Clin. Pediatr. **21**:156, 1982.

APPENDIX A

Definitions and terms

abortion termination of pregnancy before the fetus becomes viable (prior to the twenty-fourth week). An early abortion is one that occurs before the sixteenth week; a late abortion is one that occurs from the sixteenth to the twenty-fourth week.

dysmature refers to infants of any gestational age who show malnutrition at birth, with evidence of dry and scaly skin.

early neonatal period the time interval from birth through 7 days of age.

excessive-sized neonate a newborn who weighs more than 4,500 gm (over 9 lb 15 oz).

fetal death the death of a product of conception prior to its complete expulsion (stillbirth), irrespective of the duration of the pregnancy.

    early fetal death death with a pregnancy duration of less than 20 weeks' gestation.

    intermediate fetal death death in which duration of the pregnancy was between 20 and 28 weeks.

    late fetal death death that occurs from the twenty-eighth week of gestation on.

gestational period the number of completed weeks of pregnancy, calculated from the first day of the last menstrual period to the date of delivery. Since conception occurs approximately 2 weeks after the first day of the last menstrual period, the definition of gestational period includes these 2 prior weeks.

gravida a pregnant woman. The term is often combined with a prefix to indicate the number of times a patient has been pregnant.

immature infant a live-born preterm infant with a weight at birth of 1,000 gm (2 lb 3 oz) or less.

live birth the complete expulsion or extraction of a product of conception from its mother, irrespective of the duration of pregnancy, which after such separation breathes or shows any other evidence of life such as beating of the heart, pulsation of the umbilical cord, or definite movement of the voluntary muscles, whether or not the umbilical cord has been cut or the placenta is attached; each product of such a birth is considered live-born.*

low birth weight infant any live-born infant with a weight at birth of 2,500 gm (5½ lb) or less.

neonatal death the death of an infant within the first 27 days of life.

neonatal mortality the number of neonatal deaths per 1,000 live births.

neonatal period the time interval from birth through the first 27 days of life.

parity the number of infants (live or dead) that a woman has delivered, excluding abortions.

perinatal mortality the combined fetal and neonatal death rates per 1,000 live births.

perinatal period I the time interval from 28 weeks of completed gestation through the first 7 days of life.

perinatal period II the time interval from 20 weeks of completed gestation through 27 days of age.

postmenstrual age the gestational period (fetal), as measured from the first day of the last menstrual period, plus the postnatal age (neonatal). Postmenstrual allows comparisons of infants on the basis of their total life (fetal and neonatal) independent of the time of birth.

postterm infant (postmature) a live-born infant of over 42 completed weeks of gestation.

preterm infant (premature) a live-born infant of less than 38 completed weeks of gestation, regardless of birth weight. Some definitions place this period below 37 weeks.

term infant a live-born infant of 38 to 42 completed weeks of gestation.

undergrown, small-for-dates, and intrauterine growth-retarded infants infants who are significantly undersized for their period of gestation.

---

*Statistical paper, Series M, No. 19, New York, 1953, Statistical Office of the United Nations.

APPENDIX B

Equipment for endotracheal intubation and umbilical vessel catheterization

EQUIPMENT FOR ENDOTRACHEAL INTUBATION OF NEONATE

Laryngoscope with nos. 0 or 1 blade (check light)
Wire stylet
Portex E-T tubes (2.5, 3, 3.5, and 4 mm) with adapters
Lubricant
Elastoplast
Scissors
Tincture of benzoin
Cotton-tip applicators
4-0 silk suture with taper needle
Needle holder
½-inch adhesive tape
Measuring tape
DeLee suction set
Suction source, nos. 5 and 8 Fr catheters
Neonatal bag and mask connected to oxygen source
Heat lamp or radiant warmer
Heart rate monitor

EQUIPMENT FOR UMBILICAL VESSEL CATHETERIZATION

Umbilical artery catheter insertion tray contains the following preparation set:
  1 ring forceps
  1 3½-inch stainless bowl
  4 prep sponges
  1 straight suture scissors
  1 curved Mayo scissors
  2 curved mosquito hemostats
  1 curved iris forceps
  1 Hudson forceps without teeth
  1 small needle holder
  4 muslin towels
  1 small circumcision drape
  2 8-inch umbilical ties
  6 4 × 4 gauze pads
  1 3 × 3 gauze pad
  1 package of 4-0 silk with cutting needle
Measuring tape
Sterile gloves
Masks
Betadine
1 each: umbilical artery catheters, 3½ and 5 Fr
1 each: blunt needles, 18 and 20 gauge
1 no. 11 blade
1 6 ml syringe
1 3 ml syringe
1 three-way stopcock
1 20 gauge by 1-inch needle
1 30 ml bottle heparinized normal saline solution (0.03 ml heparin added to 30 ml of normal saline [1:1,000])
2 cotton-tipped applicators
Tincture of benzoin
1- or ½-inch clear tape
1 tongue blade covered with adhesive tape
Intravenous setup infusion pump

APPENDIX C

Neonatal emergency transport equipment

MEDICATIONS

Ampicillin, 500 mg
Atropine sulfate, 0.5 mg/ml
Calcium gluconate, 100 mg/ml
Dexamethasone (Decadron), 4 mg/ml
50% dextrose in water (D50W), 50 ml
Diazepam (Valium), 5 mg/ml
Epinephrine (Adrenaline), 1 mg/ml
Glucagon, 10 mg/ml
Heparin, 1,000 U/ml
Hydrocortisone succinate (Solu-Cortef), 50 mg/ml
Isoproterenol (Isuprel), 0.2 mg/ml
Gentamicin, 10 mg/ml
Nafcillin, 250 mg/ml
Naloxone hydrochloride (Narcan), 0.02 mg/ml
Phenobarbital, 65 mg/ml
Phytonadione (AquaMephyton), 10 mg/ml
Plasma protein fraction (Plasmanate), 50 ml
Sodium bicarbonate, 1 mEq/ml
Sterile normal saline solution, 30 ml
Sterile water, 30 ml
Tolazoline hydrochloride (Priscoline), 25 mg/ml
d-Tubocurarine chloride (chloride of active principle of curare), 3 mg/ml

INTRAVENOUS EQUIPMENT

Blunt needles, 18 gauge
D10W 250 ml and D5W 250 ml
4-0 silk suture with cutting needle
Holter pump tubing (A, B, C)
Intravenous extension set
Metriset
Razor and blades
Scalp-vein set, 25 and 27 gauge
Three-way stopcocks
Umbilical artery catheter insertion tray
Umbilical artery catheters, 3½ and 5 Fr

SUCTIONING EQUIPMENT

Clear tubing
DeLee suction sets
Sterile examination gloves
Suction catheters, 5 and 8 Fr

CHEST-DRAINAGE EQUIPMENT

Angiocaths, 18 gauge
Chest tubes, nos. 10 and 12
Curved hemostat
Heimlich valves
Intracaths, size 16, 8-inch, 14-gauge needle

RESUSCITATION EQUIPMENT

Airway, no. 00
Elastoplast
Endotracheal tubes with adapters, 2.5, 3.0, 3.5, and 4.0 mm
4-0 silk suture with taper needle
Laryngoscope with blades, nos. 0 and 1, with extra bulbs and batteries
Needle holder
Neonatal resuscitation bag and masks
Scissors
Wire stylet

RESPIRATORY CARE EQUIPMENT

Crescent wrench, 12 inch
Elbow and male adapters
Nasal prongs, large and small
Oxygen nipple adapter
Oxygen wrench
Travel CPAP
Travel ventilator
Universal oxygen tubing
Wall oxygen and air adapters (several brands, for use in referring and referred hospitals)

APPENDIX B

Equipment for endotracheal intubation and umbilical vessel catheterization

EQUIPMENT FOR ENDOTRACHEAL INTUBATION OF NEONATE

Laryngoscope with nos. 0 or 1 blade (check light)
Wire stylet
Portex E-T tubes (2.5, 3, 3.5, and 4 mm) with adapters
Lubricant
Elastoplast
Scissors
Tincture of benzoin
Cotton-tip applicators
4-0 silk suture with taper needle
Needle holder
½-inch adhesive tape
Measuring tape
DeLee suction set
Suction source, nos. 5 and 8 Fr catheters
Neonatal bag and mask connected to oxygen source
Heat lamp or radiant warmer
Heart rate monitor

EQUIPMENT FOR UMBILICAL VESSEL CATHETERIZATION

Umbilical artery catheter insertion tray contains the following preparation set:
   1 ring forceps
   1 3½-inch stainless bowl
   4 prep sponges
   1 straight suture scissors
   1 curved Mayo scissors
   2 curved mosquito hemostats
   1 curved iris forceps
   1 Hudson forceps without teeth
   1 small needle holder
   4 muslin towels
   1 small circumcision drape
   2 8-inch umbilical ties
   6 4 × 4 gauze pads
   1 3 × 3 gauze pad
   1 package of 4-0 silk with cutting needle
Measuring tape
Sterile gloves
Masks
Betadine
1 each: umbilical artery catheters, 3½ and 5 Fr
1 each: blunt needles, 18 and 20 gauge
1 no. 11 blade
1 6 ml syringe
1 3 ml syringe
1 three-way stopcock
1 20 gauge by 1-inch needle
1 30 ml bottle heparinized normal saline solution (0.03 ml heparin added to 30 ml of normal saline [1:1,000])
2 cotton-tipped applicators
Tincture of benzoin
1- or ½-inch clear tape
1 tongue blade covered with adhesive tape
Intravenous setup infusion pump

APPENDIX C

Neonatal emergency transport equipment

MEDICATIONS

Ampicillin, 500 mg
Atropine sulfate, 0.5 mg/ml
Calcium gluconate, 100 mg/ml
Dexamethasone (Decadron), 4 mg/ml
50% dextrose in water (D50W), 50 ml
Diazepam (Valium), 5 mg/ml
Epinephrine (Adrenaline), 1 mg/ml
Glucagon, 10 mg/ml
Heparin, 1,000 U/ml
Hydrocortisone succinate (Solu-Cortef), 50 mg/ml
Isoproterenol (Isuprel), 0.2 mg/ml
Gentamicin, 10 mg/ml
Nafcillin, 250 mg/ml
Naloxone hydrochloride (Narcan), 0.02 mg/ml
Phenobarbital, 65 mg/ml
Phytonadione (AquaMephyton), 10 mg/ml
Plasma protein fraction (Plasmanate), 50 ml
Sodium bicarbonate, 1 mEq/ml
Sterile normal saline solution, 30 ml
Sterile water, 30 ml
Tolazoline hydrochloride (Priscoline), 25 mg/ml
d-Tubocurarine chloride (chloride of active principle of curare), 3 mg/ml

INTRAVENOUS EQUIPMENT

Blunt needles, 18 gauge
D10W 250 ml and D5W 250 ml
4-0 silk suture with cutting needle
Holter pump tubing (A, B, C)
Intravenous extension set
Metriset
Razor and blades
Scalp-vein set, 25 and 27 gauge
Three-way stopcocks
Umbilical artery catheter insertion tray
Umbilical artery catheters, 3½ and 5 Fr

SUCTIONING EQUIPMENT

Clear tubing
DeLee suction sets
Sterile examination gloves
Suction catheters, 5 and 8 Fr

CHEST-DRAINAGE EQUIPMENT

Angiocaths, 18 gauge
Chest tubes, nos. 10 and 12
Curved hemostat
Heimlich valves
Intracaths, size 16, 8-inch, 14-gauge needle

RESUSCITATION EQUIPMENT

Airway, no. 00
Elastoplast
Endotracheal tubes with adapters, 2.5, 3.0, 3.5, and 4.0 mm
4-0 silk suture with taper needle
Laryngoscope with blades, nos. 0 and 1, with extra bulbs and batteries
Needle holder
Neonatal resuscitation bag and masks
Scissors
Wire stylet

RESPIRATORY CARE EQUIPMENT

Crescent wrench, 12 inch
Elbow and male adapters
Nasal prongs, large and small
Oxygen nipple adapter
Oxygen wrench
Travel CPAP
Travel ventilator
Universal oxygen tubing
Wall oxygen and air adapters (several brands, for use in referring and referred hospitals)

MISCELLANEOUS

Alcohol swabs
Applicators
Band-Aids
Betadine, (1.67%)
Betadine swabs
Catheter adapter
Cotton balls
Chemstrip
Extra monitor cable
Flashlight
4 × 4 inch gauze pads
Lancets
Lubricant packets
Measuring tape
Needles and syringes (variety)
Pen
Rubber bands
Safety pins
Sterile drape
Sterile gloves (small, medium, large)
Stethoscope
Thermometer
Tincture of benzoin
Umbilical ties

APPENDIX D

Newborn transfer record

```
                              PERINATAL HISTORY

NAME _____ HOSPITAL # _____ HOSPITAL PHONE: _____
HOSPITAL _____ CITY: _____ STATE: _____
ATTENDANT AT BIRTH _____ INFANT'S PHYSICIAN: _____ PHONE: _____
MOTHER'S NAME _____ HOSPITAL # _____ AGE ____ PHONE: _____
MARITAL STATUS: _____ RACE: _____ RELIGION: _____  PRIVATE ☐   CLINIC ☐
FATHER'S AGE _____ OCCUPATION _____  LABOR  Spontaneous ☐  Induced ☐
RELEVANT FAMILY HISTORY (RE BABY)
                                            Induction indication _____

                                            Method _____
                                            DRUGS GIVEN    DOSE    ROUTE   TIME




TYPE ____ Rh ____ ANTIBODIES _____
PAST OBSTETRIC HISTORY
                                            ANESTHESIA         AGENTS USED/DETAILS
GRAV ____ LOW BIRTH WT. (<2500g) ____       None          ☐
                                            Pudendal      ☐
PARA ____ PREMATURES (<37 wks) ____         Paracervical  ☐
                                            Spinal        ☐
AB. _____ FETAL DEATHS (>20 wks) ____       Epid./Caudal  ☐
NEONATAL DEATHS ____ CONGEN. ANOM ____      Inhalation    ☐

LIVING CHILDREN ____                        FIRST STAGE          ____ HOURS
DETAIL ABNORMALITIES:                       SECOND STAGE         ____ MINUTES
                                            MEMBRANES RUPTURED   ____ HOURS/DAYS

                                            FETAL DISTRESS           MONITOR
                                            Not Noted ☐  Meconium ☐  Yes ☐  No ☐
                                            Heart <100 ☐ Acidosis ☐  Decelerations:
                                            Heart >160 ☐ Nuchal cord ☐ Type:
                                            Heart Irreg ☐ Prolapsed cord ☐

                                            DELIVERY  Time _____ Date _____
CURRENT PREGNANCY        L.M.P. _____     Presentation _____
SEROLOGY                 E.D.C. _____     Spontaneous ☐    Operative ☐
    Rubella ____ S.T.S. ____                Breech Ext. ☐  Forceps: Mid ☐   C Section ☐
Cigarettes/D ____                           Breech Assist. ☐         Low ☐  Vacuum Ext. ☐
COMPLICATIONS
Include details of all drugs/meds  dose, duration and gestational period;
recent infections (state bacterial, viral); other prenatal complications.   Indication:
DETAILS:




                                            AMNIOTIC FLUID  Appearance: _____
°This record was modified by Dr. Joseph Butterfield,
Director, Department of Neonatology, Children's Hos-   Volume ____ ml. Normal ☐   Reduced ☐
pital, Denver, from his manual on newborn transport    Excessive ☐    Not noted ☐
services used in the state of Colorado.
                                            PLACENTA  Weight _____ Vessels _____
                                            Abnormalities:
```

Newborn transfer record—cont'd

NEONATAL

Singleton ☐
Multiple (Birth Order) _____

APGAR SCORE

Min.	H	R	T	S	C	Score
1						
5						
10						

First gasp _____ min.

Regular resps. established _____ min.

RESUSCITATION

Nil required ☐
O₂ Mask/Catheter ☐
O₂ with Pos Press
  by Mask ☐
  Endotracheal ☐

Antagonist ☐
Alkali ☐
Cardiac Massage ☐

DETAILS AND RESPONSE:

INITIAL EXAMINATION *   At Age _____

Weight _____   Gestation _____

Length _____   Clin. Gest _____

Head C. _____   Sex _____

DETAIL ABNORMALITIES

- Nutrition ☐
- Color ☐
- Tone ☐
- Reflexes ☐
- Resps ☐
- Head/Face ☐
- Eyes ☐
- Palate ☐
- Chest ☐
- Heart ☐
- Abdomen ☐
- Umbilicus ☐
- Hips ☐
- Femorals ☐
- Genitalia ☐
- Limbs ☐
- Skin ☐

Vitamin K given: Yes ☐   No ☐
* (√) indicates item normal to exam.

PROGRESS
Please include all medications and fluids

First Feeding: Age (Hours) _____
Route: _____
Fluid/Formula _____
Last voided _____
Last stooled _____

Signed: _____
ATTENDING PHYSICIAN

REMINDER: We will require
1. Mother's blood (5 - 10 ml clotted)
2. Cord blood (when available)
3. Placenta (when available)
4. Relevant X-rays, Lab. data, Xerox copies of case notes, mother and baby
5. This Transfer Record completed in DETAIL.
6. Consent for Transport.

Adapted from a form in use at National Women's Hospital, Auckland, New Zealand.

APPENDIX
E

Neonatal transfer log

APPENDIX F

Respiratory flow sheet for all infants receiving oxygen or assisted ventilation

SIDE 1	Date															
	Time															
BLOOD GASES	Source															
	pH															
	PCO$_2$															
	PO$_2$															
	HCO$_3$/B.E.															
SETTINGS	FiO$_2$															
	ImV															
	PIP/PEEP															
	Insp Time															
	NaHCO$_3$(mEq)															
ORDERS	Time															
	FiO$_2$															
	ImV															
	PIP/PEEP															
	Insp Time															
	Next Blood Gases At															
	OTHER															
	ORDERED BY															
	CARRIED BY															

University of Oregon Health Sciences Center
Hospital and Clinics
Portland, Oregon

RESPIRATORY FLOW SHEET

APPENDIX G

Drug dosages

Drug	Dosage	Route
Antibiotics (p. 238)		
Acetaminophen	10 mg/kg/dose every 4 to 6 hr	PO or PR
Adrenergics		
Dopamine	5-15 µg/kg/min	IV
Dobutamine	5-20 µg/kg/min	IV
Epinephrine (1:10,000 solution)	0.5 ml in single dose; repeat as indicated	IV, IM, or per endotracheal tube
Isoproterenol	0.2-0.4 µg/kg/min	IV
Aminophylline	5 mg/kg loading dose; 2 mg/kg every 6-8 hr maintenance dose	IV
Anticonvulsants		
Phenobarbital	10 mg/kg loading dose, 2 mg/kg every 12 hr maintenance dose	IV or PO
Phenytoin	10 mg/kg loading dose, 2.5 mg/kg every 12 hr maintenance dose	IV
Diazepam	0.1 mg/kg every 4 hr as needed	IV
Atropine	0.01 mg/kg/dose (0.1 mg maximum dose)	IV, SQ, PO
Blood derivatives		
Whole blood	10-15 ml/kg	IV (slowly)
Packed cells	5-10 ml/kg	IV (slowly)
Plasma	10-15 ml/kg	IV (slowly)
Albumin	1 gm/kg	IV (slowly)
Plasmanate	10-15 ml/kg	IV (slowly)
Calcium gluconate	1-2 ml/kg, diluted 1:1 with sterile H_2O	IV (slowly)
Chloral hydrate	30-50 mg/kg every 4-6 hr as needed	PO
Dexamethasone	0.5-1.0 mg/kg/24 hr in divided doses	IV or PO
Digoxin	Total digitalizing dose: 0.02 mg/kg, give half of total dose immediately, the rest in quarter doses every 8 hr, maintenance dose 0.002 mg/kg/every 12 hr	IV or PO
Furosemide	1-3 mg/kg/dose	IV or PO
Indomethacin	Give in 1 to 3 doses every 12-24 hr (mg/kg/dose) dose 1 dose 2 dose 3 Infants <48 hr 0.2 0.1 0.1 Infants 2-7 days 0.2 0.2 0.2 Infants >7 days 0.2 0.25 0.25	IV
Morphine	0.05-0.1 mg/kg	IV, IM, SQ
Naloxone	0.01 mg/kg/dose	IV, IM
Pancuronium	0.05-0.1 mg/kg/dose for muscle relaxation	IV
Tolazoline	1 mg/kg test dose; infusion, 1 mg/kg/hour	IV
Sodium bircarbonate	2-4 mEq/kg (diluted)	IV

APPENDIX H

Screening of all pregnancies

Screening of all pregnancies and determination of therapy for those with significant antibody levels
1. First visit
   a. Document blood group and Rh type.
   b. Screen blood serum for antibodies with the Hemantigen type of screening test.
2. At 28 to 36 weeks of gestation
   a. Repeat antibody screening test.
   b. If no antibody is demonstrated, no further studies are needed.

If antibody is demonstrated
1. Obtain the gravida's serum for the following:
   a. Identification of the antibody by testing with a known panel of red cells
   b. Measurement of serum titer by anti–human globulin test
2. Perform amniocentesis after 23 weeks of gestation and repeat as indicated by the following:
   a. Serum titer over 1:8 or presence of Rh antibodies
   b. Previous erythroblastotic infant

TECHNIQUE OF AMNIOCENTESIS AND SPECTROPHOTOMETRY

1. Locate placenta. Use of ultrasonic B-scan is ideal.
2. Have patient void bladder; check FHR.
3. Prepare area determined best for amniocentesis with suitable antiseptic.
4. Raise a skin wheal and anesthetize a tract to the uterus with an appropriate local anesthetic.
5. Perforate amniotic cavity with a 20- or 22-gauge spinal needle.
6. Withdraw approximately 5 to 10 ml of fluid. If it is grossly bloody, obtain fluid from another puncture site.
7. Centrifuge fluid for 10 minutes at 14,000 rpm and decant if it is cloudy or bloody; store in a dark bottle in refrigerator; filter supernatant fluid if not clear. Centrifugation may be delayed up to 48 hours, while fluid is protected from light.
8. Place clear fluid in a cuvette in a spectrophotometer and obtain at least 15 optical density values from 350 to 700 nm; plot these values on two-cycle semilogarithmic graph paper, using optical density as the ordinate and decreasing wavelength as the abscissa (Fig. H-1).

Interpretation of spectral absorption curve of amniotic fluid
1. Three grades of severity
   a. A mildly affected fetus for which a term delivery is recommended
   b. A moderately affected fetus with a good chance of survival if delivered when physiologic maturity testing indicates fetal capability to survive outside the uterus
   c. A severely affected fetus, which, if immature by physiologic maturity testing, may require an intrauterine transfusion to avoid fetal death
2. Errors in interpretation
   a. False negatives—usually mild cases with no harm done
   b. False positives in a pregnancy with an Rh-negative fetus, indicating the possibility of a previous severely affected infant

Fetal transfusion
Fetal transfusion is indicated for the early treatment of pronounced degrees of fetal isoimmunization (severely affected zone, see Fig. H-1) prior to the thirty-second to thirty-fourth week of pregnancy. Once fetal hydrops has developed, however, intrauterine transfusion usually will not save the offspring. Intrauterine transfusion, generally every 7 to 10 days, is

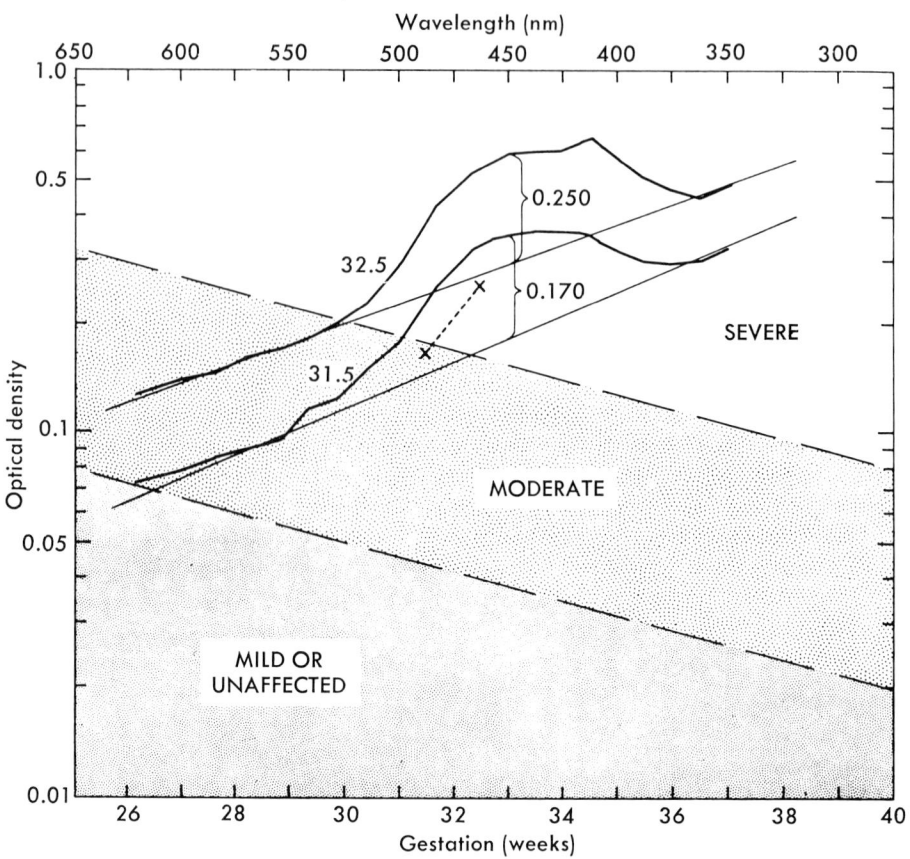

Fig. H-1. Spectrophotometric analysis of amniotic fluid surrounding an erythroblastotic fetus. Amniocentesis was performed at 31½ and at 32½ weeks of gestation. The spectral absorption curve was obtained by plotting of the optical densities at various wavelengths on two-cycle semilogarithmic graph paper. A tangential line joining the lowest portions of this curve approximates unstained amniotic fluid and is the baseline for calculations. The difference between the involved and uninvolved curves is measured at 450 nm. (Maximum absorption by bilirubin or bilirubin-like products occurs at 450 nm.) This difference is plotted at the appropriate number of weeks of gestation, as illustrated by the *dotted line*. This case reveals rapid progression from moderate to severe disease. Under such conditions fetal death often is imminent; prompt delivery usually must be accomplished if gestational age will permit; otherwise, intrauterine fetal transfusion may be considered.

required to prevent fetal exodus before early delivery can be accomplished. Once the fetus is delivered, replacement transfusion and specific supportive measures are possible.

Fetal transfusion requires percutaneous catheterization of the fetal peritoneal space. Packed red blood cells (0-negative blood) are then injected into the peritoneal cavity of the fetus. The erythrocytes soon pass into the fetal bloodstream. Techniques vary with local preference and equipment, but the procedure and complications are hazardous and warrant transfer of such affected pregnancies to a specialized center.

Prevention

For suppression of Rh immunization, 300 μg of Rh immunoglobin (RhoGAM) is given promptly to all unimmunized Rh-negative women who (1) deliver Rh-positive babies, (2) abort, or (3) undergo amniocentesis, unless the husband is Rh negative.

Index

A

A-II; *see* Angiotensin II
Abdomen of newborn, examination of, in birth room, 89
Abdominal distention, intestinal obstruction and, 306
Abdominal masses, 311
Abdominal wall defects, 309-310
ABO incompatibility, 277
Abortion, 333
   diabetes and, 230
   midtrimester, 171
   multiple pregnancy and, 193
   therapeutic, 330-331
Abortogenic infections, 331
Abruptio placentae, 160, 169, 194, 199, 209, 211, 212, 213, 214, 215-216
Abscesses, 239
Abuse, child, 321
Acardiac amorphous fetus, 191, 193
Accelerations of fetal heart rate, 48-49
Accidental pregnancy, irresponsible parenthood and, 7
Acetone, 125
Achondrogenesis, 310
Acid-base nomogram, 257
Acidosis, 253
   fetal, 53
   metabolic, 253, 256
   respiratory, 253, 256
   respiratory distress and, 256
Acyclovir, 243
ADH; *see* Antidiuretic hormone
Adolescent medicine, 330
Adrenergic drugs, 285
Adrenocorticotropic hormone, 298
Age
   fetal; *see* Fetal age
   gestational, 32-33, 317
   menstrual, 32-33
Alarm settings on heart rate monitors, 125, 126
Albumin
   factors interfering with binding of, 277
   pregnancy and, 6

Alcohol, 14, 15-16, 331
   ethyl, 162
Aldomet, 202
Alkaline phosphatase, 187
Alpha-fetoprotein, 11, 30, 310
Ambiguous genitalia, 311
American College of Obstetricians and Gynecologists, 10
American Committee on Maternal Welfare, 197
American Medical Association, 323
Amino acids, 153, 154
Aminophylline, 268
Amnesics, 76
Amniocentesis, 28-30, 40, 67, 168, 192, 211, 343-344
Amniography, 43-44
Amnion nodosum, 90
Amnionitis, 168-170
Amnioscopy, 42-43, 67
Amniotic fluid
   assessment of, 39-41, 66-67
   color of, 41-42, 67
   meconium staining of, 66, 67, 84-85, 175, 269
   osmolarity of, 41
   visual inspection of, 41-42
Amniotomy, 83
Amorphous fetus, acardiac, 191, 193
Amphetamines, 14
Amphotericin, 238
Ampicillin, 39, 170, 237, 238, 240, 247
Amyl nitrate, 83
Analgesia, 72-78; *see also* Anesthesia
   for fetus at risk in premature labor, 72-76
   hypertensive states in pregnancy and, 205
   multiple pregnancy and, 189
Anaphylactic shock, anesthesia and, 78
Anemia, 113, 192, 213, 293-295
   delayed, 294
   dilution, multiple pregnancy and, 192
   early, 293-294
   Fanconi's, 21
   multiple pregnancy and, 192
Anencephaly, 310

345

Anesthesia, 72-78; *see also* Analgesia
  for cesarean section, 77-78
  general, 76
  hypertensive states in pregnancy and, 205
  paracervical, 73-74, 75
  for patient in shock, 78
  regional, 73, 77-78
Anesthetics, 162
  breech presentation and, 224-225
  inhalation, 76-77
  parenteral, 77
Aneuploidy, 21
Angio-Conray; *see* Iothalamate acid
Angiography, placenta previa and, 217
Angiotensin, 197
Angiotensin II (A-II), 197
Antenatal diagnosis, 28-30
Antenatal visits, standard, 11
Antepartum testing, 54-58
Antibiotic therapy, 170, 171, 238-239, 240, 285, 295
Antibody, hemagglutinin-inhibition, 241-242
Anticonvulsants, 296
Antidiuretic hormone (ADH), 141
Antigen, human lymphocyte, 229
Antihypertensives, 201, 205, 206
Anus, imperforate, 308-309
Aortic blood gas samples, 255
Apgar, V., 87
Apgar score, 87-88
Apnea, 113, 125, 253
  continued, with assisted ventilation, 94
  of prematurity, 261, 268
Apt test, 136, 211
AquaMephyton; *see* Vitamin K_1
Ara-A; *see* Vidarabine
Arborization test, 168
Arrest disorders of labor, 66
Artificial pancreas, 233
Ascites, 192
Asphyxia, 93, 320
  perinatal, 92
  placenta previa and, 218
Asphyxia neonatorum, 185
Aspiration of tension pneumothorax, 136
Aspirin, 197
Assisted breech presentation, 224
Assisted ventilation; *see* Ventilation
Ataractics, 76
Atelectasis, pulmonary, 269
ATN; *see* Tubular necrosis, acute
Atresia
  choanal, 117, 303
  duodenal, 307
  esophageal, 117, 304-305
  ileal, 308
  jejunal, 308
Atropine, 285
Atropine sulfate, 78
Autoimmunity, diabetes and, 229
Automobile lap belt restraints, 212
Autosomal dominantly inherited diseases, 22, 29
Autosomes, 21

Avery, G.B., 311
Azotemia, 143

B

Backward somersault, breech presentation and, 222
Bacterial septicemia and other severe infections, 237-239
Bag
  infant, 99
  and mask, ventilation with, 260
Ballottement, internal, 36
Barbiturates, 14, 162
Basal body temperature record, calculation of pregnancy duration from, 33-34
Bathing infant, 133
Beat-to-beat variability of fetal heart rate, 46, 47-48
Bed rest, 188, 331
Behavior disorders in low birth weight infant, 321, 322
Behrman, R.E., 311
Benzathine penicillin, 245
Benzoin, tincture of, 98
Bergsma, D., 310
Beta-blockers, 203
Betadine; *see* Povidone-iodine
Beta-glucuronidase, 275
Beta-hemolytic streptococci, group B, 239-240
Betamethasone (Celestone), 166, 170
Beta-mimetic agents, 192, 250
Bile-stained vomitus, intestinal obstruction and, 306
Bilirubin, 275-276
Bilirubin encephalopathy, 277
Bilirubinemia, excessive, 279
Biochemical monitoring
  in assessment of fetal well-being, 38-39
  by fetal scalp blood sampling, 52-54
Biologic factors in screening, 16-17
Biophysical profile score, fetal, 58, 59
Biostator, 233
Birth, 70
  change of blood gases at, 91
  circulation of blood before and after, 90
  risk categories of, classification of, 103-107
Birth room
  examination of newborn in, 89
  initial care of infant in, 87-92
  parent-infant bonding in, 89
  physical observations of newborn in, 88-89
  placental observations in, 89-90
  team care in, 70-72
Birth weight, 5
Bishop score, 81
Bladder, exstrophy of, 309
Bladder tap, 136
Blastocyst, 23
Blastula, 23
Bleeding, 295-296
  placental, 209-210
  third trimester; *see* Hemorrhage, late pregnancy
  uterine, 209-210
  vaginal, premature labor and, 160
Bleeding diathesis, 113
Block
  caudal, 75

Block—cont'd
   lumbar epidural, 75
   paracervical, 73-74, 75
   spinal, 75-76
Blood, circulation of, before and after birth, 90, 91
Blood gas changes, 91, 253
Blood gas sampling, 255-256
Blood glucose screening, technique for, 136
Blood loss, fetal, 211
Blood oxygenation, insufficient, 71
Blood pressure, measurement of, 126-127, 128
Blood sampling, fetal, 53
Blood smear, bacterial septicemia and, 237
Blood volume in fetus at term, 92
Bloody show, 208
Bloom's dwarfism, 21
Blueberry muffin baby, 241
Body measurement in evaluation of risk groups, 105-106
Body temperature of newborn, maintenance of, 88
Body temperature record, basal, in calculation of pregnancy duration, 33-34
Bonding, parent-infant, 89
Bottle feeding, 133, 148
BPD; *see* Bronchopulmonary dysplasia
Bradycardia, 46, 49, 94, 149
Braxton-Hicks' contractions, 61
Breast milk, 144, 145
Breast stimulation, 57-58
Breathing devices, positive-pressure, 99
Breathing effort, increasing, 111
Breathlessness, sensation of, multiple pregnancy and, 192
Breech extraction, total, 224
Breech presentation, 84, 220-226
   anesthetics and, 224-225
   assisted, 224
   backward somersault, 222
   cesarean section and, 222, 223
   complete, 220
   correlations predisposing to, 220-225
   criteria for scoring, 223
   diagnosis of, 221
   differential diagnosis of, 221
   double footling, 220
   external cephalic version, 221-222
   forward somersault, 222
   frank, 220, 222
   incomplete, 220
   large-for-dates infant and, 181
   management of, 221-225
   maternal and perinatal complications of, 225
   neonatal care and, 225-226
   placenta previa and, 216
   premature rupture of membranes and, 225
   single footling, 220
   spontaneous expulsion, 224
   total breech extraction, 224
   type of, by fetal weight, 220-225
   vaginal delivery and, 222-225
Broad-spectrum antibiotics, 239
Bronchopulmonary dysplasia (BPD), 262-263, 271-272
Brow presentation, 226
Brown fat, 122

Bubble test, 159, 168
Butterfly, Elastoplast, 98
Burping infant, 133

C

Calcium, 143, 154, 155, 188, 206
Calcium chloride, 201
Calcium gluconate, 201, 206
Caloric density, 143
Caloric expenditure of low birth weight infant, 142
Caloric requirements for low birth weight infant, 141-142
Candidal infections, 239
Carbohydrate, 4, 140
   needs for, of preterm infant, 143
   in total parenteral nutrition, 153-154
Carbon dioxide, 268
Carcinoma of cervix, invasive, 208
Cardiac failure, 283-284
Cardiac massage, external, 94
Cardiac monitors, 125
Cardiogenic shock, 78, 284
Cardiovascular changes at birth, 90-92
Cardiovascular problems, 282-287
Casein, 153
Catheterization, umbilical vessel, 99-102
Caudal block, 75
CDP; *see* Continuous transpulmonary distending pressure
Cefotaxime, 238
Celestone; *see* Betamethasone
Cellular growth, 317-318
Central cyanosis, 252, 282-283, 306
Central nervous system disorders, 288-289
Central nervous system injury, multiple pregnancy and, 193
Central vein as site for total parenteral nutrition, 155
Cephalic version, external, breech presentation and, 221-222
Cerclage, cervical, 171-173, 192
Cerebral palsy, multiple pregnancy and, 185, 193
Cervical cerclage, 171-173, 192
Cervical dilatation and effacement, 61-63
Cervical lesions, 208
Cervical mucus, extrusion of, 208
Cervicitis, 169, 211
Cervix
   incompetent, 160-161, 169, 171-173
   invasive carcinoma of, 208
Cesarean section, 214, 331
   anesthesia for, 77-79
   breech presentation and, 222, 223
   diabetes mellitus and, 78-79
   emergency, 79
   fetal distress and, 78
   isoimmunization and, 79
   large-for-dates infant and, 181
   multiple pregnancy and, 189-190, 191, 193
   placenta previa and, 216, 217, 218
CHD; *see* Congenital heart disease
Chemstrip, 116, 136
Chest of newborn, examination of, in birth room, 89
Chest illumination, 135
Chest tube placement for pneumothorax, 264-265

Chest-drainage equipment for neonatal emergency transport, 336
Child abuse, 321
Child neglect, 321
Childbirth, prepared, 72-73; *see also* Birth
Chlordiazepoxide (Librium), 162
Chlorhexidine, 120
Chlorhexidine gluconate, 122
2-Chloroprocaine, 73
Chlorothiazide diuretics, 39
Choanal atresia, 117, 303
Cholestasis, total parenteral nutrition and, 157
Chondrodystrophies, 310
Chorea, Huntington's, 29
Choriocarcinoma, 38, 197
Chorionic gonadotropin, 187
Chorionic villi sampling (CVS), 29-30
Chromium, 154
Chromosomal aberrations and genetic transmissions, 21-22
Chromosomal breakage, 21
Cigarette smoking, effect of, on fetus, 15, 212, 215, 331
Circulation of blood before and after birth, 90, 91
Circummarginate placenta, 218-219
Circumvallate placenta, 160, 169, 209, 218-219
Cleavage, 23
Cleft lip, 311
Cleft palate, 311
Clinitest, 136
Cloaca, exstrophy of, 309
Clostridium, 149
Clothing, 133
Clothing transfer for premature infant, 130
CMV infection; *see* Cytomegalovirus infection
CNP; *see* Continuous negative pressure
Coagulase-negative staphylococci, 236
Coagulation, disseminated intravascular, 192, 208, 213, 295-296
Coagulopathy, 208-209, 214
  consumption, 192, 213, 215-216
Coitus, single, calculation of pregnancy duration from, 33-34
Collaborative Perinatal Study of the National Institute of Neurological Diseases and Stroke, 226, 227
Committee on Perinatal Welfare of the Massachusetts Medical Society, 329
Community health nurse, 132
Community hospital
  intermediate or larger, 323, 325-326
  small, 323-325
Complete breech presentation, 220
Complete placenta previa, 216
Complete prolapse of umbilical cord, 226
Completed weeks in calculation of pregnancy duration, 33
Concealed hemorrhage, 215-216
Congenital abnormalities associated with hydramnios, 183
Congenital anomaly(ies)
  abdominal masses as, 311
  abdominal wall defects as, 309-310
  ambiguous genitalia as, 311
  cleft lip as, 311
  cleft palate as, 311
  cyanosis and congenital heart disease as, 306
  diabetes and, 230

Congenital anomaly(ies)—cont'd
  dislocated hips as, 311
  fetal alcohol syndrome as, 312
  fetal heart rate tracings in fetuses with, 59
  hypothyroidism as, 311
  intestinal obstruction as, 117, 306-309
  major, and developmental defects, 303-312
  metabolic, endocrine, and miscellaneous defects as, 310-312
  multiple, 21-30, 310
  respiratory distress associated with, at birth, 303-306
  of respiratory tree, 272
  subluxated hips as, 311
Congenital heart disease (CHD), 252-253, 282, 306
Congenital infections, 240-247
Congenital rubella, 242
Congenital syphilis, 245
Congenital toxoplasmosis, 246
Congenital tuberculosis, 246
Conjoined twins, 193
Conjunctivitis, inclusion, 239
Consumption coagulopathy, 192, 213, 215-216
Continuous negative pressure (CNP), 258
Continuous positive airway pressure (CPAP), 257, 258-259, 261
Continuous transpulmonary distending pressure (CDP), 256-259
Contraction stress testing (CST), 54, 56-57
Contractions, 159
  assessment of, 63-66
  Braxton-Hicks', 61
  premature labor and, 159, 160-161, 162
Cooling of high-risk infant, hazards from, 123
Coombs' test, 277
Copper, 154
Cor pulmonale, 215
Cord, umbilical
  clamping of, timing of, 92
  prolapse of, multiple pregnancy and, 194
  two-vessel, 89
  velamentous insertion of, 227-228
Cord accidents, malpresentation and, 220-228
Cord entanglement, multiple pregnancy and, 194
Cortical necrosis, renal, 214-215
Corticosteroids, 39, 78, 163, 203-204
Coumadin derivatives, 296
Couvelaire uterus, 212
Coxsackievirus disease, 246
CPAP; *see* Continuous positive airway pressure
Creatinine, 41
Crib deaths, 321
Crib transfer for premature infants, 130
Cryoprecipitate, 215
CST; *see* Contraction stress testing
Cuffed flashlight, 135
Cultural factors influencing perinatal morbidity and mortality, 7-9
CVS; *see* Chorionic villi sampling
Cyanosis, 111, 252-253, 282-283, 306
  central, 252, 282-283, 306
  increasing, 95-96
  peripheral, 282
  of pulmonary origin, 252

Cyclopropane, 77, 78
Cyst, lutein, multiple pregnancy and, 192
Cysteine, 153
Cysteine hydrochloride, 153, 154
Cystine, 143, 187
Cytomegalovirus (CMV) infection, 244

D

Daily feeding requirements for low birth weight infant, 143
Death
   crib, 321
   fetal; *see* Fetal death
   neonatal, multiple pregnancy and, 193
   perinatal; *see* Perinatal death
Deceleration
   of fetal heart rate; *see* Fetal heart rate, deceleration of
   of labor, prolonged phase of, 66
Decidua, bleeding from, 211
Deep cephalic curve forceps, 79
Defibrination syndrome, 215
Dehydration of low birth weight infant, 250-251
Dehydroepiandrosterone sulfate (DHEA-S), 197
Deletion, 21
Delivery
   acute emergencies during, 71
   cesarean section; *see* Cesarean section
   diabetes and, 234
   emergency, in home, 85-86
   fetal distress with, chronic factors predisposing to, 71
   of fetus at risk, 70-86
   forceps, 79-80
   hypertensive states in pregnancy and, 205
   methods of, 79-80
   multiple pregnancy and, 188-191
   perinatal infections acquired during, 236
   perinatal risk associated with, 70, 71, 84-86
   of twins, 189, 190
   vaginal; *see* Vaginal delivery
Denver Developmental Screening Test, 322
Denver weight grid, 179
Dependent edema, 4
Depressed infant, resuscitation and stabilization of, 93-96
Depression
   narcotic, 93, 94
   neonatal, 207
   respiratory, 253
Descent of presenting part, 63, 64, 65, 66
Dexamethasone, 268
Dextrose, 153, 154
Dextrostix, 136, 147
DH; *see* Diaphragmatic hernia
DHEA-S; *see* Dehydroepiandrosterone sulfate
Diabetes, 181, 182-183, 229-235
   abortion and, 230
   autoimmunity and, 229
   cesarean section and, 78-79
   classification of, 230
   congenital anomalies and, 230
   control of, 232-233
   delivery and, 234
   detection of, 231-232
   diet in control of, 232-233, 235
   drug-induced, 229

Diabetes—cont'd
   effects of, on pregnancy, 230-231
   effects of pregnancy on, 229, 230
   excessive-sized infants and, 230
   fetal death in utero and, 230
   gestational, 181, 192, 298-299
   human lymphocyte antigen and, 229
   hypertensive states of pregnancy and, 230
   increased complications of pregnancy and, 230
   increased neonatal morbidity and mortality and, 230-231
   infants of mothers with, 298-299
   infertility and, 230
   inheritance of, 229
   insulin guidelines for control of, 233, 235
   insulin-dependent, 229
   insulin-independent, 229
   intrauterine growth retardation and, 230
   juvenile-onset, 229
   macrosomia and, 230
   management of, 232-235
   maternal evaluation and, 233-234
   maturity-onset, 229
   polyhydramnios and, 230
   premature labor and delivery and, 230
   Priscilla White classification of, 230
   screening method for, 231-232
   timing of delivery in relation to fetal and placental evaluation in, 234
   treatment of ketoacidosis with, 233
   type I, 229
   type II, 229
   upper limits of normal blood glucose values for detection of, in pregnancy, 232
Diabetic retinitis, 230
Diagnosis
   antenatal, 28-30
   and management of high-risk fetus and neonate, 1-219
Diamine oxidase, 39
Diamniotic pregnancy, 187, 194
Diaphragmatic hernia (DH), 117, 305-306
Diarrhea, 149
Diathesis, bleeding, 113
Diatrizoate sodium (Hypaque-M), 44
Diazepam (Valium), 162, 204
Diazoxide, 202, 205
Diet, 232-233, 235, 331
Digitalis, 191, 203
Dilatation, 61-63, 64, 65, 66
Dilution anemia, multiple pregnancy and, 192
Diplococcus pneumoniae, 236
Dislocated hips, 311
Disproportionate fetouterine growth, 177-184
Disseminated intravascular coagulation, 192, 208, 213, 295-296
Distention, 146
Distress
   fetal; *see* Fetal distress
   maternal, multiple pregnancy and, 192
Diuresis, osmotic, 140
Diuretics, 183, 206
   chlorothiazide, 39
   thiazide, 203, 205, 207, 295
Dizygotic twins, 185, 194

D5/lactated Ringer's solution, 162
D5/0.5NS, 162
Dobutamine, 285
Dominantly inherited autosomal diseases, 22
Dopamine, 210-211, 285
Doppler principle, 34, 68
Doppler ultrasonography, transcutaneous, 126
Double footling breech presentation, 220
Down's syndrome, 310, 331
Driver in transport team, 115
Drop ether, 83
Drug addiction, maternal, effects of, on fetus and neonate, 14-15
Drug dosage, 342
Drug-induced diabetes, 229
Dry labor, 167
Dührssen incisions, 214
Duodenal atresia, 307
Dwarfism
   Bloom's, 21
   thanatophoric, 310
Dye test, 168
Dysplasia, bronchopulmonary, 262-263, 271-272

E

ECG strip recorder, 125, 126
Eclampsia, 196, 198, 204, 207
   multiple pregnancy and, 192
   superimposed chronic hypertension with, 199
Economic factors influencing perinatal morbidity and mortality, 7-9
Edema, 139
   dependent, 4
   generalized, 4
   gestational, 196
   pathologic, 4
   physiologic, 4
   pregnancy and, 4
Educational states, perinatal morbidity and mortality and, 8
Effacement, 61-63
Elastoplast butterfly, 98
Electrocardiography, fetal, multiple pregnancy and, 187
Electrodes on heart rate monitors, 125
Electrolytes, 138-139
   parenteral administration of, 138-140
   for short-term needs, 138-139
   in total parenteral administration, 154
Electronic detection of fetal heart tones, 34-35
Electronic fetal heart rate monitoring, 125
   indications for, 45-46, 47
   by indirect methods, 68
   methods of, 46
   pitfalls of, 51-52
Electrophoresis, hemoglobin, 211
Elliott forceps, 79
Embryo, effect of radiation on, 26
Embryonic phase, 24
Emergency, acute, during delivery, 71
Emergency cesarean delivery, 79
Emergency delivery in home, 85-86
Emergency karyotyping, 310
Emotional stress, pregnancy and, 6-7
Emphysema, 269, 272

Encephalopathy, bilirubin, 277
Endocrine defects, 310-312
Endotheliosis, glomerular capillary, 198
Endotracheal intubation, 260
   equipment for, 335
   laryngoscopy and, 97-99
Energy, pregnancy and, 3
Enfamil Premature, 144
Enflurane, 77
Enteral feedings
   combined parenteral feedings and, 156
   schedule of, for preterm infant, 146
Enterobacter, 149, 236
Enterocolitis, necrotizing, 113, 146, 149-152, 153
Epidural block, lumbar, 75
Epinephrine, 78, 83, 94, 162, 285
Episiotomy, multiple pregnancy and, 190
Equipment
   for endotracheal intubation and umbilical vessel catheterization, 335
   neonatal emergency transport, 336-337
Ergot, 190
Errors of metabolism, inborn, 22
Erythroblastosis fetalis, 16, 276-277, 279, 298, 344
Erythromycin, 239
Escherichia coli, 239
Esophageal atresia, 117, 304-305
Estimation of fetal age, 31-34
Estriol, 38-39, 187
Ethanol, 16, 165-166
Ether, 83
Ethiodan; *see* Iophendylate
Ethyl alcohol, 162
Ethyl ether, 77
Excessive-sized infant, diabetes and, 230; *see also* Large-for-dates infant
Exchange transfusions, 279-280, 295
Exercise
   curtailment of, multiple pregnancy and, 188
   extraordinary, high-risk pregnancy and, 16
Expiration, time of inspiration and, 261
Exstrophy of bladder and cloaca, 309
External cardiac massage, 94
External cephalic version, breech presentation and, 221-222
Extrachorial placenta, 218-219
Extraction, vacuum, 80
Extrusion of cervical mucus, 208
Extubation, mechanical ventilation and, 262
Eyes of infant
   care of, in intensive care unit, 130
   discharges from, 239

F

Face presentation, 226
Factor VIII, 215
FAD; *see* Fetal activity-acceleration determination
False labor, differentiation of, from true labor, 61
Family planning, 330
Fanconi's anemia, 21
Fat
   brown, 122
   needs for, of preterm infant, 143
   pregnancy and, 4

Fat—cont'd
  saturated, 143
  in total parenteral nutrition, 154
Father, occupation of, perinatal morbidity and mortality and, 8
Fatty acid deficiency, 154
Feeding, 133-134
  bottle, 148
  nasogastric, 148
  oral, low birth weight infant and, 141-152
  problems of, 113
  transpyloric, 148-149
Ferro drops, 144
Fetal acidosis, 53
Fetal activity-acceleration determination (FAD), 154-156
Fetal age
  estimation of, 31-44
    postnatal, 104
    by ultrasonography, 36, 37
Fetal alcohol syndrome, 16, 312, 331
Fetal assessment, 42-44
Fetal biophysical profile score, 58, 59
Fetal blood, method of obtaining, 53
Fetal blood loss, 211
Fetal blood sampling, 53
Fetal bradycardia, 46, 49
Fetal circulation, 71
Fetal compromise, confirmation of, 52-54
Fetal death, 66, 191-192, 329
  determination of, 44
  diabetes and, 230
  multiple pregnancy and, 193
  twins and, 193
Fetal deprivation
  chronic, of small-for-dates neonate, 179
  of dysmaturity, subacute, of small-for-dates neonate, 180
Fetal development, interference with, 31
Fetal distress, 54
  absence of, 54
  cesarean section and, 78
  critical, 54
  with delivery, chronic factors predisposing to, 71
  of small-for-dates neonate
    acute, 180
    chronic, 179
  suspicion of, 54
  treatment of, from interpretation of fetal heart rate patterns, 54
Fetal electrocardiography, multiple pregnancy and, 187
Fetal growth, 31
  interference with, 31
  laboratory parameters of, 36-38
Fetal growth curves, 31, 32
Fetal health, detection of risk factors of, 31-44
Fetal heart rate (FHR), 45
  abnormalities of, 46-48
  acceleration of, 48-49
  beat-to-beat variability of, 46, 47-48
  combined patterns of, 51
  deceleration of, 49-51
    early, 49, 54
    late, 49-51, 54
    variable, 51, 54

Fetal heart rate (FHR)—cont'd
  early signs of fetal compromise in, 51
  indirect monitoring of, 67-68
  in intensive care unit, 125-127
  irregularity of, 46
  long-term variability of, 46
  monitoring of, 47
  normal, 46
  patterns of, interpretation of, 51
  periodic changes in, 48-51
  short-term variability of, 46
  sinusoidal patterns of, 48
  tracing of, in fetuses with congenital anomalies, 59
  treatment of fetal distress from interpretation of, 54
Fetal heart tones, 34-35
Fetal infant growth graph, 106
Fetal jeopardy, indicators of, 45-59
Fetal lie, determination of, 36
Fetal lung maturity tests, 40
Fetal maturity, methods of determining, 42-44
Fetal mortality, 313, 314
Fetal motion, calculation of pregnancy duration from, 35-36
Fetal nursing care, 68-69
Fetal phase, 24
Fetal position, determination of, 36
Fetal scalp blood sampling, biochemical monitoring by, 52-54
Fetal size, estimation of, in utero, 182
Fetal tachycardia, 46-47
Fetal transfusion, 343-344
Fetal transport, 114; see also Transport
Fetal weight
  correlations of uterine fundal measurement with, 34
  estimation of, 34, 36, 37
  in intensive care unit, 131
  occurrence of onset of labor after premature rupture of membranes related to, 167
  type of breech presentation by, 220-221
Fetal well-being, laboratory parameters of, 38-42
Fetopelvic disproportion, 182
Fetoscopy, detection of fetal heart tones by, 35
Fetotoxic compounds, human, 26-27
Fetouterine growth, disproportionate, 177-184
Fetus(es)
  acardiac amorphous, 191, 193
  average duration of gestation and perinatal deaths related to number of, 193
  with congenital anomalies, fetal heart rate tracings in, 59
  early development and growth of, 22-24
  growth-retarded, 177-179; see also Growth retardation, intrauterine
  high-risk, diagnosis and management of, 1-219
  large-for-dates, 85, 181-183
  nutrition and, 5-6
  overactivity of, 67
  oversized, 85, 181-183
  physiologic maturity determinations of, 39-42
  at risk, delivery of, 70-86
  at term, blood volume in, 92
Fetus papyraceus, 185, 192
Fetus-to-fetus transfusion, 191
FHR; see Fetal heart rate

Fiberoptic light, 135
Fibrin, 153
Fibrindex test, 213
Fibrinogen, 215
Fibroplasia, retrolental, 262
Fistula, tracheoesophageal, 304-305
Flaring of nares, 252
Flashlight, cuffed, 135
Fluid and electrolytes, parenteral administration of, 138-140
Fluid requirements, assessment of, 138-139
Fluid support of high-risk infant, 116-117
Fluorescence microviscosity, 42
Fluorescent treponemal antibody-absorption (FTA-ABS) test, 245
Fluroxene, 78
Flush method of measuring blood pressure, 126
Folic acid, 6, 188
Forceps delivery, 79-80, 190, 214
Formulas for preterm infant, 142-145
Forward somersault, breech presentation and, 222
Frank breech presentation, 220, 222
Fraternal twins, 194
FTA-ABS test; see Fluorescent treponemal antibody-absorption test
Fundal height, calculation of pregnancy duration from, 34
Fundal measurement, correlations of fetal weight with, 34
Fundus, relationship of, to landmarks on abdominal wall, 35
Furosemide (Lasix), 263, 287

G

Galactosemia, 276
Gamma globulin, 242
Gastric aspirate
  bacterial septicemia and, 237
  excessive, intestinal obstruction and, 306
Gastroschisis, 117, 309
Gastrulation, 23
Gavage, intermittent, 147-148
General anesthesia, 76
Generalized edema, 4
Genetic and congenital defects, 21-30
Genetic syndromes, 229
Genetic transmissions and chromosomal aberrations, 21-22
Genital tract abnormalities, premature labor and, 160
Genitalia, ambiguous, 311
Gentamicin, 170, 237, 238, 240
Gentian violet, 239
Germ cell, 24-25
German measles, 240-242
Gestation, assessment of infants by, 103-106
Gestational age, 32-33, 317
Gestational diabetes, 181, 192, 298-299
Gestational edema, 196
Gestational hypertension, 196
Gestational hypoglycemia, multiple pregnancy and, 192
Gestational proteinuria, 196-197
Girth measurement, calculation of pregnancy duration from, 34
Glomerular capillary endotheliosis, 197
Glomerulonephritis, 198
Glucocorticoid therapy, 166, 170

Glucose, 138-139, 143
  imbalances of, 140
  for short-term needs, 138-139
Glucose intolerance, multiple pregnancy and, 192
Glucose support of high-risk infants, 116-117
Glucosuria, 153
Glucuronide, 275
Glucuronyl transferase, 275
Gonorrheal ophthalmia, 239
Gravimetric test, 213
Group B beta-hemolytic streptococci, 239-240
Growth
  and development of low birth weight infant, 317-322
  disproportionate fetouterine, 177-184
  neonatal, and development of low birth weight infant, 317-319
  postnatal, and development of low birth weight infant, 329
Growth retardation, intrauterine, 177-179
  diabetes and, 230
  multiple pregnancy and, 185, 188, 193
  of small-for-dates neonate, 181
Growth-retarded fetus, 177-179
Growth-retarded term infants, comparison of clinical features of, with those of large premature babies, 112
Grunting, 252

H

Halothane, 77, 78
Handwashing in nursery, 122
HCG; see Human chorionic gonadotropin
HCS; see Human chorionic somatomammotropin
Head chamber for continuous positive airway pressure, 258
Head circulation, 106, 317
Head-to-length ratio, 106
Health of low birth weight infant, 321
Hearing in low birth weight infant, 321
Heart disease, congenital, 252-253, 282, 306
Heart failure, 283-284
Heart rate, fetal; see Fetal heart rate
Heat-stable alkaline phosphatase, 39
Heel-stick blood gas samples, 255
Height and weight of women, standard, 2
Helmet cells, 215
Hemagglutinin-inhibition (HI) antibody, 241-242
Hematologic problem(s), 293-296
  anemia as; see Anemia
  bleeding or skin hemorrhage as, 295-296
  disseminated intravascular coagulation as, 295-296
  neonatal hyperviscosity as, 294-295
  thrombocytopenia as, 295
  vitamin K deficiency as, 296
Hemoglobin electrophoresis, 211
Hemoglobin-oxygen dissociation curve, 91-92
Hemorrhage
  concealed, 215-216
  intraventricular, 289-290
  late pregnancy, 208-219, 331
    cervical and vaginal lesions and, 208
    circummarginate placenta and, 218-219
    circumvallate placenta and, 160, 169, 209, 218-219
    coagulopathies and, 208-209

Hemorrhage—cont'd
  late pregnancy—cont'd
    extrachorial placenta and, 218-219
    laboratory evaluations of, 210
    life support measures for, 210
    placenta previa and; *see* Placenta previa
    placental and uterine bleeding as, 209-210
    symptoms of acute blood loss in, 210
    vasa previa and, 209, 211, 213, 219, 227-228
  occult, 211
  periventricular, 250, 289-290
  postpartum, multiple pregnancy and, 192-193
  pulmonary, respiratory distress and, 271
  skin, 295-296
Hemorrhagic shock, 211
Heparin, 203, 216
Hepatitis, serum, 215
Hernia, diaphragmatic, 117, 305-306
Heroin, 14
Herpes simplex virus infection, 242-243
Herpesvirus infection, 242-243
Herpesvirus type 1, 243
Herpesvirus type 2, 242, 243
HI antibody; *see* Hemagglutinin-inhibition antibody
High altitude exposure, high-risk pregnancy and, 16
High-risk infant, 1-9
  care and stabilization of, transport and, 116-118
  diagnosis and management of, 1-219
  intensive care of; *see* Intensive care of high-risk infant
  parents of, 117-118
  transport of, 114-119
High-risk pregnancy; *see* Pregnancy, high-risk
Hips, dislocated and subluxated, 311
Hirschsprung's disease, 307, 308
HLA; *see* Human lymphocyte antigen
HMD; *see* Hyaline membrane disease
Home, emergency delivery in, 85-86
Homeostatic imbalance, 139-140
Homologous serum jaundice, 215
Hormonal abnormalities, 229
Hormonal insufficiency, high-risk pregnancy and, 16
Hospital
  community; *see* Community hospital
  rural, 323-325
HPL; *see* Human placental lactogen
Human chorionic gonadotropin (HCG), 38-39
Human chorionic somatomammotropin (HCS), 39
Human fetotoxic compounds, 26-27
Human lymphocyte antigen (HLA), 229
Human milk, 144, 145
Human placental lactogen (HPL), 39, 187
Humidification, intensive care unit and, 124-125
Huntington's chorea, 29
Hyaline membrane disease (HMD), 252, 253, 257-258, 261, 262, 298-299
  placenta previa and, 218
  respiratory distress and, 266-268
Hydatidiform mole, 197
Hydralazine, 202, 205, 214-215
Hydramnios, 183-184
  intestinal obstruction and, 306
  multiple pregnancy and, 193
Hydrocephalus, 106, 290-291, 317

Hydrocortisone, 298
Hydrorrhea gravidarum, 169
Hydroxyzine pamoate (Vistaril), 76
Hypaque-M; *see* Diatrizoate sodium
Hyperbilirubinemia, 299
  prevention of kernicterus and, 275-281
  nonhemolytic, 278
Hypercarbia, 78, 253, 258
Hyperfibrinogenemia, 208
Hyperglycemia, 139, 140, 153, 299-300
  total parenteral nutrition and, 157
  very low birth weight infant and, 250
Hyperinsulinism, temporary, hypoglycemia caused by, 299
Hyperkalemia, 299
Hyperlipemia, 154
Hypermagnesemia, 207, 301
Hypernatremia, 139-140, 300
Hyperoxia, very low birth weight infant and, 250
Hyperphosphatemia, 299
Hypertension
  persistent pulmonary, 270-271
  in pregnancy, 196, 207
    acute, 205
    chronic, 197, 198-199, 204-205, 206
    gestational, 196
  primary pulmonary, 253
Hypertensive states in pregnancy, 196-207, 230
Hyperviscosity, neonatal, 294-295
Hypnotics, 76
Hypocalcemia, 140, 145, 299, 300-301
Hypocarbia, 271
Hypofibrinogenemia, 213
Hypoglycemia, 109, 111, 140
  caused by temporary hyperinsulinism, 299
  with erythroblastosis fetalis, 298
  gestational, multiple pregnancy and, 192
  of newborn, 297-299
  persistent, 297
  rebound, 147, 157, 297
  symptomatic, 297
  total parenteral nutrition and, 157
  very low birth weight infant and, 250
Hypomagnesemia, 299, 301
Hyponatremia, 139-140, 142, 300
Hypoplastic small-for-dates neonate, 179
Hypotension, 78, 192
Hypothermic infant, rewarming of, 124
Hypothyroidism, 311
Hypotonia, 113, 207
Hypoventilation, 125
Hypovolemia, 92, 218
Hypovolemic shock, 78, 284
Hypoxemia, 253, 260
Hypoxia, 250, 320
Hysterectomy, 214

I

Identical twins, 194
I:E ratio; *see* Time of inspiration and expiration
Ileal atresia, 308
Ileus, 146, 149
  meconium, 308

Illness
  of low birth weight infant, 321
  protection against, 133
Immune serum globulin, 242
Imperforate anus, 308-309
Inborn errors of metabolism, 22
Inclusion conjunctivitis, 239
Incompetent cervix, 169, 171-173
  cervical cerclage in treatment of, 171-173
  differential diagnosis of midtrimester abortion and, 171
  premature labor and, 160-161
Incomplete breech presentation, 220
Incomplete twins, 24, 187
Incubator, closed, 123-124
Indomethacin, 197, 287
Induction of labor, 80-84, 331
  combined, 83
  contraindications to, 81
  elective, 81
  hazards of, 81
  indications for, 80-81
  medical procedural recommendations for, 81-83
  pelvic score for, 82
  prognosis for, 83-84
  surgical, 83
Infa-Length, 106
Infant(s); *see also* Neonate; Newborn; Perinate
  assessment of, by weight and gestation, 103-106
  depressed, resuscitation and stabilization of, 93-96
  excessive-sized, diabetes and, 230
  high-risk; *see* High-risk infant
  hypothermic, rewarming of, 124
  initial care of, in birth room, 87-92
  large-for-gestational age, 105, 110-111
  low birth weight; *see* Low birth weight infant
  at medium risk and their specific care, 108-113
  nonbreathing, ventilation for, 94
  postmature, 173-174
  postterm, 105, 110
  premature; *see* Premature infant
  preterm; *see* Preterm infant
  small-for-dates; *see* Small-for-dates infant
  small-for-gestational age, 105, 111
  term; *see* Term infant
  very low birth weight; *see* Very low birth weight infant
Infant bag, 99
Infant-parent relationships in intensive care unit, 131
Infection, 113
  abortogenic, 331
  candidal, 239
  congenital, 240-247
  cytomegalovirus, 244
  herpes simplex virus, 242-243
  local, 239
  minor, 239
  nursing regulations for control of, 122
  perinatal; *see* Perinatal infections
  premature labor and, 160
  severe, 237-239
  total parenteral nutrition and, 157
  viral, 240-247
Infertility, diabetes and, 230
Influenza, 26

Inhalants, 76
Inhalation anesthetics, 76-77
Initial care of infant in birth room, 87-92
Injections, intramuscular, in intensive care unit, 131
INPV; *see* Intermittent negative pressure ventilation
Insensible water loss (IWL), 138
Inspiration and expiration, time of, 261
Insulin, 230, 233, 235
Insulin receptor abnormalities, 229
Insulin-dependent diabetes, 229
Insulin-independent diabetes, 229
Intellectual deficits of low birth weight infant, 319-321
Intensive care of high-risk infant, 120-137
  admission care in, 127
  aspiration of tension pneumothorax in, 136
  blood pressure monitoring in, 126-127
  clothing and crib transfer for premature infant in, 130
  discharge from, 130, 131-132
  humidification and, 124-125
  intramuscular injections in, 131
  intubation in, 136
  monitoring heart rate and respirations in, 125-127
  nose, eyes, and mouth care in, 130
  nursery facilities for, 120-122
  nursing notes and recording of data in, 130
  nursing regulations for control of infections in, 122
  parent-infant relationships in, 131
  peripheral vein infusion in, 135
  positioning of infant in, 127-130
  procedures in, 134-136
  responsibilities in
    of community health nurse, 132
    of neonatal nurse, 134
    of social worker, 132-133
  retinal examination in, 135
  skin care in, 130
  spinal fluid tap in, 135
  temperature control in, 122-124
  transillumination in, 135
  urine and stool care in, 130-131
  weighing and measuring infant in, 131
Intercostal retractions, 252
Intercourse, isolated, calculation of pregnancy duration from, 33-34
Intermediate care, 325-326
Intermittent gavage, 147-148
Intermittent negative pressure ventilation (INPV), 260
Intermittent positive pressure ventilation (IPPV), 260
Internal ballottement, 36
Internal podalic version and extraction, 80
Intestinal obstruction, 117, 306-309
Intestine, perforation of, 149
Intoxication, water, 81
Intraarterial measurement, direct, of blood pressure, 126-127
Intralipid, 154, 155
Intramuscular injections in intensive care unit, 131
Intrapartum screening, 18-19
Intrauterine growth retardation; *see* Growth retardation, intrauterine
Intrauterine jeopardy, factors relating to, 11-12
Intravascular coagulation, disseminated, 192, 208, 213, 295-296

Intravenous equipment for neonatal emergency transport, 336
Intraventricular hemorrhage (IVH), 289-290
Intubation, 136
  continuous positive airway pressure by, 259
  endotracheal
    equipment for, 335
    laryngoscopy and, 97-99
  problems of, 98-99
Invasive carcinoma of cervix, 208
Iodine
  organic, 125, 136
  pregnancy and, 6
Iophendylate (Ethiodan), 44
Iothalamate acid (Angio-Conray), 44
Iowa trumpet, 73
IPPV; *see* Intermittent positive pressure ventilation
Iron, 6, 188
Iron medications, 134
Iron needs of preterm infant, 143-144
Irresponsible parenthood, accidental pregnancy and, 7
Island, resuscitation, 93
Isoimmunization, cesarean section and, 79
Isolated intercourse, calculation of pregnancy duration from, 33-34
Isoniazid, 247
Isoproterenol, 211, 285
IVH; *see* Intraventricular hemorrhage
IWL; *see* Insensible water loss

J

Jaundice, 113, 275
  excessive, diagnostic approach to, 276
  homologous serum, 215
  when to investigate, 276
Jejunal atresia, 308
Jitteriness, 288
Johnson, R.W., 34
Juvenile-onset diabetes, 229

K

Kanamycin, 240
Karyotyping, emergency, 310
Ketoacidosis, 233
Klebsiella, 149, 236
Kleihauer-Betke test, 211
Kleihauer's stain, 40, 218

L

Labor, 159
  abnormal, multiple pregnancy and, 192
  abnormal patterns of, 66
  arrest disorders of, 66
  assessment of, 60-69
    clinical parameters of, 60-68
  definition of, 61
  dry, 167
  false, differentiation of, from true labor, 61
  first stage of, 61
  indications for elective fetal monitoring in, 45-46
  induction of; *see* Induction of labor
  multiparous, 62, 63, 65
  nulliparous, 62, 63, 64

Labor—cont'd
  occurrence of onset of, after premature rupture of membranes, related to fetal weight, 167
  placental stage of, 61
  premature; *see* Premature labor
  prodromal, 61
  progress in, assessment of, 61-63
  prolongation disorders of, 66
  prolonged deceleration phase of, 66
  prolonged latent phase of, 66
  protraction disorders of, 66
  second stage of, 61
  stages of, 61
  third stage of, 61
  true, differentiation of, from false labor, 61
Laboratory screening, routine, 11
Lactation, recommended daily dietary allowances for, 3
Lactobezoar, 144, 146
Lactogen, human placental, 39, 187
Large-for-dates infant, 181-183
Large-for-gestational age (LGA) infant, 105, 110-111
Largon; *see* Propiomazine
Laryngoscopy and endotracheal intubation, 97-99
Lasix; *see* Furosemide
Last menstrual period (LMP), calculation of pregnancy duration from, 32-33, 317
Late pregnancy hemorrhage; *see* Hemorrhage, late pregnancy
Lecithin/sphingomyelin (L/S) ratio, 40-41, 159, 168, 179, 211
Left-to-right shunt, 90
Length, 6, 106, 317
Leopold's maneuvers, 35, 36, 55, 221
Lesions, cervical and vaginal, 208
Lethargy, 113
Leucine aminopeptidase, 187
Leukomalacia, periventricular, 320
Levarterenol bitartrate, 211
LGA infant; *see* Large-for-gestational age infant
Librium; *see* Chlordiazepoxide
Lidocaine, 73
Light, fiberoptic, 135
Linoleic acid, 143
Lip, cleft, 311
Lipids, 154
Liposoluble contrast media, 44
Listeria monocytogenes, 247
Listeriosis, 247
LMP; *see* Last menstrual period
Longitudinal assessment
  of fetal health, 31-44
  of low birth weight infant, 319, 321-322
Long-term variability of fetal heart rate, 46
Low birth weight infant, 159; *see also* Preterm infant; Very low birth weight infant
  association between prepregnancy weight, maternal weight, and birth weight and, 5
  behavior disorders of, 321, 322
  child abuse and, 321
  child neglect and, 321
  growth and development of, 317-322
  health of, 321
  hearing of, 321

Low birth weight infant—cont'd
    illness of, 321
    intellectual deficits of, 319-321
    longitudinal assessments of, 321-322
    longitudinal growth of, 319
    mortality and, 314-315
    motor delay of, 322
    multiple pregnancy and, 193
    neonatal growth and development of, 317-319
    neurologic defects of, 317-322
    neuromuscular responses of, 319
    nutritional requirements and oral feedings of, 141-152
    postnatal growth and development of, 319
    sensory responses of, 319
    social responses of, 319
    temperature control of, 124
    vision of, 321
    weight loss of, 141
Low forceps, 79
L/S ratio; see Lecithin/sphingomyelin ratio
Lumbar epidural block, 75
Lung maturity, fetal, 40
Lutein cysts, multiple pregnancy and, 192

M

Macrosomia, diabetes and, 230
Magnesium sulfate, 162, 166, 201, 204, 205, 206, 207
Males, incidence of, in multiple pregnancy, 186
Malformations, multiple pregnancy and, 193
Malnutrition, pregnancy and, 2-6
Malposition, multiple pregnancy and, 193
Malpresentation and cord accidents, 220-228
Malrotation of volvulus, 307-308
Manganese, 154
Mannitol, 214
Manometer, pressure, 99
Marfan's syndrome, 29
Marginal sinus, ruptured, 209
Mask
    and bag, ventilation with, 260
    for continuous positive airway pressure, 258
Masses, abdominal, 311
Maternal age, fetal chromosomal abnormalities and, 22
Maternal drug addiction, effects of, on fetus and neonate, 14-15
Maternal nutritional risk identification, 4-5
Maternal weight gain, 2-3, 5
Maturity determination, physiologic, of fetus, 39-42
Maturity-onset diabetes, 229
McDonald's maneuver, 34, 35, 172
MCT oil, 149
Measles, German, 240-242
Mechanical ventilation; see Ventilation
Meconium, 43, 87
Meconium aspiration syndrome, 84-85, 175, 269-270
Meconium ileus, 308
Meconium peritonitis, 308
Meconium plug syndrome, 309
Meconium staining of amniotic fluid, 66, 67, 84-85, 175, 269
Medical history in screening, 17-18

Medications
    for neonatal emergency transport, 336
    to be used with caution in high-risk pregnancy, 76-77
Medicine, adolescent, 330
Medium-chain triglycerides, 143, 149
Megacolon, 308
Megadose vitamin and mineral supplementation, pregnancy and, 6
Membranes, premature rupture of; see Premature rupture of membranes
Menstrual age, 32-33
Menstrual period, last, calculation of pregnancy duration from, 32-33, 317
Mental retardation, multiple pregnancy and, 193
Meperidine, 76
Mepivacaine, 73
Mersilene, 172
Metabolic acidosis, 253, 256
Metabolic assessment of infant receiving total parenteral nutrition, 155
Metabolic problems, 297-302, 310-312
Metabolic support of high-risk infants, 116-117
Metabolism, inborn errors of, 22
Metaraminol bitartrate, 211
Methadone, 14
Methemoglobinemia, 207
Methicillin, 238
Methoxyflurane, 77
Methyldopa, 203, 205
Microcephalus, 106, 290-291
Microcolon, 308
Microphene, 122
Microviscosity, fluorescence, 42
Midtrimester abortion, 171
Milk, breast, 144, 145
Minerals
    needs for, of preterm infant, 143
    supplementation of, pregnancy and, 6-7
Miniheparin, 170
Minimal brain syndrome, 321
Mole, hydatidiform, 197
Monitor
    cardiac, 125
    electronic fetal heart rate; see Electronic fetal heart rate monitoring
    respiratory-apnea, 125
Monoamniotic twins, 187, 189, 194
    monochorionic, 24
Monosomy, 21
Monozygotic twins, 24, 185, 186, 187, 191, 193, 194
Morbidity and mortality
    classification of newborn infants by birth weight and gestation and, 105
    very low birth weight infant and, 249
    perinatal; see Perinatal morbidity and mortality
Morphine sulfate, 162
Mortality; see also Morbidity and mortality
    fetal, 313, 314
    low birth weight infant and, 314-315
    neonatal, 313-314, 315
    perinatal, 313-316, 329

Mosaic, 21
Motor delay of low birth weight infant, 322
Mouth care in intensive care unit, 130
Mouth-to-mouth ventilation, 99
Mouth-to-tube ventilation, 99
Mucus, cervical, extrusion of, 208
Mucus vomiting, 147
Multiparous labor, 62, 63, 65
Multiple gestation, 84
Multiple pregnancy, 185-195
    analgesia and, 189
    antepartum care and, 188
    bed rest and, 188
    benefits of early detection of, 188
    cerebral palsy and, 185
    cesarean section and, 189-190, 191, 193
    complications and sequelae of, 192-194
        fetal, 193
        maternal, 192-193
        placental and related to cord, 194
    delivery and, 188-191
    diagnosis of, by laboratory procedure, 187-188
    differential diagnosis of, 187-188
    episiotomy and, 190
    exercise curtailment and, 188
    fetal electrocardiography in diagnosis of, 187
    forceps and, 190
    growth retardation and, 185, 188
    human placental lactogen assay in diagnosis of, 187
    identification of, by clinical associations and observations, 186-187
    incidence and associations of, 185-186
    maternal risk and, 185
    nutrition and, 188
    prematurity and, 185, 188
    quadruplets in; *see* Quadruplets
    radiography in diagnosis of, 187
    special care during, 188
    special perinatal considerations of, 191-192
    triplets in; *see* Triplets
    twins in; *see* Twins
    ultrasonography in diagnosis of, 187-188
    vaginal delivery and, 190-191
Multivitamin mixtures, 144
Muscle relaxant, 77
Mutagen, 24-25
Mutagenesis, 24-26
MVI-Pediatric, 154
Mycostatin; *see* Nystatin
Mydriacyl; *see* Tropicamide
Myelomeningocele, 309-310

N

NaHCO$_3$; *see* Sodium bicarbonate
Naloxone (Narcan), 76
Narcan; *see* Naloxone
Narcotic depression, 93, 94
Narcotic drugs, 76
Narcotic withdrawal, 14
Narcotics, injectable, 76
Nares, flaring of, 252
Narrow-shank forceps, 79
Nasal prongs, continuous positive airway pressure by, 258, 259
Nasal stuffiness, 207
Nasogastric feeding, 148
Nasopharyngeal tube, continuous positive airway pressure by, 258-259
National Committee on Radiation Protection, 26
National Diabetes Data Group (NDDG), 229, 230
National Fertility Study, 332
National Institute of Neurological Diseases and Stroke (NINDS), 226
NDDG; *see* National Diabetes Data Group
Nebulization, ultrasonic, 124-125
Necrosis
    acute tubular, 142
    renal cortical, 214-215
    tissue, total parenteral nutrition and, 157
Necrotizing enterocolitis, 113, 146, 149-152, 153
Needle aspiration of pneumothorax, 264
Needle electrodes on heart rate monitors, 125
Negative nitrogen balance, 138
Neglect, child, 321
Neonatal death, multiple pregnancy and, 193
Neonatal depression, 207
Neonatal emergency transport equipment, 336-337
Neonatal growth and development of low birth weight infant, 317-319
Neonatal hyperbilirubinemia; *see* Hyperbilirubinemia
Neonatal hyperviscosity, 294-295
Neonatal intensive care unit; *see* Intensive care of high-risk infant
Neonatal morbidity and mortality, 230-231, 313-314, 315
Neonatal nurse
    in intensive care unit, 134
    in transport team, 115
Neonatal purpura, 241
Neonatal transfer log, 340
Neonatal transport; *see* Transport
Neonate; *see also* Infant(s); Newborn; Perinate
    born after premature rupture of membranes, management of, 170-171
    breech presentation and, 225-226
    high-risk, diagnosis and management of, 1-219
    hypertensive states in pregnancy and, 207
    placenta previa and, 218
    respiratory distress in, 266-272
    small-for-dates, 89, 179-181
    specific problems of, 249-316
Neosporin, 239
Neo-Synephrine; *see* Phenylephrine
Neural tube defect, 29-30
Neurogenic shock, anesthesia and, 78
Neurologic defects
    low birth weight infant and, 317-322
    small-for-dates infant and, 181
Neurologic disorder(s), 288-292
    central nervous system disorders as, 288-289
    hydrocephalus as, 290-291
    intraventricular hemorrhage as, 289-290
    microcephalus as, 290-291

Neurologic disorder(s)—cont'd
  periventricular hemorrhage as, 289-290
  seizures as, 288-289
Neurologic examination of newborn in birth room, 89
Neuromuscular responses of low birth weight infant, 319
Neutral zone of temperature, 123
Newborn; see also Infant(s); Neonate; Perinate
  examination of, in birth room, 89
  factors placing, at increased jeopardy, 12-14
  hypoglycemia of, 297-299
  maintenance of body temperature of, 88
  neurologic examination of, in birth room, 89
  physical observations of, in birth room, 88-89
  physiologic assessment of, 87-88
  transient tachypnea of, 271
Newborn transfer record, 338-339
NINDS; see National Institute of Neurological Diseases and Stroke
Nitrites, 207
Nitrogen, 153
Nitrogen balance
  negative, 138
  positive, 153
Nitroprusside, 205
Nitrous oxide, 76-77, 78
Nonbreathing infant, ventilation for, 94
Nondisjunction, 21
Nonhemolytic hyperbilirubinemia, 278
Nonstress test, 54-56
Normoglycemia, 157
Nose, care of, in intensive care unit, 130
Noxious habits, 14-16
Nulliparous labor, 62, 63, 64
Nurse
  charge, in nursery, responsibilities of, 122
  neonatal; see Neonatal nurse
  transport, training of, 119
Nursery
  equipment and cleaning of, 122
  perinatal infections acquired in, 236-238
  responsibilities of charge nurse in, 122
  technique in, 122
  technique to be used before entering, 122
Nursing notes in intensive care unit, 130
Nutrients, pregnancy and, 3-4
Nutrition, 331
  fetus and, 5-6
  multiple pregnancy and, 188
  pregnancy and, 2-6
  total parenteral; see Total parenteral nutrition
Nutritional impairment of small-for-dates neonate, 179-181
Nutritional requirements of low birth weight infant, 141-152
Nutritional risk, maternal, identification of, 4-5
Nystatin (Mycostatin), 238, 239

O

Observation, physical, of newborn in birth room, 88-89
Obstetric forceps, 79
Obstetric history
  previous, premature labor and, 160
  in screening, 17
Obstetric measures, high-risk pregnancy and, 330-332

Obstetric problems, serious, and perinate, 220-248
Obstipation, intestinal obstruction and, 306
Occult hemorrhage, 211
Occult prolapse of umbilical cord, 226, 227
Occupational states, perinatal morbidity and mortality and, 8
OCT; see Oxytocin challenge test
OD^{650nm}, 42
Oligohydramnios, 66, 89, 183-184
Oliguria, 141
Omphalocele, 117, 309
Ophthalmia, gonorrheal, 239
Opiates, 76
Oral feedings
  of low birth weight infants, 141-152
  of premature infants, 145-147
Organic iodine, 125, 136
Organogenesis, 23, 25
Oscilloscope, 125, 126
Osmotic diuresis, 140
Osteogenesis imperfecta, 310
Ototoxic drugs, 321
Overactivity of fetus, 67
Overgrown fetus, 85, 181-183
Overt prolapse of umbilical cord, 226, 227
Ovular phase, 23
Oxygen, 77, 78, 83, 96, 203, 268
  administration of, 254
  blood level of, monitoring of, in infant, 254-255
  respiratory flow sheet for infants receiving, 341
Oxygen therapy
  complications arising from, 262-266
  respiratory distress and, 254-255
Oxygenation
  of high-risk infants, 116
  physiologic aspects of, 91-92
Oxyhood, 116
Oxytocin, 57-58, 65, 81, 82, 83, 190-191, 212, 218, 224
Oxytocin challenge test (OCT), 54, 55, 56-57
Oxytocinase, 39

P

Palate, cleft, 311
Pallor, 113
Pancreas, artificial, 233
Pancreatic disease, 229
Para-aminosalicylic acid, 247
Paracervical block, 73-74, 75
Paraldehyde, 76
Paralytic ileus, 207
Paregoric, 14
Parent support group, 131
Parenteral administration of fluid and electrolytes, 138-140
Parenteral anesthetics, 77
Parenteral feedings, combined enteral feedings and, 156
Parenteral nutrition, total; see Total parenteral nutrition
Parenthood, irresponsible, accidental pregnancy and, 7
Parent-infant bonding in birth room, 89
Parent-infant relationships in intensive care unit, 131
Parents
  of high-risk infant, 117-118
  teenage and unwed, perinatal morbidity and mortality and, 8-9

Paroxysmal supraventricular tachycardia, 286
Patent ductus arteriosus (PDA), 286-287
Pathologic edema, 4
PDA; *see* Patent ductus arteriosus
Peak inspiratory pressure (PIP), 261
PEEP; *see* Positive end-expiratory pressure
Penicillin, 170, 237, 239, 245, 247
Penicillin G, 238, 245
Penis, urine collection from, 136
Pentothal Sodium; *see* Thiopental sodium
Peptides, 153
Perinatal asphyxia, 92
Perinatal center, regional, 323, 326-327, 331
Perinatal death, multiple pregnancy and, 193
Perinatal jeopardy, 2, 72
Perinatal morbidity and mortality, 313-316, 329
    high-risk pregnancy and, 13
    social, cultural, and economic factors influencing, 7-9
Perinatal outcome, 317-328
Perinatal viral infections, 25
Perinate; *see also* Infant(s); Neonate; Newborn
    high-risk; *see* High-risk infant
    infections of, 236-248
    serious obstetric problems and, 220-248
Period, last menstrual, calculation of pregnancy duration from, 32-33, 317
Peripheral arterial blood gas samples, 255-256
Peripheral cyanosis, 282
Peripheral vein as site of total parenteral nutrition, 155
Peripheral vein infusion, 135
Peritonitis, meconium, 308
Periventricular hemorrhage (PVH), 250, 289-290
Periventricular leukomalacia, 320
Persistent hypoglycemia, 297
PG; *see* Phosphatidylglycerol
PGI$_2$; *see* Prostacyclin
pH, reasons for discrepancies between levels of fetal acidosis as measured by, 53
Phenobarbital, 14, 201, 278, 289
Phenylephrine (Neo-Synephrine), 135, 211
Phenytoin, 289
pHisoHex, 130, 239
Phonocardiography, 68
Phosphatidylglycerol (PG), 41, 159, 161, 168, 179, 211
Phosphorus, 143, 154, 155
Phototherapy, 278-279
Physical observations of newborn in birth room, 88-89
Physician in transport team, 115
Physiologic assessment of newborn, 87-88
Physiologic edema, 4
Physiologic maturity determination of fetus, 39-42
Pierre Robin syndrome, 117
Pilot in transport team, 115
PIP; *see* Peak inspiratory pressure
Piper forceps, 79-80
Placenta
    circummarginate, 218-219
    circumvallate, 160, 169, 209, 218-219
    examination of, multiple pregnancy and, 194
    extrachorial, 218-219
    observations of, in birth room, 89-90
    slight premature separation of, 211-215
Placenta accreta, 216, 217, 218
Placenta previa, 160, 194, 209, 211, 213, 216-218
Placental bleeding, 209-210
Placental perfusion, 71
Placental stage of labor, 61
Placental transfusion, 92
Plasma protamine paracoagulation test, 213
Plasmanate, 218
Platelet counts, 113
Pneumatosis intestinalis, 150
Pneumomediastinum, 265
Pneumonia, sepsis without, 261
Pneumopericardium, 265-266
Pneumoperitoneum, 265
Pneumothorax, 117, 135, 136, 263-265, 269
Podalic version, internal, and extraction, 80
Polycythemia, 113
Polyhydramnios, 89, 183-184
    diabetes and, 230
    multiple pregnancy and, 193
Polyuria, 142
Ponderal index, 180
Positioning of infant in intensive care unit, 127-130
Positive end-expiratory pressure (PEEP), 261
Positive nitrogen balance, 153
Positive-pressure breathing devices, 99
Postmature infant, 173-174
Postmenstrual age, 317
Postnatal criteria for risk, 19-20
Postnatal estimation of fetal age, 104
Postnatal growth and development of low birth weight infant, 329
Postpartum hemorrhage, multiple pregnancy and, 192-193
Postreceptor defect, 229
Postterm infant, 105, 110
Potter's syndrome, 90, 167
Povidone-iodine (Betadine), 101, 130, 264
PPH; *see* Pulmonary hypertension, persistent
Preconceptual care, 330
Preeclampsia, 196, 197-198
    mild, 198, 200
    severe, 198, 200-204
    superimposed, chronic hypertension with, 199
Preeclampsia-eclampsia, 192, 197
Pregnancy
    accidental, irresponsible parenthood and, 7
    diabetes and, 229, 230-231
    diamniotic, 187, 194
    duration of, 31-36
    edema and, 4
    emotional stress and, 6-7
    energy and, 3
    first half of, intrauterine growth retardation during, 177
    future, counseling for, 331-332
    high-risk
        medications to be used with caution in, 76-77
        mortality and, according to diagnosis, 13
        prevention of, 329-333
    last half of, intrauterine growth retardation during, 177
    malnutrition and, 2-6
    megadose vitamin and mineral supplementation and, 6
    monoamniotic, 187, 189, 194
    multiple; *see* Multiple pregnancy
    normal, average estriol excretion in, 39

Pregnancy—cont'd
  nutrients and, 3
  prolonged, 173-174
  recommended daily dietary allowances for, 3
  sample diet for, 4
  screening of, 343-344
  untimely termination of, 159-176
  unwanted, prevention of, 332-333
  vitamin and mineral supplementation and, 6-7
  weight gain in, 2-3, 5
Pregnanediol, 39, 187, 276
Prelabor rupture of membranes, 166
Premature infant, 103, 314
  hyperglycemia and, 299
  large, comparison of clinical features of growth-retarded term infants with those of, 112
  medical care for, 134
  multiple pregnancy and, 185, 188, 193
Premature labor, 159-166
  analgesia and anesthesia for, 72-76
  clinical correlates of, 160
  contractions and, 159, 160-161, 162
  definition of, 159
  diabetes and, 230
  diagnosis of, 160-161
  exclusions to treatment of, 161
  general medical complications of, 160
  genital tract anomalies and, 160
  iatrogenic, 159
  incompetent cervix and, 160-161
  infection and, 160
  multiple pregnancy and, 192
  pharmacologic control of, 161-166
  placenta previa and, 218
  premature rupture of membranes and, 160, 166-171
  previous obstetric history and, 160
  signs and symptoms of, 160
  vaginal bleeding and, 160
Premature rupture of membranes (PROM), 160, 166-171
  breech presentation and, 225
  multiple pregnancy and, 194
  twins and, 194
Prematurity
  apnea of, 261, 268
  retinopathy of, 262, 321
Prenatal care, 10-20, 330
Prenatal visit screening, 18
Prepared childbirth, 72-73
Prepregnancy weight, association between birth weight and percentage of low birth weight infants and, 5
Presentation
  breech; *see* Breech presentation
  brow, 226
  face, 226
  transverse, 216, 226
  of twins, combinations of, 190
Presenting part
  descent of, 63, 64, 65
  determination of, 36
Pressure
  continuous negative, 258
  continuous positive airway, 257, 258-259, 261

Pressure—cont'd
  continuous transpulmonary distending, 256-259
  flush, 126
  peak inspiratory, 261
Pressure manometer, 99
Pressure-controlled ventilator, 260
Preterm infant, 105, 110; *see also* Low birth weight infant
  delivery of, 84
  enteral feeding schedule for, 146
  total parenteral nutrition for, 156
  weight loss of, 141
Preterm rupture of membranes, 166
Prilocaine, 73
Primary care, 323-325
Priscilla White classification of diabetes, 230
Procaine, 73, 78
Prodromal labor, 61
Progesterone, 162, 192
Progress in labor, assessment of, 61-63
Prolapse of umbilical cord, 226-227
Prolongation disorders of labor, 66
Prolonged pregnancy, 173-174
Prolonged premature rupture of membranes, 167
Promazine (Sparine), 76
Promethazine, 76
Prophylactic forceps, 79
Propiomazine (Largon), 76
Propranolol, 205
Prostacyclin (PGI$_2$), 197
Prostaglandin, 191, 197
Prostaglandin E, 287
Prostaglandin synthetase inhibitors, 197
Protamine sulfate, 216
Protein, 188
  insufficiency of, pregnancy and, 4
  needs for, of preterm infant, 143
  pregnancy and, 4
  in total parenteral nutrition, 153
  whey, 145
Proteinuria, gestational, 196-197
Protraction disorders of labor, 66
Psychoanalgesia, 72-73
Pudendal nerve block, 74-75
Pulmonary atelectasis, 269
Pulmonary dysmaturity, 262, 271-272
Pulmonary hemorrhage, respiratory distress and, 271
Pulmonary hypertension
  persistent, 270-271
  primary, 253
Purpura, neonatal, 241
Pustules, 239
PVH; *see* Periventricular hemorrhage
Pyridoxine, 144
Pyrimethamine, 246
Pyuria, 136

Q
Quadruplets, 185, 193
  delivery of, 189
  premature rupture of membranes and, 194
Quickening, calculation of pregnancy duration from, 35-36

R

Race, perinatal morbidity and mortality and, 7-8
Radiant warmer, open, 124
Radiation, effect of, on embryo, 26
Radiographic pelvimetry, 60, 61
Radiography
　in assessment of fetal growth, 38
　multiple pregnancy and, 187
Radioimmunoassay, 38
Rapid Plasma Reagin (RPR), 244-245
Rapid surfactant test, 40, 159, 161, 179, 211
RDS; *see* Respiratory distress syndrome
Real-time ultrasonography, 40
Rebound hypoglycemia, 147, 157, 297
Recessively inherited autosomal diseases, 22
Recommended daily dietary allowances for nonpregnant, pregnant, and lactating women, 3
Recording of data in intensive care unit, 130
Records, standard, 10-11
Rectal temperature, 123
Refractive errors in low birth weight infant, 321
Regional anesthesia, 73, 77-78
Regional perinatal center, 111-113, 323, 326-327, 331
Regionalization and guidelines for perinatal care, 323-328
Rehydration, 140
Renal agenesis, 90
Renal cortical necrosis, 214-215
Renal solute load, 141-142
Reserpine, 207
Respiration
　monitoring, in intensive care unit, 125-127
　onset of, 90-91
　seesaw pattern of, 252
Respiratory acidosis, 253, 256
Respiratory care equipment for neonatal emergency transport, 336
Respiratory changes at birth, 90-92
Respiratory depression, 253
Respiratory difficulty at birth, 95
Respiratory distress, 116-118, 266-268, 303-306
　acidosis and, 256
　blood gas sampling and, 255-256
　causes of, in neonate, 266-272
　congenital anomalies of respiratory tree and, 272
　hyaline membrane disease and, 266-268
　management of, 253-256
　mechanical ventilation and; *see* Ventilation, mechanical
　meconium aspiration syndrome and, 269-270
　oxygen therapy for, 254-255
　persistent pulmonary hypertension and, 270-271
　pulmonary dysmaturity and, 271-272
　pulmonary hemorrhage and, 271
　recognition of, 253
　transient tachypnea of newborn and, 271
　ventilatory assistance for, 256-260
Respiratory distress syndrome (RDS), 95, 142, 166, 185, 266-268
Respiratory flow sheet for infants receiving oxygen or assisted ventilation, 341
Respiratory problems, identification and management of, 252-274
Respiratory therapist in transport team, 115
Respiratory tree, congenital anomalies of, 272
Respiratory-apnea monitors, 125
Resuscitation
　perinatal infections acquired during, 236
　and stabilization of depressed infants, 93-96, 97-102
Resuscitation equipment for neonatal emergency transport, 336
Resuscitation island, 93
Retardation, intrauterine growth; *see* Growth retardation, intrauterine
Retinal examination, 135
Retinitis, diabetic, 230
Retinopathy of prematurity, 262, 321
Retractions, intercostal, 252
Retrolental fibroplasia (RLF), 262
Rewarming of hypothermic infant, 124
Rhinitis, 149
RhoGAM, 276-277, 344
Right-to-left shunt, 90, 92, 252-253, 266
Ringer's solution, 165
Risk categories
　body measurement in evaluation of, 105-106
　classification of, 103-107
　fetal health and, 31-44
　identification of, 16-20
Risk perinate, 1-9; *see also* High-risk infant
Ritodrine, 162-165
Ritodrine hydrochloride, 162
Ritodrine *p*-hydroxyphenylethyl-*p*-hydroxy-norepinephrine, 162-165
RLF; *see* Retrolental fibroplasia
Room temperature, control of, 133
RPR; *see* Rapid Plasma Reagin
Rubella, 240-242
Rubella syndrome, 241
Rupture of membranes
　prelabor, 166
　premature; *see* Premature rupture of membranes
　preterm, 166
　spontaneous, multiple pregnancy and, 192
Ruptured marginal sinus, 209
Rural hospital, 323-325

S

Safflower oil, 149
Sahling, Erich, 52
Salicylates, 277
Saturated fats, 143
Schistocytes, 215, 296
Scopolamine, 76
Screening of pregnancies, 16-18, 343-344
　for diabetes, 231-232
　intrapartum, 18-19
　laboratory, routine, 11
　prenatal, 18
Sector scan ultrasonography, 40
Sedatives, 76, 207
Seesaw pattern of respirations, 252
Seizures, 111, 113, 288-289
Selenium, 154
Sensory responses of low birth weight infant, 319

Sepsis
    clinical signs suggestive of, 237
    of high-risk infant, 117
    without pneumonia, 261
Septic shock, 78, 284
Septicemia, bacterial, 237-239
Serial measurement, abnormal, 34
Serum alpha fetoprotein measurement, 11
Serum hepatitis, 215
Servo control, 123-124
Sex chromosomal abnormalities, 21
Sex-linked dominant inherited diseases, 22
Shock, 95, 126, 284-286
    anaphylactic, 78
    anesthesia for patient in, 78
    cardiogenic, 78, 284
    hemorrhagic, 211
    high-risk infant and, 117
    hypovolemic, 78, 284
    management of, 284-286
    neurogenic, 78
    septic, 78, 284
    signs of, 284
Short-term variability of fetal heart rate, 46
Shunt
    left-to-right, 90
    right-to-left, 90, 92, 252-253, 266
Siamese twins, 24
SIDS; see Sudden infant death syndrome
Similac Special Care, 144
Single coitus, calculation of pregnancy duration from, 33-34
Single footling breech presentation, 220
Sinusoidal fetal heart patterns, 48
Skin care in intensive care unit, 130
Skin hemorrhages, 295-296
SMA Premie, 144
Small-for-dates infant, 89, 179-181
Small-for-gestational age (SGA) infant, 105, 111
Smith, D.W., 310
Smoking, cigarette, effect of, on fetus, 15, 212, 215, 331
Snuffles, 245
Social class, perinatal morbidity and mortality and, 8
Social factors influencing perinatal morbidity and mortality, 7-9
Social responses of low birth weight infant, 319
Social worker, 132-133
Socioeconomic improvement for prevention of high-risk pregnancy, 330
Sociomedical measures for presentation of high-risk pregnancy, 330
Sodium
    imbalances of, 139-140
    pregnancy and, 4
Sodium bicarbonate (NaHCO$_3$), 256
Sodium nitroprusside, 202-203
Somatic cell, 24-25
Somersault, backward and forward, breech presentation and, 222
Sparine; see Promazine
Sparteine sulfate, 83
Spaulding's sign, 44
Spectrophotometry, 41, 42, 343-344

Spherocytosis, 276
Spinal block, 75-76
Spinal fluid examination, bacterial septicemia and, 237
Spinal fluid tap, 135
Spontaneous expulsion, breech presentation and, 224
Stabilization and resuscitation of depressed infant, 93-96, 97-102
Stain, Kleihauer's, 40
Staphylococci, 236
Staphylococcus aureus, 130
Starvation, 138, 250-251
Steroids, 166, 168, 203-204, 246
Stomach, emptying, of high-risk infant, 117
Stool Clinitest, 136
Stool guaiac, 136
Strabismus, 321
Streptococci, beta-hemolytic, group B, 239-240
Stress, emotional, pregnancy and, 6-7
Stress test, contraction, 54, 56-57
Subluxated hips, 311
Succinylcholine, 77, 78
Suctioning equipment for neonatal emergency transport, 336
Sudden infant death syndrome (SIDS), 15
Surface adhesive electrodes on heart rate monitors, 125
Sulfadiazine, 246
Sulfonamides, 246, 277
Supplemental total parenteral nutrition, 157
Surgical history in screening, 17-18
Surgical problems of high-risk infant, 117
Surital; see Thiamylal sodium
Synthetic opiates, 76
Syphilis, 26, 244-245
Systemic circulation, inadequate, 71

T

Tachycardia
    fetal, 46-47
    paroxysmal supraventricular, 286
Tachypnea, 252, 299
    increasing, 111
    transient, of newborn, 90, 271
TcP$_{O_2}$; see Transcutaneous oxygen monitor
Team care in birth room, 70-72
Teenage parents, perinatal morbidity and mortality and, 8-9
TEF; see Tracheoesophageal fistula
Temperature
    basal body, calculation of pregnancy duration from, 33-34
    body, of newborn, maintenance of, 88
    control of, 123-124
        of high-risk infants, 116
        in intensive care nursery, 122-124
    excessive, of high-risk infant, hazards from, 123
    neutral zone of, 123
    rectal, 123
    room, control of, 133
Tension pneumothorax, 136, 264
Teratogen, 24-25
Teratogenesis, 24-26
Term infant, 103, 314
    growth-retarded, comparison of clinical features of, with those of large premature infants, 112

Term infant—cont'd
 total parenteral nutrition for, 156
 weight loss of, 141
Tertiary care, 323, 326-327
Tetracaine, 73
Thalidomide, 179
THAM; see Tromethamine
Thanatophoric dwarfism, 310
Theophylline, 197, 268
Therapeutic abortion, 330-331
Therapist, respiratory, in transport team, 115
Thermistor, 123, 124
Thermometer, clinical, 123
Thiamylal sodium (Surital), 77
Thiazide diuretics, 203, 205, 207, 295
Thiocyanate, 203
Thiopental sodium (Pentothal Sodium), 77, 78
Third trimester bleeding; see Hemorrhage, late pregnancy
Three-day measles, 240-242
Thrombocytopenia, 207, 295
Thromboxane (TXA_2), 197
Thrush, 239
Time
 of inspiration and expiration (I:E ratio), 261
 of insult, potential adverse effects and malformations related to, 24
Time-cycled ventilator, 260
Tincture of benzoin, 98
Tissue necrosis, total parenteral nutrition and, 157
Tocolysis, 162-166
Tocolytics, 162, 170, 222
Tokodynamometer, 46
Tolazoline, 271
TORCH, 26
Total parenteral nutrition (TPN), 153-158
Toxemia, 4, 196, 197, 206, 207
Toxoplasma gondii, 245
Toxoplasmosis, 245-246
TPN; see Total parenteral nutrition
Trace elements in total parenteral nutrition, 154
Tracheoesophageal fistula (TEF), esophageal atresia and, 304-305
Tranquilizers, 207
Transabdominal amniocentesis, 28
Transcutaneous Doppler ultrasonography, 126
Transcutaneous oxygen monitor (TcP_{O_2}), 254-255
Transfer log, neonatal, 340; see also Transport
Tranfusion
 exchange, 279-280, 295
 fetal, 343-344
 fetus-to-fetus, 191
 twin-to-twin, 191, 193
Transient tachypnea of newborn, 90, 271
Transillumination, 135, 264
Translocation, 21, 310
Transport, 114-119
 care of infant during, 118
 equipment and supplies for, 115-116, 336-337
 fetal, 114
 of high-risk perinate, 114-119
 modes of, 115-118
 to regional center, 111-113
Transport nurses, training of, 119

Transport team, 115
Transpyloric feeding, 148-149
Transverse lie, 226
Transverse presentation, placenta previa and, 216
Trasylol, 213, 214, 216
Tremulousness, 288
Treponema pallidum, 245
Trichloroethylene, 77
Triglycerides, medium-chain, 143, 149
Triplets, 185, 193
 delivery of, 189
 premature rupture of membranes and, 194
Trisomy, 21
Tromethamine (THAM), 256
TrophAmine, 153
Tropicamide (Mydriacyl), 135
True labor, differentiation of, from false labor, 61
Tuberculosis, 246-247
Tubular necrosis, acute (ATN), 142
Tucker-McLean forceps, 79
Twins, 12, 185, 193, 331
 combinations of presentation of, 190
 conjoined, 193
 diamniotic, 187, 194
 dizygotic, 185, 194
 fetal death and, 193
 fraternal, 194
 identical, 194
 incomplete, 24, 187
 mode of delivery of, 189, 190
 monoamniotic, 187, 189, 194
 monochorionic monoamniotic, 24
 monozygotic, 185, 186, 187, 191, 193, 194
 parental influence on incidence of, 186
 premature rupture of membranes and, 194
 Siamese, 21
Twin-to-twin transfusion, 187, 191, 193
Two-vessel cord, 89
TXA_2; see Thromboxane

U

Ultrasonic devices in detection of fetal heart tones, 34-35
Ultrasonic monitoring, 68
Ultrasonic nebulization, 124-125
Ultrasonography, 11, 159
 amniocentesis and, 28
 fetal age assessment by, 36, 37
 fetal growth assessment by, 36-38
 fetal weight assessment by, 36, 37
 multiple pregnancy and, 187-188
 placenta previa and, 217
 real-time, 40
 sector scan, 40
 slight premature separation of placenta and, 213
 transcutaneous Doppler, 126
Umbilical artery
 single, multiple pregnancy and, 194
 as site for total parenteral nutrition, 155
Umbilical artery catheterization, 100-101
Umbilical cord; see Cord, umbilical
Umbilical vein as site for total parenteral nutrition, 155
Umbilical vein catheterization, 102
Umbilical vessel catheterization, 99-102

Unconjugated bilirubin, factors leading to overproduction of, 275-276
Undernutrition, 331
Untimely termination of pregnancy, 159-176
Unwanted pregnancy, prevention of, 332-333
Unwed parents, perinatal morbidity and mortality and, 8-9
Urethra, urine collection from, 136
Urinary tract complications, multiple pregnancy and, 192
Urine collection, technique of, 136
Urine specimen, bacterial septicemia and, 237
Uterine bleeding, 209-210
Uterine contractions; *see* Contractions
Uterine fundal measurement, 34
Uterine rupture, 63, 209, 211
Uterine size, measurement of, calculation of pregnancy duration from, 34
Uterus, Couvelaire, 212

V

Vacuum extraction, 80
Vaginal bleeding, premature labor and, 160
Vaginal delivery
  breech presentation and, 222-225
  of large-for-dates infants, complications of, 182
  multiple pregnancy and, 190-191
Vaginal lesions, 208
Vaginitis, 169
Valium; *see* Diazepam
Vancomycin, 238
Variable decelerations of fetal heart rate, 51
Vasa previa, 209, 211, 213, 219, 227-228
Vasoactive drugs, 210-211
Vasopressor drugs, 78
Velamentous insertion of cord, 194, 227-228
Vena cava syndrome, 212
Ventilation
  assisted
    continued apnea with, 94
    methods of, 99
    respiratory distress and, 256-260
    respiratory flow sheet for infants receiving, 341
  with bag and mask, 260
  of high-risk infants, 116
  intermittent negative pressure, 260
  intermittent positive pressure, 260
  mechanical, 260-266
  mouth-to-mouth, 99
  mouth-to-tube, 99
  for nonbreathing infant, 94
Ventilator, 260
Vernix, 41
Version, internal podalic, and extraction, 80
Very low birth weight infant, 249-251
Vidarabine (Ara-A), 243

Vigor of newborn at birth, reasons for discrepancies between levels of fetal acidosis as measured by, 53
Viral infections, 25, 240-247
Visceral pressures, multiple pregnancy and, 192
Vision of low birth weight infant, 321
Vistaril; *see* Hydroxyzine pamoate
Vitamin(s)
  A, 6
  B_{12}, 154
  D, 6
  E, 144, 154
  K, 6, 127, 154, 295
    deficiency of, 296
  K_1 (AquaMephyton), 127, 143, 296
  and mineral supplementation, pregnancy and, 6-7
  in total parenteral nutrition, 154
Vitamin mixtures, 134
Vitamin needs of preterm infant, 143-144
Volume expanders, 210
Volume-controlled ventilator, 260
Volvulus, malrotation of, 307-308
Vomiting, mucus, 147
Vomitus, bile-stained, intestinal obstruction and, 306

W

Water, 138-139
  for short-term needs, 138-139
  in total parenteral nutrition, 154
Water balance in low birth weight infant, 141-142
Water imbalances, 139
Water intoxication, 81
Water loss, insensible, 138
Water requirements, basal, 138
Weaning from mechanical ventilation, 261-262
Weeks, completed, in calculation of pregnancy duration, 33
Weight, 317
  assessment of infant by, 103-106
  fetal; *see* Fetal weight
  for height of women, standard, 2
  prepregnant, 5
Weight gain in pregnancy, 2-3, 5
Weight grid, Denver, 179
Weight loss in term and preterm infants, 141
Weinberg's formula, 185
Wharton's jelly, 90
Whey protein, 145
Wilson-Mikity syndrome, 262
Withdrawal reaction, 14
World Health Organization, 33, 314
Würm procedure, 172

Z

Ziegler-Fomon formula, 142
Zinc, 154